GW00367278

Paediatric Haematology

Dedicated to Elizabeth, Alistair, Eleanore and Tricia

For Churchill Livingstone
Publisher: Mike Parkinson
Project Editor: Dilys Jones
Editorial Co-ordination: Editorial Resources Unit
    Indexer: June Morrison
Production Controller: Lesley W. Small
Design: Design Resources Unit
Sales Promotion Executive: Marion Pollock

Paediatric Haematology

Edited by

John S. Lilleyman FRCP FRCPath
Consultant Haematologist, The Children's Hospital, Sheffield

Ian M. Hann MD FRCP MRCPath
Consultant Haematologist, The Hospitals for Sick Children, London

CHURCHILL LIVINGSTONE
EDINBURGH LONDON MADRID MELBOURNE NEW YORK AND TOKYO 1992

CHURCHILL LIVINGSTONE
Medical Division of Longman Group UK Limited

Distributed in the United States of America by Churchill
Livingstone Inc., 650 Avenue of the Americas, New York,
N. Y. 10011, and by associated companies, branches and
representatives throughout the world.

© Longman Group UK Limited 1992

All rights reserved. No part of this publication may be
reproduced, stored in a retrieval system, or transmitted in any
form or by any means, eletronic, mechanical, photocopying,
recording or otherwise, without either the prior written
permission of the publishers (Churchill Livingstone, Robert
Stevenson House, 1-3 Baxter's Place, Leith Walk, Edinburgh
EH1 3AF), or a licence permitting restricted copying in the
United Kingdom issued by the Copyright Licensing Agency
Ltd, 90 Tottenham Court Road, London W1P 9HE.

First published 1992

ISBN   0-443-04366-3

British Library Cataloguing in Publication Data
A catalogue record for this book is available from the British
Library.

Library of Congress Cataloging in Publication Data
Paediatric haematology/edited by John S. Lilleyman and I. M. Hann.
      p.   cm
    Includes index.
    ISBN 0–443–04366–3
    1. Pediatric hematology.   I. Lilleyman, J. S. II. Hann, Ian M.
    [DNLM: 1. Hematologic Diseases—in infancy & childhood. WS 300
P126]
RJ411.P34   1992
618.92' 15—dc20
DNLM/DLC
for Library of Congress   92–4139

The
publisher's
policy is to use
**paper manufactured
from sustainable forests**

Produced by Longman Singapore Publishers (Pte) Ltd
Printed in Singapore

Preface

It is now 15 years since Michael Willoughby's compact treatise on paediatric haematology appeared. Other, larger, more comprehensive texts have been written both before and since, as have atlases and books dealing with laboratory investigation, neonatal haematology and childhood cancer, not to mention several dedicated issues of haematology review journals. Despite all this competition, Willoughby's book remained enormously popular long after its shelf life because it hit the right pitch. It did not contain any excess basic haematology, which could be found in standard adult-based texts, nor was it selected, as a compilation of review articles has to be. What it did was to give both expert and inexpert a succinct and balanced overview of childhood blood disorders and, being fully referenced, allowed them easy access to the relevant source literature.

There has long been a demand for a second edition, but the task, especially for a single author, proved daunting. When Churchill Livingstone approached us about the possibility of a multi-author book as a substitute, we had our doubts as multi-author texts have obvious strengths and weaknesses and it might be hard to achieve the same pitch and style. But we finally agreed to take the task on. Our first job was to persuade a number of eminent colleagues to write for us and somehow cram that extra burden into their overcommitted lives. The fact that all did so, and willingly, is a cause for gratitude which we freely express. We hope the result will successfully fill the gap and that we have managed to create a surrogate 'Willoughby II'.

The layout of the book is slightly unconventional. It does not begin with a chapter on normal haemopoiesis containing the traditional diagram of stem cell maturation, but launches straight into a comprehensive compilation of paediatric reference ranges for haematological variables which we assume could be the section most frequently used in day-to-day clinical practice. We also decided against including separate sections on neonatal blood disorders or bone marrow transplantation, as both are covered, where relevant, in the other chapters. We have tried, as far as possible, to allocate emphasis and space on the basis of clinical importance rather than academic interest, and in so doing hope to have avoided producing a stamp collector's catalogue. Inevitably, with several authors, there has been some overlap and duplication, some of which has been removed by the editors; but much has been deliberately retained in order to avoid loss of perspective.

The book is designed to be useful to all haematologists and paediatricians, at whatever stage of training and experience, and to be helpful to those taking postgraduate examinations in haematology or paediatric internal medicine. We would like to think that laboratory scientists will also find the contents valuable, but above all we hope that, whoever buys it, the book becomes as well-thumbed and dog-eared as most copies of Willoughby's original. That would be a true measure of success.

Apart from our co-authors, we would like to acknowledge the encouragement and patience of the publishers, particularly Dilys Jones, and the uncomplaining cheerfulness and hard work of Sonia Taylor and Marie Elliott who put up with far more secretarial abuse than could remotely be considered reasonable.

J.S.L.
I.M.H.

Contributors

Judith M. Chessells MD FRCP FRCPath
Leukaemia Research Fund Professor of
Haematology and Oncology
Institute of Child Health and The Hospitals for
Sick Children
London

G. Dolan MBChB MRCP MRCPath
Consultant Haematologist
University Hospital
Nottingham

O. B. Eden MB BS FRCPE
Professor of Paediatric Oncology
St Bartholomew's Hospital
London

D. I. K. Evans MA MB FRCPE DCH
Consultant Haematologist
Royal Manchester Children's Hospital and Booth
Hall Children's Hospital
Manchester

Jane P. M. Evans MB BS MRCP MRCPath
Consultant Haematologist
The Hospitals for Sick Children
London

Brenda E. S. Gibson MB ChB FRCP MRCPath
DFM
Consultant Haematologist
Royal Hospital for Sick Children
Glasgow

I. M. Hann MD FRCP MRCPath
Consultant Haematologist
The Hospitals for Sick Children
London

R. M. Hardisty MD FRCP FRCPath
Emeritus Professor of Haematology
University of London
Royal Free Hospital School of Medicine
London

R. F. Hinchliffe FIMLS
Senior Chief Medical Laboratory Scientific Officer
The Children's Hospital
Sheffield

Barbara M. Holland MB ChB BAO FRCP
Consultant Paediatrician
Department of Child Health
Queen Mother's Hospital, University of
Glasgow
Glasgow

J. G. Jones BPharm PhD
Senior Lecturer
Department of Biochemistry
University of Wales College of Cardiff
Cardiff

J. S. Lilleyman FRCP FRCPath
Consultant Haematologist
The Children's Hospital
Sheffield

M. J. Pippard BSc MB ChB MRCPath FRCP
Professor of Haematology
Ninewells Hospital and Medical School
University of Dundee
Dundee

Elaine M. Simpson MRCP MRCPath
Consultant Haematologist
Royal Hospital for Sick Children
Glasgow

R. F. Stevens BSc MB ChB FRCP MRCPath
Consultant Haematologist
Royal Manchester Children's Hospital
Manchester

S. Strobel MD PhD MRCP
Senior Lecturer and Honorary Consultant in
Paediatric Immunology
The Hospitals for Sick Children and Institute of
Child Health
London

C. A. J Wardrop MB FRCPE FRCPath
Senior Lecturer and Honorary Consultant
University of Wales College of Medicine
Cardiff

Contents

1. Reference values

R. F. Hinchliffe

The values of many haematological variables change rapidly in the first few weeks and months of life, and it is essential that reference data are available to enable the correct interpretation of laboratory results, both in infancy and until such time as normal adult ranges can be applied.

In preparing this chapter, the aim has been to provide data for a wide range of clinically important haematological variables by combining recently published work using modern technology with older information which has stood the test of time. It must be borne in mind, however, that all reference values are affected to some degree by factors such as race, diet and drug intake, and by statistical interpretation of the data. The analytical method used presents another important variable, and is referred to wherever possible when alternative methods are in widespread use for the commoner haematological tests.

Contents

Table 1.1 Normal blood count values in childhood*

Age	Hb (g/dl)	RBC ($\times 10^{12}$/1)	Hct	MCV (fl)	WBC ($\times 10^9$/1)	Neutrophils ($\times 10^9$/1)	Lymphocytes ($\times 10^9$/1)	Monocytes ($\times 10^9$/1)	Eosinophils ($\times 10^9$/1)	Platelets ($\times 10^9$/1)
Birth	14.9–23.7	3.7–6.5	0.47–0.75	100–135	10.0–26.0	2.7–14.4	2.0–7.3	0–1.9	0–0.84	
2 weeks	13.4–19.8	3.9–5.9	0.41–0.65	88–120	6.0–21.0	1.8–5.4	2.8–9.1	0.1–1.7	0–0.84	
2 months	9.4–13.0	3.1–4.3	0.28–0.42	84–105	6.0–18.0	1.2–7.5	3.0–13.5	0.1–1.7	0.1–0.8	150–450
6 months	11.1–14.1	3.9–5.5	0.31–0.41	68–82	6.0–17.5	1.0–8.5	4.0–13.5	0.2–1.2	0.3–0.8	at all ages
1 year	11.3–14.1	4.1–5.3	0.33–0.41	71–85	6.0–17.5	1.5–8.5	4.0–10.5	0.2–1.2	0.3–0.8	
2–6 years	11.5–13.5	3.9–5.3	0.34–0.40	75–87	5.0–17.0	1.5–8.5	1.5–9.5	0.2–1.2	0.3–0.8	
6–12 years	11.5–15.5	4.0–5.2	0.35–0.45	77–95	4.5–14.5	1.5–8.0	1.5–7.0	0.2–1.0	0.1–0.5	
12–18 years										
Female	2.0–16.0	4.1–5.1	0.36–0.46	78-95	4.5-13.0	1.8–8.0	1.2- 6.5	0.2-0.8	<0.1 -0.5	
Male	13.0–16.0	4.5–5.3	0.37–0.49	78-95						

* Data given as approximate ranges, compiled from various sources.
Red cell values at birth derived from skin puncture blood; most other data from venous blood.

Table 1.2 Red cell values (mean ± 1 SD) on the first postnatal day from 24 weeks' gestational age*

Gestational age (weeks) (No. of infants)	24–25 (n = 7)	26–27 (n = 11)	28–29 (n = 7)	30–31 (n = 35)	32–33 (n = 23)	34–35 (n = 23)	36–37 (n = 20)	Term (n = 19)
RBC ($\times 10^{12}$/1)	4.65 ± 0.43	4.73 + 0.45	4.62 ± 0.75	4.79 ± 0.74	5.0 ± 0.76	5.09 ± 0.5	5.27 ± 0.68	5.14 ± 0.7
Hb (g/dl)	19.4 ± 1.5	19.0 ± 2.5	19.3 ± 1.8	19.1 ± 2.2	18.5 ± 2.0	19.6 ± 2.1	19.2 ± 1.7	19.3 ± 2.2
Haematocrit	0.63 ± .04	0.62 ± .08	0.60 ± .07	0.60 ± .08	0.60 ± .08	0.61 ± .07	0.64 ± .07	0.61 ± .074
MCV (fl)	135 ± 0.2	132 ± 14.4	131 ± 13.5	127 ± 12.7	123 ± 15.7	122 ± 10.0	121 ± 12.5	119 ± 9.4
Reticulocytes (%)	6.0 ± 0.5	9.6 ± 3.2	7.5 ± 2.5	5.8 ± 2.0	5.0 ± 1.9	3.9 ± 1.6	4.2 ± 1.8	3.2 ± 1.4
Weight (g)	725 ± 185	993 ± 194	1174 ± 128	1450 ± 232	1816 ± 192	1957 ± 291	2245 ± 213	

* Counts performed on heel-prick blood using an electronic counter.
(Reproduced from Zaizov & Matoth 1976, by permission of Alan R Liss Inc.)

Table 1.3 Mean haematological values in the first 2 weeks of life in the term infant*

Haematological Value	Cord blood	Day 1	Day 3	Day 7	Day 14
Hb (g/dl)	16.8	18.4	17.8	17.0	16.8
Haematocrit	0.53	0.58	0.55	0.54	0.52
Red cells ($\times 10^{12}$/1)	5.25	5.8	5.6	5.2	5.1
MCV (fl)	107	108	99.0	98.0	96.0
MCH (pg)	34	35	33	32.5	31.5
MCHC (%)	31.7	32.5	33	33	33
Reticulocytes (%)	3–7	3–7	1–3	0–1	0–1
Nucleated RBC (mm³)	500	200	0–5	0	0
Platelets ($\times 10^9$/1)	290	192	213	248	252

* (Reproduced from Oski 1982, by permission of Dr F Oski and W B Saunders Co.)

Table 1.4 Normal haemoglobin (Hb) and red blood cell (RBC) values in the first year of life*

Hb/RBC value	Age (months)						
	0.5 (n = 232)	1 (n = 240)	2 (n = 241)	4 (n = 52)	6 (n = 52)	9 (n = 56)	12 (n = 56)
Hb(g/dl) (mean ± SE)	16.6 ± 0.11	13.9 ± 0.10	11.2 ± 0.06	12.2 ± 0.14	12.6 ± 0.10	12.7 ± 0.09	12.7 ± 0.09
−2 SD	13.4	10.7	9.4	10.3	11.1	11.4	11.3
Hct (mean ± SE)	0.53 ± 0.004	0.44 ± 0.003	0.35 ± 0.002	0.38 ± 0.004	0.36 ± 0.003	0.36 ± 0.003	0.37 ± 0.003
−2 SD	41	33	28	32	31	32	33
RBC(× 10^{12}/1)(mean ± SE)	4.9 ± 0.03	4.3 ± 0.03	3.7 ± 0.02	4.3 ± 0.06	4.7 ± 0.05	4.7 ± 0.04	4.7 ± 0.04
−2 SD, +2 SD	3.9–5.9	3.3–5.3	3.1–4.3	3.5–5.1	3.9–5.5	4.0–5.3	4.1–5.3
MCH (pg) (mean ± SE)	33.6 ± 0.1	32.5 ± 0.1	30.4 ± 0.1	28.6 ± 0.2	26.8 ± 0.2	27.3 ± 0.2	26.8 ± 0.2
−2 SD	30	29	27	25	24	25	24
MCV (fl) (mean ± SE)	105.3 ± 0.6	101.3 ± 0.3	94.8 ± 0.3	86.7 ± 0.8	76.3 ± 0.6	77.7 ± 0.5	77.7± 0.5
−2 SD	88	91	84	76	68	70	71
MCHC(g/dl) (mean ± SE)	31.4 ± 1.1	31.8 ± 1.2	31.8 ± 1.1	32.7 ± 2.7	35.0 ± 1.7	34.9 ± 1.6	34.3 ± 1.5
−2 SD	28.1	28.1	28.3	28.8	32.7	32.4	32.1

* Values after the age of 2 months were obtained from an iron-supplemented group in whom iron deficiency was excluded. Counts performed on venous blood.
(Reproduced from Saarinen & Siimes 1978, by permission of the C. V. Mosby Co.)

Table 1.5 Haemoglobin values (median and 95% range) in the first 6 months of life in iron-sufficient (serum ferritin ≥ 10 µg/1) preterm infants*

Age	Birth weight (g)			
	1000–1500	No. tested	1501–2000	No. tested
2 weeks	16.3 (11.7–18.4)	17	14.8 (11.8–19.6)	39
1 month	10.9 (8.7–15.2)	15	11.5 (8.2–15.0)	42
2 months	8.8 (7.1–11.5)	17	9.4 (8.0–11.4)	47
3 months	9.8 (8.9–11.2)	16	10.2 (9.3–11.8)	41
4 months	11.3 (9.1–13.1)	13	11.3 (9.1–13.1)	37
5 months	11.6 (10.2–14.3)	8	11.8 (10.4–13.0)	21
6 months	12.0 (9.4–13.8)	9	11.8 (10.7–12.6)	21

*All had an uncomplicated course in the first 2 weeks of life and none received exchange transfusion. Counts obtained from venous and skin-puncture blood.
(Reproduced from Lundstrom et al 1977, by permission of the C. V. Mosby Co.)

Table 1.6 Haemoglobin (Hb), haematocrit (Hct) and red blood cell (RBC) counts in term African neonates*

	No. Tested	Mean ± 1 SD		
		Hb	Hct	RBC
Day 1	304	15.6 ± 2.0	0.450 ± 0.065	4.00 ± 0.67
3	261	15.5 ± 2.1	0.442 ± 0.062	3.91 ± 0.61
7	249	14.2 ± 2.3	0.413 ± 0.063	3.67 ± 0.55
Week 2	233	13.1 ± 1.9	0.391 ± 0.043	3.45 ± 0.56
3	145	11.7 ± 1.8	0.356 ± 0.050	3.27 ± 0.47
4	117	10.6 ± 1.6	0.325 ± 0.044	3.01 ± 0.48

*Values are lower than those reported in neonates from Europe and North America, and may be intrinsic to this group. Other variables (RBC indices, reticulocytes) do not differ from those in other populations studied. Hb measured as oxyhaemoglobin, Hct by centrifuged microhaematocrit and RBC by haemocytometry, using venous blood.
(Summarized from Scott-Emuakpor et al 1985a.)

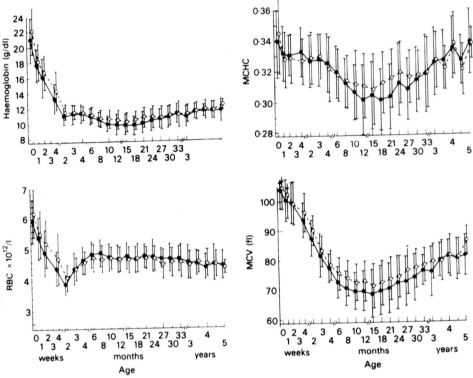

Fig. 1.1 Hb (**1**) MCHC (**2**), RBC (**3**) and MCV (**4**) values (mean ± 1SD) in Jamaican children aged from 1 day to 5 years. ● = boys; ○ = girls. A cohort of 243 children were studied, although the data at each point are derived from varying numbers. Regular iron and folate supplements were not given. Both venous and skin puncture samples were used, and counting was performed by semi-automated methods. (Reproduced from Serjeant et al 1980 by permission of Blackwell Scientific Publications.)

Table 1.7 The reticulocyte count – range (%) and (× 10⁹/l) in the first 3 months of life in term infants*

Age	%	× 10⁹/l
1 day	3.0–7.0	110–450
7 days	< 0.1–1.3	< 10–80
4 weeks	< 0.1–1.2	< 10–65
8 weeks	0.1–2.9	< 10–125
12 weeks	0.4–1.6	15–75
>12 weeks	0.2–2.0	10–105

*Data from various sources, based on microscope counts.

Table 1.8 The percentage of haemoglobin F in the first year of life*

Age	No. tested	Mean	2 SD	Range
1–7 days	10	74.7	5.4	61–79.6
2 weeks	13	74.9	5.7	66–88.5
1 month	11	60.2	6.3	45.7–67.3
2 months	10	45.6	10.1	29.4–60.8
3 months	10	26.6	14.5	14.8–55.9
4 months	10	17.7	6.1	9.4–28.5
5 months	10	10.4	6.7	2.3–22.4
6 months	15	6.5	3.0	2.7–13.0
8 months	11	5.1	3.6	2.3–11.9
10 months	10	2.1	0.7	1.5–3.5
12 months	10	2.6	1.5	1.3–5.0
1–14 years and adults	100	0.6	0.4	–

*HbF measured by alkali denaturation.
(Data from Schröter & Nafz 1981.)

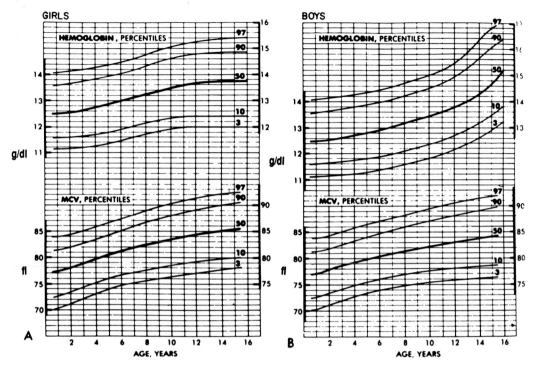

Fig. 1.2 Hb and MCV percentiles for girls (**A**) and boys (**B**) derived from non-indigent white children in California and Finland. Hb values obtained from 9946 children, MCV values from 2314; none had laboratory evidence of iron deficiency or haemoglobinopathy. Counts performed on venous blood using Coulter Model S Counters.
(Reproduced from Dallman & Siimes 1979 by permission of the C V Mosby Co.)

Table 1.9 The percentage of haemoglobin A_2 in the first two years of life*

Age (months)	A No. tested	Mean	SD	B No. tested	Mean	SD	Range
Birth	16	0.4	0.2				
1	6	0.8	0.3	5	0.8	0.4	0.4–1.3
2	7	1.3	0.7	9	1.3	0.5	0.4–1 9
3	8	1.7	0.3	8	2.2	0.6	1.0–3.0
4	9	2.1	0.3	3	2.4	0.4	2.0–2.8
5	8	2.3	0.2				
5–6				15	2.5	0.3	2.1–3.1
6	8	2.5	0.3				
7–8	6	2.5	0.4				
7–9				22	2.7	0.4	1.9–3.5
9–10	6	2.5	0.4				
10–12				14	2.7	0.4	2.0–3.3
12	5	2.5	0.3				
13–16				13	2.6	0.5	1.6–3.3
17–20				13	2.9	0.4	2.1–3.6
21–24				15	2.8	0.4	2.0–3.6

*Data derived from two studies: A = Galanello et al 1981 measured by microcolumn chromatography; B = Metaxotou-Mavromati et al 1982 measured by elution following electrophoresis

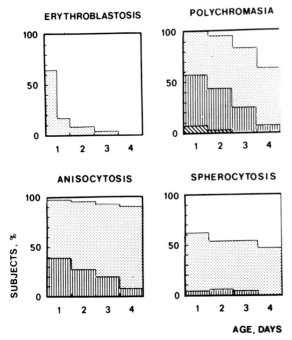

Fig. 1.3 RBC morphology in the first 4 days of life in 138 healthy term infants. Findings are graded from normal (white area) to mild, moderate and marked change (the last only in the case of polychromasia). Erythroblastosis: mild = 1–2 cells/10–15 fields; moderate = 1–5 cells/100 WBC. Polychromasia: mild = 1 cell in every or every other field; moderate = 1–3 cells/field; marked = > 3 cells/field. Anisocytosis: mild = c. 5 cells/field differ in size from normal; moderate = the variation is more marked. Spherocytosis: mild = 1 spherocyte in every or every other field; moderate = on average more than 1 spherocyte/field.
(Reproduced from Hovi & Siimes 1983 by permission of Acta Paediatrica Scandinavica.)

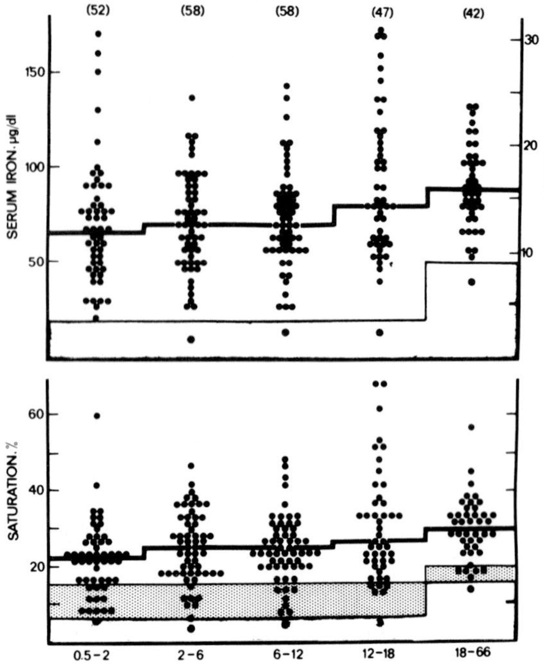

Fig. 1.4 Normal values for serum iron and transferrin saturation in individuals with normal levels of Hb, MCV, serum ferritin and free erythrocyte protoporphyrin. The heavy horizontal lines indicate the median values, the lower lines the lower limit of the 95% range, and the stippled area an intermediate zone of overlap between iron-deficient and normal subjects. Number of subjects in parentheses.
(Reproduced from Koerper & Dallman 1977 by permission of the C V Mosby Co.)

Table 1.10 Methaemoglobin levels in children and adults*

Subjects	Methaemoglobin (g/dl)				Methaemoglobin (% of total Hb)			
	No. tested	Mean	SD	Range tested	No.	Mean	SD	Range
Prematures, birth–7 days	29	0.43	0.07	0.02 –0.83	24	2.3	1.26	0.08–4.4
Prematures, 7–72 days	21	0.31	0.19	0.02–0.78	18	2.2	1.07	0.02–4.7
Newborns, 1–10 days	39	0.22	0.17	0–0.58	25	1.5	0.81	0–2.8
Infants, 1 month–1 year	8	0.14	0.09	0.02–0.29	8	1.2	0.78	0.17–2.4
Children, 1–14 years	35	0.11	0.09	0–0.33	35	0.79	0.62	0–2.4
Adults, 14–78 years	30	0.11	0.09	0–0.28	27	0.82	0.63	0–1.9

*(Summarized from Kravitz et al 1956)

Table 1.11   A comparison of enzyme activities and glutathione content in newborn and adult red blood cells*

Enzyme	Activity in normal adult RBC in IU/gHb (mean ± 1 SD at 37°)	Mean activity in newborn RBC as percentage of mean (100%) activity in normal adult RBC
Aldolase	3.19 ± 0.86	140
Enolase	5.39 ± 0.83	250
Glucose phosphate isomerase	60.8 ± 11.0	162
Glucose-6-phosphate dehydrogenase	8.34 ± 1.59	174
WHO method	12.1 ± 2.09	
Glutathione peroxidase	30.82 ± 4.65	56
Glyceraldehyde phosphate dehydrogenase	226 ± 41.9	170
Hexokinase	1.78 ± 0.38	239
Lactate dehydrogenase	200 ± 26.5	132
NADH-methaemoglobin reductase	19.2 ± 3.85 (at 30°C)	Increased
Phosphofructokinase	11.01 ± 2.33	97
Phosphoglycerate kinase	320 ± 36.1	165
Pyruvate kinase	15.0 ± 1.99	160
6-Phosphogluconate dehydrogenase	8.78 ± 0.78	150
Triose phosphate isomerase	211 ± 397	101
Glutathione	6570 ± 1040 nmol/g Hb	156

*The percentage activity in newborn RBC compared to mean adult (100%) values is presented with quantitative data from studies on adult RBC. Newborn data from Konrad et al 1972; quantitative date from Beutler 1984
(Reproduced from Hinchliffe & Lilleyman 1987 by permission of John Wiley & Sons Ltd.)

Table 1.12   Values of serum iron (SI), total iron-binding capacity (TIBC) and transferrin saturation (S%) from a group of 47 infants*

		Age (months)						
		0.5	1	2	4	6	9	12
SI: µmol/l	Median	22	22	16	15	14	15	14
	(95% range)	11–36	10–31	3–29	3–29	5–24	6–24	6–28
µg/dl	Median	120	125	87	84	77	84	78
	(95% range)	(63–201)	(58–172)	(15–159)	(18–164)	(28–135)	(35–155)	
TIBC (Mean ± SD):	µmol/l	34 ± 8	36 ± 8	44 ± 10	54 ± 7	58 ± 9	61 ± 7	64 ± 7
	µg/dl	191 ± 43	199 ± 43	246 ± 55	300 ± 39	321 ± 51	341 ± 42	358 ± 38
S%	Median	68	63	34	27	23	25	23
	(95% range)	(30–99)	(35–94)	(21–63)	(7–53)	(10–43)	(10–39)	(10–47)

*Not all infants were tested on each occasion, and those with Hb < 11 g/dl, MCV <71 fl or serum ferritin < 10 µg/l were excluded
(Reproduced from Saarinen & Siimes 1977, by permission of the C. V. Mosby Co.)

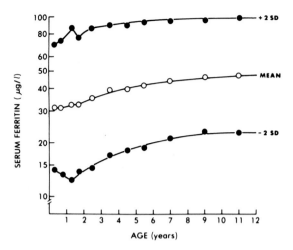

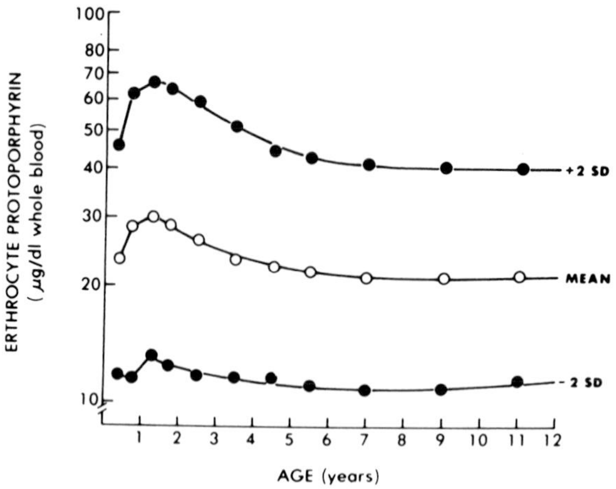

Fig. 1.5   Serum ferritin concentration (mean ± 2SD) in 3819 children aged 6 months to 12 years. Subjects with low haematocrit and evidence of increased iron absorption were excluded. Mean values for boys and girls were similar in each age group and there was no significant difference between blacks, whites and American Indians in age-matched samples. Ferritin measured by a two-site radioimmunometric assay (Reproduced from Deinard et al 1983 by permission of Dr A S Deinard and the American Society for Clinical Nutrition.)

Fig. 1.6   Erythrocyte protoporphyrin concentration (Mean ± 2 SD) measured in the same children as in Figure 1.5. Mean values for boys and girls were similar in each age group and there was no significant dirrerence between blacks, whites and American Indians in age-matched samples. Protoporphyrin measured as 'free' + zinc protoporphyrins. (Reproduced from Deinard et al 1983 by permission of Dr A S Deinard and the American Society for Clinical Nutrition.)

Table 1.13   Range of serum vitamin B_{12} levels (ng/l)*

Newborn	160–1300
Children and adults	160–925

*(Data from Tierz & Blackburn 1981, Dacie & Lewis 1984)

Table 1.14   Serum and red cell folate levels in µg/l (mean and range) obtained by microbiological assay*

Age	Serum folate Term (n = 24)	Premature (n = 20)	Red cell folate Term (n = 24)	Premature (n = 20)
Birth	24.5 (3–59)	19.2 (10–41)	315 (100–960)	689 (88–1291)
2–3 months		4.8 (1–11)		164 (26–394)
3–4 months	12.2 (5–30)		283 (110–489)	
6–8 months	7.7 (3.5–16)	8.9 (4.1–28)	247 (100–466)	299 (139–558)
1 year	9.3 (3–35)		277 (74–995)	
> 1 year	10.3 (6.1–16.5) (n = 22)			

*Values in first year of life from Vanier & Tyas 1966, 1967; other data from Dormandy et al 1963
(Reproduced from Hinchliffe & Lilleyman 1987, by permission of John Wiley & Sons Ltd)

Table 1.15 Mean red cell, plasma and total blood volume (ml/kg) measurements in children*

Age	Red cell volume	Plasma volume	Total blood volume	Study
Newborn	(43.4)	41.3	84.7	1
3 days	31**	51**	82**	2
	49†	44†	93†	2
1–7 days	37.9	(39.8)	77.7	3
1 week–30 months	29.5	(48.5)	78.0	3
3 months–11 months	(32.7)	46.0	78.7	4
3 months–1 year	23.3	(45.4)	68.7	3
1–2 years	24.1	(43.6)	67.7	3
1–3 years	(34.9)	47.9	82.8	4
2–4 years	22.9	(40.0)	62.9	3
3–5 years	(36.0)	48.4	84.4	4
4–6 years	26.7	(42.9)	69.6	3
5–7 years	(34.9)	48.9	83.8	4
6–8 years	23.3	(42.8)	66.1	3
7–9 years	(35.9)	47.8	83.7	4
8–12 years	25.9	(40.8)	66.7	3
9–11 years	(38.0)	48.5	86.5	4
11–13 years	(37.4)	46.4	83.8	4

* Bracketed data calculated from the measured variables.
** No placental transfusion at birth
† Placental transfusion at birth
  Total blood volume derived from measurement of RBC volume in study 3, and from plasma volumes in other studies. Data from: 1 = Mollison et al 1950; 2 = Usher et al 1963; 3 = Sukarochana et al 1961; 4 = Russell 1949.
  (Reproduced from Hinchliffe & Lilleyman 1987 by permission of John Wiley & Sons Ltd.)

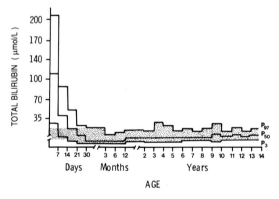

Fig. 1.7 Total bilirubin (μmol/l) measured in 2099 children. The 3rd, 50th and 97th percentiles and the adult normal range (stippled area) are shown. Bilirubin measured using a Technicon SMAC analyser.
(Reproduced from Gomez et al 1984 by permission of the American Association for Clinical Chemistry, Inc.)

Table 1.16 Red blood cell T_{50} ^{51}Cr survival in term and premature infants*

Study	Number	Range (days)	Mean (days)
Term infants			
Foconi & Sjolin 1959	10	17–25	22.8
Kaplan & Hsu 1961	11	21–35	28.5
Premature infants			
Foconi & Sjolin 1959	6	10–18	15.8
Kaplan & Hsu 1961	6	9–20	15.2

* (Reproduced from Hinchliffe & Lilleyman 1987 by permission of John Wiley & Sons Ltd.)

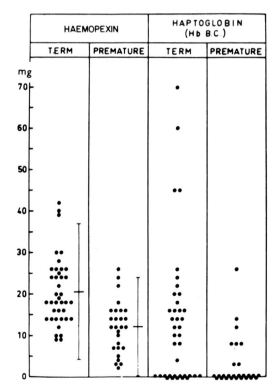

Fig. 1.8 Plasma haemopexin (mg/dl) and haptoglobin (mg/dl) of Hb binding capacity, HbBc) in 39 term and 27 premature infants on the first day of life. The mean ± 2 SD range is given for haemopexin. Measurements obtained by electroimmunodiffusion.
(Reproduced from Lundh et al 1970 by permission of Acta Paediatrica Scandinavica.)

Table 1.17   Serum haptoglobin (as haemoglobin binding capacity in mg/dl) in term infants and children*

Age	No. tested	Mean	SD	Range
At delivery, (cord blood)	21	0	0	0
1–7 days	24	10	11.7	0–41
1–4 weeks	23	28.2	15.7	0–45
1–3 months	8	59.4	16.9	41–95
3–6 months	13	91	21.1	64–134
6–12 months	17	114.9	33.5	43–160
1–5 years	28	108.7	25.5	51–160
5–10 years	37	107	25.5	62–186
over 10 years	16	110	35.1	41–165

*Measured as peroxidase activity of haptoglobin–
  haemoglobin complex
  (Summarized from Khalil et al 1967.)

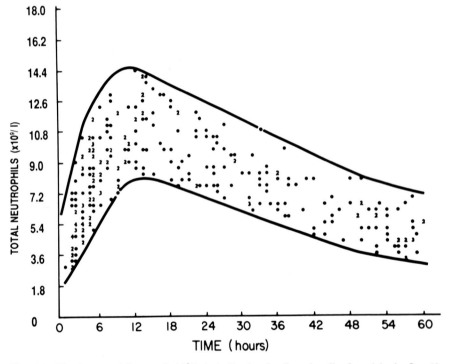

Fig. 1.9   Total neutrophil count (× 10⁹/1; including band cells and earlier forms) in the first 60 hours of life. Each dot represents a single value and numbers represent the number of values at the same point. Data based on automated leucocyte count and 100-cell differential. (Reproduced from Manroe et al 1979 by permission of the C V Mosby Co.)

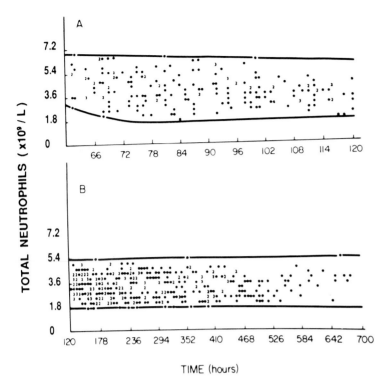

Fig. 1.10 Neutrophil count ($\times 10^9/1$) between 60–120 hours (**A**) and 120 hours–28 days (**B**). Data obtained and expressed as in Figure 1.9.
(Reproduced from Manroe et al 1979 by permission of the C V Mosby Co.)

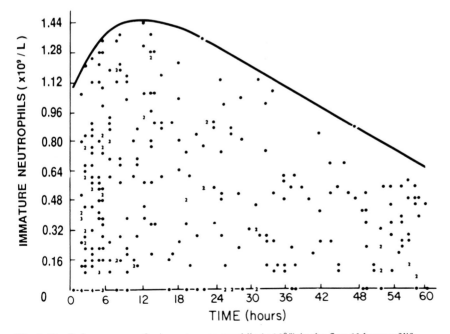

Fig. 1.11 Reference range for immature neutrophils ($\times 10^9/l$) in the first 60 hours of life. Data obtained and expressed as in Figure 1.9.
(Reproduced from Manroe et al 1979 by permission of the C V Mosby Co.)

Table 1.18   Normal values for lymphocytes, monocytes and
eosinophils ($\times 10^9/1$) from birth to 28 days of age based on a
study of 393 infants*

Cells	Age (hours)			
	Percentile	0.60	61–120	121–720
Lymphocytes	95	7.26	6.62	9.13
	50	4.19	8.66	5.62
	5	2.02	1.92	2.86
Monocytes	95	1.91	1.74	1.72
	50	0.6	0.53	0.67
	5	0	0	0.10
Eosinophils	95	0.84	0.81	0.84
	50	0.14	0.18	0.24
	5	0	0	0

*Data based on 100-cell differential count.
  (Reproduced from Weinberg et al 1985, by permission of
  the C. V. Mosby Co.)

Table 1.19   Mean and range of values for neutrophils, band forms and
lymphocytes ($\times 10^9/1$) in African neonates*

	Day 1	Day 7	Day 28
Neutrophils	5.67 (0.98–12.9)	2.01 (0.57–6.5)	1.67 (0.65–3.2)
Band forms	1.16 (0.16–2.3)	0.55 (0–1.5)	0.36 (0–0.39)
Lymphocytes	5.10 (1.4–8.0)	5.63 (2.2–15.5)	0.55 (3.2–9.9)

*Data based on 100-cell differential count
  The lower range of neutrophil values known to occur in negroes is evident in the
  neonatal period.
  (Summarized from Scott-Emuakpor et al 1985b; reproduced from Hinchliffe &
  Lilleyman 1987, by permission of John Wiley & Sons Ltd.)

Table 1.20   Normal limits of the immature/total and immature/segmented granulocyte ratios in
healthy neonates*

	Day 1	Day 7	Day 28	Reference
Immature/total	0.16	0.12	0.12	Manroe et al 1979
Immature/total (African)	0.22	0.21	0.18	Scott-Emuakpor et al 1985b
Immature/segmented	0.3			Zipursky & Jaber 1978
		(neonatal period)		

* (Reproduced from Hinchliffe & Lilleyman 1987, by permission of John Wiley & Sons Ltd.)

Table 1.21 Values for mature and immature neutrophils and the immature/total neutrophil ratio in 24 infants of < 33 weeks' gestation*

Age	Mature neutrophils ($\times 10^9/1$) Median (range)	Mean	Immature neutrophils ($\times 10^9/1$) Median (range)	Mean	Immature/total ratio Median (range)	Mean
1 (n = 10)	4.64 (2.20–8.18)	4.57	0.11 (0–1.5)	0.30	0.04 (0–0.35)	0.09
12 (n = 17)	6.80 (4.0–22.48)	8.61	0.27 (0–1.6)	0.48	0.04 (0–0.21)	0.06
24 (n = 17)	5.60 (2.61–21.20)	7.64	0.14 (0–3.66)	0.47	0.03 (0–0.17)	0.05
48 (n = 20)	4.98 (1.02–14.43)	6.24	0.13 (0–2.15)	0.44	0.02 (0–0.17)	0.05
72 (n = 22)	3.19 (1.28–13.94)	4.63	0.16 (0–2.42)	0.38	0.3 (0–0.25)	0.05
96 (n = 21)	3.44 (1.37–16.56)	5.33	0.23 (0–3.95)	0.45	0.05 0–0.37)	0.07
120 (n = 17)	3.46 (1.27–15.00)	4.98	0.25 (0–2.89)	0.44	0.05 (0–0.21)	0.07

* (Reproduced from Lloyd & Oto 1982, by permission of the editor of Archives of Disease in Childhood.)

Table 1.22 Normal progenitor cell numbers during development*

Age	PB BFU-E	BM BFU-E	BM CFU-E	PB CFU-GM	BM CFU-GM	PB CFU-Meg	BM CFU-Meg
Fetuses 18–20 weeks	75–1500			20–700		1–10	
Birth, term	40–100			10–200		5–20	
Adults	5–40	10–150	25–150	5–20	15–100	2–10	1–30

* Data shown are approximate ranges derived from various sources, and indicate numbers of progenitor cells per 10^5 mononuclear cells plated.
  Abbreviations: PB = peripheral blood; BM = bone marrow; BFU-E = burst-forming-unit-erythroid; CFU-E = colony-forming-unit-erythroid; CFU-GM = colony-forming-unit-granulocyte-macrophage; CFU-Meg = colony-forming-unit-megakaryocyte.
  (Reproduced from Auerbach & Alter 1989, by permission of Churchill Livingstone.)

Table 1.23 Mean and 95% range of total leucocyte count ($\times 10^9/1$), and mean, 95% range and mean percentage values for neutrophils, lymphocytes, monocytes and eosinophils*

Age	Total leucocytes Mean	Range	Neutrophils Mean	Range	%	Lymphocytes Mean	Range	%	Monocytes Mean	%	Eosinophils Mean	%
1 month	10.8	5.0–19.5	3.8	1.0–9.0	35	6.0	2.5–16.5	56	0.7	7	0.3	3
6 months	11.9	6.0–17.5	3.8	1.0–8.5	32	7.3	4.0–13.5	61	0.6	5	0.3	3
1 year	11.4	6.0–17.5	3.5	1.5–8.5	31	7.0	4.0–10.5	61	0.6	5	0.3	3
2 years	10.6	6.0–17.0	3.5	1.5–8.5	33	6.3	3.0–9.5	59	0.5	5	0.3	3
4 years	9.1	5.5–15.5	3.8	1.5–8.5	42	4.5	2.0–8.0	50	0.5	5	0.3	3
6 years	8.5	5.0–14.5	4.3	1.5–8.0	51	3.5	1.5–7.0	42	0.4	5	0.2	3
8 years	8.3	4.5–13.5	4.4	1.5–8.0	53	3.3	1.5–6.8	39	0.4	4	0.2	2
10 years	8.1	4.5–13.5	4.4	1.8–8.0	54	3.1	1.5–6.5	38	0.4	4	0.2	2
16 years	7.8	4.5–13.0	4.4	1.8–8.0	57	2.8	1.2–5.2	35	0.4	5	0.2	3
21 years	7.4	4.5–11.0	4.4	1 8–7.7	59	2.5	1.0–4.8	34	0.3	4	0.2	3

* Data based on 100-cell differential count
  (Summarized from Dallman 1977, by permission of Appleton-Century-Crofts.)

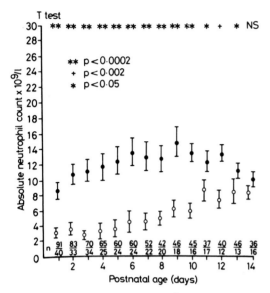

Fig. 1.12   Neutrophil count ($\times 10^9/1$, bar indicates ± 1 SD) during the first 14 days of life in babies of appropriate weight for gestational age (●) and babies who were small for gestational age (○).
(Reproduced from McIntosh et al 1988 by permission of Professor N McIntosh and the editor of Archives of Disease in Childhood.)

Table 1.24   Lymphocyte subsets (mean ± 1 SD, % and $\times 10^9/1$) in term and preterm infants*

	Total T cells	Suppressor T cells	Helper T cells	B cells
Term (n = 10)				
% total leucocytes	34(± 17)	13(± 7)	24(± 13)	5(± 4)
Absolute number $\times 10^9/1$	5.2(± 2.7)	1.9(± 1.3)	3.8(± 2.4)	0.9(± 0.9)
Preterm (n = 38)				
% total leucocytes	34(± 15)	11(± 6)	25(± 13)	8(± 6)
Absolute number $\times 10^9/1$	4.5(± 2.1)	1.5(± 0.8)	4.7(± 0.8)	1.3(± 1.2)

*Counted using indirect immunofluorescence on a fluorescence-activated cell sorter
 (Reproduced from Thomas & Linch 1983, by permission of the editor of the
 Archives of Disease in Childhood.)

Table 1.25 Lymphocyte subsets (25th, 50th and 75th centile) in children and adults

Subset	Percentage T cells				Percentage B cells			Percentage Natural Killer (NK) cells		
CD numbers	CD3				CD19			CD16$^+$/CD56$^+$,CD3$^-$		
Reagent	Leu 4				Leu 12			Leu 11$^+$/19$^+$,Leu4$^-$		
Percentile		P_{25}	P_{50}	P_{75}	P_{25}	P_{50}	P_{75}	P_{25}	P_{50}	P_{75}
Age group	Number									
Cord blood	24	49	55	62	14	20	23	14	19.5	30
1 day–11 months	31	55	60	67	19	25	29	11	15	19
1–6 years	54	62	64	69	21	25	28	8	11	15
7–17 years	31	64	70	74	12	16	23	8.5	11	15.5
18–70 years	300	67	72	76	11	13	16	10	14	19

Subset	Percentage T helper cells				Percentage T suppressor cells			Helper/suppressor (CD4/CD8) Ratio		
CD number	CD4				CD8			CD4, CD8		
Reagent	Leu 3				Leu 2			Leu 3 Leu 2		
Percentile		P_{25}	P_{50}	P_{75}	P_{25}	P_{50}	P_{75}	P_{25}	P_{50}	P_{75}
Age group	Number									
Cord blood	24	28	35	42	26	29	33	0.80	1.15	1.75
1 day–11 months	31	35	41	48	18	23	28	1.35	1.80	2.55
1–6 years	54	32	37	40	25	32	36	1.00	1.20	1.60
7–17 years	31	33	36	40	28	31	36	1.05	1.20	1.40
18–70 years	300	38	42	46	31	35	40	1.00	1.20	1.50

Data obtained using flow cytometry. Kindly supplied by Dr F Hulstaert, Becton Dickinson Immunocytometry Systems Medical Department.

Table 1.26 Reference values for coagulation tests in the healthy full-term infant during the first 6 months of life*

Tests	Day 1 (n)	Day 5 (n)	Day 30 (n)	Day 90 (n)	Day 180 (n)	Adult (n)
PT(s)	13.0 ± 1.43(61)**	12.4 ± 1.46(77)**†	11.8 ± 1.25(67)**†	11.9 ± 1.15(62)**	12.3 ± 0.79(47)**	12.4 ± 0.78(29)
APTT(s)	42.9 ± 5.80(61)	42.6 ± 8.62(76)	40.4 ± 7.42(67)	37.1 ± 6.52(62)**	35.5 ± 3.71(47)**	33.5 ± 3.44(29)
TCT(s)	23.5 ± 2.38(58)**	23.1 ± 3.07(64)†	24.3 ± 2.44(53)**	25.1 ± 2.32(52)**	25.5 ± 2.86(41)**	25.0 ± 2.66(19)
Fibrinogen (g/l)	2.83 ± 0.58(61)**	3.12 ± 0.75(77)**	2.70 ± 0.54(67)**	2.43 ± 0.68(60)**†	2.51 ± 0.68(47)**†	2.78 ± 0.6l(29)
II(U/ml)	0.48 ± 0.11(61)	0.63 ± 0.15(76)	0.68 ± 0.17(67)	0.75 ± 0.15(62)	0.88 ± 0.14(47)	1.08 ± 0.19(29)
V(U/ml)	0.72 ± 0.18(61)	0.95 ± 0.25(76)	0.98 ± 0.18(67)	0.90 ± 0.21(62)	0.91 ± 0.18(47)	1.06 ± 0.22(29)
VII(U/ml)	0.66 ± 0.19(60)	0.89 ± 0.27(75)	0.90 ± 0.24(67)	0.91 ± 0.26(62)	0.87 ± 0.20(47)	1.05 ± 0.19(29)
VIII(U/ml)	1.00 ± 0.39(60)**†	0.88 ± 0.33(75)**†	0.91 ± 0.33(67)**†	0.79 ± 0.23(62)**†	0.73 ± 0.18(47)†	0.99 ± 0.25(29)
vWF(U/ml)	1.53 ± 0.67(40)†	1.40 ± 0.57(43)†	1.28 ± 0.59(40)†	I.18 ± 0.44(40)†	1.07 ± 0.45(46)†	0.92 ± 0.33(29)†
IX(U/ml)	0.53 ± 0.19(59)	0.53 ± 0.19(75)	0.51 ± 0.15(67)	0.67 ± 0.23(62)	0.86 ± 0.25(47)	1.09 ± 0.27(29)
X(U/ml)	0.40 ± 0.14(60)	0.49 ± 0.15(76)	0.59 ± 0.14(67)	0.71 ± 0.18(62)	0.78 ± 0.20(47)	1.06 ± 0.23(29)
XI(U/ml)	0.38 ± 0.14(60)	0.55 ± 0.16(74)	0.53 ± 0.13(67)	0.69 ± 0.14(62)	0.86 ± 0.24(47)	0.97 ± 0.15(29)
XII(U/ml)	0.53 ± 0.20(60)	0.47 ± 0.18(75)	0.49 ± 0.16(67)	0.67 ± 0.21(62)	0.77 ± 0.19(47)	1.08 ± 0.28(29)
PK(U/Ml)	0.37 ± 0.16(45)†	0.48 ± 0.14(51)	0.57 ± 0.17(48)	0.73 ± 0.16(46)	0.86 ± 0.15(43)	1.12 ± 0.25(29)
HMW-K(U/ml)	0.54 ± 0.24(47)	0.74 ± 0.28(63)	0.77 ± 0.22(50)**	0.82 ± 0.32(46)**	0.82 ± 0.23(48)**	0.92 ± 0.22(29)
XIIIa(U/ml)	0.79 ± 0.26(44)	0.94 ± 0.25(49)**	0.93 ± 0.27(44)**	1.04 ± 0.34(44)**	1.04 ± 0.29(41)**	1.05 ± 0.25(29)
XIIIb(U/ml)	0.76 ± 0.23(44)	1.06 ± 0.37(47)**	1.11 ± 0.36(45)**	1.16 ± 0.34(44)**	1.10 ± 0.30(41)**	0.97 ± 0.20(29)
Plasminogen (CTA, U/ml)	1.95 ± 0.35(44)	2.17 ± 0.38(60)	1.98 ± 0.36(52)	2.48 ± 0.37(44)	3.01 ± 0.40(47)	3.36 ± 0.44(29)

* All values expressed as mean ± 1 SD. All factors except fibrinogen and plasminogen are expressed as units/ml where pooled plasma contains 1.0 units/ml. Plastinogen units are those recommended by the Committee on Thrombolytic Agents (CTA). n = numbers studied
**Values that do not differ statistically from the adult values.
† These measurements are skewed because of a disproportionate number of high values.
PT = prothrombin time; APTT = activated partial thromboplastin time; TCT = thrombin clotting time; VWF = von Willebrand factor; PK = prekallikrein; HMW-K = high molecular weight kininogen.
Note: longer APTT and TCT values may be obtained in newborns and infants using reagent combinations other than those used in this study.
(Reproduced from Andrew et al 1987, by permission of Dr M Andrew and Grune & Stratton.)

Table 1.27   Reference values for coagulation tests in healthy premature infants (30 to 36 weeks gestation) during the first 6 months of life*

	Day 1 M	Day 1 B	Day 5 M	Day 5 B	Day 30 M	Day 30 B	Day 90 M	Day 90 B	Day 180 M	Day 180 B	Adult M	Adult B
PT(s)	13.0	(10.6–16.2)**	12.5	(10.0–15.3)**†	11.8	(10.0–13.6)**	12.3	(10.0–14.6)**	12.5	(10.0–15.0)**	12.4	(10.8–13.9)
APTT(s)	53.6	(27.5–79.4)†	50.5	(26.9–74.1)†	44.7	(26.9–62.5)	39.5	(28.3–50.7)	37.5	(21.7–53.3)**	33.5	(26.6–40.3)
TCT(s)	24.8	(19.2–30.4)**	24.1	(18.8–29.4)**	24.4	(18.8–29.9)**	25.1	(19.4–30.8)**	25.2	(18.9–31.5)**	25.0	(19.7–30.3)
Fibrinogen (g/l)	2.43	(1.50–3.73)**†+	2.80	(1.60–4.18)**†+	2.54	(I.50–4.14)**†	2.46	(1.50–3.52)**†	2.28	(1.50–3.60)†	2.78	(1.56–4.00)
II(U/ml)	0.45	(0.20–0.77)†	0.57	(0.29–0.85)†	0.57	(0.36–0.95)†+	0.68	(0.30–1.06)	0.87	(0.51–1.23)	1.08	(0.70–1.46)
V(U/ml)	0.88	(0.41–1.44)**†+	1.00	(0.46–1.54)	1.02	(0.48–1.56)	0.99	(0.59–1.39)	1.02	(0.58–1.46)	1.06	(0.62–1.50)
VII(U/ml)	0.67	(0.21–1.13)	0.84	(0.30–1.38)	0.83	(0.21–1.45)	0.87	(0.31–1.43)	0.99	(0.47–1.51)**	1.05	(0.67–1.43)
VIII(U/ml)	1.11	(0.50–2.13)**†	1.15	(0.53–2.05)**†+	1.11	(0.50–1.99)**†+	1.06	(0.58–1.88)**†+	0.99	(0.50–1.87)**†+	0.99	(0.50–1.49)
vWF(U/ml)	1.36	(0.78–2.10)†	1.33	(0.72–2.19)†	1.36	(0.66–2.16)†	1.12	(0.75–1.84)**†	0.98	(0.54–1.58)**†	0.92	(0.50–1.58)
IX(U/ml)	0.35	(0.19–0.65)†+	0.42	(0.14–0.74)†+	0.44	(0.13–0.80)†	0.59	(0.25–0.93)	0.81	(0.50–1.20)†	1.09	(0.55–1.63)
X(U/ml)	0.41	(0.11–0.71)	0.51	(0.19–0.83)	0.56	(0.20–0.92)	0.67	(0.35–0.99)	0.77	(0.35–1.19)	1.06	(0.70–1.52)
XI(U/ml)	0.30	(0.08–0.52)†+	0.41	(0.13–0.69)+	0.43	(0.15–0.71)+	0.59	(0.25–0.93)+	0.78	(0.46–1.10)	0.97	(0.67–1.27)
XII(U/ml)	0.38	(0.10–0.66)+	0.39	(0.09–0.69)+	0.43	(0.11–0.75)	0.611	(0.15–1.07)	0.82	(0.22–1.42)	1.08	(0.52–1.64)
PK(U/ml)	0.33	(0.09–0.57)	0.45	(0.28–0.75)†	0.59	(0.31–0.87)	0.79	(0.37–1.21)	0.78	(0.40–1.16)	1.12	(0.62–1.62)
HMWK (U/ml)	0.49	(0.09–0.89)	0.62	(0.24–1.00)+	0.64	(0.16–1.12)+	0.78	(0.32–1.24)	0.83	(0.41–1.25)**	0.92	(0.50–1.36)
XIIIa(U/ml)	0.70	(0.32–1.08)	1.01	(0.57–1.45)**	0.99	(0.51–1.47)**	1.13	(0.71–1.55)**	1.13	(0.65–1.61)**	1.05	(0.55–1.55)
XIIIb(U/ml)	0.81	(0.35–1.27)	1.10	(0.68–1.58)**	1.07	(0.57–1.57)**	1.21	(0.75–1.67)	1.15	(0.67–1.63)	0.97	(0.57–1.37)
Plasminogen (CTA, (U/ml)	1.70	(1.12–2.48)†+	1.91	(1.21–2.61)+	1.81	(1.09–2.53)	2.38	(1.58–3.18)	2.75	(1.91–3.59)+	3.36	(2.48–4.24)

* All values are given as a mean (M) followed by lower and upper boundaries (B) encompassing 95% of the population.
  Between 40 and 96 samples were assayed for each value for newborns
** Values indistinguishable from those adults
† Measurements are skewed owing to a disproportionate number of high values. Lower limit which excludes the lower 2.5% of the population is given (B)
+ Values different from those of full-term infants
  Other data as stated in footnotes to Table 1.26
  (Reproduced from Andrew et al 1988, by permission of Dr M Andrew and Grune & Stratton.)

Table 1.28   Reference values for the inhibitors of coagulation in the healthy full-term infant during the first 6 months of life*

Inhibitors	Day l(n)	Day 5(n)	Day 30(n)	Day 90(n)	Day 180(n)	Adult(n)
AT-III(U/ml)	0.63 ± 0.12(58)	0.67 ± 0.13(74)	0.78 ± 0.15(66)	0.97 ± 0.12(60)**	1.04 ± 0.10(56)**	1.05 ± 0.13(28)
α_2-M(U/ml)	1.39 ± 0.22(54)	1.48 ± 0.25(73)	1.50 ± 0.22(61)	1.76 ± 0.25(55)	1.91 ± 0.21(55)	0.86 ± 0.17(29)
α_2–AP(U/ml)	0.85 ± 0.15(55)	1.00 ± 0.15(75)**	1.00 ± 0.12(62)**	1.08 ± 0.16(55)**	1.11 ± 0.14(53)**	1.02 ± 0.17(29)
C_1E-INH(U/ml)	0.72 ± 0.18(59)	0.90 ± 0.15(76)**	0.89 ± 0.21(63)	1.15 ± 0.22(55)	1.41 ± 0.26(55)	1.01 ± 0.15(29)
α_1–AT(U/ml)	0.93 ± 0.22(57)**	0.89 ± 0.20(75)**	0.62 ± 0.13(61)	0.72 ± 0.15(56)	0.77 ± 0.15(55)	0.93 ± 0.19(29)
HCII(U/ml)	0.43 ± 0.25(56)	0.48 ± 0.24(72)	0.47 ± 0.20(58)	0.72 ± 0.37(58)	1.20 ± 0.35(55)	0.96 ± 0.15(29)
Protein C(U/ml)	0.35 ± 0.09(41)	0.42 ± 0.11(44)	0.43 ± 0.11(43)	0.54 ± 0.13(44)	0.59 ± 0.11(52)	0.96 ± 0.16(28)
Protein S(U/ml)	0.36 ± 0.12(40)	0.50 ± 0.14(48)	0.63 ± 0.15(41)	0.86 ± 0.16(46)**	0.87 ± 0.16(49)**	0.92 ± 0.16(29)

* All values expressed in units/ml as mean ± 1 SD. n = numbers studied
** Values indistinguishable from those of adults
  AT-III = antithrombin III; α_2-M = alpha$_2$ macroglobulin; α_2–AP = alpha$_2$ antiplasmin; C_1E-INH = C_1 esterase inhibitor; α_1-AT = alpha$_1$ antitrypsin; HCII = heparin cofactor II.
  (Reproduced from Andrew et al 1987 by permission of Dr M Andrew and Grune & Stratton.)

Table 1.29 Reference values for inhibitors of coagulation in healthy premature infants during the first 6 months of life*

	Day 1		Day 5		Day 30		Day 90		Day 180		Adult	
	M	B	M	B	M	B	M	B	M	B	M	B
AT–III(U/ml)	0.38	(0.14–0.62)[+]	0.56	(0.30–0.82)**	0.59	(0.37–0.81)[+]	0.83	(0.45–1.21)[+]	0.90	(0.52–1.28)[+]	1.05	(0.79–1.31)
α_2-M(U/ml)	1.10	(0.56–1.82)[†+]	1.25	(0.71–1.77)**	1.38	(0.72–2.04)	1.80	(1.20–2.66)[†]	2.09	(1.10–3.21)[†]	0.86	(0.52–1.20)
α_2-AP(U/ml)	0.78	(0.40–1.16)	0.81	(0.49–1.13)**	0.89	(0.55–1.23)[+]	1.06	(0.64-1.48)**	1.15	(0.77–1.53)	1.02	(0.68–1.36)
C_1E–INH (U/ml)	0.65	(0.31–0.99)	0.83	(0.45–1.21)	0.74	(0.40–1.24)[††]	1.14	(0.60–1.68)**	1.40	(0.96–2.04)[†]	1.01	(0.71–1.31)
α_1-AT(U/ml)	0.90	(0.36–1.44)**	0.94	(0.42–1.46)[+]	0.76	(0.38–1.12)[+]	0.81	(0.49–1.13)***[+]	0.82	(0.48–1.16)**	0.93	(0.55–1.31)
HCII (U/ml)	0.32	(0.00–0.80)[+]	0.34	(0.00–0.69)	0.43	(0.15–0.71)	0.61	(0.20–1.11)[†]	0.89	(0.45–1.40)**[††+]	0.96	(0.66–1.26)
Protein C (U/ml)	0.28	(0.12–0.44)[+]	0.31	(0.11–0.51)	0.37	(0.15–0.59)[+]	0.45	(0.23–0.67)[+]	0.57	(0.31–0.83)	0.96	(0.64–1.28)
Protein S (U/ml)	0.26	(0.14–0.38)[+]	0.37	(0.13–0.61)	0.56	(0.22–0.90)	0.76	(0.40–1.12)[+]	0.82	(0.44–1.20)	0.92	(0.60–1.24)

  * All values are expressed in units/ml, where pooled plasma contains 1.0 U/ml. All values are given a mean (M) followed by lower and upper
    boundaries encompassing 95% of the population (B). Between 40 and 75 samples were assayed for each value for the newborn.
 ** Values indistinguishable from those of adults.
  [†] Measurements are skewed owing to a disproportionate number of high values. Lower limit which excludes the lower 2.5% of the population is
    given (B).
  [+] Values different from those of full-term infants.
    Other data as stated in footnote to Table 1.28.
    (Reproduced from Andrew et al 1988 by permission of Dr M Andrew and Grune & Stratton.)

Table 1.30 Range of values for fibrin/fibrinogen
degradation products (FDP) in µg/ml in the first week of life*

N	FDP
25	0–16

  * Measured by latex particle agglutination.
    (Data from Stuart et al 1973.)

Table 1.31 Vitamin $K_{1(20)}$ levels (pg/ml) in formula-fed and breast-fed infants with
(K^+) and without (K^-) vitamin $K_{1(20)}$ prophylaxis

Age	1–4 days				29–35 days			
	Mean	Median	No. used	< DL[a]	Mean	Median	No. used	< DL[a]*
Breast-fed (K^-)	280	249	12	2	913	646	10	1
Breast-fed (K^+)	32711	24446	13	–	697	535	9	–
Formula-fed	1900	1515	5	2	2890	2827	6	–

 * < DL[a] = below detection limit of 60 pg/ml
    (Reproduced from Lambert et al 1987, by permission of Dr W. Lambert and Elsevier
    Science Publishing.)

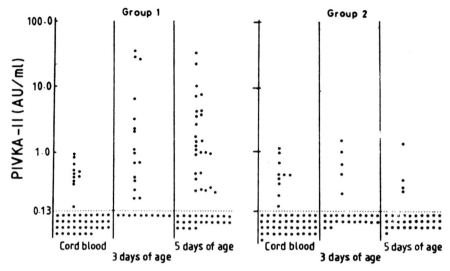

Fig. 1.13 Protein induced by vitamin K absence or antagonist-II (PIVKA–II) levels in cord blood and blood samples obtained at 3 or 5 days of age. Group 1 did not receive vitamin K; group 2 received vitamin K. (The dotted line indicates the lower limit of sensitivity of the assay.) One arbitrary unit (AU) of PIVKA II corresponds to 1 μg of purified prothrombin. (Reproduced from Motohara et al 1985 by permission of the Lancet Ltd.)

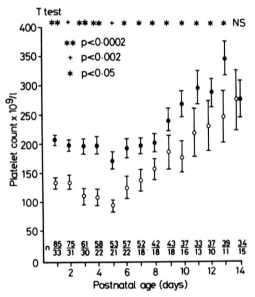

Fig. 1.14 Platelet count (× 10⁹/1; bar indicates ± 1 SD) during the first 14 days of life in babies of appropriate weight for gestational age (●) and babies who were small for gestational age (○).
(Reproduced from McIntosh et al 1988 by permission of Professor N McIntosh and the editor of Archives of Disease in Childhood.)

Table 1.32 Bleeding time (minutes) in newborns and children*

Subjects	No. tested	Sphygmomanometer pressure (mmHg)	Mean	Range
Term newborn	30	30	3.4	1.9–5.8
Preterm newborn:				
< 1000 g	6	20	3.3	2.6–4.0
1000–2000 g	15	25	3.9	2.0–5.6
> 2000 g	5	30	3.2	2.3–5.0
Children	17	30	3.4	1.0–5.5
Adults	20	30	2.8	0.5–5.5

*Bleeding time performed using a template technique, with incision 5 mm long and 0.5 mm deep. All subjects had normal platelet counts.
(Summarized from Feusner 1980.)

Table 1.33 Bleeding time (minutes) in children and adults

Subjects	No. tested	Mean	SD	Range
Children	36	4.6	1.4	2.5–8.5
Adults	48	4.6	1.2	2.5–6.5

Bleeding time performed using a template technique, with incision 6 mm long and 1 mm deep and sphygmomanometer pressure 40 mmHg.
(Data from Buchanan & Holtkamp 1980)
N.B. Using this technique, bleeding times up to 11.5 minutes have been observed in apparently healthy children tested in the author's laboratory.

Table 1.34 The properties of cord blood platelets compared to mature platelets

Parameter	Response compared to mature platelets	References
Sensitive to ADP, collagen, adrenaline, thrombin	↓	Mull & Hathaway 1970 Ts'ao et al 1976 Corby & Zuck 1976
Sensitivity to ristocetin	↑	Ts'ao et al 1976
Lag phase to collagen, ADP, thrombin	↑	Mull & Hathaway 1970
Maximal aggregatory response	↓	Mull & Hathaway 1970
Adhesiveness to glass fibres	↓	Hrodek 1964
Content of ADP and ATP	↓	Corby & Zuck 1976
Release of ^{14}C-5-hydroxytryptamine	↓	Ts'ao et al 1976 Whaun 1973
Lipid peroxidation	↓	Stuart 1978 Stuart et al 1979
Availability of PF3	↓	Hrodek 1964

(Reproduced from Hinchliffe & Lilleyman 1987, by permission of Dr M. Greaves and John Wiley & Sons Ltd.)

Table 1.35 Serum immunoglobulin levels in UK caucasians (–2 SD, meridian, +2 SD by log-Gaussian)*

Age		IgG(g/l)	IgA(g/l)	IgM(g/l)
	Cord	10.8 (5.2–18.0)	< 0.02	0.1 (0.02–0.2)
Weeks	0–2	9.4 (5.0–17.0)	0.02 (0.01–0.08)	0.1 (0.05–0.2)
	2–6	7.1 (3.9–13.0)	0.05 (0.02–0.15)	0.2 (0.08–0.4)
	6–12	3.9 (2.1–7.7)	0.15 (0.05–0.4)	0.4 (0.15–0.7)
Months	3–6	4.6 (2.4–8.8)	0.2 (0.1–0.5)	0.6 (0.2–1.0)
	6–9	5.2 (3.0–9.0)	0.3 (0.15–0.7)	0.8 (0.4–1.6)
	9–12	5.8 (3.0–10.9)	0.4 (0.2–0.7)	1.2 (0.6–2.1)
Years	1–2	6.4 (3.1–13.8)	0.7 (0.3–1.2)	1.3 (0.5–2.2)
	2–3	7.0 (3.7–15.8)	0.8 (0.3–1.3)	1.3 (0.5–2.2)
	3–6	9.9 (4.9–16.1)	1.0 (0.4–2.0)	1.3 (0.5–2.0)
	6–9	9.9 (5.4–16.1)	1.3 (0.5–2.4)	1.2 (0.5–1.8)
	9–12	9.9 (5.4–16.1)	1.4 (0.7–2.5)	1.1 (0.5–1.8)
	12–15	9.9 (5.4–16.1)	1.9 (0.8–2.8)	1.2 (0.5–1.9)
	15–45	9.9 (5.4–16.1)	1.9 (0.8–2.8)	1.2 (0.5–1.9)
	>45	9.9 (5.3–16.5)	1.9 (0.8–4.0)	1.2 (0.5–2.0)

*Determined in 53 males and 54 females above 15 years and in groups of at least 30 subjects for the other age groups
(Reproduced from Ward 1988, by permission of Protein Reference Unit Publications.)

Table 1.36 Mean and 5th–95th centile ranges (g/l) for IgG subclasses at various ages*

Age	IgG$_1$	IgG$_2$	IgG$_3$	IgG$_4$
Cord blood	4.7 (3.6–8.4)	2.1 (1.2–4.0)	0.6 (0.3–1.5)	0.2 (< 0.5)
6 months	2.3 (1.5–3.0)	0.4 (0.3–0.5)	0.3 (0.1–0.6)	< 0.1
2 years	3.5 (2.3–5.8)	1.1 (0.3–2.9)	0.4 (0.1–0.8)	< 0.1 (< 0.5)
5 years	3.7 (2.3–6.4)	2.0 (0.7–4.5)	0.5 (0.1–1.1)	0.3 (< 0.1–0.8)
10 years	5.2 (3.6–7.3)	2.6 (1.4–4.5)	0.7 (0.3–1.1)	0.4 (< 0.1–1.0)
15 years	5.4 (3.8–7.7)	2.6 (1.3–4.6)	0.7 (0.2–1.2)	0.4 (< 0.1–1.1)
Adult	5.9 (3.2–10.2)	3.0 (1.2–6.6)	0.7 (0.2–1.9)	0.5 (< 0.1–1.3)

* In adults IgG$_3$ levels are higher in females than in males, and IgG$_4$ higher in males than in females. No sex difference is seen before the age of 15 years.
(Reproduced from Ward 1988, by permission of Protein Reference Unit Publications.)

Table 1.37 Serum IgD levels (g/l)

No. tested	Age	IgD
23	6 weeks–19 months	< 0.01–0.016
105	3–14 years	< 0.01–0.036

Data from Buckley & Fiscus 1975.
(Reproduced from Hinchliffe & Lilleyman 1987, by permission of John Wiley & Sons Ltd.)

Table 1.38 Total serum IgE levels*

Age	Median	95th centile
Newborn	0.5	5
3 months	3	11
1 year	8	29
5 years	15	52
10 years	18	63
Adult	26	120

*Expressed in units in relation to the first British Standard for human serum IgE 75/502.
(Reproduced from Ward 1988, by permission of Protein Reference Unit Publications.)

Table 1.39 Erythrocyte sedimentation rate (mm/h) in healthy children

Method	No. tested	Age (years)	Mean	Range	% above 20 mm
Wintrobe					
	245	4–11	12.0	1–41	9
	169	12–15	7.5	< 1–34	7
Westergren (read at 45min)					
	78	4–7	13	< 1–55	
	153	8–14	10.5	1–62	

Data from Hollinger & Robinson 1953; Osgood et al 1939a, b

Table 1.40 Isohaemagglutinin titre in relation to age

Age	Isohaemagglutin titre (IHA) mean and range
Cord blood	0*
1–3 months	1:5[+]
	(0–1:10)
4–6 months	1:10[+]
	0–1:160)
7–12 months	1:80**
	(0–1:640)
13–24 months	1:80**
	(0–1:640)
25–36 months	1:160[†]
	(1:10–1:640)
3–5 years	1:80
	(1:5–1:640)
6–8 years	1:80
	(1:5–1:640)
9–11 years	1:160
	(1:20–1:640)
12–16 years	1:160
	(1:10–1:320)
Adult	1:160
	(1:10–1:640)

 * IHA activity is rarely detectable in cord blood
 [+] 50% of normal infants will not have IHA at this age
** 10% of normal infants will not have IHA at this age
 [†] Beyond this age all normal individuals have IHA with the exception of those of blood group AB.
Summarized from Ellis & Robbins 1978
(Reproduced from Hinchliffe & Lilleyman 1987, by permission of John Wiley & Sons Ltd.)

REFERENCES

Andrew M, Paes B, Milner R, et al 1987 Development of the human coagulation system in the full-term infant. Blood 70: 165–172

Andrew M, Paes B, Milner R, et al 1988 Development of the coagulation system in the healthy premature infant. Blood 72: 1651–1657

Auerbach A D, Alter B P 1989 Prenatal and postnatal diagnosis of aplastic anaemia. In: Alter B P (ed) Perinatal Haematology. Methods in Haematology 19. Churchill Livingstone, Edinburgh, p 225–251

Beutler E 1984 Red cell metabolism 3rd edn. Grune & Stratton, New York

Buchanan G R, Holtkamp C A 1980 Prolonged bleeding time in children and young adults with hemophilia. Pediatrics 66: 951–955

Buckley R H, Fiscus S A 1975 Serum IgD and IgE concentrations in immunodeficiency diseases. Journal of Clinical Investigation 55: 157–165

Corby D G, Zuck T F 1976 Newborn platelet dysfunction: a storage pool defect. Thrombosis and Haemostasis 36: 200–207

Dacie J V, Lewis S M 1984 Practical haematology, 6th edn. Churchill Livingstone, Edinburgh

Dallman P R 1977 Blood and blood forming tissues. In: Rudolph A M (ed) Pediatrics, 16th edn. Appleton Century-Crofts, New York, p 1109–1222

Dallman P R, Barr G D, Allen C M, Shinefield H R 1978 Hemoglobin concentration in white, black and oriental children: is there a need for separate criteria in screening for anaemia? American Journal of Clinical Nutrition 31: 377–380

Dallman P R, Siimes M A 1979 Percentile curves for hemoglobin and red cell volume in infancy and childhood. Journal of Pediatrics 94: 26–31

Deinard A S, Schwartz S, Yip R 1983 Developmental changes in serum ferritin and erythrocyte protoporphyrin in normal (non-anemic) children. American Journal of Clinical Nutrition 38: 71–76

Dormandy K M, Waters A H, Mollin D L 1963 Folic acid deficiency in coeliac disease. Lancet 1: 632–635

Ellis E F, Robbins J B 1978 In Johnson T R, Moore W M (eds) Children are different: developmental physiology. Ross Laboratories, Columbus Ohio

Feusner J H 1980 Normal and abnormal bleeding times in neonates and young children using a fully standardised template technic. American Journal of Clinical Pathology 74: 73–77

Foconi S, Sjolin S 1959 Survival of Cr-labelled red cells from newborn infants. Acta Paediatrica 48 (suppl 117): 18–23

Galanello R, Melis M A, Ruggeri R, Cao A 1981 Prospective study of red blood cell indices, hemoglobin A_2 and hemoglobin F in infants heterozygous for β-thalassaemia. Journal of Pediatrics 99: 105–108

Gomez P, Coca C, Vargas C, Acebillo J, Martinex A 1984 Normal reference-intervals for 20 biochemical variables in healthy infants, children, and adolescents. Clinical Chemistry 30: 407–412

Hinchliffe R F, Lilleyman J S (eds) 1987 Practical paediatric haematology. John Wiley & Sons, Chichester

Hollinger N, Robinson S J 1953 A study of the erythrocyte sedimentation rate for well children. Journal of Pediatrics 42: 304–319

Hovi L M, Siimes M A 1983 Red blood cell morphology in healthy full-term newborns. Acta Paediatrica Scandinavica 72: 135–136

Hrodek O 1964 Les Fonctions des plaquettes sanguines chez le nouveau-né. Hemostase 4: 55–62

Kaplan E, Hsu K S 1961 Determination of erythrocyte survival in newborn infants by means of Cr-labelled erythrocytes. Pediatrics 27: 354–361

Khalil M, Badr-El-Din M K, Kassem A S 1967 Haptoglobin level in normal infants and children. Alexandria Medical Journal 13: 1–9

Koerper M A, Dallman P R 1977 Serum iron concentration and transferrin saturation in the diagnosis of iron deficiency in children: normal developmental changes. Journal of Pediatrics 91: 870–874

Konrad P M, Valentine W M, Paglia D E 1972 Enzymatic activities and glutathione content of erythrocytes in the newborn: comparison with red cells of older normal subjects and those with comparable reticulocytosis. Acta Haematologica 48: 193–201

Kravitz H, Elegant L D, Kaiser E, Kagan B M 1956 Methemoglobin values in premature and mature infants and children. American Journal of Diseases of Children 91: 1–5

Lambert W, De Leenheer A, Tassaneeyakul W, Widdershoven J 1987 Study of Vitamin $K_{1(20)}$ in the newborn by HPLC with wet-chemical post-column reduction and fluorescence detection. In: Suttie J W (ed) Current advances in vitamin K research. Elsevier, New York, p 509–514

Lloyd B W, Oto A 1982 Normal values for mature and immature neutrophils in very preterm babies. Archives of Disease in Childhood 57: 233–235

Lundh B, Oski F, Gardner F H 1970 Plasma haemopexin and haptoglobin in haemolytic disorders of the newborn. Acta Paediatrica Scandinavica 59: 121–126

Lundstrom U, Siimes M A, Dallman P R 1977 At what age does iron supplementation become necessary in low-birth-weight infants? Journal of Pediatrics 91: 878–883

McIntosh N, Kempson C, Tyler R M 1988 Blood counts in extremely low birthweight infants. Archives of Disease in Childhood 63: 74–76

Manroe B L, Weinberg A G, Rosenfeld C R, Browne R 1979 The neonatal blood count in health and disease 1. Reference values for neutrophilic cells. Journal of Pediatrics 95: 89–98

Metaxotou-Mavromati A D, Antonopoulo H K, Laskari S S, Tsiarta H K, Ladis V A, Kattamis C A 1982 Developmental changes in Hemoglobin F levels during the first two years of life in normal and heterozygous β-thalassemia infants. Pediatrics 69: 734–738

Mollison P L, Veall N, Cutbush M 1950 Red cell and plasma volume in newborn infants. Archives of Disease in Childhood 25: 242–253

Motohara K, Endo F, Matsuda I 1985 Effect of vitamin K administration on acarboxy prothrombin (PIVKA-II) levels in newborns. Lancet ii: 242–244

Mull M M, Hathaway W E 1970 Altered platelet function in newborns. Pediatric Research 4: 229–237

Osgood E E, Baker R L, Brownlee I E, Osgood M W, Ellis D M, Cohen W 1939a Total, differential and absolute leukocyte counts and sedimentation rates of healthy children four to seven years of age. American Journal of Diseases of Children 58: 61–70

Osgood E E, Baker R L, Brownlee I E, Osgood M W, Ellis M, Cohen W 1939b Total, dffferential and absolute leukocyte counts and sedimentation rates for healthy children. Standards for children eight to fourteen years of age. American Journal of Disease of Children 58: 282–294

Oski F A 1982 Normal blood values in the newborn period. In: Oski F A, Naiman J L (eds). Hematologic problems in the newborn. W B Saunders, Philadelphia, p 1–31

Russell S J M 1949 Blood volume studies in healthy children. Archives of Disease in Childhood 24: 88–98

Saarinen U M, Siimes M A 1977 Developmental changes in serum iron, total iron-binding capacity, and transferrin saturation in infancy. Journal of Pediatrics 91: 875–877

Saarinen U M, Siimes M A 1978 Developmental changes in red blood cell counts and indices of infants after exclusion of iron deficiency by laboratory criteria and continuous iron supplementation. Journal of Pediatrics 92: 412–416

Schröter W, Nafz C 1981 Diagnostic significance of hemoglobin F and A_2 levels in homo- and heterozygous β-thalassaemia during infancy. Helvetica Paediatrica Acta 36: 519–525

Scott-Emuakpor A B, Okolo A A, Omene J A, Ukpe S I 1985a Normal hematological values of the African neonate. Blut 51: 11–18

Scott-Emuakpor A B, Okolo A A, Omene J A, Ukpe S I 1985b Pattern of leukocytes in blood of healthy African neonates. Acta Haematologica 74: 104–107

Serjeant G R, Grandison Y, Mason K, Serjeant B, Sewell A, Vaidya S 1980 Haematological indices in normal negro children: a Jamaican cohort from birth to five years. Clinical and Laboratory Haematology 2: 169–178

Stuart J, Breeze G R, Picken A M, Wood B S B 1973 Capillary-blood coagulation profile in the newborn. Lancet ii: 1467–1471

Stuart M J 1978 The neonatal platelet: evaluation of platelet malonyl dialdehyde formation as an indicator of prostaglandin synthesis. British Journal of Haematology 39: 83–90

Stuart M J, Elrad H, Graeber J E, Hakanson D O, Sunderji S G, Barvinchak M K 1979 Increased synthesis of prostaglandin endoperoxides and platelet hyperfunction in infants of mothers with diabetes mellitus. Journal of Clinical and Laboratory Medicine 94: 12–17

Sukarochana K, Parenzan L, Thalurdas N, Kieswelter W B 1961 Red cell mass determinations in infancy and childhood, with the use of radioactive chromium. Journal of Pediatrics 59: 903–908

Thomas R M, Linch D C 1983 Identification of lymphocyte subsets in the newborn using a variety of monoclonal antibodies. Archives of Disease in Childhood 58: 34–38

Tietz N W, Blackburn R H (eds) 1981 Reference values and general information. Lexington Kentucky. Clinical Laboratories, A B Chandler Medical Center, University of Kentucky

Ts'ao C-H, Green D, Schultz K 1976 Function and ultrastructure of platelets of neonates: enhanced ristocetin aggregation of neonatal platelets. British Journal of Haematology 32: 225–233

Usher R, Shephard M, Lind J 1963 The blood volume of the newborn infant and placental transfusion. Acta Paediatrica Scandinavica 52: 497–512

Vanier T M, Tyas J F 1966 Folic acid status in newborn infants during the first year of life. Archives of Disease in Childhood 41: 658–665

Vanier T M, Tyas J F 1967 Folic acid status in premature infants. Archives of Disease in Childhood 42: 57–61

Ward A M (ed) 1988 Protein Reference Unit handbook of clinical immunochemistry, 2nd edn. PRU Publications, Sheffield

Weinberg A G, Rosenfeld C R, Manroe B L, Browne R 1985 Neonatal blood cell count in health and disease. II: Values for lymphocytes, monocytes, and eosinophils. Journal of Pediatrics 106: 462–466

Whaun J M 1973 The platelet of the newborn infant. Thrombosis et Diathesis Haemorrhagica 30: 327–333

Zaisov R, Matoth Y 1976 Red cell values on the first postnatal day during the last 16 weeks of gestation. American Journal of Hematology 1: 272–278

Zipursky A, Jaber H M 1978 The haematology of bacterial infection in newborn infants. Clinics in Haematology 7: 175–193

2. Aplastic anaemia

D. I. K. Evans

INTRODUCTION

Shahidi & Diamond (1961) defined aplastic anaemia as a 'physiological and anatomical failure of the bone marrow with marked decrease or absence of blood-forming elements in the marrow, peripheral pancytopenia and no splenomegaly, hepatomegaly or lymphadenopathy'. The statement still applies although we now know much more about the aetiology; it serves to remind us that the prime feature of bone marrow aplasia is failure of blood production with no evidence of extramedullary disease. Whereas cases may from time to time present with an enlarged liver, enlarged spleen or lymphadenopathy, due to disease which may or may nor be associated with the aplastic process, the enlargement of any one or more of these organs with a pancytopenia should initially suggest an alternative diagnosis, such as leukaemia or lymphoma.

Marked decrease of blood-forming elements in the bone marrow is a feature of severe aplastic anaemia, the type which is most common in childhood; but moderately affected cases may show only slight changes in blood and bone marrow, which may be overlooked unless the diagnosis is kept in mind. Cases presenting with thrombocytopenia, and only slight or absent anaemia, and a total leucocyte count in the normal range, but with a modest neutropenia, are sometimes misdiagnosed as acute thrombocytopenia. To exclude a diagnosis of marrow aplasia, rather than one of leukaemia, is one of the main reasons for undertaking bone marrow examination in children presenting with thrombocytopenia.

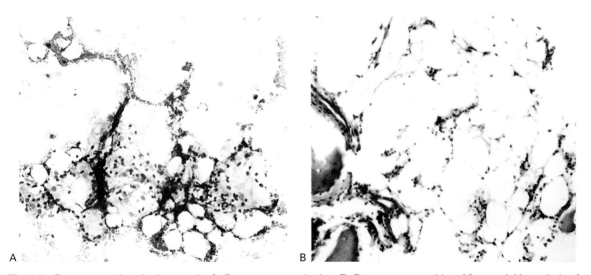

A   B

Fig. 2.1 Bone marrow in aplastic anaemia. **A.** Bone marrow aspiration. **B.** Bone marrow trephine. Note markd hypoplasia of all marrow elements

Pathologically, the characteristic lesion is replacement of the haemopoietic marrow elements by hypocellular fatty tissue containing reticulum cells, lymphocytes, plasma cells and, usually, tissue mast cells (Fig. 2.1). In severe cases, there is always a marked reduction or absence of megakaryocytes, myeloid cells and normoblasts.

Knospe & Crosby (1971) put forward the hypothesis that the primary cause of marrow depopulation is damage to the sinusoidal microcirculation of the marrow with secondary effects upon the haemopoietic cells. Such vascular lesions can be produced by large doses of localized X-irradiation in rats. However, the discovery that some patients treated by cytotoxic immunosuppressive drugs in preparation for bone marrow transplant recovered their own bone marrow function, with and without a transplant of normal marrow, suggested that in some patients, there might

Table 2.1 Aplastic anaemia in childhood

1. Constitutional
    Fanconi's anaemia
    –with other congenital defects (classical type)
    –without other defects (Estren-Dameshek type)
    –without chromosome changes
    Dyskeratosis congenita
    Shwachman's syndrome
    Other rare types – radio-ulnar fusion, Scandinavian type, etc.
2. Acquired
    Idiopathic
    Post-infectious
    –hepatitis
    –other infections
    Due to drugs
    –chemotherapy
    –other drugs
    Due to radiation
    Due to chemicals and toxins
    With paroxysmal nocturnal haemoglobinuria
    Pre-leukaemia

Table 2.2 Investigation of suspected bone marrow aplasia in children*

Group I	Group II—Aplasia confirmed
Aplasia suspected	Tests for haemolysis
Full blood counts including	Autohaemolysis
Haemoglobin and red cell count	Red cell enzymes
Red cell indices	Red cell survival (^{51}Cr)
Reticulocytes	
Total white cell count and differential counts	Tests for constitutional aplasias
Bone marrow aspiration	Height and weight
Blood group and Rhesus type	Head circumference
Direct Coombs' test	X-ray forearms and wrists for bone age and bone defects
	Intravenous pyelography
Aplasia probable	Urine and plasma amino-acids
Repeat bone marrow at second site	IQ assessment
Haemoglobin electrophoresis	Electroencephalography
Alkali denaturation test	Endocrine studies
Kleihauer test and test for HbH	
HLA typing	Tests for PNH
Chromosome analysis (blood and bone marrow)	Ham's acid serum test
Urea/creatinine	Sugar water test
Direct and indirect serum bilirubin	
Liver function tests	Test for Shwachman's syndrome
Proteins and electrophoresis	Faeces – trypsin and faecal fat
Immunoglobulins	Fat loading test
Hepatitis serology	Pancreatic function tests/duodenal intubation
Virus isolation–throat, urine and faeces	Urine sugar chromatography (galactose)
Urine-bilirubin, urobilin and urobilinogen, haemosiderin	
Family–full blood counts and HLA typing	Miscellaneous tests
	Leucocyte alkaline phosphatase
Group I tests are desirable in all cases	Serum B$_{12}$
	Red cell and serum folate
	Serum iron and iron-binding capacity
	Serum ferritin
	Full red cell antigens
	CFU–bone marrow and blood
	Group II tests may help with specific diagnosis, and may be selected for specific cases

* (Adapted from Evans 1979)

be immunological damage to the bone marrow. Subsequently it has been shown that lymphocytes or plasma constituents may be responsible for bone marrow suppression, and that in these cases, aplastic anaemia may be regarded as an autoimmune disease.

Immunosuppressive treatment with high doses of methyl prednisolone and or anti-lymphocyte globulin may be curative. Not all patients respond to treatment of this sort, and bone marrow failure is likely to be the end result of a variety of mechanisms.

CLASSIFICATION

In children and young people, aplastic anaemia may be *constitutional*, as shown by a familial tendency or associated congenital defects, or *acquired*. If acquired, there may be an identifiable cause, toxic or infective, or no such identifiable cause, when it is classified as being 'idiopathic'. The aplastic anaemia of childhood is usually a pancytopenic disorder with all three haemopoietic lines involved. On rare occasions only one cell line is predominantly affected, and changes in the others are only slight and not always consistent in the same case. Isolated aplastic and hypoplastic cytopenias should, strictly speaking, not be classified as aplastic anaemia, and are dealt with elsewhere in this book. Table 2.1 gives a general classification of aplastic anaemia, and Table 2.2 lists the investigations which are helpful in the diagnosis.

CONSTITUTIONAL APLASTIC ANAEMIA

Fanconi's anaemia

Introduction

Fanconi (1927) made the original description of the anaemia associated with his name. He described a pancytopenia with macrocytosis resembling pernicious anaemia. Patients also have multiple congenital abnormalities which may be apparent at birth although the blood and bone marrow changes may not become detectable until several years later (Table 2.3). Nilsson's (1960) paper summarized 82 reported cases. There was a familial background in 62, occurring in 30

families, usually as siblings. The disease is inherited in an autosomal recessive manner. There is no suggestion that either sex is predisposed to the disease. In one family both mother and child were affected (Imerslund 1953). It was suggested in this case that the inheritance was dominant. However, in the same family, the manifestations of the disease may vary considerably, and it may be difficult to distinguish patients with minor manifestations from carriers. At one time a distinction was made between constitutional aplastic anaemia associated with other congenital defects (known as Fanconi's anaemia) and constitutional aplastic anaemia lacking other congenital defects which was known as the Estren–Dameshek variant (Estren & Dameshek 1947). Now that both types have been recognized in the same family, it has to be acknowledged that the two presentations are the same disease, but with different manifestations.

There is an associated predisposition to leukaemia, usually of the myelomonocytic variety, which seems likely to be related to the chromosome de-

Table 2.3 Physical abnormalities in Fanconi's anaemia (data from 68 published cases) (adapted from Nilsson (1960))

Abnormal pigmentation	51	Mental backwardness	14
Skeletal deformities	40†	Microphthalmia	9
Stunted growth	38	Exaggerated reflexes	9
Small head	29	Deafness	7
Renal anomalies	19	Cryptorchism	5
Renal aplasia	(10)	Adiposity	5
Double pelvis		Congenital heart disease	4
and/or ureters	(5)	Ear deformities	3
Horseshoe kidney	(3)	Hypospadias	3
Hydronephrosis	(2)	Ptosis	2
Abnormally low		Epicanthus	2
kidney	(2)	Nystagmus	2
Congenital renal cyst	(1)	Transposition of	
Cardiac murmurs	19	penis & scrotum	1
Strabismus	18		
Hypogenitalism	15		

† The skeletal deformities in these 40 cases comprised:

Thumb deformities	28	Congenital dislocation	
Reduced number of		of the hip	3
ossification centres at		Syndactyly	3
the wrist	17	Absence of lower	
Aplasia of first		arm	1
metacarpal	7	Sprengel's deformity	1
Aplasia of the radius	7	Scoliosis	1
Generalised		Cervical rib	1
osteoporosis	5	Hip disease of	
Increased impressiones		Perthe's type	1
digitatae in cranium	4	Club foot	1
Hypoplasia of radius	3		
Broad base in proximal			
phalanges	3		

fects. Occasionally, leukaemia may be the initial presenting feature of the disease, and the possibility of Fanconi's anaemia should be considered in any child presenting with congenital defects and this type of leukaemia. Other malignant disorders have been described, including carcinoma, hepatoma, lymphoblastic leukaemia and lymphoma. In some cases who have survived many years, the malignant disease has presented very late, as in the case of Smith et al (1989) who presented with acute lymphoblastic leukaemia at the age of 45, and that of Rogers et al (1989) who died of carcinoma of the breast 20 years after diagnosis.

The chromosome defect of Fanconi's anaemia

Structural chromosome aberrations in cultured peripheral blood lymphocytes were first described in Fanconi's anaemia by Schroeder et al (1964). The abnormalities include chromatid exchanges, chromatid breaks and endoreduplication (Fig. 2.2). Apart from endoreduplication, the number of chromosomes remains normal.

Similar morphological changes of the chromosomes have been found in several childhood diseases, notably Bloom's syndrome, a disease characterized by failure to thrive, telangiectatic ery-

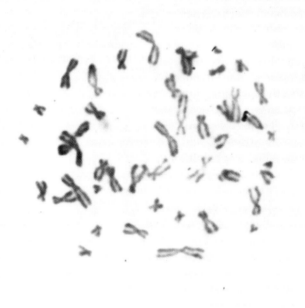

Fig. 2.2   Chromosome abnormalities in Fanconi's anaemia—multiple breaks and constrictions. (Reprinted from Evans 1979 with permission of Bailliere Tindall.)

thema of the face, molar hypoplasia, short stature and predisposition to leukaemia (Sawitsky et al 1966). They have also been found in ataxia telangiectasia (Louis-Bar syndrome), in which a progressive cerebellar ataxia is associated with capillary telangiectasia and a variable immune defect, and xeroderma pigmentosum, a rare autosomal recessive disease with skin sensitivity to sunlight. The patients are unable to repair DNA damaged by ultraviolet light, and develop erythema, scaling, telengiectasia, scarring and malignant changes in exposed areas. Such chromosome changes have also been reported in a case of infantile genetic agranulocytosis (Matsaniotis et al 1966), a condition in which the aplasia is restricted to the myeloid series.

The chromosome defect affects tissues other than the lymphocytes, and has also been demonstrated in the bone marrow and cultured skin fibroblasts (Swift & Hirshhorn 1966). Hirshhorn (1968) suggested that it is possible to explain all the manifestations of Fanconi's anaemia on the basis of a hereditary susceptibility to chromosome breakage: 'Many of the cells with broken chromosomes would be lost during development, causing the developmental anomalies, and during haemopoiesis causing aplastic anaemia, but some of the remaining cells would be more susceptible to neoplastic transformation'. Fibroblast cultures from patients with Fanconi's anaemia, as well as heterozygous carriers, are more easily transformed in vitro by a variety of agents, including cross-linking agents such as mitomycin C, cyclophosphamide, nitrogen mustard, cis-platinum, isonicotinic acid hydrazide and diepoxybutane, as well as irradiation, and the oncogenic simian virus, SV40. It may be relevant that the most frequently involved organ systems undergo embryonic differentiation at a similar time, the 25th to 34th day of fetal life (Althoff 1953).

Clinical features

The clinical features of Fanconi's anaemia may be extremely diverse, so that a diagnosis based

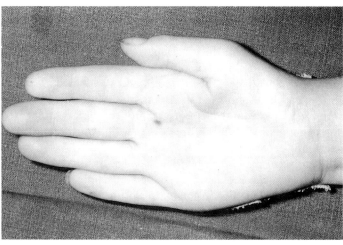

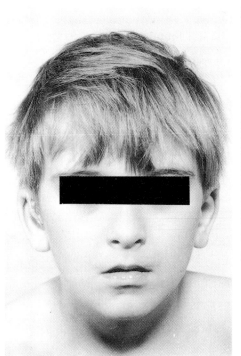

B

A

Fig. 2.3 Clinical features of Fanconi's anaemia. **A.** Shows pointed chin and elf-like facies. **B.** Shows hypoplasia of thenar and hypothenar eminences.

on clinical manifestations alone may be difficult and is often unreliable (Auerbach et al 1989). These authors have pointed out that cases reported in the literature are biased towards the most severe clinical cases which typically showed the most severe clinical manifestations, so that cases which do not fit this preconceived picture are not diagnosed. Many malformations are associated with the bone marrow disorder. Common findings include a low birth weight, poor stature, microcephaly, abnormal pigmentation, skeletal and renal deformities (Fig. 2.3). Some cases have responded to growth hormone; others have been resistant. The skin lesions comprise brown spots or hypopigmented areas at birth, and more deeply pigmented areas on the neck and axillae which darken progressively. Deformities of the hands and forearms are common, usually affecting the pre-axial border, such as hypoplasia of the thumb or first metacarpal. The kidney abnormalities include ectopia, aplasia, double kidney or ureter and malrotation. Exaggerated reflexes and osteoporosis are not uncommon. The face is often small with a pointed chin which, together with microphthalmia, gives the face an elfin appearance. X-rays of the long bones may show retardation of bone growth; and X-rays of the wrists may show abnormalities of the ossification centres. A very wide variety of defects have been described, and it is reasonable to assume that, owing to the random nature of the chromosome defects, any combination of congenital disorders are possible. The most frequently reported defects are listed in Table 2.3.

The disease may affect all racial groups. In different series, the incidence of associated clinical defects has varied. For instance, in South Africa, Rogers et al (1989) commented on the 20% incidence of gastrointestinal disease, which is higher than other series. The incidence of renal disorders, hyperreflexia and malignant disease is very variable. The clinical features of Fanconi's anaemia are compared with those of acquired aplastic anaemia in Table 2.4.

There is no enlargement of the liver or spleen, and the lymph nodes are not normally enlarged. Cervical lymphadenopathy may, however, develop secondary to infection in the upper respiratory tract. Susceptibility to infection is seen only rarely, and may be associated with neutropenia

or treatment with corticosteroids. Children who receive multiple transfusions over many years may develop generalized skin pigmentation due to haemosiderosis, and this should be distinguished from localized pigmentation due to the disease.

The Estren-Dameshek syndrome was the term used to describe patients with congenital aplastic anaemia who lacked the other congenital defects described in 'classical' Fanconi's anaemia. However, such cases have now been described in families with other children who show the typical Fanconi features (Glanz & Fraser 1982), so it appears that the Estren-Dameshek syndrome is simply another manifestation of Fanconi's anaemia, and not a separate clinical syndrome.

In spite of the familial pattern and associated clinical abnormalities, the cytopenias do not usually appear for several years, and purpura due to thrombocytopenia is frequently the initial presenting feature. Girot & Buriot (1980) reported on 45 cases; most presented between the ages of 3 and 10 years, although one case presented in the first year of life, and four were over 20 years old, the oldest being 28. Thrombocytopenia by itself, with neutropenia or anaemia, or as part of a pancytopenia was found in 41 cases (91%).

Table 2.4 Comparison of features of constitutional and acquired aplastic anaemia*

Feature	Constitutional	Acquired
Age of onset	4–7 years in boys 6–10 years in girls	Any age
Sex ratio	61% male	Equal
Neutropenia	Moderate 0.25–0.95 $\times 10^9/1$	Severe
Marrow cellularity	Hypocellular	Aplastic
Erythropoiesis	Dyserythropoiesis	Virtually absent
Reticulocytes	Up to 3%	Usually less than 1%
Fetal haemoglobin	6–12%	3–15%
i-antigen	Usually present	Present in approx. 50%
Aminoaciduria	May be present in 50%	Absent
Retarded bone growth	Present	Absent
Response to androgens	Good but temporary	Approx. 50%
Effect of withdrawal of androgens	Usually rapid relapse	Transitory drop of Hb but no relapse

* (Adapted from Willoughby 1977)

Clinical examination. The clinical examination of a suspected case should include a careful search for the less obvious features of the disease such as hyperreflexia, deafness, cardiac murmur, mental retardation, and abnormalities of the ears, eyes and feet. The two hands should be carefully compared for differences in the size of the digits and muscles. Radiological investigations should include examination of the vertebrae and ribs as well as the lung fields and heart shadows, and the forearm and hand bones. The kidneys should be examined by ultrasound and by intravenous pyelography if necessary.

Differential diagnosis

A diagnosis of Fanconi's anaemia should be considered in any child presenting with a cytopenia and poor growth. The latter may not always be very obvious and, in the author's experience, many cases have been misdiagnosed as idiopathic thrombocytopenic purpura. It is necessary to distinguish the anaemia and poor growth that goes with chronic renal disease and chronic infection, particularly if the child is admitted with a temporary neutropenia or thrombocytopenia due to an acute exacerbation of infection.

Shwachman's syndrome (p. 33) leads to poor growth and is associated with defective pancreatic function which usually, but by no means invariably, is associated with neutropenia. The neutropenia is usually part of a more extensive bone marrow dysplasia, which can be complicated by either aplasia or leukaemia. Some cases of Diamond-Blackfan anaemia (p. 231) may show short stature, congenital defects such as thumb and foot deformities, and neutropenia together with anaemia. They may be very difficult to distinguish from Fanconi's anaemia. Examination of the peripheral blood chromosomes, including the susceptibility to stress by cross linking agents, may be necessary. Dyskeratosis congenita (p. 32) is an extremely rare disease with poor growth, congenital defects and bone marrow failure, also complicated by a predisposition to malignant disease. Other rare congenital marrow aplasias are described below.

Laboratory features

In the advanced stage of the disease there is pancytopenia. The red cells are macrocytic and well haemoglobinized, with poikilocytosis, anisocytosis and reticulocytopenia. The haemoglobin level is of the order of 5–9 g/dl with an MCV of 105–115 fl. The neutrophil count is of the order of $0.25–1.0 \times 10^9/1$ and the neutrophils may show toxic granulation. The lymphocytes and monocytes are normal in number and appearance. The platelet count is low at less than $10–30 \times 10^9/1$. In the early stages of the disease, the haemoglobin may be normal, and the red cells may be normocytic or macrocytic. There may sometimes be a reticulocytosis, with features of a mild haemolytic state, often associated with dyserythropoiesis, which can precede the overt aplastic or hypoplastic stage. Anaemia is often the last defect to show in the blood count. Blast cells are not usually seen. If present, they indicate the development of leukaemia.

There is an increase of fetal haemoglobin, usually to between 3 and 15%, and a Kleihauer test may show its presence in only a selection of red cells, suggesting the presence of an abnormal clone. Various enzymopathies have been reported, including deficiency of hexokinase, pyruvate kinase, phosphofructokinase and diphosphoglycerate mutase, with increased activity of glucose-6-phosphate dehydrogenase and aldolase, as seen in the refractory anaemias of adults (Girot & Buriot 1980).

Bone marrow examination is necessary for the confirmation that pancytopenia is due to reduced bone marrow activity. Although increased erythropoiesis has been noted in the early stages of the disease, in most cases the marrow is hypoplastic. Dyserythropoiesis may be noted with megaloblastic changes, binuclear chromatin bridges, degenerate nuclei and defective haemoglobinization. However, the giant metamyelocytes seen in megaloblastic anaemia due to B_{12} or folate deficiency are not seen, and the serum B_{12} and red cell folate levels are normal. As with other aplastic disorders, the bone marrow may show an increase of tissue mast cells and histiocytes, and occasionally of plasma cells, and aspiration may sometimes draw marrow from an active area which is not representative of the marrow overall. Trephine biopsy is recommended to avoid sampling error of this sort, and to confirm hypoplasia.

The liver function tests, serum urea and electrolytes are normal unless liver or renal disease co-exist. The serum iron is likely to be low at diagnosis, due to thrombocytopenic bleeding, but rises if blood transfusions become necessary as a result of depressed erythropoiesis. Growth hormone deficiency has been documented, but treatment with growth hormone has not always proved effective, indicating an inability of tissues to respond.

Bone marrow culture for granulocyte-macrophage colony-forming units (GM-CFUs) and other similar techniques show defective in vitro growth, but with normal production of growth factors, suggesting a stem cell defect (Saunders & Freedman 1978). Such studies give valuable information about the nature of the disease but are not essential for diagnosis.

Cytogenetic studies

There is a normal karyotype, with an increased number of spontaneous chromatid and isochromatid breaks and gaps, rearrangements, chromatid interchange figures and endoreduplication. Ten to 70% of the patients' cells were affected compared to less than 10% of control cells in the series of 40 cases from the Netherlands reviewed by Kwee & Kuyt (1989). Five of their patients showed chromosomal abnormalities before the onset of pancytopenia. A similar number of abnormalities were found in the 44 cases reported from South Africa by Smith et al (1989). In all cases of Fanconi's anaemia, the number of chromosome abnormalities is significantly increased by incubating peripheral blood lymphocytes or skin fibroblasts in the presence of the cross-linking agents described above. The usual agents used are diepoxybutane or mitomycin C. With these agents, the number of chromosome breaks is increased considerably to over 10 per cell (Schroeder-Kurth et al 1989), even for the minority of cases with Fanconi's anaemia who show no spontaneous chromosome breakage. The breakage rate varies from case to case and with different agents. The parents of children with Fanconi's anaemia are heterozygote carriers. Their spontaneous chromosome breakage rate is usually normal, but most show increased breakages if their lymphocytes are incubated with mitomycin C or diepoxybutane, but not to the same extent as shown by Fanconi cases. This test enables normal siblings to be distinguished from carriers.

Antenatal diagnosis

The sensitivity of lymphocytes and fibroblasts from cases of Fanconi's anaemia to increased breakage after stress with cross-linking agents has been successfully used for antenatal diagnosis. Auerbach et al (1989) have examined the amniotic fluid cells of 42 cases at risk of Fanconi's anaemia. The seven affected cases showed a 5-fold increase of sensitivity to diepoxybutane. Two newborns and two fetuses diagnosed antenatally as affected were examined clinically and all showed signs and symptoms of Fanconi's anaemia. In 14 pregnancies at risk, cultured trophoblast cells obtained by chorionic villus biopsy were similarly stressed. Three affected cases showed an over 10-fold increase of breakages. The three cases were aborted, and although the fetuses showed no obvious malformations, their tissues showed a markedly raised breakage rate. These tests give reliable results and enable early diagnosis to be made in pregnancies at risk; the parents can then be offered termination of the pregnancy.

Treatment

Bone marrow transplantation. The only curative treatment for the pancytopenia of Fanconi's anaemia is bone marrow transplantation. It has now been successfully undertaken in a number of cases. Because of the abnormal sensitivity of the cells to cross-linking agents and irradiation, the pre-transplant cytoreductive and immunosuppressive regimen requires that drugs are given in lower doses than are used in other patients. Before this was recognized, patients died of the side-effects of chemotherapy together with the effects of graft-versus-host disease, comprising mucosal damage, diarrhoea, haemorrhagic cystitis, cardiac failure and fluid overload. Cyclophosphamide, which has been widely used as preparation for acquired aplastic anaemia, is particularly dangerous. Transplants have been successfully achieved with the dose reduced from 150 or 200 mg/kg body weight to 20 mg/kg, together with total body or thoracoabdominal irradiation at a dose of around 5 Gy instead of the more usual dose of 8 Gy or so. With these lower doses, the success rate exceeds 80% (Gluckman et al 1987, 1989; Hows et al 1989; Ebell et al 1989). A 5-year-old boy was successfully transplanted using stored umbilical cord blood cells from a matched sibling (Gluckman et al 1989). Successful transplants have also been achieved using matched unrelated donors, but the failure rate is high (Sokal et al 1987, Hows et al 1989).

Standard treatment. For patients with bone marrow failure the standard treatment comprises androgens, steroids, and transfusion with red cells or platelets, and the administration of antibiotics as required. Fanconi patients usually show a good initial response to androgens. The haemoglobin rises, and there may be a modest increase of the platelet count, both increases being adequate to avoid the need for transfusion. Unfortunately, the

initial response is not always maintained, and increasing doses may be needed to maintain the patient's condition. Eventually, most cases become refractory, and transfusions of blood and platelets are left as the only way to maintain the blood count.

As for other aplasias, the androgen most widely used has been oxymetholone, at a dose of 2–5 mg/kg, or 50 mg/m². Ebell et al (1989) reported a response rate of around 50%, which is the same as that reported earlier by Alter & Potter (1983). The side-effects of androgen treatment include increased growth, virilization (Fig. 2.4) and, rarely, peliosis hepatis or hepatoma, which in at least one case was reversed by stopping the androgen. Cramps are not uncommon. The side-effects of androgen treatment are more fully discussed under acquired aplastic anaemia (p. 45). Corticosteroids have also been used, usually low-dose prednisone, i.e. 1–2 mg/kg daily, either with a view to encouraging bone marrow recovery and supporting platelet survival, or of antagonizing

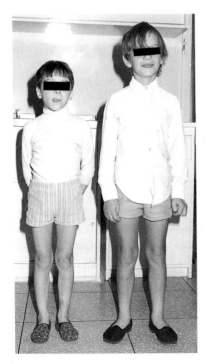 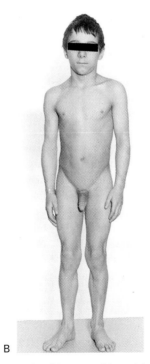 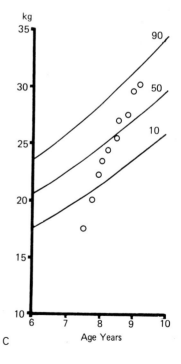

Fig. 2.4 A. The patient (left) with Fanconi's anaemia with a normal boy of the same age (7½ years) to show small stature at presentation. **B.** Same patient after treatment with oxymetholone 50 mg/m² for 20 months, showing muscular development, penile hypertrophy and pubic hair. **C.** The patient's growth chart showing height increase after treatment. (Reprinted from Evans 1979 with permission of Churchill Livingstone.)

the possible effects of androgens on premature fusion of the epiphyses with limitation of the final body height. In the author's experience, corticosteroids have not proved effective for the former use, and are unnecessary for the latter. The use of corticosteroids in neutropenias runs the risk of increasing infection by depressing immunity further, and Ebell et al (1989) reported severe bacterial infections in Fanconi patients thus treated, even though the granulocyte counts were almost normal. Abnormalities of chemotaxis and phagocytosis were demonstrated. The author's preference is to use androgens and avoid the use of corticosteroids. Occasionally, it is possible to stop androgen treatment, and the patient will remain in remission. Two cases of Rogers et al (1989) remained in remission for 18 and 20 years after stopping treatment, although the latter died of metastatic carcinoma of the breast.

An increased neutrophil count in a 9-year-old girl with Fanconi's anaemia was attributed to treatment with lithium citrate 10 mg/kg (Barrios et al 1989), but two patients given lithium by Chan et al (1981) showed no response.

OTHER CONGENITAL DISORDERS ASSOCIATED WITH APLASTIC ANAEMIA

Dyskeratosis congenita

This is a rare hereditary disease characterized by an ectodermal dystrophy which presents as a reticular skin pigmentation, leucokeratosis of the mucosal membranes, and nail dystrophy in the first decade although the time of onset is not constant. In 30–50% of cases, these signs are followed by a bone marrow defect which usually develops in the second or third decade, and carcinomas may appear in the leucokeratotic areas from the third decade onwards. The disease was first described by Zinsser (1906); it is usually inherited in a sex-linked recessive manner, but a dominant inheritance has been described.

Clinical features

Skin changes. These comprise linear, brown areas of hyperpigmentation surrounded by non-pigmented circular or oval areas. They form a reticular pattern, and are most prominent, at least in the early stages, over the neck and the dorsum of the hands and feet. On the neck they may extend over the upper trunk giving a décolleté distribution. As the nail changes progress, the nails develop longitudinal ridging followed by crumbling and shortening of the nails. The nails may disintegrate and disappear. The normal dermatoglyphics may be lost. The palms of the hands and soles of the feet may have abnormally thin skin. The leukokeratotic areas in the mouth and elsewhere may in time develop the changes of squamous cell carcinoma.

Other clinical features. Patients may also show a tendency to opportunistic infections, leucoplakia of the tongue, lacrimation due to blockage of the lacrimal ducts, aseptic necrosis of bone, hair loss and prematurely grey hair, abnormal dentition, and strictures of internal organs such as the urethra, ureter, oesophagus, anus and vagina. Growth retardation, testicular hypoplasia, osteoporosis and mental retardation have also been described. The clinical picture varies considerably from case to case. Some features, such as osteoporosis may be secondary to treatment. Because of the relatively late presentation of symptoms, few reports have appeared in the paediatric literature: most have appeared in dermatological journals.

Laboratory features

The haematological changes resemble those of Fanconi's anaemia. In general, there are progressive anaemia and pancytopenia. There may be a suggestion of haemolysis with reticulocytosis of around 5% and macrocytosis of 105–110 fl. The white cell and platelet counts drop. The patient described by Inoue et al (1973) showed a shortened red cell survival with a half-life of ^{51}Cr-tagged red cells of 18 days compared to the normal of 25–27 days, and a low serum haptoglobin. The bone marrow changes include progressive aplasia with an increase of mast cells and plasma cells. There may be dyserythropoiesis and reduction of megakaryocytes. Most cases have developed haematological changes after the skin disorder has been recognized; but the case of De Boeck et al (1981) presented with isolated thrombocytopenia at the age of 5 years and the skin changes did not develop until 3 years later. A stem cell defect was proposed by Friedland et al (1985), as their patient showed a decrease of erythroid precursor cells in both blood and bone marrow. The chromosome changes found in Fanconi's anaemia have not been detected in dyskeratosis congenita.

Treatment

Treatment comprises support with blood and platelet transfusions. The rarity of the disease means that few cases have received treatment of an up-to-date type. Many have received long-term corticosteroids which may have accounted for some of the symptoms, such as osteoporosis, bone necrosis and infection. Unlike Fanconi's anaemia, the response to androgens has been disappointing. Bone marrow transplantation has been attempted, but the first patient showed a sensitivity to high-dose alkylating agents, similar to that of patients with Fanconi's anaemia, and died with complications (Conter et al 1988).

Shwachman's syndrome

This disorder comprises a constitutional bone marrow disorder which commonly, but not invariably, presents with neutropenia. The main features comprise poor growth, predisposition to infection and malabsorption due to exocrine pancreatic failure. The patients superficially resemble children with cystic fibrosis and were first described from a clinic dealing with the latter disease (Shwachman et al 1964). Some cases have shown severe pancytopenia and present as aplastic anaemia with decreased CFU-C (Woods et al 1981). One of the two cases described by these authors responded to corticosteroids and later transformed to a myelomonocytic leukaemia.

Amegakaryoctic thrombocytopenia and aplastic anaemia

Thrombocytopenia with deficient megakaryocytes presenting at birth or in early infancy has been followed by aplastic anaemia after months or years (O'Gorman Hughes & Diamond 1964). A few children have also had mental retardation and other disorders, but most have been normal, apart from aplasia (O'Gorman Hughes 1974). The changes found in Fanconi's anaemia have not been pre-sent, and the family history, apart from one case, has not suggested a genetic predisposition. (See also Ch. 6)

Other disorders

Two families, one English and one Portuguese, have been reported with late onset of bone marrow failure associated with proximal fusion of the radius and ulna (Dokal et al 1989). Three boys from two Scandinavian families have been described with progressive pancytopenia, microcephaly, cerebellar hypoplasia and growth failure (Høyeraal et al 1970, Hreidarsson et al 1988). Alter et al (1989) described a dominantly inherited stem cell disorder with immune dysfunction, poor dentition, hyperpigmented skin, warts, midterm abortions and one case of acute myelomonocytic leukaemia. The patients lacked the typical chromosome changes of Fanconi's anaemia which the disease otherwise resembled.

A defect of folate metabolism was reported in a child with aplastic anaemia who responded to high doses of folic acid (Branda et al 1978). The family showed a high incidence of leucopenia and leukaemia.

ACQUIRED APLASTIC ANAEMIA

Epidemiology

Geographical incidence

The incidence of acquired aplastic anaemia varies with age and in different parts of the world. It appears to be low in Western countries and high in Asian countries (Aoki et al 1980). In California (Wallerstein et al 1969) the incidence of fatal aplastic anaemia was approximately 1.1 per million per year for children up to the age of 9. In Baltimore, USA, it was 4.6 for males and 1.7 for females under the age of 19 (Sklo et al 1985). In Denmark, the annual incidence of severe aplastic anaemia in children aged 0–14 years was 2.2 cases per million (Clausen 1986), and in Sweden 4–5 per million in children under 15 years of age (Böttiger & Westerholm 1972). By contrast, in Japan, for children under the age of 15 it was 22 per million (Nakayama & Nagakawa 1978).

Precise figures for the incidence of aplastic anaemia in underdeveloped countries are difficult to obtain. The difference is likely to be due to poorer control of toxic insecticides and contaminated foodstuffs. Garewal et al (1981) in a report on hypoplastic anaemia commented that 'it is almost certain that the incidence of indiscriminate use of potentially myelotoxic drugs is high in India'. Nevertheless, identifiable causes account for only one-third or so of cases.

There may also be genetic differences in susceptibility, as it has been noted that, in a group of individuals all exposed at work to similar concentrations of benzene, only a minority developed bone marrow damage (Ronchetti 1922). Mice homozygous for the Ah^d locus were susceptible to aplastic anaemia in less than 4 weeks after daily exposure to oral benzo(a)pyrene, whereas siblings who were heterozygous, or homozygous for Ah^b remained healthy for six months while continuously receiving the same dose (Nebert et al 1977).

It is interesting that, in Hawaii, the incidence of aplastic anaemia between 1968 and 1976 was 0.30 per 100 000 for Japanese Hawaiians, one-third that of indigenous Japanese, compared with 0.43 per 100 000 for caucasian Hawaiians (Aoki et al 1980). The differences for the two groups of Hawaiians are not statistically significant, but the figures suggest that external factors operate in Japan which are absent in Hawaii. A genetic difference is unlikely. The acquired forms of pancytopenia are several times more frequent than the constitutional (congenital) forms. Most of the latter are cases of Fanconi's anaemia.

Age and sex differences

In the Far East, cases of aplastic anaemia show a disproportionately large number of young males with male:female ratios of 2 or 4:1 (Young et al 1986). Two-thirds of cases are less than 30 years old. The figures may reflect greater exposure of males to bone marrow toxins, as the male:female ratio in the West is 1:1. An alternative explanation is that there may be a sex difference in susceptibility to drugs which harm the bone marrow. It has been shown that male rats are more susceptible to the toxic effects of organophosphorus compounds (DuBois 1971), and although these chemicals are rare causes of aplastic anaemia, a similar sex difference may apply in the case of other toxins. In the West, the increase of aplastic anaemia with advancing age may be due to a progressive age-dependent deterioration of renal function, leading to higher blood levels of toxic drugs for a given dose; but a different explanation is needed for the relatively higher incidence in young people in the East. However, the statistics reflect the local customs for consulting a doctor and not necessarily the true incidence.

Classification of severity

Because of the need to identify clearly the patients with the poorest prognosis, whose illness is sufficiently severe to justify the risks of bone marrow transplantation, several authors have produced formulae to calculate a prognosis. The first was introduced by Lynch et al (1975), but the formula of Camitta et al (1982) has the virtue of brevity and is widely used (Table 2.5). It has subsequently been modified to include a very severe group with neutrophils less than $0.2 \times 10^9/1$. Najean & Pecking (1979) proposed a formula which took more factors into consideration, but it is more difficult to calculate and little used. There is no difficulty identifying severe and mild cases by any of these formulae; it is the calculation of the prognosis in intermediate cases which presents the most difficulty and in which the formulae are of least help.

Aetiology

For many cases of acquired aplastic anaemia in childhood, no specific aetiology can be found. In 39 cases from Denmark, a probable cause was found in 21 (54%) including five due to

Table 2.5 Criteria for severe aplastic anaemia (Camitta et al 1982)

Blood	–Neutrophils less than $0.5 \times 10^9/1$ –Platelets less than $20 \times 10^9/1$ –Reticulocytes less than 1% (corrected for haematocrit)
Marrow	–Severe hypocellularity –Moderate hypocellularity with less than 30% of residul cells being haematopoietic

Severe aplastic anaemia is defined by any two blood criteria and either marrow criterion.

pesticides, two following hepatitis, six following other infections and five from drugs or chemicals (Clausen 1986). On the other hand, of 36 cases from the Hospital for Sick Children in Toronto, the cause was unknown in 34 (94%) of cases (Halperin et al 1989). The disorder may develop as a complication of graft-versus-host disease, and immune mechanisms appear to be responsible for marrow aplasia in many cases considered to be idiopathic in origin (Cline & Golde 1978).

Acquired aplastic anaemia is the commonest form of bone marrow failure. It can present at any age, and becomes more common with increasing age. There are many agents that can damage the bone marrow and cause aplasia. The association between aplastic anaemia and drugs is well known, but because of the large number of drugs which may cause bone marrow aplasia, many physicians who are not blood specialists are unaware that drugs which they prescribe may occasionally damage bone marrow. In developed countries, steps are taken to avoid the use of these drugs; for instance, in the United Kingdom, phenylbutazone was withdrawn because of an unacceptable incidence of neutropenia. Thus, aplasia due to drug use occurs rarely; but in underdeveloped countries their use is unrestricted, and they are sometimes available without a doctor's prescription.

Bone marrow growth in vitro

There are three requirements for blood cells to develop normally in the bone marrow:

1. stem cells of normal number and function
2. a normal marrow micro-environment
3. normal growth factors.

Laboratory techniques have been developed which enable each of these factors to be examined. Bone marrow from patients with aplastic anaemia grows poorly in culture (Kern et al 1977) with poor stem cell proliferation (Juneja & Gardner 1985). There is a defective response to growth factors, including granulocyte-macrophage colony-stimulating factor (GM-CSF) and interleukin-3 (IL-3). In a few cases, bone marrow cultures may develop into clusters instead of colonies, comprising macrophages or fibroblasts (Nissen-Druey 1989). This pattern is usually seen in patients with pre-leukaemic disorders.

When bone marrow is grown in long-term culture (Dexter et al 1977), there is little evidence of production of primitive progenitor cells. The defect persists even after recovery. Cross-over experiments showed a stromal defect in only one case, a 60-year-old woman with ulcerative colitis. In 22 other cases, including two children, the defect of blood cell production was due to a stem cell defect, independent of the degree of haematological recovery after treatment with anti-lymphocyte globulin (Marsh et al 1990). On the basis of this work, the hypothesis of Knospe & Crosby (1971), that aplastic anaemia is due to a stromal defect, can only occasionally be true. The defect appears to lie in the stem cell itself.

Drugs and chemicals and aplastic anaemia

Drugs that cause aplastic anaemia are of two types. The first group includes those drugs which are regularly used for chemotherapy in the treatment of leukaemia and cancer, or as immunosuppressants. They are given with a view to suppressing the growth of malignant cells, or of depressing lymphocyte reactions. They show variable activity on normal bone marrow cells, but if given in sufficiently large doses, will depress the bone marrow of everyone receiving them. The second group comprises drugs used to depress the activity of a cell or tissue system, and which in normal doses affect the bone marrow of only a minority of individuals. This group includes the anti-thyroid drugs, anti-inflammatory agents, and anticonvulsants. Antibacterial and antiviral drugs, both antibiotics and chemotherapeutic agents such as sulphonamides, come into the latter group; but instead of being used to depress activity of the patient's tissues, they are used to affect the metabolism of bacteria.

It is not always easy to prove that a drug is a cause of bone marrow failure; drugs are often given in combination, making it difficult to identify which particular drug may be responsible. Aplastic anaemia is a serious disease and it is unethical to try to reproduce bone marrow failure by re-exposing a patient who has recovered to the drug suspected of causing the illness. It is sometimes possible to demonstrate drug toxicity in vitro, by culturing the patient's bone marrow for colony-forming units (CFU-C and/or CFU-E) in the presence of the suspected drug. In this way, Kelton et al (1979) were able to demonstrate that both a transient serum factor and quinidine were responsible for marrow aplasia in a 66-year-old man. Similar techniques have been used to diagnose agranulocytosis due to amidopyrine (Barrett et al 1976) and to diphenylhydantoin (Tactle et al 1979). A list of drugs associated with acquired aplastic anaemia is given in Table 2.6.

Chloramphenicol

Chloramphenicol has been thoroughly studied. The incidence of aplastic anaemia secondary to chloramphenicol is rare and develops in 1 in 24 500–40 800 cases (Wallerstein et al 1969). In over 25 years of practice at the Royal Manchester Children's Hospital, which acts as a centre for blood diseases in a population of around 4.5 million, this author has never seen a case.

The reaction is idiopathic, and there may be a genetic element in its aetiology as the association occurred in identical twins (Nagao & Mauer 1969). Aplasia occurs after both oral and intravenous use; and has also been recognized after use in eye-drops (Stevens & Mission 1987). It may develop up to 9–12 months after stopping treatment, and the prognosis is worst when aplasia develops 2 or more months after cessation (Polak et al 1972). There is an association with liver damage due to chloramphenicol and marrow aplasia; if a patient on chloramphenicol develops abnormal liver function, the drug should be stopped. This idiopathic reaction is rare, irreversible, and frequently fatal. The complication appears to be less common in the UK than in the USA. In the 1960s there were 24 cases of aplastic anaemia in a period when 1,000,000 prescriptions were issued by general practitioners in the UK, plus an unknown number in hospitals, while in Philadelphia, one teaching hospital was using 0.84 kg of the drug per month, and in five hospitals, chloramphenicol accounted for a large proportion, up to one half, of all antibiotics prescribed (Reimann & D'Ambola 1966, British Medical Journal 1967). The use of chloramphenicol in the USA fell considerably in the 1970s and 80s (Feder 1986), and now that a wider range of antibiotics is available, and the dangers of chloramphenicol are better recognized, aplastic anaemia due to chloramphenicol should become very rare indeed. Unfortunately, the rarity of the complication encourages a false sense of security, and the drug may be prescribed for conditions other than those for which it is still generally accepted to be indicated (shown in Table 2.7). Regular blood counts will not prevent the development of aplastic anaemia with chloramphenicol.

A dose-related, reversible depression of erythropoiesis is a more common finding with chloramphenicol. It is seen when serum levels are greater than 25 µg/ml or when treatment is prolonged. The mitochondrial enzyme ferrochelatase is inhibited,

Table 2.6   Drugs and chemicals reported to have caused aplastic anaemia*

Drugs

Antibacterial drugs	Antidiabetic drugs
chloramphenicol	chlorpropamide
sulphonamides	tolbutamide
methicillin	Anaesthetic agents
organic arsenicals	nitrous oxide
Anticonvulsants and drugs	Miscellaneous drugs
acting on the CNS	quinidine
phenytoin and other	acetazolamide
hydantoins	dinitrophenol
carbamazepine	
promazine, chlorpromazine	*Chemicals*
meprobromate	Insecticides
chlordiazepoxide	gammabenzene hexachloride
Analgesic and anti-	(Lindane)
inflammatory drugs	chlordane
phenylbutazone and	dichlorodiphenothane
oxyphenbutazone	(DDT)
gold	Solvents
indomethacin	benzene
diclophenac	carbon tetrachloride
Antimalarial drugs	model airplane glue
chloroquine	glue solvents
mepacrine	Stoddard solvent
trimethoprim	Others
pyrimethamine	thiocyanate
Antithyroid drugs	
propyl thiouracil	
potassium perchlorate	
methimazole	

* (Updated and modified from Nieweg 1973 and Williams et al 1973)

Table 2.7   Clinical indications for the use of chloramphenicol (Smyth & Pallett 1988)

Meningitis in children up to age of school entry
Brain abscess
Invasive *Haemophilus influenzae* infections
Chronic granulomatous disease
Rickettsial infection in patients unable to take tetracycline
Eye infection

leading after 5–7 days to diminished uptake of iron by the normoblasts, which become vacuolated, resulting in anaemia with reticulocytopenia and a raised serum iron level. Neutropenia and thrombocytopenia may also develop. At therapeutic doses there is a 60–90% inhibition of colony growth of bone marrow cells in vitro (Ratzen et al 1974). The changes resolve when the drug is stopped, so regular monitoring of the serum level and blood count of patients on chloramphenicol should reduce the possibility of serious toxicity due to this type of reaction.

The grey baby syndrome is a side effect of chloramphenicol of particular paediatric interest. It may also affect older children and adults receiving large doses, and is therefore more properly called the 'grey syndrome'. The patients develop vomiting, abdominal distension, respiratory distress, hypotension, shock and a peculiar grey colour due to a pallid cyanosis. Unless the drug is stopped, about 40% of cases die. The effects are due to high levels of the drug, above 40 µg/ml, interfering with mitochondrial electron transport (Leitman 1979). Neonates are particularly susceptible because their immature glucuronyl transferase system and reduced renal clearance lead to prolonged high levels of the drugs. Treatment is supportive. Charcoal column haemoperfusion or exchange transfusion may be helpful.

Other drugs

Many of the drugs that are well-known causes of aplastic anaemia in adults are not given to normal healthy children, and it is the normal healthy child who most frequently develops aplastic anaemia. Even when there is a history of exposure to a drug which has been reported to cause aplastic anaemia, it is difficult to prove a direct link between exposure and the disease. The drugs most frequently involved are listed in Table 2.6. They include anticonvulsants, anti-inflammatory agents, tranquillizers, analgesics, antibiotics and antidiuretics. They fall into the second group described in the introductory section. Most of these drugs, starting as they do with the prefix 'anti', exercise a depressant action on some aspect of cell activity, so, for some individuals with idiosyncracy they are also anti-bone-marrow.

Cytotoxic drugs usually cause bone marrow depression while they are given or shortly afterwards. The blood count usually recovers within a few days of stopping the drug. However, some patients who have had prolonged chemotherapy, such as for leukaemia and cancer, may recover much more slowly than others. This picture is commonly seen in patients treated by bone marrow autotransplantation after leukaemia relapse. After prolonged chemotherapy to induce remission, the bone marrow is harvested and re-infused after further high doses of cytotoxic drugs. In these patients, it frequently take several weeks for their bone marrow to recover, whereas patients given a transplant from a healthy matched sibling donor recover much more quickly. We may conclude that the autotransplanted marrow has suffered stem cell loss and damage as result of the earlier chemotherapy. Occasionally, patients may develop aplastic anaemia some time after a course of chemotherapy and/or radiation; for instance, the two patients of Lishner & Curtis (1989) developed aplasia 3 and 4 years after treatment for cancer, having recovered from the immediate effects of treatment in the interval. In these cases it seems unlikely that the stem cells have been damaged, as the delay is too great; it is more likely that the cytotoxic treatment has altered immune function in such a way as to predispose the patients to an immunological effect (see below).

Prolonged exposure to *nitrous oxide* as occurs during the treatment of tetanus, causes temporary bone marrow depression. At lower doses, it produces megaloblastic changes (Lancet 1978).

Chemicals

Benzene has been known to cause bone marrow disease, both aplasia and leukaemia, for many years (Saita 1973). Most cases are due to exposure at work. Insecticides may be a more common cause of so-called idiopathic aplastic anaemia in childhood than is generally recognized, possibly as a result of contamination with benzene. Reeves et al (1981) reported nine children seen over 8 years in California, USA, in whom aplastic anaemia was attributed to insecticides. All had been exposed by inhalation of organophosphates. These drugs inhibit cholinesterase, and aplastic anaemia is usually considered to be a rare side-effect of exposure. In six cases, DDT was combined with propoxur. One frequently inhaled pyrethrin. Weanling rats are more susceptible to organo-phosphates than adults (Du Bois 1971) and it is possible that children may be more susceptible to their effects too. Inhalation is more toxic than skin exposure (Gosselin et al 1976).

Glue-sniffing may cause aplastic anaemia (Massengale et al 1963) and has been responsible for at least one fatal case (Powars et al 1965).

Mechanisms of drug action

Nieweg (1973) and Benestad (1979) have described three types of drug action on the bone marrow. They may be:

1. dose-dependent
2. conditional (i.e. idiosyncratic)
3. immunologic

The dose-dependent effects are exemplified by the action of cytotoxic drugs: although there is individual variation in the bone-marrow-suppressant activity of a cytotoxic drug, there is a standard dose which gives acceptable bone-marrow toxicity. Any increase of the dose increases bone-marrow suppression. A conditional or idiosyncratic effect is similar in principle to the haemolysis shown by patients with red cell glucose-6-phosphate dehydrogenase deficiency who haemolyse after treatment with primaquine, a drug which is harmless to individuals with normal enzyme levels.

The occasional patient who develops aplastic anaemia after a low exposure to benzene (Ronchetti 1922) may be an example of the second type. This is a true allergy or idiosyncracy.

The third type is more a 'high-dose allergy', which Nieweg (1973) attributes to antibodies dependent on cell membrane damage due to -SH inhibition; he calls this 'spoiled membrane allergy', while Benestad simply refers to it as immunological. The immunologic effects can be due to:

1. hapten mechanisms
2. immune complex mechanisms
3. auto-immune mechanisms
4. mechanisms involving altered regulatory lymphocytes.

It is also important to consider the level at which the pathological process acts. Does it affect the bone marrow environment, the stem cells, or the transit cell population? The irreversible idiosyncratic effect which results in aplastic anaemia with chloramphenicol is a direct action on the marrow stem cell. The reversible, dose-dependent effect on erythropoiesis is an action on the developing normoblasts. Other drugs acting on the stem cell include phenylbutazone and gold; whereas benzene and chlorpromazine act on the transit cell compartment.

Immunological aspects

That aplastic anaemia may be due to immunological effects has become apparent as a result of attempts to treat the disease. Patients prepared for bone marrow transplantation with high doses of cytotoxic drugs such as busulphan and cyclophosphamide have shown recovery before the transplant was given (Sensenbrenner et al 1977), or have recovered after bone marrow transplantation but with repopulation by their own bone marrow, not the donor bone marrow (Jeannet et al 1976, Territo et al 1977). Treatment with antilymphocyte globulin has been effective. These results led to investigation for possible immune-mediated bone marrow depression, and poor bone marrow growth has been shown to be associated with humoral and cellular mechanisms. Humoral factors both stimulating and depressing the growth of bone marrow in vitro were described by Karp et al 1978; and in one case described by Freedman et al 1979 there was suppression of bone marrow erythroid and granulocyte colonies by IgG separated from the patient's serum. Aplastic anaemia is rarely associated with thymoma (Lyonnais 1988).

Humoral factors may be provoked by transfusion of blood and platelets (Singer et al 1978). Tests were therefore done on untreated patients. Although Sullivan et al (1980) were unable to demonstrate any cell-mediated autoimmune suppression of myeloid stem cell proliferation in aplastic anaemia, other workers have been able to demonstrate depression of normal bone marrow growth with patient's lymphocytes or T-cells (Torok-Storb et al 1980, Bacigalupo et al 1981). It has been suggested that this suppressant activity is mediated by gamma-interferon (Zoumbos et al 1984, Mangan et al 1985), and that granulocyte colony-stimulating factors may interfere with laboratory assays in such tests (Young 1987). On the other hand, Torok-Storb (1987) was unable to demonstrate inhibition of erythroid colonies with gamma-interferon, and Hanada et al (1987) found no evidence that it was gamma-interferon which mediated bone marrow depression by T-cells.

The peripheral blood lymphocytes may show changes. There is an increase in single-strand breaks in DNA, suggesting that the repair processes are disturbed (Hashimoto et al 1975). Some patients have hypogammaglobulinaemia (Mir et al 1977, Elfenbein et al 1979), and the differentiation of lymphoid cells is impaired in some cases with this complication (Uchiyama et al 1978). The peripheral blood cells stimulated with phytohaemagglutinin produce less colony-stimulating activity than normal cells (Weatherly et al 1979). In idiopathic acquired aplastic anaemia the serum contains a migration inhibitory factor which is not present in normal individuals or patients with Fanconi's anaemia (Fassas & Bruley-Rosset 1979). The lymphocyte count is usually reduced, cutaneous hypersensitivity reactions are impaired, and there is a marked monocytopenia. Some of these effects on the lymphocytes can be attributed to corticosteroid treatment (Elfenbein et al 1979); but in addition to their low number, the monocytes show delayed maturation in vitro (Andreesen et al 1989). In nearly half the 117 patients studied by Warren et al (1980) the lymphocytes reacted against the lymphocytes of HLA-matched compatible siblings, compared to only 4% of controls. The T-cell helper/suppressor ratio may be reversed, and the response to poke-weed mitogen may be reduced. The patients with a low number of T-cells may show a better response to treatment (Ruiz-Argüelles et al 1984).

Growth factors may be involved. There may be reduced production of interleukin-1 (Nakao et al 1989); but production of gamma-interferon and tumour necrosis factor-α are increased (Hinterberger et al 1989). The changes reported here have been studied in patients of all ages. They have not been restricted to children, but there is no reason to suspect that children's lymphocytes will give different responses from adults. The problem is to know how far these changes are in some way secondary to the stem cell defect, and to what extent they are responsible for the disease itself. It seems probable that monocytopenia is linked to neutropenia, as the two types of cell originate from a common precursor cells, and both are stimulated by a growth factor (GM-CSF). The lymphocyte originates from a different stem cell, and it is tempting to think that the lymphocyte changes are in some way responsible for the aplasia rather than part of a common stem cell defect. Immunosuppressive treatment may improve the bone marrow suppression without altering these lymphocyte changes.

Infection and aplastic anaemia

Infection is a rare cause of aplastic anaemia. In different series, the incidence varies from 0.3% in Korea (Whang 1978) to 5% in Sweden (Böttiger & Westerholm 1972), and 15% in the Australian/ American series of O'Gorman Hughes (1966). The association of aplastic anaemia and infection was originally recognized with tuberculosis (Dyke 1924).

Hepatitis has been well known as a cause of aplastic anaemia since the 1950's (Lorenz & Quaiser 1955). The prognosis is generally poor, with mortality as high as 88% (Aljouni & Doeblin 1974). Some patients may, however, recover spontaneously (Dhingra et al 1988); others may respond to immunosuppressive treatment (Liang et al 1990). Subclinical hepatitis may be a more common cause of aplastic anaemia than is generally recognized. No test exists to identify previous non-A, non-B, non-C infections, which may have recovered by the time aplastic anaemia is identified. This may partly explain the increased incidence of aplastic anaemia in the Far East, where hepatitis of all types is more common, and where widespread testing for hepatitis C is not yet available.

Other infections which have been considered to have caused aplastic anaemia include infectious mononucleosis and dengue. About a dozen cases of the former have been reported (Kurtzman & Young 1989). Cases have also followed measles and mumps (Evans 1979). Babies with congenital rubella have developed transient bone marrow hypoplasia (Horstmann et al 1965, Lafer & Morrison 1966).

HIV infection leads to marrow suppression and is a particular problem for patients treated with zidovudine.

Transient bone marrow depression is found in many viral diseases. Children with dengue and Thai haemorrhagic fever showed severe myelosuppression affecting particularly megakaryocytes in the acute stages, followed in most cases by haematological recovery (Bierman & Nelson 1965). The tick-borne rickettsial organism, *Ehrlichia canis* causes an illness with pancytopenia in dogs and has caused bone marrow hypoplasia in man (Pearce et al 1988). Parvovirus Bl9 often causes acute suppression of haemopoiesis, but may cause aplastic anaemia in normal (Hamon et al 1988) and immune-deficient patients (Kurtzman et al 1987).

Whereas temporary bone marrow suppression may be caused by direct viral inhibition of cell proliferation, perhaps by production of interferons, the reason why infection in a small number of cases is followed, often after an interval of weeks, by marrow aplasia is more difficult to understand. In patients with immune deficiency, persisting virus infection can lead to chronic disease; but no evidence of long-term virus infection is found in most cases of acquired aplasia and it seems likely that the infection may trigger an immune mechanism: patients with aplastic anaemia secondary to hepatitis have responded to immunosuppressive treatment.

Other causes

Pregnancy is a rare but well recognized cause of aplastic anaemia but the subject is not appropriate for a paediatric text book. *Leukaemia* rarely presents as aplastic anaemia. The complication is covered in Chapters 3, 4 and 12. *Starvation* and *anorexia nervosa* lead to pancytopenia and bone marrow necrosis with gelatinous transformation (Smith & Spivak 1985) which may also be associated with blood disease, sepsis, toxaemia and drugs (Conrad & Carpenter 1979).

Down's syndrome and aplastic anaemia have been described twice (Weinblatt et al 1981, Hanukoglu et al 1987) but, unlike leukaemia, too few cases have been identified for this to be more than a chance association.

Idiopathic aplastic anaemia

The onset may be acute or chronic. The former is more common. Occasionally, patients present with neutropenia and thrombocytopenia, but with minimal anaemia. However, there is reticulocytopenia and a very flat bone marrow. The haemoglobin level soon falls, and it is apparent that the aplasia is of recent onset. The incidence of severe aplastic anaemia is higher in children than adults. In a large European study 52% of children had severe aplastic anaemia with three or more of Camitta's indicators of a bad prognosis (Camitta et al 1982), compared to 25% of adults (Najean et al 1982).

One group of children with pancytopenia may show a slow onset and a chronic benign course (Schröter 1970). The anaemia is severe with a haemolytic element, a modest neutropenia and variable thrombocytopenia. The red cell pyruvate kinase is low, and the haemoglobin F level is high. The bone marrow shows erythroid hyperplasia rather than erythroid depression. This disorder is not completely characteristic of aplastic anaemia; it has a resemblance to the early stages of Fanconi's anaemia without being congenital in origin, and appears to be a variant of chronic bone marrow hypoplasia.

The prognosis is poor. In the European study (Najean et al 1982), the results of treatment of 48 children were compared with the results of treatment of 483 adults and 23 children with genetic aplasia. All received treatment with androgens. At 20 months of age, approximately 23% of children with acquired aplastic anaemia were alive, compared to 89% of children with Fanconi's anaemia and 45% of adults.

The presence of a raised level of fetal haemoglobin was at one time thought to be a good prognostic factor (Bloom & Diamond 1968). However, severe cases require blood transfusions, so patients with raised fetal haemoglobin who are not transfused, are the patients who are the less severely affected cases. Subsequent studies failed to support the hypothesis (Li et al 1972, Najean et al 1982). A raised haemoglobin F is only one of the characteristics of fetal erythropoiesis seen in aplastic anaemia. There are changes in the amounts of haemoglobin A_2, carbonic anhydrase B, hexokinase isoenzymes, and the red cell antigens I and i and ABH (Gahr & Schröter 1982). These authors found that patients with aplastic anaemia showed only slight increases of fetal haemoglobin, which was thought to be a stress reaction. A reversal to fetal erythropoiesis was found only in juvenile chronic myeloid leukaemia and erythroleukaemia.

Paroxysmal nocturnal haemoglobinuria

Paroxysmal nocturnal haemoglobinuria (PNH) tends to occur in young adult men, and is extremely rare in childhood. As the name implies, there is a haemolytic anaemia and the urine often contains haemosiderin and may contain haemoglobin. It is characterized by a clone of defective blood cells of all three lines. The membrane is abnormal. There is usually a pancytopenia and incomplete reticulocytosis, and a normocellular marrow with relative increase of erythropoiesis. The red cells are very sensitive to complement and lyse in solutions of low ionic strength (the sugar-water test) and in acidified serum (Ham's test). There is a tendency to thrombosis. Patients develop iron deficiency due to haemosiderinuria.

The relevance of PNH to this chapter arises from the fact that it may present de novo or develop after aplastic anaemia. In the latter case, the high neutrophil alkaline phosphatase level found in aplastic anaemia falls: a low level is a feature of PNH (Beck & Valentine 1951). An intermediate stage exists when tests for PNH are positive; but the full laboratory picture is not present. The interval between the start of aplastic anaemia and the onset of PNH is often years: the complication has been rare in children as very few children have, in the past, survived a long time. The disease may resolve spontaneously.

Dacie & Lewis (1972) reported that 29% of cases of PNH were first diagnosed as aplastic anaemia, whereas after immunosuppressive treatment, the incidence of PNH is of the order of 65% (de Planque et al 1989).

Bone marrow transplantation may be curative, and in one case was successfully undertaken between identical twins without chemotherapy or irradiation (Fefer et al 1976).

Radiation

It is well known that X-irradiation damages the bone marrow, leading to both leukaemia and aplastic anaemia. For whole-body irradiation, the fatal dose is low, because the normal bone marrow cells are very sensitive. Much higher doses can be given to localized areas because the cells recover after the initial depression, and normal stem cells are able to move into the affected site and repopulate it. Nevertheless, there is a limit to the amount of radiation bone marrow will tolerate, and with high doses no regeneration will occur. Irradiation damages not only the haemopoietic cells, but also the micro-environment, including the blood vessels.

The experiments of Knospe & Crosby (1971) nicely illustrate sensitivity to increasing doses of irradiation. One femur and tibia of rats was exposed to low doses, below 1000 rads. Aplasia occurred at 4 days but recovery followed at 14 days. With 2000–4000 rads there was again an initial recovery, but it was followed after 3 months by a secondary aplasia. This was attributed to damage to the micro-environment — the sinusoidal vascular cells — with failure to support the growth of haemopoietic cells. The secondary aplasia recovered after about 6 months. Doses of 4000–6000 rads produced permanent aplasia, but if the bone marrow was curetted before implantation of normal bone marrow, recovery was still possible with such high doses. It was proposed that curettage stimulated the micro-environment and allowed vascular cells to migrate from other areas to sustain stem cell growth.

In man, irradiation kills cells directly. It reduces the survival time of differentiated cells and prolongs interphase arrest (Cronkite 1967). A few hours following a single dose of whole body irradiation as low as 100–450 rads there is profound lymphopenia followed by granulocytopenia and thrombocytopenia. In the bone marrow, the red cell precursors show early morphological changes, although anaemia takes longer to develop, followed by the granulocyte and megakaryocyte series. The cells show chromosomal breaks, bridges and abnormal mitoses (reminiscent of the changes found in untreated Fanconi's anaemia). Cell division eventually ceases and is followed by fatty atrophy (Donati & Gartner 1973). If the patient can be kept alive, recovery follows in 6–7 weeks. Higher doses, as used for the treatment of cancer, may cause permanent aplasia of the bone marrow in the irradiated area. Even though the red cells, white cells and platelets recover, there may be a long-lasting lymphopenia. When children with acute lymphoblastic leukaemia were given cranio-spinal irradiation as prophylaxis for central nervous system leukaemia, the mean lymphocyte count was only $0.6 \times 10^9/1$ over a year later, compared to a count of $1.4 \times 10^9/1$ in children who had similar anti-leukaemia treatment omitting the cranio-spinal radiotherapy (Campbell et al 1973). Lymphocyte chromosome abnormalities may be detected many years after irradiation.

The children who were exposed to irradiation from the atomic bomb showed a higher incidence of leukaemia than of aplastic anaemia. However, irradiation accidents such as occurred at Chernobyl cause extensive burns from beta irradiation. This was the main cause of death, rather than haemopoietic failure, with the result that treatment by bone marrow transplantation was ineffective (Lancet 1986).

TREATMENT OF APLASTIC ANAEMIA

General managemant

There are two goals for the treatment of aplastic anaemia : the first is to maintain the general health of the child with pancytopenia until recovery occurs, and the second is to reverse or cure the bone marrow aplasia. The first shares many of the features of the management of leukaemia, but the second, with the exception of bone marrow transplantation, entails the use of different drugs, which in general are not cytotoxic. In the past, treatment has not been very successful, and the prognosis for children with aplastic anaemia has been worse than that of adults. Lately, the results appear to have improved, but because of the rarity of the disease, inadequate numbers of cases have received newer forms of treatment, and results of reliable series are awaited. As a result, a positive approach should be taken to treatment. Cases are best referred to a centre for paediatric haematology/oncology.

Intravenous access

Patients with aplastic anaemia may need frequent transfusions of blood and platelets, intravenous broad-spectrum antibiotics, and intravenous nutrition. The maintenance of good venous access is therefore extremely important. Venepunctures should be done by skilled staff using the smallest needle possible. We have found the use of central venous catheters, such as Hickman lines, to be extremely valuable. In toddlers and babies, the veins may be very small and easily damaged in the presence of a low platelet count. Such children become fretful and difficult to manage because of the need for frequent pricks, and the children, their parents and the staff appreciate the advantages of easy long-term venous access, which outweigh the disadvantages such as the risk of infection. We have found it helpful to make the entry site on the back, over the scapula instead of on the anterior chest wall. It is out of the way and out of the child's sight, where it can be less easily played with or pulled out. It can be draped over the edge of the bath more easily. Parents can learn the technique of looking after these lines, and patients may keep them in place at home for many months.

Thrombocytopenia

Platelet transfusions are the mainstay of management of the child with a low platelet count. Unlike leukaemia, aplastic anaemia may remain static for many months or years, and it cannot be assumed that treatment will improve the platelet count. The platelets are frequently the last component of the blood count to improve, and patients who have responded well to drugs may continue to show a subnormal platelet count after the red and white cells have returned to normal. So platelet transfusions may be needed for a long time and there is a risk of sensitization to random platelets, with failure of the platelet count to rise as expected after transfusion. It is sensible to treat children with petechiae and bruising, and essential to treat children with epistaxis, bleeding gums, haematuria, as these are signs of a more severe bleeding tendency. As a guide, the platelet count should be maintained above $20 \times 10^9/1$; but this will vary from case to case.

Platelet concentrates are 80–90% as effective as platelet rich plasma in raising the platelet count.

Four units of platelets/m² surface area twice a week will normally maintain the platelet count above $20 \times 10^9/1$ (Freireich 1966). Platelet increments may be higher if the platelet pack is warmed to 37°C for an hour before infusion (Hutchinson et al 1989). Platelets may be successfully transfused after storage for three years or more at –80°C or –120°C (Daly et al 1979).

Resistance to platelets occurs infrequently with fewer than ten transfusions; but unfortunately, as the number of platelets transfused rises, the probability of isoimmunization against platelets increases (Shulman 1966). Patients who do not respond to random platelets will respond to HLA-matched platelets (Yankee et al 1973), but some cases who fail to respond to HLA-matched platelets can respond if contaminating white cells are removed. The process also prevents transfusion reactions due to leucocyte reactions (Herzig et al 1975). The use of platelets from donors whose HLA types cross-react with the patient's is also effective, and increases the pool of potential donors (Duquesnoy et al 1977). Lymphocytotoxicity tests can help predict a poor response. Granulocyte antibodies, however, do not affect the platelet response; but they do correlate with severe transfusion reactions (Gmür et al 1978). Various tests have been introduced to screen for platelet compatibility, as full cross-matching along the lines for red cell transfusion would be cumbersome. An enzyme-linked immunosorbent assay was described by Tamerius et al (1983). A combination of lymphocytotoxicity and platelet immunofluorescence tests was recommended by Murphy & Waters (1985). McFarland & Aster (1987), who compared four tests, found a monoclonal anti-IgG assay to be the most effective, and superior to the platelet immunofluorescence test, ^{51}Cr release, and microlymphocytotoxicity. Fortunately, antibody levels may fall with time, and patients who have been refractory may later show good responses when rechallenged with random donor platelets again (Lee & Schiffer 1987).

Isoimmunization against platelets may be minimized by reducing exposure to platelet antigens. The use of single donor platelets, collected by a cell separator, may be helpful, but not completely successful. Removal of leucocytes from blood and platelet transfusions is much more effective: in one series (Eernisse & Brand 1981) only 24% of recipients of leucocyte-free donations became refractory, compared to 93% of controls. In another series, none of 26 patients given leucocyte-free blood components became refractory compared to 11 of 21 controls (Saarinen et al 1990). ABO compatibility is of slight but distinct importance (Heal et al 1987) but may increase the likelihood of developing refractoriness (Lancet 1990). Group O donors may have high titres of anti-A or anti-B, which can cause significant haemolytic reactions in patients of group A or B. Rhesus incompatibility does not affect platelet survival, but may lead to Rhesus sensitization of Rhesus-negative individuals.

Other complications include the development of antibodies linked to vancomycin (Christie et al 1990), and granulocytopenia from incompatible platelet transfusions (Herzig et al 1974).

Leucopenia

The pancytopenia comprises a reduction of all types of white cells. Granulocytopenia predisposes to bacterial infection; lymphopenia to fungal and viral infection. There is also a prominent monocytopenia, which leads to depletion of tissue macrophages and also predisposes to infection (Twomey et al 1973). The macrophages fail to mature from monocytes normally (Andreesen et al 1989).

Granulocyte transfusions can replace missing white cells, but have not proved as useful and successful as was at first hoped. There is no place for prophylactic white cell transfusions. They may be considered for bacterial infections in neutropenic cases who are not responding to antibiotics. They need to be given for at least 4 days. In the neutropenic patient with leukaemia who is not in the terminal stages of the disease, there is a chance that chemotheraphy will produce remission within a few days, and it can be anticipated that leucocyte transfusions will be needed for a finite period. No such assumption can be made for the patient with aplastic anaemia. Once started, leucocyte transfusions can only be stopped when the infection has recovered, and there is no guarantee that this will happen. Consequently, there is even less enthusiasm for their use in aplastic anaemia than there is in leukaemia. One bonus for granulocyte transfusions in childhood is that they are often contaminated with platelets, so a granulocyte transfusion may give rise to a substantial rise of the platelets as well (Fig. 2.5).

Granulocytes should ideally be collected from ABO-matched donors; and HLA-compatibility improves granulocyte survival (Hester & Rossen 1974). The donors used and the method of collection will depend on local circumstances. Better yields seem to be achieved from men than from women: in general the former have a larger blood volume and can tolerate greater blood volume depletion, and their higher PCV may make leucocyte separation more effective. As with platelet transfusions, repeated granulocyte transfusions may lead to the development of a refractory state due to the presence of antibodies.

The side-effects of granulocyte transfusion are twofold. There is often a pyrexial reaction. More severe systemic reactions may also occur, with dys- and tachypnoea, and rigors. These may be due to the effect of the infection on the transfused leucocytes, to antigen–antibody reaction or to complement damage to the leucocytes during collection (Gordon-Smith 1979). The other complication is the development of graft-versus-host disease, due to the presence of viable stem cells. The former may be helped by prophylactic prescription of hydrocortisone and antihistamines; the latter by irradiation of the leucocytes to 15 Gy. Graft-versus-host disease will only occur in the presence of profound lymphopenia. It is more likely to arise when a patient with aplastic anaemia has been prepared for bone marrow transplantation by cytotoxic chemotherapy, or has received methyl prednisone with or without anti-lymphocyte globulin. The author's practice is to irradiate all blood products in these circumstances.

Anaemia

Anaemia is usually a simple matter to control with red cell transfusions. If the white cells are removed from the red cells, there is less chance that the recipient will develop antiplatelet antibodies, so platelet transfusions will be more effective, and less chance of developing antileucocyte antibodies which may lead to pyrexial transfusion reactions. A bone marrow transplant is less likely to be rejected if fewer blood transfusions are given; but transplants

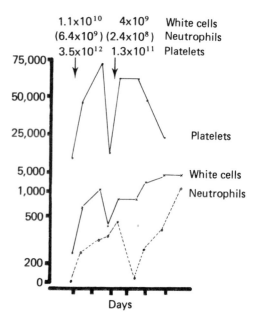

Fig. 2.5 Increments of white cells and platelets in a child after transfusion of cells from a normal adult donor collected with Haemonetics Model 30 blood cell processor. (Reprinted from Evans 1979 with permission of Churchill Livingstone.)

have been given successfully to patients who have received transfusions over many years for thalassaemia, and multiple transfusions are not a contraindication in aplastic anaemia. It is preferable to avoid using family members as blood donors, because they may share HLA antigens with the patient and cause sensitization, which could compromise the result of transplantation. Many children can tolerate levels of haemoglobin down to 7 g/dl, and it is not necessary to give a transfusion unless the patient has symptoms due to anaemia. If transfusions can be minimized, the risk of post-transfusion infection with cytomegalovirus (CMV) and hepatitis can be reduced too. Patients who lack antibodies to CMV, and who are candidates for bone marrow transplantation, should be transfused with blood from donors lacking CMV antibodies, as this reduces the chance of CMV infection developing after the transplant. The possibility that removal of leucocytes from blood by filtration will reduce the possibility of transmission of CMV from infected donors is under investigation.

Infection

The *normal childhood immunizations* can be given

to children with aplastic anaemia unless they are profoundly lymphopenic and thrombocytopenic, or on treatment with immunosuppressive drugs. The combination of antilymphocyte globulin and high dose methyl prednisolone is particularly immunosuppressive.

Lymphopenia is a feature of many aplasias, and predisposes to infections with fungi and viruses. Parents should be warned of the dangers of chicken pox and measles, but the risks of these infections are not as great as in children with leukaemia.

Bacterial infection, secondary to neutropenia, is more of a problem. Any pyrexia for which the cause is not immediately apparent calls for prompt blood culture and examination of urine and swabs from the throat and nose, followed by treatment with a broad-spectrum antibiotic. Many units have an antibiotic policy for the initial treatment of pyrexia of unknown origin in leucopenic patients. The use of an aminoglycoside plus one of the newer penicillins is popular, for example gentamicin plus carbenicillin or amikacin plus piperacillin. However, many of these drug protocols have been developed in adults. Children tend to have fewer infections with Gram-negative organisms, and more with Gram-positive cocci. Several studies have compared the use of single versus multiple antibiotics for treatment of febrile neutropenic patients; these are reviewed by Hathorn & Pizzo (1986). Many antibiotic combinations have been used, and most centres will have a policy for these cases. However, children may respond as well to one of the third generation cephalosporins such as ceftriaxone, which has the added advantage of once-daily dosage, as to an aminoglycoside-penicillin combination (Smith et al 1990). Such treatment avoids the danger of ototoxicity and the necessity for measurement of blood levels for aminoglycosides.

If the pyrexia fails to respond, a different drug combination is introduced, the assumption being that the bacterial infection is resistant to the initial combination. Vancomycin is often used, on the understanding that penicillin-resistant staphylococci may be the cause; and an aminoglycoside may be added at this stage. If this fails, treatment is started with amphotericin-B to cover the possibility of a fungal infection. It has the advantage of covering *Aspergillus* as well as *Candida* and other fungi and yeasts: its disadvantage is that it is nephrotoxic, has a high risk of side-effects, and must be given slowly over several hours, diluted in glucose.

Splenectomy and the spleen

In the past, when there were fewer options for treatment, occasional patients were treated by splenectomy. The operation was attended by a risk of haemorrhage. The only indication at present for splenectomy would be for a patient who has developed a large spleen as a sequel to multiple transfusions, and who has developed hypersplenism as a result. Splenomegaly is not a normal feature of aplastic anaemia, and the presence of a large spleen in a patient under investigation for aplastic anaemia should lead to a suspicion that the true diagnosis is myelodysplasia. Splenomegaly may also be a complication of cirrhosis, which may be a sequel to hepatitis and which itself may be the cause of aplasia.

Other measures

Poor nutrition may develop as a result of loss of appetite associated with long-term illness, recurrent infection and antibiotic treatment. Vitamin supplements by themselves do not cure aplasia, but as undernutrition may cause bone marrow failure (Smith & Spivak 1985), so adequate nutrition is even more important for the management of aplastic anaemia than it is for other chronic illnesses. Dietary supplements may be needed, and we start intravenous nutrition if there is over 10% loss of body weight.

Drug treatment

Androgens

Testosterone. The use of testosterone, first introduced by Shahidi & Diamond (1959) with five children in Boston, was the first measure substantially to affect the prognosis in aplastic anaemia. Testosterone had previously been shown to increase the haemoglobin level of patients with cancer of the breast (Kennedy & Nathanson 1953). One case was treated shortly after diagnosis. For the other four, the interval between diagnosis and start of treatment was 6 months to one year, during which time the patients were treated with cortico-steroids and transfusions. They also received corti-costeroids or ACTH concurrently with testo-sterone. One patient died, but the other four cases all responded. In an addendum, the authors commented that three of a further five cases had also responded. Shahidi & Diamond (1959) used sublingual testosterone propionate or methyl testosterone, with one case receiving intramuscular testosterone enanthate.

Oxymetholone. This 17-α alkylated androgen was introduced for the treatment of refractory anaemia in Mexico by Sanchez-Medal et al (1964), as its virilizing activity is less than that of testosterone. Ten of 19 cases responded. Three of their cases were children, and it is interesting to note that two died early before a response could be seen. The third responded, relapsing when oxymetholone was withdrawn, and responding again when oxymetholone was reintroduced. Since then, oxymetholone has been widely used for the treatment of aplastic anaemia in patients of all ages. A high dose is needed to achieve an effect, with the result that this 'non-virilizing' androgen produces virilizing effects. A customary dose is 3–5 mg/kg or 50 mg/m² per day. There is an increase of height, muscle bulk and strength, acne and a greasy flushed skin, obesity, penile and clitoral hypertrophy, increased body hair, and a hoarse voice (Fig. 2.4). Patients may complain of cramp. Cholestatic jaundice is a well-recognized complication. It is dose-related, and resolves when the drug is withdrawn or the dose reduced. The serum alkaline phosphatase is frequently raised in the presence of jaundice. There is also an increase of the serum cholesterol and triglycerides.

Initially, there was anxiety that androgen treatment would lead to premature fusion of the epiphyses, so that children who at first showed a growth spurt with treatment would end up dwarfed. Corticosteroids were sometimes prescribed to counteract this possible effect. Fortunately, it has been shown that this anxiety is not founded on fact; children treated with androgens and corticosteroids in high doses over a prolonged period do not show premature epiphyseal fusion (Shahidi & Crigler 1976). Hepatoma and peliosis hepatis appear to be more frequently associated with treatment in Fanconi's anaemia (p. 31).

The response to androgens is variable. The initial good response in Boston was not maintained: in a second report the results were inferior; 13 of 17 cases responded of whom three relapsed and later died, and another died of infection leaving only nine in remission (Shahidi & Diamond 1961). The patients who respond appear to be those with moderate disease: it is as if androgens can only stimulate a bone marrow which has been partially suppressed: a completely suppressed bone marrow is unable to respond. It takes 2 or 3 months before any response is seen, so patients need to be supported by blood and platelet transfusions while a response to androgens is anticipated. The main effect of androgens is to increase erythropoiesis. Nevertheless, two-thirds of children treated in an international cooperative trial of androgens in aplastic anaemia (Najean 1976) showed an increase of granulocytes, and one-third showed a rise of platelets. A variety of androgens are effective (Shahidi 1973). A comparative trial of four androgens given in similar doses suggested that norethandrolone was most effective (Najean 1976), but the effectiveness is probably related to dose rather than to the individual androgen. Many products formerly produced are no longer available.

The emotional effects of androgens in children should not be ignored. Children frequently show a premature interest in sexual matters. One of the author's patients, an eight-year-old boy, frequently embarrassed his mother by commenting loudly, and approvingly, in public on the size of women's breasts. Boys may become amorous with their mothers and interfere with little girls at school. Erections and masturbation may occur. Parents must be reminded that their children's physical development is artificially stimulated, and that their emotional and intellectual development is only equivalent to their true age. It is also helpful to explain that the drugs are similar to those used illegally by athletes to increase muscle mass; and whereas the athletes are at risk of complications from the treatment, their children are under constant medical supervision so that any unwelcome side-effects can be properly dealt with.

Corticosteroids

Before more effective forms of treatment became

available, low doses of oral corticosteroids were given, mainly with a view to preventing bleeding by maintaining capillary integrity. Such treatment is of doubtful benefit: it certainly does not stop bleeding in children with severe aplastic anaemia who need platelet transfusions. Furthermore, the effects of corticosteroids on resistance to infection, coupled with neutropenia, increase the number of bacteraemias and other infections: so low-dose corticosteroids in the long term may be harmful rather than beneficial. In one patient who responded to prednisone, cortisol enhanced colony growth by depleting inhibitory T-cells (Bagby et al 1979).

High-dose intravenous methyl prednisolone, on the other hand, has proved much more effective. Based on the knowledge of its effectiveness in renal graft rejection, Bacigalupo et al (1981) treated six children, three of whom showed complete remission within 3–4 weeks. In a series of 28 Turkish children, 64% responded to a regimen comprising 30 mg/kg for 3 days, 20 mg/kg for 4 days, and subsequently 10, 5, 2 and 1 mg/kg for one week each (Ozsoylu et al 1984). Methyl prednisolone is now more frequently used in conjunction with antilymphocyte globulin (see below).

Antilymphocyte globulin

The use of methyl prednisolone has coincided with the introduction of other immunosuppressive treatments, notably antilymphocyte globulin. The two agents are frequently used together, as methyl prednisolone not only aids bone marrow recovery, but also suppresses the side-effects, such as serum sickness, which may accompany the use of antilymphocyte globulin. Antilymphocyte globulin was first used as part of the conditioning programme prior to bone marrow transplantation (Mathé et al 1970). It was then found to be successful both with and without marrow infusion (Speck et al 1977) and became more widely adopted. Evidence that aplastic anaemia was in some cases due to T-cell inhibition of bone marrow growth in vitro encouraged its use (Bacigalupo et al 1981). By the early 1980s, over 60% survivals were reported in a group of 32 patients given one HLA-haplotype-matched bone marrow and androgens, compared with a 44% survival of 18 patients given

HLA-identical sibling marrow after conditioning with cyclophosphamide. All of the former group were shown to have recovered autologous bone marrow function (Speck et al 1981). Both groups included children, but the results were not analyzed by age. A study by the European Bone Marrow Transplant Group found no difference in the one-year survival of patients treated with antithymocyte globulin, antithymocyte globulin plus haplo-identical bone marrow infusion, and high-dose bolus 6-methyl prednisolone (Gluckman et al 1982). By 1982, a study of children showed that 12 of 23 cases treated with antilymphocyte globulin gave a complete or partial response, with minimal complications of urticaria or fever (Cairo & Baehner 1978). In another trial of patients of all ages, 11 of 21 treated by intravenous antithymocyte globulin given for 8 days showed sustained improvement. None of 21 controls given supportive care improved (p = 0.0005) (Champlin et al 1983). However, the results are uneven: in another group of 12 children given antithymocyte globulin with or without high dose methyl prednisolone, only 25% showed complete remission, compared with a 79% cure rate for bone marrow transplantation from a histocompatible related donor (Halperin et al 1989). Both antilymphocyte and antithymocyte globulin were used.

The *ideal dose* is not known. Daily doses of 40 mg/kg for 4 days (Speck et al 1981), 20 mg/kg for 8 days (Champlin et al 1983) and 10 mg/kg for 5 days (Gluckman et al 1978) have all been used. In a trial using horse immunoglobulin, it was shown that doses over 100 mg/kg produced better results (Coiffier et al 1983); but in a larger series of 79 cases with several disorders no difference was found between patients treated for 10 or 28 days (Young et al 1988). Clearly a minimum dose is necessary, and is likely to vary with each product.

Variation between batches is possible, as antilymphocyte globulin is prepared in animals, usually horses or rabbits. The lymphocyte preparation used for immunization, the animal used and the response of the animal could lead to slight differences in the products of the various manufacturers. Two different lots of anti-human thoracic duct lymphocyte globulin produced by the Swiss Serum Institute gave response rates of 69% and 31%. There was wide variation in the amounts of individual antibody specificity within each lot (Smith et al 1985). In a trial at the Hammersmith Hospital, London, 21 patients were treated with antilymphocyte globulin from three different sources, but the origin of the antilymphocyte globulin was without effect on survival: it was the length of time before treatment started which was significant (Fairhead et al 1983). The European group compared two preparations. 128 patients given a French preparation showed 59% survival: 136 patients given a Swiss product showed 64% survival (Bacigalupo et al 1986).

The *response to antilymphocyte globulin* depends on the severity of the disease. Studies from Seattle reported a 67% remission rate, and showed that a high granulocyte count and younger age also implied a better prognosis (Doney et al 1984). A series of 64 cases treated at the Hammersmith Hospital, London, showed a 53% six-year actuarial survival. Patients with severe aplastic anaemia showed 36% survival: the others showed 79% survival. Some idea of the likelihood of a response to antithymocyte globulin may be gained by measuring the release in vitro of colony-stimulating activity after starting treatment. Low release predicts a poor response (Nissen et al 1989). The mean red cell volume (MCV) may also be an early indicator of response (Marsh et al 1987). Four of 18 patients who failed to improve at first responded to a second course (Marsh et al 1987).

For the second course, antilymphocyte globulin from a different animal is used in order to avoid reactions which might occur from sensitization after the first course. A second dose of antilymphocyte globulin may produce a second remission in patients who have relapsed after the first course (Doney et al 1984).

The *effect of androgens combined with antilymphocyte globulin* became a matter of interest when it became apparent that its effects were not affected by the infusion of HLA-haplotype-matched bone marrow. At first, androgens were shown not to make any difference (Champlin et al 1985), but two later studies showed improved rates when the two drugs were combined (Bacigalupo et al 1986, Kaltwasser et al 1988).

The *combination of antilymphocyte globulin with corticosteroids* is frequently used, for two reasons: steroids reduce side-effects from sensitization to

animal proteins, and have an intrinsic immunosuppressive effect which may be additive. The former may in fact be important: serum sickness after antithymocyte globulin may impair recovery (Bielory et al 1986). There was no difference in the response to ALG whether low-dose (5 mg/kg/day) prednisolone or high-dose (20 mg/kg/day) was given (Bacigalupo et al 1986).

The *precise mode of action of antilymphocyte globulin* is unknown. There is no correlation between the clinical response and the lymphocyte response to pokeweed mitogen, herpes simplex virus or tetanus toxoid (Lum et al 1987). The target cells may be the lymphocytes which express activation antigen Tac (interleukin-2 receptor) (Platanias et al 1987). Antithymocyte globulin did not affect the outcome of other diseases with bone marrow failure, such as myelodysplasia, amegakaryocytic thrombocytopenia, pure red cell aplasia, myelofibrosis, cyclical neutropenia or paroxysmal nocturnal haemoglobinuria. Two of eight patients with pancytopenia and cellular bone marrows responded (Young et al 1988). One patient with paroxysmal nocturnal haemoglobinuria and aplastic anaemia, a 14-year-old boy, did respond to antilymphocyte globulin (Kusminsky et al 1988).

Late complications after recovery from aplastic anaemia treated by antilymphocyte globulin were described by the European Bone Marrow Transplantation Group. Of 223 long-term survivors, 31 developed other bone marrow diseases including paroxysmal nocturnal haemoglobinuria, myelodysplasia, and acute leukaemia (de Planque et al 1989). Most have a normal haemoglobin with a raised MCV and a normal granulocyte count with a left shift, and remain thrombocytopenic, often with impaired platelet function. Serum IgG and IgA are significantly decreased, but lymphocyte subsets are within the normal range, with a slight decrease of T4 (helper) lymphocytes.

Cyclosporin A

Once other immunosuppressive treatment was recognized to be successful, it became inevitable that cyclosporin would be tried. Initially, 12 adults with severe aplastic anaemia treated in South Africa showed a complete failure to respond

(Jacobs et al 1985). Subsequent attempts met with better success. Two patients, one a 15-year-old boy, responded within 6 weeks to 10 mg/kg per day after failing to respond to methyl prednisolone and antilymphocyte globulin (Bridges et al 1987). Eight of 21 patients, including a two-year-old boy and a 16-year-old girl with chronic severe aplastic anaemia, showed significant improvement of blood counts after 3–6 months' treatment. Fourteen similar cases, including four children of 16 years of age or less, did not. Better results were achieved when prednisolone was added. None of four cases with severe acute aplasia responded (Leonard et al 1989). There are other successful reports. The difficulty of achieving adequate blood levels may contribute to a poor response. One adult female showed a second response after a second course of treatment (Bern et al 1987).

Further trials are under way. Preliminary results showed that 43% of cases responded initially to cyclosporin, and the response rate rose to 57% when nonresponders were treated with antilymphocyte globulin. The results were as good as when the latter product was used initially, perhaps because androgens were used concurrently (Marin et al 1989). Cyclosporin was effective treatment for a 17-year-old girl with hypoplastic anaemia developing in Shwachman's syndrome (Barrios & Kirkpatrick (1990).

A reminder that long-term immunosuppressive treatment with cyclosporin may lead to infection is given by the case of Pogliani et al (1989) who developed tuberculous pericarditis after five months successful treatment for severe aplastic anaemia.

Growth factors

Many haemopoietic growth factors have been identified including granulocyte, macrophage and granulocyte-macrophage colony-stimulating factors, interleukins 1 to 11, tumour necrosis factor, and the interferons α, β and γ as well as platelet stimulating factors (for a review see Jones & Miller 1989). Interferons show inhibitory effects and have been used in the treatment of leukaemia, but the leucocyte colony stimulating factors increase the total granulocyte count in normal individuals and patients with leucopenia secondary to chemotherapy. Experience with their use in children is

at present limited. Ten of 11 adults with aplastic anaemia given recombinant granulocyte-macrophage colony-stimulating factor showed substantial increments of granulocytes, monocytes and eosinophils, but only one showed higher red cells and platelets. Three patients developed pulmonary infiltrates which responded when treatment was stopped (Champlin et al 1989). However, in another trial, in which seven patients with aplastic anaemia were treated, the granulocytes responded poorly or not at all; but there was some improvement of the signs of infection (Milne & Gordon-Smith 1990). The difference may be due to the fact that the cases in the second series were infected. Further studies are needed to see if granulocyte or other colony-stimulating factors are of value in aplastic anaemia. Their use with regulators, such as interleukin-1, which act on stem cells has already been shown to enhance haemopoietic regeneration in laboratory animals. Most experience so far has been with leukaemia. In some cases the number of blast cells has increased. One can speculate that colony stimulating factors may increase the risk of developing leukaemia after aplastic anaemia.

Other drugs

Lithium was for a time popular for the treatment of granulocytopenia. It has not been given any extensive trial in aplastic anaemia. In the mouse, lithium causes an increase of megakaryocyte colonies, and encourages stromal cells to produce substances stimulating the growth of megakaryocyte, granulocyte, monocyte, macrophage and mixed lineage colonies, inducing production of granulocyte-macrophage colony-stimulating factor (McGrath et al 1987). Some response might be expected in aplasia. Improvement was reported in three patients (Barrett et al 1977, Blum 1979).

Three of eight patients treated with *acyclovir* improved, but only one showed sustained recovery (Gomez-Almaguer et al 1988). This may be a chance association.

Intravenous immunoglobulin

An 11-year-old girl with aplastic anaemia associated with anti-neutrophil, anti-platelet and anti-erythrocyte antibodies was treated with three 4-day courses of intravenous immunoglobulin, 2g/kg, followed by maintenance of 0.5 g/kg fortnightly for 6 months. She remained in remission after treatment was stopped (Kapoor et al 1988). This case may not be typical, but a seven-year-old boy who had failed to respond to two courses of antithymocyte globulin and high-dose methyl prednisolone improved with a 6 month course of 1 g/kg every 4 weeks, and remained well after treatment was stopped (Sadowitz & Dubowy 1990). With these limited results, further studies are justified.

BONE MARROW TRANSPLANTATION IN ACQUIRED APLASTIC ANAEMIA

Bone marrow transplantation for aplastic anaemia using HLA-compatible sibling donors and conditioning with cyclophosphamide was successfully pioneered by the Seattle group (Donnall Thomas et al 1972). In Europe, the early cases were prepared by antilymphocyte globulin, but results were inferior, and it was usually their own bone marrow which recovered. More intensive chemotherapy with cyclophosphamide is now preferred for conditioning, and antilymphocyte globulin without a bone marrow transplant is used for patients who lack a histocompatible family donor.

Rejection of the grafted bone marrow is more likely in aplastic anaemia than in other diseases. Rejection rates vary between 5 and 60% (Champlin et al 1989). It is as if the defect leading to failure of growth of the patient's own bone marrow also affects the transplanted marrow. When 21 of 73 (29%) Seattle cases had rejected their grafts, an analysis showed that two factors correlated strongly with graft rejection: a reaction in mixed lymphocyte culture indicating sensitization of the patient against the donor, and a low number of marrow cells (less than 3×10^8 cells per kg) infused (Storb et al 1977). By 1982, 252 Seattle patients had been analyzed (Niederwieser et al 1988). A significant association between a high number of cells engrafted and a low rejection rate was confirmed. High doses also produced a faster recovery and better survival. Graft rejection is also related to previous transfusions. There is a reduced risk if patients have been prepared by irradiation, and if they have received cyclosporine rather than

methotrexate or T-cell depletion as prophylaxis against graft-versus-host disease (Bacigalupo et al 1988, Champlin et al 1989). Patients who have rejected the first graft may be transplanted a second time with success, using antithymocyte globulin in addition to cyclophosphamide for preparation, but only 40% are long-term survivors (Storb et al 1987).

Children showed a 70% survival rate, with some children alive 12 and 13 years after transplantation. The single factor associated with increased survival was the absence of significant graft-versus-host disease (Sanders et al 1986). Early graft failure is more common when bone marrow transplantation is delayed beyond a year from diagnosis (Hows et al 1989). Some centres have used total body irradiation, or total lymphoid irradiation as part of the conditioning regimen for children with aplastic anaemia, as well as leukaemia (McGlave et al 1987, Miyamura et al 1988). There is a high incidence of hypothyroidism (McGlave et al 1987). The potential for inducing later malignant disease, and the effects on growth, have lessened enthusiasm in most centres.

Children with no HLA-matched donor have a poor prognosis. Transplants have therefore been made using unrelated histocompatible donors or partially matched family donors. The post-transplant course is difficult and dangerous; but the European Bone Marrow Transplantation Group reported that 12 of 46 (26%) patients of all ages were alive 16–84 months after transplant (Bacigalupo et al 1988). In a smaller American series, seven of 13 children so treated were alive at 37–2692 days after transplant. They were prepared with an intensive regime including cyclophosphamide, high dose cytosine arabinoside, methyl prednisolone, and total body irradiation. The bone marrow was depleted of T-cells and the children received cyclosporin for prophylaxis against graft-versus-host disease (Camitta et al 1989).

An identical twin is the ideal donor for a patient with acquired aplastic anaemia. Such transplants given without prior immunsuppression are likely to fail, but second transplants given after immunosuppression have succeeded (Champlin et al 1984).

Bone marrow transplantation for post-hepatitic aplasia is successful, and runs the same risk of graft rejection and graft-versus-host disease as idiopathic aplasia. Survival is the same, and hepatic damage or abnormal liver function tests do not appear to increase morbidity, hepatocellular damage or the risk of veno-occlusive disease (Witherspoon et al 1984).

REFERENCES

Aljouni K, Doeblin T D 1974 The syndrome of hepatitis and aplastic anaemia. British Journal of Haematology 27: 345–355

Alter B, Potter NU 1983 Long term outcome in Fanconi's anaemia: description of 26 cases and review of the literature. In: German J (ed) Chromosome mutation and neoplasia. Liss, New York, p 43–61

Alter C L, Levine P H, Bennett J et al 1989 Dominantly transmitted hematologic dysfunction clinically similar to Fanconi's anemia. American Journal of Hematology 32: 241–247

Althoff H 1953 Zur Panmyelopathie Fanconi ab Zustandbild multipler Abartungen. Zeitschrift für Kinderheilkunde 77: 267

Andreesen R, Brugger W, Thomssen C, Rehm A, Speck B, Löhr G W 1989 Defective monocyte-to-macrophage maturation in patients with aplastic anemia. Blood 74: 2150–2156

Aoki K, Fujiki N, Shimizu H, Ohno Y 1980 Geographic and ethnic differences of aplastic anaemias in humans. In: Najean Y (ed) Medullary aplasia. Masson, New York p 79–88

Auerbach A D, Ghosh R, Pollio P C, Zhang M 1989 Diepoxybutane test for prenatal and postnatal diagnosis of Fanconi anaemia. In: Schroeder-Kurth T M, Auerbach A D, Obe G (eds) Fanconi anaemia, clinical, cytogenetic and experimental aspects. Springer, Berlin, p 71–82

Aymard J P, Guerci O, Herbeuval R 1980 Infection-induced aplastic anemia. In: Najean Y (ed) Medullary aplasia. Masson, New York, p 43–51

Bacigalupo A, Podesta M, Van Lint M T et al 1981 Severe aplastic anaemia: correlation of in vitro tests with clinical response to immunosuppression in 20 patients. British Journal of Haematology 47: 423–433

Bacigalupo A, Van Lint M T, Congiu M et al 1986 Treatment of SAA in Europe 1970–1985: a report to the SAA working party. Bone Marrow Transplantation 1 (suppl 1): 19–21

Bacigalupo A, Hows J, Gordon-Smith E C et al 1988 Bone marrow transplantation for severe aplastic anaemia from donors other than HLA identical siblings: a report of the BMT working party. Bone Marrow Transplantation 3: 531–535

Bagby G C, Goodnight S H, Mooney W M, Richert-Boe K 1979 Prednisone-responsive aplastic anemia: a mechanism of glucocorticoid action. Blood 54: 322–333

Barrett A J, Weller E, Rozengurt N, Longhurst P, Humble J G, 1976 Amidopyrine agranulocytosis: drug inhibition of granulocyte colonies in the presence of the patient's serum. British Medical Journal ii: 850–851

Barrett A J, Hugh-Jones K, Newton K, Watson J G 1977 Lithium therapy in aplastic anaemia. Lancet i: 202

Barrios N J, Kirkpatrick D V 1990 Successful cyclosporin A treatment of aplastic anaemia in Shwachman-Diamond syndrome. British Journal of Haematology 74: 540–544

Barrios N J, Kirkpatrick, D V, Stine K C, Humbert J R 1989 Lithium therapy in Fanconi aplastic anaemia. British Journal of Haematology 73: 422–423

Beck W S, Valentine W N 1951 Biochemical stidues on leucocytes II. Phosphatase activity in chronic lymphatic leukaemia, acute leukaemia and miscellaneous haematologic conditions. Journal of Laboratory and Clinical Medicine 38: 245

Benestad H B 1979 Drug mechanisms in marrow aplasia. In: Geary C G (ed) Aplastic anaemia. Bailliere Tindall, London, p 26–42

Bern M M, Roberts M S, Yoburn D 1987 Cyclosporin treatment for aplastic anaemia: a case report demonstrating a second response to a second exposure to cyclosporin. American Journal of Haematology 24: 307–309

Bernstein S E 1970 Tissue transplantation as an analytical and therapeutic tool in hereditary anaemias. American Journal of Surgery 119: 448–451

Bernstein M S, Hunter R L, Yachnin S 1971 Hepatoma and peliosis hepatitis developing in a patient with Fanconi's anaemia. New England Journal of Medicine 284: 1135–1136

Bielory L, Gascon P, Lawley T J, Nienhuis A, Frank MM, Young N S 1986 Serum sickness and haemopoietic recovery with antithymocyte globulin in bone marrow failure patients. British Journal of Haematology 63: 729–736

Bierman H R, Nelson E R 1965 Hematodepressive virus diseases of Thailand. Annals of Internal Medicine 62: 867–884

Bloom G E, Diamond L K 1968 Prognostic value of fetal hemoglobin levels in acquired aplastic anemia. New England Journal of Medicine 278: 304–307

Blum S F 1979 Lithium therapy of aplastic anemia. New England Journal of Medicine 300: 677

Böttiger L E, Westerholm B 1972 Aplastic anemia III– Aplastic anemia and infectious hepatitis. Acta Medica Scandinavica 192: 323–326

Brand A, van Leeuwen A, Eerniss J G, Van Rood J J 1978 Platelet transfusion therapy. Optimal donor selection with a combination of lymphocytotoxicity and platelet fluorescence tests. Blood 51: 781–788

Branda R F, Moldow C F, MacArthur J R, Wintrobe M M, Anthony B K, Jacob H S 1978 Folate-induced remission in aplastic anemia with familial defect of cellular folate uptake. New England Journal of Medicine 298: 469–475

Bridges R, Pineo G, Blahey W 1987 Cyclosporin A for the treatment of aplastic anemia refractory to antithymocyte globulin. American Journal of Hematology 26: 83–87

British Medical Journal 1967 Leading article: Toxicity of chloramphenicol British Medical Journal 1: 649–650

Cairo M S, Baehner R L 1982 The use of antithymocyte globulin in the treatment of severe aplastic anemia in children. Journal of Pediatrics 100: 307–311

Campbell A C, Hersey P, MacLennan I C M, Kay H E M, Pike M C, and the Medical Research Council working party on leukaemia in childhood 1973 Immunosuppressive consequences of radiotherapy and chemotherapy in patients with acute lymphoblastic leukaemia. British Medical Journal 2: 385–388

Camitta B M, Rappeport J M, Parkman R, Nathan D G 1975

Selection of patients for bone marrow transplantation in severe aplastic anaemia. Blood 45: 355–363

Camitta B M, Storb R, Donnall Thomas E 1982 Aplastic anaemia: II Pathogenesis, diagnosis, treatment and prognosis. New England Journal of Medicine 306: 712–718

Camitta B, Ash R, Menitove J et al 1989 Bone marrow transplantation for children with severe aplastic anemia: use of donors other than HLA-identical siblings. Blood 74: 1852–1857

Champlin R, Ho W, Gale R P 1983 Antithymocyte globulin treatment in patients with aplastic anemia. New England Journal of Medicine 308: 113–118

Champlin R, Feig S, Sparkes R, Gale R P 1984 Bone marrow transplantation from identical twins in the treatment of aplastic anaemia: implication for the pathogenesis of the disease. British Journal of Haematology 56: 455–463

Champlin R E, Ho W G, Winston D J, Lenarsky C, Gale R P 1985 Do androgens enhance the response to antithymocyte globulin in patients with aplastic anemia? A prospective randomized trial. Blood 66: 184–188

Champlin R E, Horowitz M M, van Bekkum D W et al 1989 Graft failure following bone marrow transplantation for severe aplastic anemia: risk factors and treatment results. Blood 73: 606–613

Champlin R E, Nimer S D, Ireland P, Oette D H, Golde D W 1989 Treatment of refractory aplastic anemia with recombinant human granulocyte-macrophage-colony-stimulating factor. Blood 73: 694–699

Chan H S, Saunders E F, Freedman M H 1981 Lithium therapy in children with chronic neutropenia. American Journal of Medicine 70: 1073–77

Christie D J, van Buren N, Lennon S S, Putnam J L 1990 Vancomycin-dependent antibodies associated with thrombocytopenia and refractoriness to platelet transfusion in patients with leukemia. Blood 75: 518–523

Clausen N 1986 A population study of severe aplastic anemia in children: incidence, etiology and course. Acta Paediatrica Scandinavica 75: 58–63

Cline M J, Golde D W 1978 Immune suppression of haematopoiesis. American Journal of Medicine 64: 301–310.

Coiffier B, Viala J J, Bryon P A, Fiere D, 1983 Antithymocyte globulin in severe aplastic anaemia: how much? Lancet ii: 100–101

Conrad M E, Carpenter J T 1979 Bone marrow necrosis. American Journal of Hematology 7: 181–189

Conter V, Johnson F L, Paolucci P, Ruggiero M, Janco R L 1988 Bone marrow transplantation for aplastic anaemia associated with dyskeratosis congenita. American Journal of Pediatric Hematology/Oncology 10: 99–102

Cronkite E P 1967 Radiation-induced aplastic anemia. Seminars in Hematology 4: 273–277

Dacie J V, Lewis S M 1972 Paroxysmal nocturnal haemoglobinuria: clinical manifestations, haematology and nature of the disease. Series Hematologica 5: 3–23

Daly P A, Schiffer C A, Aisner J, Wiernik P H 1979 Successful transfusion of platelets cryopreserved for more than 3 years. Blood 54: 1023–1027

De Boeck K, Degreef H, Verwilghen R, Corbeel L Casteels-Van Daele M 1981 Thrombocytopenia: first symptom in a patient with dyskeratosis congenita. Pediatrics 67: 898–903

de Planque M M, Bacigalupo A, Würsch A et al 1989 Long term follow-up of severe aplastic anaemia patients treated with antithymocyte globulin. British Journal of Haematology 73: 121–126

Dexter T M, Allen T D, Lajtha L G 1977 Conditions controlling the proliferation of haemopoietic cells in vitro. Journal of Cellular Physiology 91: 335–344

Dhingra K, Michels S D, Winton E F, Gordon D S 1988 Transient bone marrow aplasia associated with non-A, non-B hepatitis. American Journal of Hematology 29: 168–171

Dokal I, Ganly P, Riebero I, et al 1989 Late onset of bone marrow failure associated with proximal fusion of radius and ulna: a new syndrome. British Journal of Haematology: 71: 277–280

Donati R M, Gartner G E 1973 Haematological aspects of radiation exposure. In: Girdwood R H (ed) Blood disorders due to drugs and other agents. Excerpta Medica. Amsterdam, p 241.

Doney K, Dahlberg S J, Monroe D, Storb R, Buckner C D, Thomas E D 1984. Therapy of severe aplastic anemia with antihuman thymocyte globulin and androgens: the effect of HLA-haploidentical marrow infusion. Blood 63: 342–348

Donnall Thomas E, Buckner C D, Storb R et al 1972 Aplastic anemia treated by marrow transplantation. Lancet i: 284–289

Du Bois K P 1971 the toxicity of organophosphorus compounds to mammals. Bulletin of the World Health Organisation 44: 233–240

Duquesnoy R J, Filip D J, Rodey G E, Rimm A A, Aster R H 1977 Successful transfusion of platelets 'mismatched' for HLA antigens to alloimmunised thrombocytopenic patients. American Journal of Hematology 2: 219–226

Dyke S C 1924 Some cases of aleukia or aplastic anemia associated with thrombopenia. Lancet i: 1048–1051

Ebell W, Friedrich W, Kohne E 1989 Therapeutic aspects of Fanconi anaemia. In: Schroeder-Kurth T M, Auerbach A D, Obe G (eds) Fanconi anaemia, clinical, cytogenetic and experimental aspects. Springer, Berlin p 47–59

Eernisse J G, Brand A 1981 Prevention of platelet refractoriness due to HLA antibodies by administration of leucocyte-poor blood components. Experimental Hematology 9: 77–83

Elfenbein G J, Kallman C H, Tutschka P J et al 1979 The immune system in 40 aplastic anemia patients receiving conventional therapy. Blood 53: 652–665

Estren S, Dameshek W 1947 Familial hypoplastic anemia of childhood. Report of 8 cases in 2 families with beneficial effect of splenectomy in one case. American Journal of Diseases in Children 73: 671–687

Evans D I K 1979 Aplastic anemia in childhood. In: Geary C G (ed) Aplastic anaemia. Bailliere Tindall, London, p 161–194

Fairhead S M, Chipping P M, Gordon-Smith E C 1983 Treatment of aplastic anaemia with antilymphocyte globulin (ALG) British Journal of Haematology 55: 7–16

Fanconi G 1927 Familiäre infantile perniziosaaartige Anämie (pernizioses Blutbild und Konstitution). Jahrbuch für Kinderheilkunde 117: 257–280

Fassas A, Bruley-Rosset M 1979 Leukocyte migration-inhibitory activity in serum from patients with aplastic anemia. New England Journal of Medicine 300: 91–92

Feder H M 1986 Chloramphenicol: what we have learned in the last decade. Southern Medical Journal 79: 1129–34

Fefer A, Freedman H, Storb R et al 1976 Paroxysmal nocturnal haemoglobinuria and marrow failure treated by infusion of marrow from an identical twin. Annals of Internal Medicine 84: 692–695

Freedman M H, Gelfand E W, Saunders E F 1979 Acquired

aplastic anemia: antibody-mediated hematopoietic failure. American Journal of Hematology 6: 135–141

Freireich E J 1966 Effectiveness of platelet transfusion in leukaemia and aplastic anemia. Transfusion 6: 50–54

Friedland M, Lutton J D, Spitzer R, Levere R D 1985 Dyskeratosis congenita with hypoplastic anemia: a stem cell defect. American Journal of Hematology 20: 85–87

Gahr M, Schröter W 1982 The pattern of reactivated fetal erythropoiesis in bone marrow disorders of childhood. Acta Paediatrica Scandinavica 71: 1013–1018

Garewal G, Mohanty D, Das K C 1981 A study of hypoplastic anemia. Indian Journal of Medical Research 73: 558–70

Gascon P, Zoumbos N, Young N 1986 Analysis of natural killer cells in patients with aplastic anemia. Blood 67: 1349–1355

Gibson F M, Gordon-Smith E C 1989 Long term culture of bone marrow in aplastic anaemia. British Journal of Haematology 71 (suppl 1): 17

Gluckman E, Devergie A, Faille A et al 1978 Treatment of severe aplastic anemia with antithymocyte globulin. Experimental Hematology 6: 679–687

Gluckman E, Derogie E, Meletis J et al 1987 Bone marrow transplantation in severe aplastic anemia. Report of 100 consecutive cases. Bone Marrow Transplant 2 (suppl 2): 101

Gluckman E, Broxmeyer H E, Auerbach A D et al 1989 Hematopoietic reconstitution in a patient with Fanconi's anemia by means of umbilical-cord blood from an HLA-identical sibling. New England Journal of Medicine 321: 1174–1178

Gmür J, von Felten A, Frick P 1978 Platelet support in polysensitized patients: role of HLA specificities and crossmatch testing for donor selection. Blood 51: 903–909

Gomez-Almaguer D, Marfil-Rivera J, Kudish-Wersh A 1988 Acyclovir in the treatment of aplastic anemia. American Journal of Hematology 29: 172–173

Gordon-Smith E C 1979 Treatment of aplastic anaemia. I Conservative management. In: Geary C G (ed) Aplastic anaemia. Bailliere Tindall, London, p 108–130

Gosselin R E, Hodge H C, Smith R P, Gleason M N 1976 Clinical toxicology of commercial products 4th ed. Williams & Wilkins, Baltimore.

Grishaber J E, McClain K L, Mahoney D H, Fernbach D J 1988 Successful outcome of severe aplastic anemia following Epstein-Barr virus infection. American Journal of Hematology 28: 273–275

Groos G, Arnold O H, Brittinger G 1974 Peliosis hepatis after long-term administration of oxymetholone. Lancet i: 874

Gutmann L, Chou S M, Pore R S 1975 Fusariosis, myasthenic syndrome and aplastic anemia. Neurology (Minneapolis) 25: 922–926

Guy J T, Auslander M O 1973 Androgenic steroids and hepatocellular carcinoma. Lancet i: 148

Halperin D S, Grisaru D, Freedman M H, Saunders F 1989 Severe acquired aplastic anemia in children: 11-year experience with bone marrow transplantation and immunosuppressive therapy. American Journal of Pediatric Hematology/Oncology 11: 304–309

Hamon M D, Newland A C, Anderson M J 1988 Severe aplastic anaemia after parvovirus infection in the absence of underlying haemolytic anaemia. Journal of Clinical Pathology 41: 1242–46

Hanada T, Yamamura H, Ehara T et al 1987 No evidence for gamma-interferon mediated haematopoietic inhibition by T cells in aplastic anaemia: an observation in the course of immunosuppressive therapy. British Journal of Haematology 67: 123–127

Hanukoglu A, Meytes D, Fried D, Rosen N, Shacked N 1987 Fatal aplastic anemia in a child with Down's syndrome. Acta Paediatrica Scandinavica 76: 539–543

Hashimoto Y, Takaku F, Kosaka K 1975 Damaged DNA in lymphocytes of aplastic anemia. Blood 46: 735–742

Hathorn J W, Pizzo P A 1986 Is there a role for monotherapy with β-lactam antibiotics in the initial empirical management of febrile neutropenic cancer patients? Journal of Antimicrobial Chemotherapy 17 (suppl A): 41–54

Hattori K 1959 A clinical study on aplastic anemia. In: Japanese Medicine in 1959 4: 168 (Anemia). Proceedings of the 15th General Assembly of the Japan Medical Congress, Tokyo, Japan

Heal J M, Blumberg N, Masel D 1987 An evaluation of crossmatching, HLA and ABO matching for platelet transfusions to refractory patients. Blood 70: 23–30

Herzig R H, Poplack D G, Yankee R A 1974 Prolonged granulocytopenia from incompatible platelet transfusions. New England Journal of Medicine 290: 1220–1223

Herzig R H, Herzig G P, Bull M I et al 1975 Correction of poor platelet transfusion responses with leukocyte-poor HLA matched platelet concentrates. Blood 46: 743–750

Hester J P, Rossen R O 1974 Multiple PMN transfusions: role of HLA compatibility and leukoagglutinins. Proceedings of the American Association of Cancer Research 1974, paper 211.

Hinterberger W, Adolf G, Bettelheim P et al 1989 Lymphokine overproduction in severe aplastic anemia is not related to blood transfusions. Blood 74: 2713–2717

Hoffman R, Zanjani E D, Lutton J D, Zalusky R, Wasserman L R 1977 Suppression of erythroid-colony formation by lymphocytes from patients with aplastic anemia. New England Journal of Medicine 296: 10–13

Homans A C, Cohen J L, Barker B E, Mazur E M 1989 Aplastic presentation of acute lymphoblastic leukaemia: evidence for cellular inhibition of normal hematopoietic progenitors. American Journal of Pediatric Hematology/Oncology 11: 456–462

Horstman D M, Banatvala J E, Riordan T T et al 1965 Maternal rubella and the rubella syndrome in infants. American Journal of Diseases of Children 110: 408–415

Hows J M, Chapple M, Marsh J C W, et al 1989 Bone marrow transplantation for Fanconi's anaemia: the Hammersmith experience 1977–89. Bone Marrow Transplantation 4: 629–634

Hows J M, Marsh J C W, Liu Yin J et al 1989 Bone marrow transplantation for severe aplastic anaemia using cyclosporin: long-term follow-up. Bone Marrow Transplantation 4: 11–16

Høyeraal H M, Lamvik J, Moe P J 1970 Congenital hypoplastic thrombocytopenia and cerebral malformations in two brothers. Acta Paediatrica Scandinavica 59: 185–91

Hreidarsson S, Kristjansson K, Johannesson G, Johannsson J H 1988 A syndrome of progressive pancytopenia with microcephaly, cerebellar hypoplasia and growth failure. Acta Paediatrica Scandivanica 77: 773–775

Hughes W, Kuhn S, Chaudhary S et al 1977 Successful chemoprophylaxis for pneumocystis carinii pneumonitis (PCP) Paediatric Research 11: 501

Hutchinson R E, Kunkel K D, Schell M J et at 1989 Beneficial effect of brief pre-transfusion incubation of platelets at 37°C. Lancet i: 986–988

Imamura N, Miuta K, Kuramoto A 1985 Increment of suppressor T-cells with aplastic anaemia. British Journal of Haematology 59: 555–559

Imerslund G 1953 Hypoplastic anaemia associated with multiple deformities Nordisk Medicin 50: 1301

Inoue S, Mekanik G, Mahallati M, Zuelzer W W 1973 Dyskeratosis congenita with pancytopenia. America Journal of Diseases of Children 126: 389–396

Jacobs P, Wood L, Martell R W 1985 Cyclosporin A in the treatment of severe acute aplastic anaemia. British Journal of Haematology 61: 267–272

Jeannet M, Speck B, Rubinstein A, Pelet B, Wyss M Kummer H 1976 Autologous marrow reconstitution in severe aplastic anaemia after ALG pretreatment and HLA semicompatible bone marrow cell transfusion. Acta Hematologica 55: 129–139

Jones A L, Millar J L 1989 Growth factors in haemopoiesis. Bailliere's Clinical Haematology 2: 83–111

Juneja H S, Gardner F H 1985 Functionally abnormal marrow stromal cells in aplastic anemia. Experimental Hematology 13: 194–199

Kagan W A, Ascensao J A, Pahwa R N et al 1976 Aplastic anemia: presence in human bone marrow of cells that suppress myelopoiesis. Proceedings of the National Academy of Sciences of the USA 73: 2890–2894

Kaltwasser J P, Dix U, Schalk K P, Vogt H 1988 Effect of androgens on the response to antithymocyte globulin in patients with aplastic anaemia. European Journal of Haematology 40: 111–118

Kapoor N, Hvizdala E, Good R A 1988 High dose intravenous gammaglobulin as an approach to treatment of antibody mediated pancytopenia. British Journal of Haematology 69: 98–99

Karp J E, Schachter I P, Burke P J 1978 Humoral factors in aplastic anemia: relationship of liver dysfunction to lack of serum stimulation of bone marrow growth in vitro. Blood 51: 397–414

Keidan A J, Tsatalas C, Cohen J, Cousins S, Gordon-Smith E C 1986. Infective complications of aplastic anaemia. British Journal of Haematology, 63: 503–508

Kelton J G, Huang A T, Mold N, Logue G, Rosse W F 1979 The use of in vitro techniques to study drug-induced pancytopenia. New England Journal of Medicine 301: 621–624

Kennedy B J, Nathanson I T 1953 Effects of intensive sex steroid hormone therapy in advanced breast cancer. Journal of the American Medical Association 152: 1135–1141

Kern P, Heimpel H, Heit W, Kubanek B 1977 Granulocytic progenitor cells in aplastic anaemia. British Journal of Haematology 35: 613–623

Knospe W H, Crosby W H 1971 Aplastic anaemia: a disorder of the bone marrow sinusoidal micro-circulation rather than stem cell failure? Lancet i: 20–22

Kojima S, Matsuyama K, Kodera Y, Okada J 1989 Circulating activated suppressor T lymphocytes in hepatitis-associated aplastic anemia. British Journal of Haematology 71: 147–151

Kuriyama K, Tomonaga M, Jinnai I et al 1984 Reduced helper (OKT4+): suppressor (OKT8) T ratios in aplastic anaemia: relation to immunosuppressive therapy. British Journal of Haematology 57: 329–336

Kurtzman G J, Ozawa K, Cohen B, Hanson G, Oseas R, Young N S 1987 Chronic bone marrow failure due to persistent B19 parvovirus infection. New England Journal of Medicine 317: 287–294

Kurtzman G, Young N 1989 Viruses and bone marrow failure. Bailliere's Clinical Haematology 2: 51–67

Kusminsky G D, Barazutti L, Korin J D, Blasetti A, Tartas N E, Sanchez Avalos J C 1988 Complete response to antilymphocyte globulin in a case of aplastic anemia-paroxysmal nocturnal haemoglobinuria syndrome. American Journal of Hematology 29: 123

Kwee M L, Kuyt L P 1989 Fanconi anemia in the Netherlands. In: Schroeder-Kurth T M, Auerbach A D, Obe G (eds) Fanconi Anemia: clinical, cytogenetic and experimental aspects. Springer, Berlin, p 18–33

Lafer C Z, Morrison A N 1966 Thrombocytopenic purpura progressing to transient hypoplastic anemia in a newborn with rubella syndrome. Pediatrics 38: 499–501

Lancet editorial 1978 Nitrous oxide and the bone-marrow. Lancet ii: 613–614

Lancet editorial 1986 Living with radiation – after Chernobyl. Lancet ii: 609–610

Lancet editorial 1990 ABO incompatibility and platelet transfusion. Lancet i: 142–143

Lee E J, Schiffer C A 1987 Serial measurement of lymphocytotoxic antibody and response to nonmatched platelet transfusions in alloimmunised patients. Blood 70: 1727–1729

Leitman P S 1979 Chloramphenicol and the neonate – 1979 view. Clinics in Perinatology 6: 151–162

Leonard E, Raefsky E, Griffith P, Kimball J, Nienhuis A, Young N S 1989 Cyclosporine therapy of aplastic anaemia, congenital and acquired red cell aplasia. British Journal of Haematology 72: 278–284

Li F P, Alter B P, Nathan D G 1972 The mortality of acquired aplastic anemia in children. Blood 40: 153–162

Liang D-G, Lin K-H, Lin D-T, Yang C-P, Hung K-L, Lin K-S 1990 Post-hepatitic aplastic anaemia in children in Taiwan, a hepatitis prevalent area. British Journal of Haematology 74: 487–491

Lishner M, Curtis J E, 1989 Aplastic anaemia following successful treatment of malignant epithelial tumours with radiation and/or chemotherapy. British Journal of Haematology 73: 416–417

Lorenz E, Quaiser K 1955 Panmyelopathie nach hepatitis epidemica. Wiener medizinischer Wochenschrift 105: 19–21

Lum L G, Seigneuret M C, Doney K C, Storb R 1987 In vitro immunoglobulin production, proliferation, and cell markers before and after antithymocyte globulin therapy in patients with aplastic anemia. American Journal of Hematology 26: 1–15

Lynch R E, Williams D M, Reading J C, Cartwright G E, 1975 The prognosis in aplastic anaemia. Blood 45: 517–528

Lyonnais J 1988 Thymoma and pancytopenia. American Journal of Hematology 28: 195–196

McCulloch E A, Till J E, Siminowitch L 1965 Genetic factors affecting the control of hemopoiesis. In: Begg R W, Leblond C P, Noble R L, Rossiter R J, Taylor R M, Wallace A C (eds) Canadian Cancer Conference Pergamon Press, Oxford, p 336

McFarland J G, Aster R H 1987 Evaluation of four methods for platelet compatibility testing. Blood 69: 1425–1430

McGlave P B, Haake R, Miller W, Kim T, Kersey J, Ramsay N K C 1987 Therapy of severe aplastic anemia in young adults and children with allogeneic bone marrow transplantation, Blood 70: 1325–1330

McGrath H E, Liang C-M, Alberico T A, Quesenberry P K 1987 The effect of lithium on growth factor production in long-term bone marrow cultures. Blood 70: 1136–1142

Mangan K F, Shadduck R K, Zeigler Z, Winkelstein A 1985 Interferon-induced-aplasia: evidence for T-cell-mediated suppression of hematopoiesis and recovery after treatment with horse antihuman thymocyte globulin. American Journal of Hematology 19: 401–403

Marin P, Nomdedeu B, Rovira M, Montserrat E, Rozman C 1989 Cyclosporin A versus antilymphocytic globulin in severe aplastic anaemia. British Journal of Haematology 73: 285–286

Marsh J C W, Hows J M, Bryett K A, Al-Hashimi S, Fairhead S M, Gordon-Smith E C 1987 Survival after antilymphocyte globulin therapy for aplastic anemia depends on disease severity. Blood 70: 1046–1052

Marsh J C W, Chang J ,Testa N G, Hows J M, Dexter T M 1990 Characterisation of the haemopoietic defect in aplastic anaemia by long term bone marrow culture. British Journal of Haematology 74 (suppl 1): 1

Marsh J C W, Chang J, Testa N G, Hows J M, Dexter T M, 1990 The haemopoietic defect in aplastic anemia assessed by long term bone marrow culture. Blood 76: 1748–1757

Massengale O N, Glaser H H, LeLievre R E, Dodds J B, Klock M E 1963 Physical and psychologic factors in glue sniffing. New England Journal of Medicine 269: 1340–1344

Mathe G, Amiel J L, Schwarzenburg L et al 1970 Bone marrow graft in man after conditioning by antilymphocyte serum. British Medical Journal ii: 131–136

Matsaniotis N, Kiossoglou K A, Karpanzas J, Anastasea Vlachou K 1966 Chromosomes in Kostmann's disease. Lancet 2: 104

Milne A E, Gordon-Smith E C 1990 Treatment of infection in patients with severe aplastic anaemia with recombinant granulocyte-macrophage colony-stimulating factor. British Journal of Haematology 74 (suppl 1): 37

Mir M A, Geary C G, Delamore I W 1977 Hypoimmunoglobulinaemia and aplastic anaemia. Scandivanian Journal of Haematology 19: 225–229

Miyamura K, Kojima S, Takeyama K et al 1988 Use of cyclophosphamide and total lymphoid irradiation combined with cyclosporine in bone marrow transplantation for transfused severe aplastic anaemia. Bone Marrow Transplantation 3: 457–461

Mukherji A K, Ghosh R N, Biswas S K et al 1974 Acquired toxoplasmosis presenting with severe anaemia and pancytopenia. Journal of the Association of Physicians of India 22: 781–783

Murphy S, Gardner F H 1969 Platelet preservation: effect of storage temperature on maintenance of platelet viability – deleterious effect of refrigerated storage. New England Journal of Medicine 80: 1094–98

Murphy M F, Waters A H 1985 Immunological aspects of platelet transfusions. British Journal of Haematology 60: 409–414

Nagao T, Mauer A M 1969 Concordance for drug induced aplastic anemia in identical twins. New England Journal of Medicine 281: 7–11

Najean Y 1976 Androgen therapy in aplastic anaemia in childhood. In: Congenital disorders of erythropoiesis Ciba Foundation Symposium 37 Elsevier, Amsterdam, p 354–361

Najean Y, Pecking A 1979 Prognostic factors in acquired aplastic anaemia: a study of 352 cases. American Journal of Medicine 67: 564–571

Najean Y, Girot R, Baumelou E 1982 Prognostic factors and evolution of acquired aplastic anaemia in childhood. American Journal of Paediatric Hematology/Oncology 4: 273–283

Nakao S, Matsushima K, Young N 1989 Decreased interleukin 1 production in aplastic anaemia. British Journal of Haematology 71: 431–436

Nakayama K, Nagakawa T 1978 Prevalance and clinical states of aplastic anaemia among children in Japan. In: Hibino S, Takaku F, Shahidi N T (eds) Aplastic anaemia. University Park Press, Baltimore, p 207–223

Nebert D W, Levitt R C, Jensen N M, Lambert G H, Felton J S 1977 Birth defects and aplastic anemia: differences in polycyclic hydrocarbon toxicity associated with the Ah locus. Archives of Toxicology 39: 109–132

Niederwieser D, Pepe M, Storb R, Loughran T P, Longton G 1988 Improvement in rejection, engraftment rate and survival without increase in graft-versus-host disease by high marrow cell dose in patients transplanted for aplastic anaemia. British Journal of Haematology 69: 23–28

Nieweg H O 1973 Aplastic anaemia (panmyelopathy). A review with special emphasis on the factors causing bone marrow damage. In: Girdwood R H (ed). Blood disorders due to drugs and other agents. Excerpta Medica, Amsterdam, p 83–106

Nilsson L R 1960 Chronic pancytopenia with multiple congenital abnormalities (Fanconi's anaemia) Acta Paediatrica 49: 519–529

Nissen C, Moser Y, Dalle Carbonare V, Gratwohl A, Speck B 1989 Complete recovery of marrow function after treatment with anti-lymphocyte globulin is associated with high, whereas early failure and development of paroxysmal nocturnal haemoglobinuria are associated with low endogenous G-CSA release. British Journal of Haematology 72: 573–577

Nissen-Druey C 1989 Pathophysiology of aplastic anaemia. Bailliere's Clinical Haematology 2: 37–49

Obeid D A, Hill F G H, Harnden D, Mann J R, Wood B S B 1980 Fanconi anaemia. Oxymetholone hepatic tumors and chromosome aberrations associated with leukaemic transition. Cancer 46: 1401–1404

O'Gorman Hughes D W 1974 Aplastic anaemia in childhood III. Constitutional aplastic anaemia and related cytopenias. Medical Journal of Australia 1: 519–526

O'Gorman Hughes D W, Diamond L K 1964 A new type of constitutional aplastic anaemia without congenital anomalies presenting as thrombocytopenia in infancy. Journal of Pediatrics 65: 1060

Ozsoylu S, Coskun T, Minassazi S 1984 High dose intravenous glucocorticoid in the treatment of childhood acquired aplastic anaemia. Scandinavian Journal of Haematology 33: 309–316

Pearce C J, Conrad M E, Nolan P E, Fishbein D B, Dawson J E 1988 Ehrlichosis: a cause of bone marrow hypoplasia in humans. American Journal of Hematology 28: 53–55

Pegels J G, Bruynes E C E, Engelfriet C P, Borne A E G von dem 1982 Serological studies on platelet and granulocyte substitution therapy. British Journal of Haematology 52: 59–68

Platanias L, Gascon P, Bielory L, Griffith P, Nienhuis A, Young N 1987 Lymphocyte phenotype and lymphokines following anti-thymocyte globulin therapy in patients with aplastic anaemia. British Journal of Haematology 66: 437–443

Pogliani E M, Cortellaro M, Foa P, Iurlo A, Polli E E 1989 Cyclosporin A in the treatment of severe aplastic anemia: description of a case complicated by the development of tubercular pericarditis during treatment. American Journal of Hematology 30: 257–258

Polak B C P, Wesseling H, Schut D, Herxheimer A, Meyler L 1972 Blood dyscrasias attributed to chloramphenicol. Acta Medica Scandivanica 192: 409–414

Powars D 1965 Aplastic anemia secondary to glue sniffing. New England Journal of Medicine 273: 700–702

Ratzan R J, Moore M A S, Yunis A A 1974 Effect of chloramphenicol and thiamphenicol on the in-vitro colony-forming cell. Blood 43: 363–369

Reeves J D, Driggers D A, Kiley V A 1981 Household insecticide associated aplastic anaemia and acute leukaemia in children. Lancet ii: 300–301

Reimann H A, D'Ambola J 1966 The use and cost of antimicrobics in hospitals. Archives of Environmental Health 13: 631–636

Rogers P C J, Desai F, Karabus C D, Hartley P S, Fisher R M, 1989 Presentation and outcome of 25 cases of Fanconi's anaemia. American Journal of Pediatric Hematology/Oncology 11: 141–145

Ronchetti V 1922 Quoted in: Hunter D, The diseases of occupations, 5th ed. English Universities Press, London, p 483

Ruiz-Argüelles G J, Katzmann J A, Greipp P R, Marin-Lopez A, Gonzalez-Laven J, Cano-Castellanos R 1984 Lymphocyte subsets in patients with aplastic anemia. American Journal of Hematology 16: 267–275

Saarinen U M, Kekomäki R, Siimes M A, Myllylä G 1990 Effective prophylaxis against platelet refractoriness in multitransfused patients by use of leukocyte-free blood components. Blood 75: 512–517

Sadowitz P D, Dubowy R L 1990 Intravenous immunoglobulin in the treatment of aplastic anemia. American Journal of Pediatric Hematology/Oncology 12: 198–200

Saita G 1973 Benzene induced hypoplastic anaemias and leukaemias. In: Girdwood R H (ed) Blood disorders due to drugs and other agents. Excerpta Medica, Amsterdam, p 127–146

Sanchez-Medal L, Pizzuto J, Torre-Lopez E, Derbez R 1964 Effect of oxymetholone in refractory anemia. Archives of Internal Medicine 113: 721–729

Sanders J E, Whitehead J, Storb R et al 1986 Bone marrow transplantation experience for children with aplastic anemia. Pediatrics 77: 179–186

Saunders E F, Freedman M H 1978 Constitutional aplastic anaemia: defective haematopoietic stem cell growth in vitro. British Journal of Haematology 40: 277–287

Sawitsky A, Bloom D, German J 1966 Chromosomal breakage and acute leukaemia in congenital telangiectatic erythema and stunted growth. Annals of Internal Medicine 65: 487

Schiffer C A, Slichter S J 1982 Platelet transfusions from single donors. New England Journal of Medicine 307: 245–248

Schroeder T M, Anschütz F, Knopp A 1964 Spontane Chromosomaberrationen bei familiäre Panmyelopathie. Humangenetik 1: 194–196

Schroëder-Kurth T M, Zhu T H, Hong Y, Westphal I 1989 Variation in cellular sensitivities among Fanconi anemia patients, non-Fanconi anemia patients, their parents and siblings, and control probands. In: Schroeder-Kurth T M,

Auerbach A D, Obe G (eds) Fanconi anemia: clinical, cytogenetic and experimental aspects. Springer, Berlin, 105–136.

Schröter 1970 Chronic idiopathic infantile pancytopenia. Schweizerische Medizinische Wochenschrifte 100: 1101–1108

Sensenbrenner L L, Steel A A, Santos G W 1977 Recovery of hematologic competence without engraftment following attempted bone marrow transplantation for aplastic anaemia: a report of a case with diffusion chamber studies. Experimental Hematology 5: 51–58

Shahidi N T 1973 Androgens and erythropoiesis. New England Journal of Medicine 289: 72–80

Shahidi N T, Diamond L K 1959 Testosterone-induced remission in aplastic anemia. AMA Journal of Diseases of Children 98: 293–302

Shahidi N T, Diamond L K 1961 Testosterone-induced remission in aplastic anemia of both acquired and congenital types: further observations in 24 cases. New England Journal of Medicine 264: 953–967

Shahidi N T, Crigler J F Jr 1967 Evaluation of growth and of endocrine systems in testosterone-corticosteroid-treated patients with aplastic anemia. Journal of Pediatrics 70: 233–242

Shu X O, Gao Y T, Linet M S et al 1987 Chloramphenicol use and childhood leukaemia in Shanghai. Lancet ii: 934–937

Shulman N R 1966 Immunological considerations attending platelet transfusion. Transfusion 6: 39–48

Shwachman H, Diamond L K, Oski F A, Khaw A T 1964 The syndrome of pancreatic insufficiency and bone marrow dysfunction. Journal of Pediatrics 65: 645–663

Singer J W, Brown J E, Storb R, Thomas E D 1978 The effect of peripheral blood lymphocytes from patients with aplastic anemia on granulocytic colony growth from HLA-matched and-mismatched marrows: effects of transfusion sensitization. Blood 52: 37–46

Sklo M, Sensenbrenner L, Markowitz J, Weida S, Warm S, Linet M 1985 Incidence of aplastic anaemia in metropolitan Baltimore, a population based study. Blood 66: 115–119

Smith A G, O'Reilly R J, Hansen J A, Martin P J 1985 Specific antibody-blocking activities and antilymphocyte globulin as correlates of efficacy for the treatment of aplastic anemia. Blood 66: 721–723

Smith R R L, Spivak J L 1985 Marrow cell necrosis in anorexia nervosa and involuntary starvation. British Journal of Haematology 60: 525–530

Smith S, Marx M P, Jordaan C J, van Niekerk C H 1989 Clinical aspects of a cluster of 42 patients in South Africa with Fanconi anemia. In: Schroeder-Kurth T M, Auerbach A D, Obe G (eds) Fanconi anemia: clinical, cytogenetic and experimental aspects. Springer, Berlin, p 35–46

Smith L, Will A M, Williams R F, Stevens R F 1990 Ceftriaxone vs. azlocillin and netilmicin in the treatment of febrile neutropenic children. Journal of Infection 20: 201–206

Smyth E G, Pallett A P 1988 Clinicians guide to antibiotics: chloramphenicol. British Journal of Hospital Medicine May: 424–428

Sokal E, Michel M, Ninane J, Latine D, de Bruyere M, Cornu G 1987 Bone marrow transplantation from an unrelated donor for Fanconi's anaemia: two unusual complications. Bone Marrow Transplantation 2: 99–102

Speck B, Gluckman E, Haak H L, Van Rood J J 1977

Treatment of aplastic anemia by antilymphocyte globulin with and without allogeneic bone marrow infusions. Lancet ii: 1145–1148

Speck B, Gratwohl A, Nissen C et al 1981 Treatment of severe aplastic anaemia with antilymphocyte globulin or bone-marrow transplantation. British Medical Journal 282: 860–863

Stevens J D, Mission G P 1987 Ophthalmic use of chloramphenicol. Lancet ii: 1456

Stewart J S, Farrow L J, Clifford R E et al 1978 A three-year survey of viral hepatitis in west London. Quarterly Journal of Medicine 47: 365–384

Storb R, Prentice R L, Donnall Thomas E 1977 Marrow transplantation for treatment of aplastic anemia: an analysis of factors associated with graft rejection. New England Journal of Medicine 296: 61–66

Storb R, Weiden P L, Sullivan K M et al 1987 Second marrow transplants in patients with aplastic anemia rejecting the first graft: use of a conditioning regimen including cyclophosphamide and antithymocyte globulin. Blood 70: 116–121

Sullivan R, Quesenberry P J, Parkman R, Zuckerman K S, Levey R H, Rappepport J, Ryan M 1980 Aplastic anemia: lack of inhibitory effect of bone marrow lymphocytes on in vitro granulopoiesis. Blood 56: 625–632

Swift M R, Hirschhorn K 1966 Fanconi's anaemia: inherited susceptibility to chromosome breakage in various tissues. Annals of Internal Medicine 65: 495–503

Tactle R, Lane T A, Mendelsohn J 1979 Drug-induced agranulocytosis: in vitro evidence for immune suppression of granulopoiesis and a cross-reacting lymphocyte antibody. Blood 54: 501–512

Tamerius J D, Curd J G, Tani P, McMillan R 1983 An enzyme-linked immunosorbent assay for platelet compatibility testing. Blood 62: 744–749

Territo M C for the UCLA BMT team 1977 Autologous bone marrow repopulation following high dose cyclophosphamide and allogeneic marrow transplantation in aplastic anemia. British Journal of Haematology 36: 305–312

Torok-Storb B J, Sieff C, Storb R, Adamson J, Donnall Thomas E 1980 In vitro tests for distinguishing possible immune-mediated aplastic anemia from transfusion-induced sensitization. Blood 55: 211

Torok-Storb B 1987 Response to letter by N S Young. Blood 70: 338–339

Twomey J J, Douglass C C, Sharkey O Jr. 1973 The monocytopenia of aplastic anemia. Blood 41: 187–195

Uchiyama T, Nagai K, Yamagishi M, Takatsuki K, Uchino H 1978 Pokeweed mitogen-induced B cell differentiation in idiopathic aplastic anemia associated with hypogammglobulinaemia. Blood 52: 77–83

van't Veer-Korthof E T, van Weel-Sipman M H, Doude M, Vossen J M 1989 Aplastic anemia in children: the Leiden experience. British Journal of Haematology 71 (suppl 1): 17

Wallerstein R O, Condit P K, Kasper C K, Brown J W, Morrison F R 1969 Statewise study of chloramphenicol

therapy and fatal aplastic anaemia. Journal of American Medical Association 208: 2045–2050

Warren R P, Storb R, Donnall Thomas D, Su P J, Mickelson E M, Weiden P L 1980 Autoimmune and alloimmune phenomena in patients with aplastic anemia: cytotoxicity against autologous lymphocytes and lymphocytes from HLA identical siblings. Blood 56: 683–689

Waters A H, Minchinton R M, Bell R, Ford J M, Lister T A 1981 A cross-matching procedure for the selection of platelet donors for alloimmunized patients. British Journal of Haematology 48: 59–68

Weatherly T L, Fleisher T A, Strong D M, 1979 Reduced granulocyte-macrophage colony-stimulating activity by mitogen-stimulated lymphocytes from patients with aplastic anaemia. British Journal of Haematology 43: 335–340

Weinblatt M E, Higgins G, Ortega J A 1981 Aplastic anemia in Down's syndrome. Pediatrics 67: 896–897

Whang K S 1978 Aplastic anemia in Korea. A clinical study of 309 cases. In: Hibino S, Takaku F, Shahidi N T (eds) Aplastic anemia. University Park Press, Baltimore p 225–242

Williams D M, Lynch R E, Cartwright G E 1973. Drug-induced aplastic anaemia. Seminars in Hematology 10: 195–223

Willoughby M L N 1977 Paediatric haematology. Churchill Livingstone, Edinburgh, p 57

Witherspoon R P, Storb R, Shulman H et al 1984 Marrow transplantation in hepatitis-associated aplastic anemia. American Journal of Hematology 17: 269–278

Woods W G, Krivit W, Lubin B H, Ramsay N K C 1981 Aplastic anaemia associated with the Shwachman syndrome. American Journal of Pediatric Hematology/Oncology 3: 347–351

Yankee R A, Graff K S, Dowling R, Henderson E S 1973 Selection of unrelated compatible platelet donors by lymphocyte HLA-matching. New England Journal of Medicine 288: 760–764

Young N S, Issaragrasil S, Chieh C W, Takaku F 1986 Aplastic anaemia in the Orient. British Journal of Haematology 62: 1–6

Young N S 1987 Gamma interferon and aplastic anemia. Blood 70: 337–339

Young N, Griffith P, Brittain E et al 1988 A multicenter trial of antithymocyte globulin in aplastic anemia and related disease. Blood 72: 1861–1869

Ziegenfuss J, Carabasi R 1973 Androgens and hepatocellular carcinoma. Lancet i: 262

Zinsser F 1906 Atrophia cutis reticularis cum pigmentatione, dystrophia unguium et leukoplakia oris. Ikono Dermat Kioto 5: 219–223

Zoumbos N C, Djeu J Y, Young N S 1984 Interferon is the inhibitor of hematopoiesis generated by stimulated lymphocytes in vitro. Journal of Immunology 133: 760–774

Zoumbos N C, Gascon P, Djeu J Y, Trost S R, Young N S 1985 Circulating activated suppressor T lymphocytes in aplastic anemia. New England Journal of Medicine 312: 257–65

3. Chronic myeloid leukaemia, myeloproliferative disorders, and myelodysplasia

Judith M. Chessells

Over 95% of children with leukaemia have acute myeloid leukaemia (AML) or acute lymphoblastic leukaemia (ALL). This chapter will review the diagnosis and management of the minority with chronic disorders, either myeloproliferative or myelodysplastic. These chronic disorders predominantly involve the myeloid lineage. Chronic lymphocytosis in childhood is usually a response to infection or an immunoregulatory abnormality (see Ch. 11); there has been only a handful of case reports of chronic lymphocytic leukaemia.

The term 'myeloproliferative disorder', denoting an abnormal proliferation of the bone marrow, was coined in the 1950s by Dameshek to include a spectrum of diseases that included myeloid leukaemias, polycythaemia rubra vera, essential thrombocythaemia and myelofibrosis. In the ensuing 40 years the myeloid leukaemias have been intensively classified, but the term non-leukaemic myeloproliferative disorders has been retained in adult practice to describe the other conditions, all of which are exceptionally rare in paediatrics. Meanwhile, the concept of myelodysplasias, characterized by a cellular bone marrow with pancytopenia and/or marked morphological abnormalities in one or more cell series, has gained wide acceptance.

Both myeloproliferative (MPD) and myelodysplastic (MDS) disorders arise from an abnormal clone of cells and carry a risk of progression to acute leukaemia, albeit at a variable pace. They are well described in adults, particularly the elderly, and have been obsessionally classified in the haematology literature using all available laboratory techniques. Unfortunately for the paediatrician faced with a patient with potential MPD or MDS, diagnosis in paediatrics has not progressed to the same level of sophistication, and apart from the

Table 3.1 Chronic myeloid leukaemia, myeloproliferative disease and myelodysplasia

Myeloproliferative disorders	Primary myelodysplasia
Chronic (Ph¹ positive) Granulocytic leukaemia (CGL)	Juvenile chronic myeloid leukaemia (JCML)
Ph¹ negative CML	Infantile monosomy 7 syndrome
Essential Thrombocythaemia	Refractory anaemia (RA)
Polycythaemia rubra vera	Refractory anaemia with ringed sideroblasts (RARS)
Myelofibrosis	Refractory anaemia with excess blasts (RAEB)
Transient myeloproliferative disease of the newborn	Refractory anaemia with excess blasts in transformation (RAEB-t)
Miscellaneous others	*Secondary myelodysplasia*
Familial disorders	Familial
	Therapy-induced

common conditions identified in the next section, there are few guidelines to diagnosis, management and prognosis.

Now that effective forms of treatment are becoming available, classification of paediatric MDS/MPD is of more than theoretical interest. A tentative and personal attempt at classification is made in Table 3.1. It must be recognized that the distinction between MPD and MDS is somewhat arbitrary; for example, because juvenile chronic myeloid leukaemia resembles adult chronic myelomonocytic leukaemia morphologically and is characterized by abnormalities of all cell lines, it is included here as a type of MDS.

HISTORICAL PERSPECTIVE

Thirty years ago, Nowell & Hungerford described the Philadelphia chromosome (Nowell & Hungerford 1960), the first consistent cytogenetic change to be identified in any human cancer. This abnormal G group chromosome was found in the bone marrow of the majority of patients with chronic myeloid leukaemia (CML), and was associated with an apparent survival advantage, since patients with CML who were Ph[1] negative appeared to have a worse prognosis than those who were Ph[1] positive. Chronic leukaemias were subsequently described in childhood, although as a rare occurrence, and in 1964 Hardisty, Speed & Till distinguished two types of CML: the so-called adult type, with a relatively long survival, which resembled exactly the disease in adults, and was associated with the Ph[1] chromosome as then described; and juvenile chronic myeloid leukaemia (JCML) (Hardisty et al 1964). Juvenile chronic myeloid leukaemia is associated with suppurative infections, severe thrombocytopenia, a non-specific but characteristic skin rash, and a very poor prognosis. Further interest in this rare disorder was awakened by the reports of a consistently raised fetal haemoglobin level (Weatherall et al 1968). A third type of myeloproliferative disorder described in young infants, associated with a missing C group chromosome, was first described in 1970 by Teasdale and colleagues (Teasdale et al 1970). These three conditions are the most frequently described types of MPD/MDS in childhood.

The advent of chromosome banding was followed by the discovery in 1973 that the Ph[1] chromosome arose as a result of a translocation involving chromosomes 9 and 22 t(9;22) (q34;q11) (Rowley 1973). Further cytogenetic studies were to show a large number of nonrandom changes in leukaemias and myelodysplasias and, while no typical cytogenetic features were found in JCML, the C group abnormality in infantile myelodysplasia was characterized as a monosomy 7 (Sieff et al 1981).

Meanwhile, the morphological approach to classification of myelodysplasia was rationalized by the French-American-British (FAB) cooperative group (Bennett et al 1982) and systematic attempts to classify these disorders ensued, largely however involving adult patients. Secondary leukaemias and myelodysplasias were being described with increasing frequency in patients previously treated for Hodgkin's disease and ovarian cancer, and also occasionally in paediatric practice.

During the 1980s, understanding of these disorders progressed at the molecular level with identification of genes involved in translocations and of some of the gene products. The main advance in treatment has been the widespread introduction of allogeneic marrow transplantation for disorders hitherto incurable by conventional means. Most excitingly, analysis of this group of diseases has the potential to provide real insight into both normal haemopoiesis and leukaemogenesis.

INCIDENCE AND EPIDEMIOLOGY

All the conditions to be described in this chapter are rare, and probably do not represent more than 3% of haematological malignancies in childhood. There are, as yet, no population-based studies on the incidence of these conditions in childhood, but it seems highly likely that their frequency is greater than previously suspected. Adult (Ph[1]-positive) chronic granulocytic leukaemia (CGL) is a disease of middle-age with a peak incidence in the forties and fifties. However, it can occur at any age, even in infancy, although it is more frequently seen in older children. Ionizing radiation is the only proven factor involved in pathogenesis, as shown by the increased incidence following the atomic bombing in Japan and the development of CGL in radiologists and people who had received radiation therapy for ankylosing spondylitis.

There are no epidemiological clues in the rare JCML; it is not even clear whether the characteristic fetal haemopoeisis seen in this disorder represents a reversion to fetal pattern, or whether genetic alterations predisposing to this pattern have caused persistence of fetal haemopoeisis since birth. There appears to be a real association between JCML and the common autosomal dominant neurofibromatosis (Kaneko et al 1989), and there are reports of JCML mimicked by persistent infection with the Epstein-Barr virus (Herrod et al 1983). The syndrome of myeloproliferative disorder with monosomy 7 usually occurs sporadically, but there have been several reports of familial monosomy 7 (Carroll et al 1985).

Secondary leukaemia is virtually always myeloid, and secondary myelodysplasia is increasingly described, particularly in patients treated for Hodgkin's disease, multiple myeloma and ovarian cancer. Secondary myelodysplasia and leukaemia may be seen after treatment of many other solid tumours, and as a second haematological malignancy. The role of alkylating agents in their development appears established, but a genetic basis for some cases cannot be excluded.

A number of hereditary disorders predispose to leukaemia or myelodysplasia. These include Schwachman's syndrome of pancreatic exocrine insufficiency and neutropenia. Systematic investigation of such patients shows generalized abnormality of haemopoiesis with raised fetal haemoglobin and thrombocytopenia in many patients, together with abnormalities of neutrophil function. These patients are at increased risk of ALL, AML and myelodysplasia (Woods et al 1981). Thrombocytopenia is usually the presenting and dominant haematological symptom in Fanconi's anaemia, and precedes anaemia and neutropenia often by many years. Patients with Fanconi's anaemia are at significant risk of development of AML, but may actually present with myelodysplasia or AML (Nowell et al 1984).

Children with Down's syndrome have a 20- to 30-fold increased risk of development of acute leukaemia, usually the common subtype of ALL or the megakaryoblastic variant of AML. A transient myeloproliferative disorder has been described in newborn infants with Down's syndrome, and the blast cells have been characterized as megakaryoblasts (Eguchi et al 1989). Intriguingly, this syndrome has also been described in phenotypically normal neonates who are mosaic for trisomy 21. A recent review of transient neonatal myeloproliferative disorders discusses this problem but also confirms that some of the affected children with Down's syndrome subsequently develop acute myeloid leukemia (Barnett et al 1990). The frequency of transient MPD in both Down's syndrome and trisomy 21 mosaics is unknown at present, as is the risk of subsequent development of AML.

CLINICAL FEATURES

The symptoms and signs of MPD and MDS are not always as obvious as those of acute leukaemia, and the diagnosis may even be made incidentally. Pallor is common, bacterial infections may be a consequence of neutropenia or defective neutro-

Table 3.2   Investigations in suspected MPD or MDS

Essential	*Other investigations*
Hb and red cell indices	Neutrophil function
WBC and differential:	Platelet function
monocyte, eosinophil,	Colony assays; bone marrow
basophil count	and/or blood
Blood film	Molecular biology (see text)
Fetal haemoglobin	
Leucocyte alkaline	
phosphatase	
Immunoglobulins	
Bone marrow aspirate and	
trephine biopsy	
Cytochemistry including	
iron stain	
Bone marrow cytogenetics	

phil function, and bruising may be due to thrombocytopenia and/or abnormal platelet function. Lymph node enlargement is a feature of JCML. The liver and spleen may be impalpable in MDS or grossly enlarged in CGL or myelofibrosis. Bone pain is uncommon except in the blast crisis of CGL. A characteristic skin rash, mimicking Langerhan's cell histiocytosis, may occur on the face or trunk in JCML and, less frequently, in monosomy 7.

INVESTIGATIONS

Blood and bone marrow examination

Table 3.2 lists the recommended investigations in children with a suspected chronic leukaemia, myeloproliferative or myelodysplastic syndrome. The blood and bone marrow appearances are extremely variable, and a list of noteworthy features is shown in Table 3.3. It is essential to examine the blood and marrow in tandem, and frequently the blood film is the more helpful in diagnosis. A trephine biopsy of the bone marrow should be obtained in all cases, and important observations include: the overall cellularity of the marrow, the relative proportions of the three cell lines (erythroid, myeloid and megakaryocyte), the presence of fibrosis and reticulin and the localization of immature precursors.

Further investigations, such as measurement of fetal Hb, and/or red cell carbonic anhydrase, neutrophil function and platelet function may serve to confirm abnormalities of development of one or more cell series.

The examination of the blood and marrow, with appropriate investigations such as cytogenetics,

Table 3.3   Morphological abnormalities in MPD/MDS

Series	Blood film	Bone marrow
Erythroid	Abnormal RBC morphology	Dyserythropoiesis
	Basophilic stippling	Multinuclear normoblasts
	Poikilocytosis	Ringed sideroblasts
	Nucleated red cells	Reduced (<5%) or increased (>60%) normoblasts
Platelet	Large platelets	Reduced megakaryocytes
		Large mononuclear forms
		Multiple small nuclei
		Micromega-karyocytes
White cell	Monocytosis	Increased blasts
	Basophilia	Auer rods
	Eosinophilia	Abnormal granulation in early myeloid cells
	Hypersegmented or hyposegmented polymorphs	
	Agranular polymorphs	
	Myelocytes and metamyelocytes	
	Blasts	
	Auer rods	

should confirm a presumptive diagnosis of CGL, where the findings are typically those of a leucocytosis with normal or increased platelets, not more than 10% immature myeloid cells and basophilia. Increased monocytes are not usually seen in CGL and should lead to consideration of an alternative diagnosis.

In cases when the picture is not typical of CGL or one of the other rare proliferative disorders (see Table 3.1) an attempt should be made to classify the case with the FAB scheme as shown in Table 3.4. This classification was developed in adults, but it is important to try to apply it to all paediatric cases, the majority of which have hitherto simply been described as syndromes on the basis of clinical and basic laboratory findings.

Cytogenetics

Cytogenetic analysis of the bone marrow is an essential investigation in all these disorders. The classic specific abnormality is, of course, the Ph^1 translocation, which is only found in adult-type CGL, Ph^1-positive ALL and Ph^1-positive AML. Cytogenetic findings in the myelodysplasias have recently been reviewed by the morphologic, immunologic and cytogenetic (MIC) study group (Third MIC Cooperative Study Group 1988). An abnormal karyotype was found in 60% of patients with primary MDS, and 98% with secondary MDS. Some of the more common abnormalities are shown in Table 3.5, which is based on the analysis of the MIC group.

These cytogenetic abnormalities, unlike those found in de novo AML, are not normally specific to any morphological subtype. The main exception to this rule, in adult practice, is the 5q– syndrome; this occurs primarily in elderly females, who present with refractory macrocytic anaemia and a normal or elevated platelet count. Most of these patients have refractory anaemia with or

Table 3.4   FAB classification of myelodysplasia

Type	Blood film	Bone Marrow
Refractory anaemia (RA)	Blasts <1%	Blasts <5%
	Reticulocytopenia	Erythroid hyperplasia
	Dyserythropoiesis	Dyserythropoiesis
RA with ringed sideroblasts (RARS)	As RA, plus:	As RA, plus:
	Basophilic stippling	Ringed sideroblasts ≥ 15% nucleated cells
	Dimorphic film	
RA with excess of blasts (RAEB)	As RA, plus:	5–20% blasts
	Blasts but <5%	Dysgranulopoiesis
	Dysgranulopoiesis	Abnormal megakaryocytes
		Dyserythropoiesis
RAEB in transformation (RAEB-t)	As RAEB but > 5% blasts	As RAEB, but 20–30% blasts
	Auer rods	Auer rods
CMML	Monocytes > 1×10^9/l	As in RAEB, plus:
	Dysgranulopoiesis	Increased monocytes
	Blasts <5%	

Table 3.5 Chromosome changes in myelodysplasia

Primary MDS	Secondary MDS
−7	Single chromosome changes
+8	del (5q)
del (5) (q12–q34) and	del (7q)
translocations involving 5q	−5
del (7q)	−7
del (11q)	del (12p)
del (12) (p11p13)	t(1;7) (p11;p11)
del (13q)	
del (20) (q11q13)	Multiple chromosome
	changes
t(1;3) (p36;q21)	Any of the above plus:
t(2;11) (p21;q23)	+8
t(6;9) (p23;q34)	+21
t(11;21) (q24;q11.2)	3p (del or t),
i(17q)	17p (del or t),
	17p (del or t), −17
	6p (del or t)
	19p or q (t)
	Xq13 (t or dup)
	Xp11 (t)

* Adapted from Third MIC Study Group 1988.

without ringed sideroblasts and, provided deletion of 5q is the only abnormality, survival is prolonged.

BIOLOGY AND PATHOGENESIS

Studies of G6PD variants, and of other X-linked restriction fragment polymorphisms (Tefferi et al 1990) have shown that MPD and MDS are clonal disorders arising in a pluripotent stem cell or early progenitor cell; in some instances, the lymphoid cells may also be clonally derived, thus suggesting origin from a pluripotent stem cell. The resulting daughter cells may have a function which varies from near normal (as in the granulocytes from CGL, which have been used as a source of granulocyte transfusion) to grossly defective (as in monosomy 7 cells). Abnormalities of lymphoid regulation or lymphocyte populations may be manifest by abnormal immunoglobulin levels and formation of autoantibodies.

Further insight has been obtained by laboratory studies of bone marrow culture. Human bone marrow cells may be cultured in vitro with appropriate adjustments to the culture medium to produce various types of colony, including erythroid, macrophage, granulocyte, megakaryocyte or mixed colonies. A variety of growth factors responsible for stimulating these colonies in vitro were originally identified in urine, placenta and other tissues, and these were eventually isolated and purified. It then became possible to identify and clone the genes responsible for production of these colony-stimulating factors; recently, several of the factors have been produced using recombinant DNA technology and are becoming available for clinical use. The most widely available factors at present are granulocyte colony-stimulating factor (G-CSF) and granulocyte-macrophage colony-stimulating factor (GM-CSF).

It has become apparent that most of these factors or cytokines affect cell function as well as replication and differentiation, and that in vivo they form a complex and interactive network. It is of great interest that several of the genes responsible for production of cytokines, such as macrophage colony-stimulating factor (M-CSF), IL-3 (multi-CSF) and GM-CSF are located on the long arm of chromosome 5, a region frequently involved in both primary and secondary MDS (Kastan et al 1989).

Studies of bone marrow culture in vitro in patients with MPD and MDS may show a variety of abnormalities. There may be increased colony growth, sometimes without addition of appropriate cytokines. Thus, increased growth of erythroid colonies has been found in primary proliferative polycythaemia, and of megakaryocyte colonies in myelofibrosis. The pattern in myelodysplasia is often one of reduced or absent colony formation (List et al 1990), except in CMML and JCML where there is increased unstimulated growth of granulocyte-macrophage colonies.

A further area of very active investigation is the study of proto-oncogenes. These are genes which play an essential role in growth regulation within normal cells but which appear to be similar if not identical in structure to the transforming genes found in retroviruses, RNA tumour viruses. It must be emphasized that, except for the human T-cell lymphotrophic viruses, there is no direct evidence that retroviruses cause human neoplasia. However, it has been possible in laboratory experiments to induce malignant transformation in cultured cells by transfection of DNA fragments containing oncogenes derived from tumour lines. Many human malignancies have now been found to contain altered or abnormal levels of proto-oncogenes. It remains unclear whether such findings are primary or secondary phenomena in leukaemogenesis, but it is clear that these genes play an important part in normal cell growth and development. An example of this role in normal growth regulation is that of the c-fms proto-oncogene, the homologue of which causes fibro-sarcomas in cats. In humans, this proto-oncogene encodes the glycoprotein which acts as the receptor on cells of the macrophage system for macrophage CSF, (M-CSF), the gene itself being located on the critical region of chromosome 5. The c-sis proto-oncogene has homology with platelet-derived growth factor, which stimulates fibroblasts, smooth muscle cells and glial cells.

The most comprehensive investigations to date have involved the molecular analysis of the Ph[1] translocation in CGL, where the c-abl proto-oncogene, situated on the long arm of chromosome 9, is translocated to chromosome 22. The c-abl proto-oncogene normally codes for a 150-kD protein with tyrosine kinase activity. In CGL the gene resulting from fusion of the abl gene with the breakpoint cluster (bcr) region on chromosome 22 produces a larger chimeric mRNA and a 210-kD protein. It is as yet unclear how this abnormal gene product causes leukaemia, but it has recently been shown that transplanting mouse bone marrow infected with a retrovirus encoding the P210 bcr-abl fusion gene can cause a chronic myelo-proliferative disorder resembling CGL in the recipient (Daley et al 1990).

A more general type of study is that of onco-gene expression and mutation in myelodysplasias (Jacobs 1989). There are now over 30 oncogenes described, and among those under the most intense investigation are those of the ras gene family, thought to be involved in control of cell proliferation. Studies in a variety of human tumours have shown ras activation and/or mutation, and there is some evidence that ras mutation is associated with leukaemic progression in MDS. It is, however, unclear whether such findings are a step in the development of leukaemia or merely a hallmark of increased or disordered cellular proliferation.

TREATMENT OF MYELOPROLIFERATIVE DISORDERS

This section contains a brief résumé of the methods which have been used in treatment of MPD/MDS. The reader is referred to the excellent review by Cheson (1990) for a detailed bibliography of this subject (mostly, of course, citing experience with adults).

Leucapheresis

A long established method of reducing the cell burden in CGL is leucapheresis. The clearest indication for leucapheresis is the management of CGL in pregnancy where, particularly in the early months, it is important to avoid the potentially teratogenic effects of treatment with cytotoxic drugs. Leucapheresis may occasionally be indicated in other patients with leucocyte-induced hyperviscosity.

Splenectomy

Splenectomy has been used in CGL, but randomized trials have shown that it is of no benefit in prolonging survival. Splenectomy is obviously to be avoided whenever possible, because of the risks of later fulminating sepsis, and the operation itself is more hazardous when the spleen is massively enlarged. However, it may occasionally be helpful in patients with persistent massive splenomegaly and CGL and in myelofibrosis.

Chemotherapy

Chemotherapy is either used to achieve symptom control and reduce the cell burden in CGL, or is given intensively with the aim of achieving a haematological remission. Busulphan, hydroxyurea and thioguanine are the drugs most frequently used for stabilization of chronic phase CGL; they have also been used in other myeloproliferative disorders. Busulphan, an alkylating agent, is given orally either as a single daily dose, or every 4–6 weeks; in either case it must be used with caution since it can produce irreversible marrow aplasia. Long-term use in adults causes amenorrhoea, infertility and, sometimes, pigmentation. The syndrome of busulphan lung, an idiosyncratic pulmonary fibrosis, is characterized by fever, cough and, ultimately, respiratory failure. Hydroxyurea, an inhibitor of DNA synthesis, is well tolerated, apart from the facts that it is packaged in large capsules, and that its action is rapidly reversible.

More intensive combination chemotherapy, of the type given in AML (see Ch. 4), has been used experimentally in chronic phase CML and in MDS. Many reports of chemotherapy in MDS are derived from retrospective analysis in which patients on review were found to have evidence of myelodysplasia. In most reports, intensive chemotherapy in MDS is less successful than in AML, and is more successful in RAEB and RAEB-t than in other forms.

Low-dose cytarabine has been used in MDS as a potential differentiating agent, but review of published reports suggests that its success, if any, is probably due to a cytotoxic effect.

Differentiating agents, cytokines, biological response modifiers

Leukaemic cells in culture may be induced to differentiate by a variety of agents, which might therefore in theory have a beneficial effect in MDS; these include low dose cytarabine (see above), retinoids and vitamin D3. However, small randomized trials of 13-cis-retinoic acid and vitamin D3 have shown no real benefit from these forms of treatment, and both agents carry a theoretical risk of accelerating progression to acute leukaemia.

Interferons are glycoproteins which have antiproliferative, antiviral and immunoregulatory activity. Alpha-interferon was originally derived from leucocytes or lymphoblastoid cell lines, but is now made by recombinant DNA technology. It inhibits colony growth in vitro and has been shown to have a myelosuppressive effect in vivo; it has recently attracted considerable interest as a form of treatment for CGL, where it may induce clinical and cytogenetic remission. The precise method of action of interferon is unclear. Interferon is given daily, at first by subcutaneous injection, and many patients experience temporary side-effects such as a flu-like illness, fatigue, nausea and depression. A few patients experience more serious long-term effects, including fatigue, weight loss and neurotoxicity.

Now that recombinant colony-stimulating factors have become available for clinical use, they are being administered in every conceivable situation, most logically perhaps with the aim of ameliorating myelotoxicity after intensive chemotherapy. Preliminary reports of the use of GM-CSF and G-CSF in patients with MDS indicate that they may increase marrow cellularity and improve neutropenia, at least in the short term; there is uncertainty whether the neutrophils produced in patients with MDS in response to cytokine therapy would have normal function and whether these agents may accelerate progression to AML. Both GM-CSF and G-CSF have been given by intravenous infusion or subcutaneously. Both cause a variety of side-effects which are dose-related, including nausea, vomiting and anorexia, and fever and chills. Bone pain, bronchospasm and abdominal pain appear to be complications specific to GM-CSF.

Allogeneic bone marrow transplantation (BMT), matched unrelated donors (MUD) and autologous BMT (ABMT).

Twelve years have elapsed since the Seattle group reported the first successful syngeneic transplants in a small number of patients with CGL. Since that time, bone marrow transplantation (BMT) has been widely used in CGL and in most forms of MDS. In general, children tolerate BMT well, and it should be considered in most patients with any of these disorders. However, the short-term tolerability of BMT is accompanied by significant long-term morbidity, and careful consideration should be given to late effects of treatment when evaluating the various preparative regimens available.

This section reviews the general principles and complications of BMT; detailed recommendations and references are given in the sections dealing with individual conditions.

The HLA antigens, which constitute the major histocompatiblity complex, are located on chromosome 6. Despite their extreme polymorphism, each region is normally inherited as a single haplotype from either parent; thus there is a 25% chance that any two siblings will be HLA identical. About one in three children with leukaemia in the UK have a histocompatible sibling, and most experience has been gained with this type of

BMT. However, even when there is full HLA compatibility between siblings, graft-versus host disease (GVHD) is an important and potentially lethal complication of BMT and measures to prevent its development are essential.

GVHD is mediated by immunocompetent T-cells infused with the bone marrow which react against minor antigens in the recipient. Acute GVHD may develop up to 5–6 weeks after BMT, and the features include a skin rash, abnormal liver function and diarrhoea. A scoring system has been devised based on the number and extent of organ involvement; the severity varies from a maculopapular skin rash to exfoliation, severe jaundice, severe abdominal pain and the passage of litres of diarrhoea.

There are two approaches to the prevention of GVHD: immunosuppression of the recipient and T-cell depletion of the donor marrow. There are various protocols for immunosuppression, but the most widely used is the combination of cyclosporin for up to 6 months and a short course of methotrexate. Cyclosporin is nephrotoxic and tends to cause weight gain and hypertension; careful monitoring of the blood level is therefore essential. Depletion of T-cells in donor marrow has been performed with a variety of techniques, but is most commonly effected by incubation with monoclonal antibodies and complement before reinfusion. T-cell depletion significantly reduces the incidence of GVHD at the expense of a greater risk of graft rejection or leukaemic relapse, which, at least in CGL, outweighs its benefits (Apperley et al 1988).

Acute GVHD is usually treated with methlyprednisolone, alone or in combination with other agents such as monoclonal antibodies. Chronic GVHD, an extremely unpleasant complication, may follow acute GVHD or occur de novo. It is characterized by chronic change in the skin and mucous membranes which can resemble scleroderma, contractures, and immunodeficiency. Other features may include hepatic fibrosis, cholestasis, myositis and chronic respiratory insufficiency. Treatment is unsatisfactory and it is usual to give steroid therapy, sometimes in conjunction with azathioprine or thalidomide. The risk of GVHD is in general increased by the use of donors who are not HLA identical.

The choice of conditioning regimen for BMT will vary with the age of the patient and the diagnosis. The most widely used regimens have been various combinations of cyclophosphamide and total body irradiation (TBI), sometimes with the addition of other drugs such as cytarabine. This combination has the advantage of readily facilitating engraftment and is associated with a relatively low relapse rate, varying according to the indications for BMT and the method of prevention of GVHD. The dose of TBI varies; the original Seattle schedule was a dose of about 1000 cGy given at a dose rate of 5 cGy/minute in a single fraction, while lower doses such as 750 cGy have been successfully given at a faster rate of 25 cGy/minute. Fractionated TBI is usually given in doses of up to 200 cGy twice daily over 3–4 days.

The regimen without TBI which has been used most widely is a combination of busulphan and cyclophosphamide (Tutschka et al 1987). Unfortunately, there are no published reports of randomized trials comparing the two preparative regimens.

The risks and complications of BMT when performed for CGL and MDS are similar to those encountered in acute leukaemia. During the first 2–3 weeks after BMT the patient has severe neutropenia, frequently compounded by mucositis due to radiotherapy and chemotherapy, and is at risk of bacterial and fungal infections. Herpes simplex is an important factor in causing or exacerbating mucositis and delaying engraftment. High-dose chemotherapy and radiotherapy induce long-term immunosuppression which is exacerbated in the presence of chronic GVHD. Common viral infections after BMT include cytomegalovirus, an important cause of pneumonitis, varicella-zoster, and adenovirus. Other important infections are *Pneumocystis carinii* pneumonitis and pneumococcal sepsis; these are common in patients with chronic GVHD.

The pattern of late effects of treatment following BMT depends on the conditioning regimen and the age of the patient; in general, the younger patients will be the most vulnerable to the late effects of TBI. Children who have received TBI have growth failure which is in part due to spinal shortening and partly to hypothalamic-pituitary failure. Delayed puberty and gonadal failure are common, and there is a variable risk of hypothyroidism, cataracts and learning problems. The incidence and severity of these complications will vary according to the age of the child and the dose rate and fractionation of TBI (Sanders et al 1986, Leiper et al 1987). The combination of busulphan and cyclophosphamide may induce sterility, but is unlikely to have such a significant effect on growth or neuropsychological development. However, there is little available information on the efficacy of this preparative regimen in many conditions, and the risks of veno-occlusive disease of the liver and pulmonary toxicity are unclear at the moment.

Unfortunately, while BMT is the treatment of choice for many children with MPD/MDS, the majority of patients will not have a histocompatible sibling. Since the prognosis for most of these disorders is very poor and there are no effective alternative forms of treatment, use of alternative donors would seem entirely justifiable despite the increased risks involved. There are two possible approaches in such patients: the use of a haplo-identical family donor or a matched unrelated donor (MUD). Most studies hitherto have involved the use of MUD donors and the present state of development of such donor panels has recently been reviewed (Hows & Bradley 1990). The chance of finding a suitable donor depends on the patient's haplotype, the size of the donor pool, and the ethnic group of the patient and the pool. At present, the time between requesting and finding a donor is from 3 to 10 months. Thus, in practice, there is more time to find a donor for a patient with CGL than one with acute leukaemia, and a search seems entirely justified. The hazards of such transplants are, of course, greater than those of standard BMT, the most notable being failure of engraftment or rejection and GVHD which may be chronic and disabling. However, it seems highly likely that results of treatment, like those of standard BMT, will improve.

Autologous BMT (ABMT) has the advantages of being safer than BMT and universally applicable, and it can be used in patients who are deemed too old to receive an allograft; hence its popularity in AML. Although ABMT could not conceivably cure CGL, it was introduced as a palliative measure, albeit an intensive one, to prolong the chronic phase. Blood and/or bone marrow were harvested from patients in chronic phase, stored, and reinfused after high dose chemoradiotherapy to facilitate reversion to chronic phase after patients had developed blast crisis. Not surprisingly, this approach did not produce dramatic improvements in survival, although it produced a good quality second chronic phase in some patients. The concept of ABMT in CGL has undergone a slight resurgence in recent years, with reports that bone marrow in long-term culture or bone marrow in patients treated with alpha-interferon may become Ph[1]-negative, thus introducing the hope that it might be possible to reinfuse normal autologous marrow. Despite anecdotes and preliminary reports of success, this approach to treatment remains experimental at present and is unlikely to benefit patients with other types of MPD/MDS.

CHRONIC GRANULOCYTIC LEUKAEMIA

Clinical features and diagnosis

Chronic granulocytic leukaemia (CGL) is rare in young children (Castro-Malaspina et al 1983) but has been seen even in infants under one year. The disease in children resembles in every respect that in adults. The presenting features are usually those of an abdominal mass due to an enlarged spleen, abdominal discomfort or fatigue. The diagnosis may be a chance one on routine examination or blood count. Occasionally, patients may have a more dramatic presentation, with hyperleucocytosis causing priapism, retinal haemorrhages or a hypermetabolic state.

The blood count, as previously described, shows leucocytosis, usually in excess of $100 \times 10^9/1$, with neutrophils, basophils, myelocytes and metamyelocytes. While the morphology of the neutrophils is normal, the leucocyte alkaline phosphatase is invariably reduced. The platelet count is usually raised and anaemia is common. The bone marrow aspirate shows a cellular dense marrow with many granulocyte precursors, and trephine confirms that there is a cellular bone marrow, with increased megakaryocytes and myeloid cells, often with some increase in fibrosis. Other laboratory findings such as raised vitamin B_{12} and B_{12}-binding proteins and uric acid are secondary to the increased myeloid proliferation and, not surprisingly, the colony cultures from the blood show increased numbers of myeloid progenitor cells. There is usually little difficulty in establishing a diagnosis which is confirmed on cytogenetic analysis, when the Ph[1] translocation t(9;22) (q34;q11) or a variant thereof is almost invariably demonstrated.

In the occasional patient in whom cytogenetic analysis is negative, a careful morphological re-appraisal may suggest some other form of MPD or MDS (Pugh et al 1985). Alternatively, if the clinical and laboratory features are typical, molecular analysis may show a bcr-abl rearrangement in the presence of a normal karyotype (Ganesan et al 1986); these patients should be managed as if they had typical CGL.

Natural history

The natural history of CGL, whether treated or untreated, is one of a chronic phase of variable duration with a median of about 3.5 years. The disease then enters an accelerated phase, becoming difficult to control by standard chemotherapy. The spleen may remain enlarged, with onset of a myelofibrotic picture. Blast crisis, which is in effect development of an acute leukaemia, may follow an accelerated phase or occur abruptly. A blast crisis may be heralded by the development of lytic bony lesions, or extramedullary disease, usually in the central nervous system. Morphological and immunological characterization of the blast cells in this phase has shown that they may be myeloid, lymphoid or, indeed, of mixed lineage (Chessells et al 1979). The leukaemic cells in blast crisis show overexpression of the multi-drug resistance P-glycoprotein gene, an observation of some interest in view of the poor response to therapy. Treatment of blast crisis may induce remission and reversion to chronic phase, but survival following blast crisis is usually poor, the occasional patient experiencing a prolonged second chronic phase.

There have been a number of attempts to predict the duration of chronic phase, onset of blast crisis, or response to therapy using clinical features (Thomas & Clift 1989), cytogenetic analysis or examination of the molecular location of the bcr breakpoint (Morris et al 1990). There is evidence from multivariate analysis in adults that patients with a large spleen, low platelet count or higher number of circulating blasts, and those with additional cytogenetic abnormalities are likely to have a poor survival, but there is no evidence that location of the breakpoint may influence the duration of chronic phase. These observations may have some predictive value for prognosis, but however prolonged survival in chronic phase, CGL is an inevitably fatal disease.

The Ph[1] chromosome in acute leukaemia and in CGL; one or two diseases?

It is well known that about 1–2% of children with ALL and a small number with AML may have an acute leukaemia in association with the Ph[1] chromosome. The clinical features may be indistinguishable from those of any other acute leukaemia, save perhaps for preservation of platelet and granulocyte count during treatment and refractoriness to chemotherapy; if remission is achieved, the Ph[1] chromosome may be undetectable, but the prognosis is poor and relapse virtually inevitable.

There has been heated controversy over whether Ph[1]-positive acute leukaemias and CGL are one or two (or three) diseases; this controversy has been summarized in a recent review (Gale & Butturini 1990). In most children with Ph[1]-positive ALL, the site of translocation of the abl oncogene differs from that in CGL. Thus, the resultant mRNA is smaller and the protein product has a MW of 190 kD instead of 210 kD. There have not as yet been similar studies of Ph[1]-positive AML. This finding is of theoretical interest but no practical relevance at present, since all three diseases have a poor prognosis with conventional treatment.

Management

Conventional treatment

The typical child with CGL has significant splenomegaly, anaemia and leucocytosis, and treatment is indicated to reduce the bulk of the disease and reduce the risk of hyperviscosity. This can normally been done gradually on an outpatient basis; the very occasional patient with symptoms of hyperviscosity may need more aggressive therapy with allopurinol, hydroxyurea and even leucapheresis.

The most appropriate form of treatment is oral hydroxyurea or busulphan; hydroxyurea should be used in the first instance because it is less myelotoxic and because there is concern that busulphan may predispose to pulmonary toxicity in the event of BMT. Hydroxyurea is given at a dose of 20–30 mg/kg per day or more conveniently, since the capsules come in 500-mg doses, at 80 mg/kg 2–3 times per week. Busulphan can be given in a small daily dose of 0.06 mg/kg per day, but is more conveniently and safely given scaled down in an equivalent to the adult dose of 50–100 mg, appropriately every 3–4 weeks. The blood count should be monitored particularly carefully when using busulphan, and the drug stopped once the leucocyte count approaches $20 \times 10^9/1$. Busulphan is extremely myelotoxic and can cause irreversible marrow aplasia.

There is no evidence that more intensive combination chemotherapy during the chronic phase of the disease will prolong this phase or induce a full cytogenetic remission, although a reduction in the proportion of Ph^1-positive cells has been achieved in some patients.

Alpha-interferon either as a single agent, or in combination with other drugs such as cytosine arabinoside, is undergoing active investigation in randomized trials on both sides of the Atlantic. Treatment with alpha-interferon induces clinical and haematological remission in up to 80% of patients, and several studies have now confirmed the original report from the MD Anderson Hospital (Talpaz et al 1986) that the Ph^1 chromosome may be suppressed in possibly 10–20% of patients. The efficacy of interferon seems to be dose-dependent, and treatment is less effective in late-stage CGL. The majority of patients experience side-effects as previously described. At present, there is no clear evidence that interferon prolongs chronic phase or survival, and in view of the side-effects and need for injections it cannot be recommended in clinical practice outside the context of a clinical trial. It may be of benefit in the occasional patient in whom thrombocytosis is a dominant feature, but significant problems from thrombocytosis are rare in adults and thus presumably rarer in children.

Blast crisis of CGL is usually treated with appropriate chemotherapy, that is prednisolone and vincristine for lymphoid crisis and combination chemotherapy as used in AML for myeloid crisis. It is possible that children respond more readily to chemotherapy but, as previously indicated, survival is poor.

Bone marrow transplantation

The indications for BMT in CGL were recently reviewed by the Seattle team (Thomas & Clift 1989). Bone marrow transplantation from an HLA-compatible sibling donor is the only curative treatment for CGL and it should be considered in all patients. There has been some debate in the literature about the optimal timing of BMT, because an unsuccessful BMT may, of course, shorten life, particularly in a patient who has a good chance of a long chronic phase. However, there seems no reason to delay BMT in children, since in general they tolerate BMT better than adults. All families should be HLA-typed, and if a compatible donor is found it would seem appropriate to proceed to BMT as soon as convenient, once the chronic phase has been controlled.

A review of results from the International Bone Marrow Transplant Registry (Goldman et al 1985) shows that actuarial survival after BMT from a sibling donor is 65% for BMT in first chronic phase, 32% in accelerated phase and 14% in blast crisis. These results are similar to the more reliable ones from the Seattle group, who have also shown the benefit of BMT within a year of diagnosis. Analysis of factors associated with graft failure, GVHD and relapse both from a large French study and a multinational group (Apperley et al 1988, Devergie et al 1990), has shown that relapse is less likely when BMT is performed in first chronic phase using non-T-depleted bone marrow. Since CGL in childhood is so rare, most of these observations were, of course, derived from adults; however, they support the use of BMT in first chronic phase in childhood, and a recent small study comparing outcome in children receiving BMT and conservative treatment confirms this finding (Klingebiel et al 1990).

A search for a MUD donor seems justified in children who do not have a histocompatible sibling; the long chronic phase means that there is more time to find a donor than, for example, in relapsed acute leukaemia. Analysis of results of BMT using MUD donors in 102 consecutive patients (McGlave et al 1990) showed an actuarial event-free survival of 29% at 2.5 years; the major problems were failure of engraftment, and acute and chronic GVHD. It is to be hoped that these results will improve with more effective treatment and prevention of GVHD.

A debatable issue, especially in the young child, is whether the preparative regimen should comprise the more commonly used cyclophosphamide and TBI, or whether a regimen without irradiation, such as busulphan and cyclophosphamide, as used by the Baltimore Group (Tutschka et al 1987), is preferable. Most published reports have involved TBI, but encouraging results have been claimed for the alternative regimen; there are as yet no randomized comparisons of the two treatments. Perhaps an empirical approach in the paediatric patient would be to use chemotherapy alone in the young child, for example the under-threes, to avoid the late effects of irradiation, but to use the standard approach in older children.

In summary, the management of the child with CGL should comprise confirmation of the diagnosis, stabilization with oral drugs, and a search for a suitable donor. If an HLA-compatible sibling or close relative is identified, then BMT should be performed avoiding T-cell depletion. If there is no family donor, a search for a MUD donor is justified; the results of randomized trials involving treatment with alpha-interferon with or without other agents are eagerly awaited and could conceivably provide justification for other approaches, such as long-term treatment in chronic phase or autologous transplantation.

ESSENTIAL THROMBOCYTHAEMIA

Primary or essential thrombocythaemia (see also Ch. 6) is a myeloproliferative disease of clonal origin characterized by a persistently elevated platelet count for which there is no other obvious cause. The diagnosis and management of this condition has recently been reviewed (Pearson 1991). The condition is very rare in children, and a recent review (Schwartz & Cohen 1988) reported only 10 cases.

Diagnosis and differential diagnosis

The proposed diagnostic criteria for primary thrombocythaemia are: a persistently raised platelet count in excess of $600 \times 10^9/l$, no evidence of raised red cell mass, (taking into account the possibility of polycythaemia masked by iron deficiency), no Ph[1] chromosome, no supportive evidence for primary myelofibrosis and no demonstrable cause for secondary thrombocytosis. It is, of course, apparent that these criteria are designed for adult practice. Nevertheless, they indicate the need for trephine biopsy of the marrow, obtaining a sample for cytogenetics and actively looking for a cause for the raised platelet count. More useful observations, if available and positive, are the establishment of clonality in female patients if a suitable X-linked probe is available, and the finding of unstimulated colonies of erythroid precursors (burst-forming units) or megakaryocyte colonies in blood or marrow.

The causes of thrombocytosis are discussed in Chapter 6, and this differential diagnosis should be considered in every child with a raised platelet count.

Natural history and management

Essential thrombocythaemia in adults is a chronic disease with median survival of around 8–10 years. The complications of primary thrombocythaemia include thrombosis and haemorrhage. These are more common in patients with a count in excess of $1000 \times 10^9/l$, but bear no relationship to the abnormalities of platelet function characteristic of this disorder. The most common thrombotic symptoms are digital ischaemia and transient cerebral ischaemia, while cutaneous and mucous membrane bleeding or bruising are the most common haemorrhagic symptoms. It is probable that young people and children have a low frequency of complications.

Review of adult patients shows that a few develop polycythaemia, thus indicating the overlap between these two conditions and that myelofibrosis is a common complication. There are a number of reports of development of leukaemia possibly related to therapy. A review of outcome in 10 paediatric cases showed that one, who had been treated with ^{32}P died of leukaemia and one had developed myelofibrosis (Schwartz & Cohen 1988).

There is thus little evidence to make recommendations about treatment, but this would not seem to be necessary in the asymptomatic patient. The choice of drug is between busulphan and hydroxyurea; while episodic busulphan therapy may achieve good control of the platelet count, hydroxyurea is probably to be preferred as less toxic. Alpha-interferon may achieve control of the platelet count, but the indications for its use remain to be determined.

POLYCYTHAEMIA RUBRA VERA

Polycythaemia rubra vera is a clonal myeloproliferative disorder, most common in the over-50s, characterized by a raised red cell mass and a variable degree of leucocytosis, thrombocytosis and splenomegaly. The symptoms include plethora, dyspnoea, hypertension, giddiness and headache. Pruritus and gout are additional complications. The raised platelet count and abnormal platelet function may, as in thrombocythaemia, cause vaso-occlusive symptoms or haemorrhage.

Diagnosis and differential diagnosis

The diagnostic criteria, as described by the Polycythaemia Study Group (Hocking & Golde 1989) are an absolute polycythaemia with raised red cell mass and arterial SO_2 >92%. The presence of splenomegaly in addition is sufficient to establish the diagnosis. If the spleen is not enlarged there must be two of the following additional criteria: thrombocytosis $> 400 \times 10^9$/l, leucocyte count greater than 12.0×10^9/l, raised neutrophil alkaline phosphatase, raised serum B_{12} or B_{12}-binding capacity. These criteria are rarely met in children, and there are very few fully documented cases (Schwartz & Cohen 1988).

Children with presumed polycythaemia should be fully investigated to exclude other causes of absolute polycythaemia (i.e. a raised red cell mass) such as hypoxia and inappropriate erythropoietin secretion.

Patients with true polycythaemia vera normally have other evidence of a myeloproliferative disorder, such as a raised platelet and leucocyte count. The bone marrow is densely cellular, and cytogenetic abnormalities are found in about 15% of cases. Some patients exhibit spontaneous growth of erythroid colonies in the absence of erythropoietin; plasma erythropoietin levels are low.

Natural history, treatment and prognosis

The median reported survival of adults with polycythaemia vera is between 10 and 15 years. The risk of complications is in part related to the type of treatment. Thus, patients treated with phlebotomy tend to develop thrombotic complications, whereas ^{32}P therapy increases the risk of leukaemia. About one-fifth of adult patients develop myelofibrosis with massive splenomegaly and pancytopenia. The methods of treatment available are venesection, ^{32}P, and chemotherapy with hydroxyurea or busulphan. Treatment is usually necessary because of the symptoms associated with a raised red cell mass and the risk of complications which cannot however be quantified because of the rarity of the disease in paediatrics. The recommended method of treatment in children is phlebotomy.

MYELOFIBROSIS

Acute myelofibrosis was originally described as an illness associated with fever, weight loss, pancytopenia, absence of splenomegaly, but a fibrotic bone marrow with an increase of blast cells and abnormal megakaryocytes. The illness was rapidly fatal and occasionally seen in childhood. It is now apparent that most, if not all, of such patients, had acute megakaryoblastic leukaemia and that they respond to intensive chemotherapy as given for other forms of acute myeloid leukaemia (See Ch. 4).

By contrast, chronic myelofibrosis is a well recognized myeloproliferative disease of the middle-aged and elderly, presenting with massive splenomegaly, a leucoerythroblastic blood film with teardrop poikilocytes, and a bone marrow which is difficult to aspirate. Trephine biopsy shows a hyperplastic bone marrow with prominent megakaryocytes and increased reticulin and fibrosis demonstrated on silver stain. Platelet function is defective in many patients, and colony culture shows increased CFU-GM and megakaryocyte colonies. The median survival is about 3 years from diagnosis.

Diagnosis and differential diagnosis

Chronic myelofibrosis is virtually never seen in childhood and there are no case reports studied with modern techniques or since the recognition of megakaryoblastic leukaemia. The author had one such patient treated with bone marrow transplantation but, in retrospect, this boy might have had a subacute megakaryoblastic leukaemia and no attempt was made to induce remission with chemotherapy prior to bone marrow transplantation. Patients with a leucoerythroblastic blood film and a marrow that is difficult to aspirate may have infections such as tuberculosis or toxoplasmosis, lymphomas, leukaemia, or disseminated tumours such as neuroblastoma. Myelofibrosis may also be a presenting feature of Ph^1-positive CGL. In all such secondary cases, the fibrosis responds to appropriate treatment. A leucoerythroblastic marrow in the young child is also a feature of osteopetrosis, but here the radiological appearances are diagnostic.

In summary, the finding of a leucoerythroblastic blood film and a marrow that is difficult to aspirate is an indication for a trephine biopsy and a search for possible causes of myelofibrosis. Primary myelofibrosis is excessively rare in childhood, and it remains unclear whether all such cases are variants of megakaryoblastic leukaemia, but the majority are.

TRANSIENT MYELOPROLIFERATIVE DISORDER OF THE NEWBORN ASSOCIATED WITH DOWN'S SYNDROME.

The infant with Down's syndrome may develop a myeloproliferative disorder in the neonatal period (Barnett et al 1990). The clinical findings are of enlargement of the liver and spleen without the lymphadenopathy and skin infiltration characteristic of neonatal leukaemia. A recent report summarized the haematological findings in 12 cases of transient MPD (Eguchi et al 1989). All infants had a leucocytosis with a variable number of blasts in the blood; the haemoglobin was normal and the platelet count increased in some cases, and moderately reduced in others. Infants with transient MPD do not develop progressive marrow failure, and the blast cells disappear from the blood after a variable time; in the report cited, this varied from 7 to 56 days, but the author has known of some patients in whom blasts persisted for months. This syndrome has also been described in babies who were phenotypically normal but who, on investigation, proved to be trisomy 21 mosaics.

Morphologically, cytochemically and with immunophenotyping, the blasts in transient myeloproliferative disease resemble those of acute megakaryoblastic leukaemia. Eguchi et al (1989) recently attempted to distinguish the blasts of transient MPD from those of Down's syndrome patients who had developed acute megakaryoblastic leukaemia. In both instances, the blasts reacted with platelet peroxidase and monoclonal antibodies to megakaryocytes. However, on electron microscopy the blasts from the transient disorder exhibited positivity with myeloperoxidase and showed some tendency to differentiation. Clonal chromosomal abnormalities were only seen in the samples from patients with frank leukaemia.

These observations are of great theoretical interest and much remains to be learned about the relationship between these two conditions. The frequency of transient myeloproliferative disease in Down's syndrome is unknown and will only be learned by a prospective study. It also seems apparent that a number of Down's infants with megakaryoblastic AML have had a preceding myeloproliferative disorder, and that there is a risk of development of AML following neonatal MPD, although a review of the literature suggests that this risk is confined to the first three years of life. However the pattern of evolution of this syndrome, like the incidence, awaits clarification.

Diagnosis and management

The transient neonatal myeloproliferative syndrome must be distinguished from true neonatal leukaemia and from other causes of neonatal hepatosplenomegaly such as congenital infection. The distinction is usually apparent, and confirmed by full haematological and cytogenetic investigation. Once the diagnosis is confirmed, no specific treatment should be necessary. Continued observation of affected babies would appear wise, although it must be admitted that counselling of parents in this situation of uncertain risk is particularly difficult. There is evidence (see Ch. 4) that children with Down's syndrome who do develop frank AML respond well to treatment.

OTHER RARE MYELOPROLIFERATIVE DISORDERS

There have been reports of a number of myeloproliferative disorders in infants and young children which do not fit the generally recognized categories. We have seen two infants with hepatosplenomegaly, marked eosinophilia and chromosome analysis showing a t(l;5)(q23;q33); one was refractory to chemotherapy while the other had a more prolonged course responding to oral drugs (Darbyshire et al 1987). The author has since heard of a couple of similar cases.

There has also been a recent description of a myeloproliferative disease in childhood with clinical features of chronic myeloid leukaemia associated with translocations involving chromosome 11p15 (Inaba et al 1988).

Thus, patients with a myeloproliferative disorder whose condition is not readily categorized should have full investigations as suggested in Table 3.2. The presence of a cytogenetic abnormality in the bone marrow is supportive of the diagnosis of a clonal disorder and would indicate that prognosis is likely to be poor.

FAMILIAL MYELOPROLIFERATIVE DISEASE OR MYELODYSPLASIA

When a young child develops a potentially fatal disorder, there is naturally extreme anxiety on the part of the parents lest there be a risk to other siblings. In most cases of acute leukaemia, this risk is negligible. The risk also appears to be insignificant in most cases of more chronic leukaemias and myelodysplasias, but in this section the evidence about familial disorders is reviewed.

As previously mentioned, there are a number of congenital bone marrow disorders, most notably Fanconi's anaemia and Shwachman's syndrome, which carry an increased risk of myelodysplasia as well as leukaemia. Both are inherited as autosomal recessive disorders and both are reviewed in Chapter 2. It is now recognized that the clinical spectrum of Fanconi's anaemia is wide and that patients may present with variants in which there are virtually no phenotypic abnormalities. The sine qua non for a diagnosis of Fanconi's anaemia is the presence of an increased number of chromosomal rings and breaks, indicative of a disorder of DNA repair and now best demonstrated by culture of blood lymphocytes with diepoxybutane. This investigation should be mandatory in all children presenting with marrow aplasia, particularly those with a chronic onset.

The syndrome of juvenile monosomy 7 (see below) has been documented in at least 11 families, and it has been claimed that up to one-third of cases are familial (Brandwein et al 1990). This has not been the experience of the author, and while there is no doubt that such cases occur, the frequency is at present uncertain. Monosomy 7 has also been found when leukaemic or preleukaemic transformation has occurred in familial hypoplastic anaemia in non-Fanconi families (Paul et al 1987).

There are a number of other case reports in the literature, usually of single families, where the myeloproliferative disorder has often been imperfectly studied with modern techniques, and/or does not fit any recognized category. Thus, a large kindred was described by Randall et al (1965) in which children presented at up to 4 years of age with anaemia, leucocytosis and a leucoeythroblastic blood film together with marked splenomegaly. The bone marrow was hyperplastic with no evidence of fibrosis. Long term follow-up showed reversion of blood and marrow to normal in some cases, some died and four underwent splenectomy with improvement of their symptoms of hypersplenism. Review of chronic myeloproliferative disorders seen both at St Jude (Smith & Johnson 1974) and Texas Children's Hospital (Nix & Fernbach 1981) have found similar families. We have observed a similar picture in two siblings; in neither were the morphological appearances those of CGL, and cytogenetic analysis of the bone marrow was normal. Both improved after splenectomy.

Familial myelofibrosis was seen in two infant siblings with pancytopenia and a leucoerythroblastic blood film accompanied by marked bone marrow fibrosis; the diagnosis of familial erythrophagocytic lymphohistiocytosis (FEL; see Ch. 5) was strongly considered, but not supported by histological appearances at post mortem (Sieff & Malleson 1980).

There are also a number of families in whom AML or MDS occurs in more than one member and the pattern of inheritance appears variable. So, in summary, there are several instances in which obscure or not so obscure disorders occur in more than one family member. In some of these, such as Fanconi's anaemia, there is some understanding of the genetic basis. In others, such as the obscure myeloproliferative disorders, it could be that some hitherto unexplained abnormality of the regulation of haemopoiesis might play a part and that these are not truly clonal disorders. A conservative approach to treatment would seem appropriate in this uncertain situation.

JUVENILE CHRONIC MYELOID LEUKAEMIA

Clinical features and diagnosis

Juvenile chronic myeloid leukaemia (JCML), one of the classic MPD/MDS of childhood, is more common in boys. Patients usually present with bleeding due to thrombocytopenia, pallor and splenomegaly. Progression of the disease is accompanied by wasting, lymphadenopathy and bacterial infections. The typical skin rash varies in extent and severity, but normally has a 'butterfly' facial distribution, sometimes also involving the trunk. It may precede other symptoms by several months. Biopsy of the skin rash shows a nonspecific infiltrate with lymphocytes and histiocytes. There appears to be an increased frequency of JCML in neurofibromatosis (Freedman et al 1988); certainly, there are several reports of the two conditions occurring together but the nature of this association is not yet clear.

The laboratory findings are in marked contrast to those of Ph^1-positive CGL. There are no specific diagnostic features, particularly if by chance the diagnosis is made early in the clinical course.

The morphological findings in most cases would probably be best described as consistent with CMML in the FAB classification. Indeed, the French have always described this condition as CMML of infancy, and the largest published series of JCML is that published from the Hôpital St-Louis in Paris (Castro-Malaspina et al 1984). A leucocyte count greater than $100 \times 10^9/l$ was present in only 6 of 38 cases; the majority had counts of less than $50 \times 10^9/l$. Anaemia was usual, thrombocytopenia common, and the blood film showed monocytes, eosinophils, abnormal granulocytes and some blast cells. The appearances of the blood film are more diagnostic than those of the bone marrow, where monocytes may predominate with some increase in blast cells and myelodysplasia in all cell lines.

The classification as a CMML is supported by the characteristic finding on colony cultures of spontaneous growth of macrophage colonies without addition of GM-CSF; this growth can be inhibited by the addition of neutralizing antisera to GM-CSF to the culture medium, but not by antibodies to other cytokines (Gualtieri et al 1989). However, JCML is truly a trilineage myelodysplasia, and a hallmark of the disease is the raised fetal haemoglobin associated with a fetal pattern of gamma globin chain synthesis and even synthesis of embryonic epsilon chains. The fetal haemoglobin level becomes progressively higher as the disease progresses. Further evidence for the truly fetal haemopoesis is the erythroid colony pattern, which resembles that of fetal and neonatal red cells (Weinburg et al 1990), the fetal pattern of 2,3-DPG and red cell enzymes (Travis 1983), red cell i/I antigen and carbonic anhydrase. Like adult CMML, JCML is often associated with a number of immunological abnormalities, such as antinuclear antibodies and anti Ig antibodies (Cannat & Seligman 1973).

Cytogenetic analysis of the bone marrow in JCML may show a variety of abnormalities or may be normal; there are no pathognomonic findings. The differential diagnosis includes the other types of paediatric myelodysplasia, and the distinction from monosomy 7 is sometimes a fine one (see below).

Some patients with the clinical features of JCML, including the grossly raised fetal haemoglobin, have a blood film with dominant normoblasts which is suggestive of erythroleukaemia. Two patients have been described with some features of JCML in association with infection with Epstein-Barr virus (Herrod et al 1983); notable atypical features were bone marrow lymphocytosis and absence of progressive thrombocytopenia. Thus, a search for possible viral infection is indicated in children with possible JCML, particularly if the clinical picture is not typical.

Natural history and prognosis: are there two types of JCML?

The diagnosis of JCML is a clinical one and there is a degree of clinical overlap between these patients and those with other types of MDS, most notably monosomy 7 syndrome. Indeed, a recent review (Brandwein et al 1990) emphasized that the two conditions were not mutually exclusive, but it is important to distinguish the two conditions if possible because of the different prognosis and response to therapy in typical cases.

The French series of JCML (Castro-Malaspina et al 1984) included a multivariate analysis of factors influencing prognosis; the most important variables were age, the presence of bleeding and the platelet count. The median survival for children over 2 years of age at diagnosis was 12 months, whereas younger children had a median survival of over 4 years. At the Hospital for Sick Children (HSC) we have used strict diagnostic criteria for the diagnosis of JCML, including a fetal haemoglobin in excess of 10% and progressive thrombocytopenia. In our series of 14 children seen over the last 20 years (11 male), the median age at diagnosis was 3 years (range 1–6 years) and the median survival was 7 months.

In summary, the prognosis for older children is extremely poor, younger children may survive longer and the clinical pictures of monosomy 7 and JCML are sometimes difficult to distinguish.

A terminal blast crisis in JCML has been described by some authors but this event occurs rarely, if ever, in the author's experience. The inevitable deterioration is marked by progressive bleeding, weight loss, enlargement of lymph nodes and anaemia; although the blood film may show more abnormal cells and blast cells, and some-

times a predominance of normoblasts, a true blast crisis as seen in Ph^1-positive CGL does not occur.

Management

It may be appropriate in young children with atypical features to adopt a conservative approach to management, but typical JCML is refractory to chemotherapy, even to the most intensive combinations used in acute myeloid leukaemia. There have been reports that the combination of cytosine arabinoside (Lilleyman et al 1977) or intensive combination chemotherapy (Chan et al 1987) may be effective treatment, but close analysis of the results obtained shows that a true remission is not achieved; at best, this approach produces some reduction in disease bulk. In view of the reports of abnormal cytokine production and regulation in JCML, there may conceivably be a role for some form of treatment with inhibitors or regulators of cytokines if this treatment were to become available.

Allogeneic BMT is the treatment of choice for JCML. A report from Seattle (Sanders et al 1988) showed that 3 out of 6 children receiving BMT from an HLA-identical sibling, and 3 out of 8 children transplanted from a donor with a 1–3 antigen mismatch, were alive and in remission after a conditioning programme including cyclophosphamide and total body irradiation. There was recurrence of the leukaemia in 3 of the 14 children. There has been a recent report that the combination of busulphan and cyclophosphamide was ineffective in eradicating JCML (Urban et al 1990). Since JCML is so refractory to treatment, a preparative regimen including total body irradiation should probably be used. Since there is no alternative effective treatment, a search for a MUD donor if time permits, or the use of a haplo-identical donor, would seem justifiable in cases where no matched sibling is available.

MONOSOMY 7 AND THE JUVENILE MYELODYSPLASTIC SYNDROME

Clinical features and diagnosis

Monosomy 7 is a common cytogenetic finding in primary and secondary leukaemias but also occurs in association with a chronic myeloproliferative or myelodysplastic syndrome in young children, with a marked predominance of males. The median age of 11 children (10 boys) with this juvenile syndrome seen at the Hospital for Sick Children (Evans et al 1988) was 10 months; all had hepatosplenomegaly and one a facial rash. Infections were a common symptom, with staphylococcal sepsis predominating in some. The blood and bone marrow appearances in our cases and others reported (Brandwein et al 1990, Weiss et al 1987) were those of RAEB or CMML; thrombocytopenia was not an early or dominant finding, and the fetal haemoglobin was rarely greater than 10%.

As mentioned previously, a number of cases of this disorder have occurred in siblings (Carroll et al 1985, Brandwein et al 1990), but we have encountered no such families in our practice and the true frequency of the familial syndrome is unknown.

Analysis of bone marrow chromosomes shows a variable number of cells lacking a chromosome 7 but these usually predominate. Neutrophil function in these, as in other patients with monosomy 7 is impaired, with defective chemotaxis and killing. Bone marrow culture studies show some autonomous growth of macrophage granulocyte colonies (Weiss et al 1987).

Natural history and prognosis: relationship to JCML

A recent report from Vancouver has emphasized the problems in making a distinction between monosomy 7 and JCML, and emphasized the heterogeneity of childhood myelodysplasia (Brandwein et al 1990). It is important to recognize that monosomy 7 is a common finding in both myelodysplasia and AML, and the term monosomy 7 syndrome should be reserved for those children, usually under 2 years of age, who fulfil the diagnostic criteria. The clinical evolution seen in our patients at the Hospital for Sick Children (Evans et al 1988) and in those elsewhere (Weiss et al 1987) is distinct; 3 of our 11 patients and 5 of 8 from St Jude developed frank AML, and one in each series developed massive splenomegaly and myelofibrosis. The time to evolution of AML varied from 3 months to 2 years and in a survey of

previously published cases (Sieff et al 1981) we found that several patients had survived more than 2 years from diagnosis. Thus, this syndrome, unlike JCML, is compatible with longer survival and carries a predilection to the development of frank acute myeloid leukaemia.

Management

Acute myeloid leukaemia with monosomy 7 is less responsive to induction chemotherapy than are other types (Woods et al 1985), and our original experience with infantile MDS suggested that this was also refractory. However, we have now treated a total of six children having this syndrome with intensive chemotherapy as used in AML, and three achieved clinical and cytogenetic remission; two remain in remission 4 and 5 years from presentation.

The role of bone marrow transplantation is uncertain, and in view of the young age of most of the patients it is desirable to avoid TBI. One of our original patients, who had been in a stable state for 4 years following diagnosis, was treated with cytosine arabinoside, cyclophosphamide TBI and BMT from a histocompatible sibling at the age of four, and remains well 5 years later. Patients receiving BMT after the development of acute leukaemia appear to have a high risk of relapse.

Thus, it seems appropriate in patients with myelodysplasia and monosomy 7 to look for an HLA-compatible sibling donor with a view to BMT. If there is no compatible donor available, chemotherapy alone carries a chance of long-term remission; alternatively, a search may be made for a MUD donor.

OTHER PRIMARY MYELODYSPLASIAS

This section reviews the diagnosis and management of children who present with apparent primary myelodysplasia that is not classed as JCML or infantile monosomy 7. It is extremely difficult to obtain any idea as to the incidence of these disorders. Attempts to estimate the frequency of a preleukaemic phase in AML, such as the survey from Philadelphia (Blank & Lange 1981), postulating that 17% of cases of AML had a preleukaemic phase are obviously biased towards ascertainment of more aggressive forms of MDS; we have no idea how often children develop refractory anaemia (RA) or refractory anaemia with ringed sideroblasts (RARS). The category of CMML in adults is not considered here, since such cases in childhood have been classed as JCML.

Clinical features and diagnosis

Children with MDS are likely to present with refractory anaemia and or thrombocytopenia, with perhaps a history of repeated infections.

Blood and bone marrow will show features suggestive of MDS (see Tables 3.3 and 3.4), and an attempt should be made to classify the findings accordingly. The differential diagnosis depends on the category of MDS; the distinction between refractory anaemia with excess blasts (RAEB), particularly refractory anaemia with excess blasts in transformation (RAEB-t) and acute leukaemia, notably M6 AML, is a nice one, and is not important in practice. The differential diagnosis of the less aggressive forms of MDS, RA and RARS includes other causes of sideroblastic anaemia and megaloblastic anaemia.

Sideroblasts (i.e. normoblasts containing prominent siderotic granules) may occur in the bone marrow in anaemia from many causes (see Ch. 8), and ringed sideroblasts are found in the marrow in MPD and MDS; but in refractory anaemia with ringed sideroblasts, by definition they comprise 15% or more erythroblasts. The blood film in RARS is usually dimorphic with a raised MCV and there may be some abnormalities in the white cell series. By contrast, in congenital sideroblastic anaemia (Ch. 8) the film is hypochromic and abnormalities are confined to the erythroid series.

Megaloblastic anaemia (Ch. 8) is rare in childhood, at least in developed countries, and is characterized by ineffective haemopoeisis and marked myelodysplasia. Paediatricians have a low index of suspicion of megaloblastic anaemia, which can in a hasty moment resemble an acute leukaemia or MDS, particularly in the presence of thrombocytopenia and gross changes in the white cell series. Megaloblastic anaemia in infancy may be due to defective transport of folate or B_{12}, or to other metabolic abnormalites as well as dietary lack or malabsorption of these vitamins.

Chromosome analysis is helpful in this context, the finding of a clone of cells being supportive of myelodysplasia, although absence of any abnormality does not exclude this diagnosis. The common cytogenetic abnormalities are shown in Table 3.5.

Natural history and prognosis

There have been many attempts to assess prognosis in adult MDS. These have been largely based on FAB morphology and variants thereof, and the degree of bone marrow failure supplemented by the results of cytogenetics. There have been several scoring systems, usually modelled on the so-called Bournemouth score (Mufti et al 1985); their relevance to paediatrics becomes even more dubious when it is noted that the median age of such patients is about 70, and that many patients succumb from bone marrow failure or non-haematological disease rather than from progression to myeloid leukaemia. In these scoring systems, important adverse prognostic factors have been anaemia, thrombocytopenia and the proportion of bone marrow blasts.

The recent MIC report reviewed the risk of leukaemic progression in primary MDS as 12% in RA, 8% if sideroblasts were present and, not surprisingly, as higher in RAEB (44%) and RAEB-t (60%).

How relevant is this information to paediatric practice? Wegelius (1986) in a review of 26 cases of MDS in childhood commented on the rarity of sideroblastic anaemia and the high frequency of progression to AML, at a median time in the cases reviewed of 12 months. Similarly, in a report from Italy and Germany (Creutzig et al 1987) the more aggressive forms of MDS predominated. We may conclude that in children, as in adults, RAEB and RAEB-t tend to progress to AML; we do not really have any information about the natural history of the more indolent disorders.

Treatment

Intensive chemotherapy, as used in AML, has in

our experience and that of others (Creutzig et al 1987) achieved true remission in some cases of MDS; however, as in adults, response is less likely than in AML. Long-term remission is probably unlikely in most cases, and the treatment of choice is BMT. The 3-year event-free survival in a group of 59 patients with MDS treated with BMT was 45% (Appelbaum et al 1990). The patients all received cyclophosphamide and total body irradiation, and 45 of 59 donors were HLA identical. The commonest causes of death were disease recurrence, interstitial pneumonitis and GVHD. In multivariate analysis, younger age and karyotypic abnormalities were independently predictive of good survival; recurrence was less likely in patients with fewer marrow blasts. Children are thus the group most likely to benefit from BMT, which should be considered at an early stage. Whilst most patients have received TBI, there are no comparative studies of radiotherapy and chemotherapy-based regimens, and it would seem worth considering chemotherapy conditioning particularly in the younger child.

A search for an MUD donor would be appropriate in patients with no sibling donor.

The place of cytokine therapy in MDS is unclear at present but should be resolved by the many trials at present in progress. While both G-CSF and GM-CSF may induce differentiation of myelodysplastic cells, they may also accelerate progression to leukaemia. The evidence at present is that both cytokines produce an improvement in neutrophil count, but that continued treatment is necessary for this to be sustained. It is uncertain whether neutrophil function is affected, and neither agent produces any improvement in platelet count. The risk of progression to leukaemia is not predictable on the basis of bone marrow blast or FAB morphology, but assays of response in vitro could be helpful in determining sensitivity. A review of data from 83 reported cases showed that increase in marrow blasts occurred in 22, often with rapid progression to leukaemia (Cheson 1990). The next few years should see results of prospective randomized trials of these and other cytokines, both as single agents and in combination. Meanwhile, there would seem to be no indication for cytokine therapy in paediatric MDS outside of the context of a clinical trial.

SECONDARY MYELODYSPLASIA

Congenital bone marrow disorders

Myelodysplasia and myeloid leukaemia may occur in patients with congenital bone marrow diseases (Ch. 2), most notably Fanconi's anaemia and Shwachman's syndrome. In both, the development of more profound anaemia or thrombocytopenia with appearance of blast cells in the blood should prompt bone marrow examination. The bone marrow appearances in this situation may be hard to classify.

The management of such patients once myelodysplasia has developed is extremely difficult and often no specific treatment is possible. Trials of recombinant G-CSF in Shwachman's syndrome, as in other congenital neutropenias, are in progress. However, even if cytokines are found to be effective in the chronic phase of neutropenia, the risk of accelerating leukaemic progression particularly during a myelodysplastic phase will still remain. Patients with Fanconi's anaemia and MDS or AML are resistant to chemotherapy, and the treatment of choice for Fanconi's anaemia is BMT using a suitably modified preparative regimen (see Ch. 2). Once patients have developed AML or MDS transplantation will be less effective.

Treatment-related MDS

Background and clinical features

Secondary MDS and AML have been most comprehensively studied in Hodgkin's disease, where the advent of a second cancer in a highly curable condition is a tragedy to be prevented if at all possible. Secondary MDS has also been reported with variable frequency in nonHodgkin's lymphoma (NHL), myeloma, ovarian cancer and a variety of other solid tumours. While a genetic association between the two types of cancer cannot be excluded in all cases, there is a strong association between the form of treatment given and the risk of secondary MDS/AML. The drugs most clearly implicated are the alkylating agents, including cyclophosphamide, chlorambucil, procarbazine and nitrosoureas. Naturally, most of the published information concerns adult patients. A recent international case control study (Kaldor et al 1990) confirmed that the use of chemotherapy in Hodgkin's disease increased the risk of leukemia by a factor of 9 compared with radiotherapy, that the risk was related to total drug dosage and that it was not significantly increased by the addition of radiotherapy to chemotherapy. It must be emphasized that the risk of treatment-related leukaemia/MDS is outweighed by the benefit of improved survival associated with combination chemotherapy. However, the need for equally effective but less toxic regimens is clear. The first United Kingdom Childrens Cancer Study Group (UKCCSG) protocol for non-Hodgkin's lymphoma was associated with an actuarial risk of secondary leukaemia of 7.8% at 7 years; the protocol comprised rotating chemotherapy including nitrosoureas (Ingram et al 1987).

The risk of secondary AML/MDS following treatment for ALL, particularly with newer regimens, is unknown, but in a recent report from St Jude Children's Research Hospital children treated for ALL had a cumulative risk of development of secondary AML of 4.7% at 6 years, the risk being greater in patients with T-ALL. There was no obvious explanation for this finding except that the protocols contained high and repeated doses of epipodophyllotoxin (Pui et al 1989).

The symptoms of secondary MDS are those of bone marrow failure; the median time to development of secondary MDS in one group of 39 patients was 58 months with a range of 11–92 months. Evolution from MDS to AML occurred in 11 of 39 patients in a median of 3 months (Michels et al 1985).

The morphological characteristics of secondary MDS do not always conform to FAB subtypes. There is often a relatively low proportion of blasts at the time of diagnosis and this is accompanied by marked morphological change in all cell lines. There may be basophilia in both blood and marrow, and cellularity is variable with fibrosis in some cases, thus producing a dilute aspirate (Third MIC Cooperative Study Group 1988).

Cytogenetics

Cytogenetic abnormalities, which may be multiple, are found in 98% of cases of secondary MDS, and in 94% there is some abnormality of chromosomes 5 or 7. It is significant that these chromosomes are also involved in leukaemias

developing after exposure to toxins, and that this type of cytogenetic abnormality is associated with leukaemias which is resistant to treatment.

Careful examination of chromosome 5 in a group of 17 patients showed that there was a critical region of 5q23–q32 which was deleted in all cases; this region contains the genes for many haemopoietic growth factors and differentiating agents (Le Beau et al 1986). There may also be a number of genes involved in haemopoiesis on chromosome 7 in addition to the erythropoietin gene. Thus, it seems very likely that deletion of such genes plays a critical part in development of secondary leukaemia.

An interesting exception to these typical findings is the report from St Jude mentioned previously (Pui et al 1989) in which the secondary AML was associated not with changes in chromosome 5 or 7 but with 11q23, a region frequently involved in malignant transformation of pluripotent stem cells, as in the mixed leukaemias of infancy.

Treatment of secondary MDS

There is little paediatric experience in this difficult field. Treatment of secondary leukaemia and MDS in adults using regimens designed for AML does not yield encouraging results; prolonged marrow hypoplasia and drug resistance are the main obstacles. Bone marrow transplantation has been used in secondary AML and MDS with some success, and would seem at present to be the treatment of choice. Two-year survival figures of 50–60% were quoted in a recent multicentre European survey (de Witte et al 1990) and there was some evidence that patients with secondary AML fared better if an attempt was made to induce remission before transplant.

In summary, children with secondary AML or MDS need full clinical and haematological appraisal. If they are in good health and the prognosis of the primary disorder is good, then it would seem appropriate to proceed to BMT if a donor is available; this should probably be preceded by one or more courses of intensive chemotherapy at least in children with excess of marrow blasts. There is little reason to think that intensive chemotherapy, in the absence of high dose chemoradiotherapy is likely to produce sustained remission.

REFERENCES

Appelbaum F R, Barrall J, Storb R et al 1990 Bone Marrow transplantation for patients with myelodysplasia. Pretreatment variables and outcome. Annals of Internal Medicine 112: 590–597

Apperley J F, Mauro F R, Goldman J M et al 1988 Bone marrow transplantation for chronic myeloid leukaemia in first chronic phase: importance of a graft-versus-leukaemia effect. British Journal of Haematology 69: 239–245

Barnett P L J, Clark A C L, Garson O M 1990 Acute nonlymphocytic leukemia after transient myeloproliferative disorder in a patient with Down syndrome. Medical and Pediatric Oncology 18: 347–353

Bennett J M, Catovsky D, Daniel M T et al 1982 Proposals for the classification of the myelodysplastic syndromes. British Journal of Haematology 51: 189–199

Blank J, Lange B 1981 Preleukemia in children. Journal of Pediatrics 98: 565–568

Brandwein J M, Horsman D E, Eaves A C et al 1990 Childhood myelodysplasia: suggested classification as myelodysplastic syndromes based on laboratory and clinical findings. American Journal of Pediatric Hematology/Oncology 12: 63–70

Cannat A, Seligmann M 1973 Immunological abnormalities in juvenile myelomonocytic leukaemia. British Medical Journal 1: 71–74

Carroll W L, Morgan R, Glader B E 1985 Childhood bone marrow monosomy 7 syndrome: a familial disorder? Journal of Pediatrics 107: 578–580

Castro-Malaspina H, Schaison G, Briere Jean et al 1983 Philadelphia chromosome-positive chronic myelocytic leukemia in children. Cancer 52: 721–727

Castro-Malaspina H, Schaison G, Passe S et al 1984 Subacute and chronic myelomonocytic leukemia in children (juvenile CML). Cancer 54: 675–686

Chan H S L, Estrov Z, Weitzman S S, Freedman M H 1987 The value of intensive combination chemotherapy for juvenile chronic myelogenous leukemia. Journal of Clinical Oncology 5: 1960–1967

Cheson B D 1990 The myelodysplastic syndromes: current approaches to therapy. Annals of Internal Medicine 112: 932–941

Chessells J M, Janossy G, Lawler S D, Secker Walker L M 1979 The Ph' chromosome in childhood leukaemia. British Journal of Haematology 41: 25–41

Creutzig U, Cantu-Rajnoldi A, Ritter J et al 1987 Myelodysplastic syndromes in childhood. Report of 21 patients from Italy and West Germany. American Journal of Pediatric Hematology/Oncology 9: 324–330

Daley G Q, Van Etten R A, Baltimore D 1990 Induction of chronic myelogenous leukemia in mice by the P210 bcr/abl gene of the Philadelphia chromosome. Science 247: 824–830

Darbyshire P J, Shortland D B, Swansbury J G, Sadler J, Lawler S D, Chessells J M 1987 A myeloproliferative disorder in two infants associated with eosinophilia and chromosome t(l;5) translocation. British Journal of Haemotology 6: 483–486

Devergie A, Reiffers J, Vernant J P et al 1990 Long-term follow-up after bone marrow transplantation for chronic myelogenous leukemia: factors associated with relapse. Bone Marrow Transplant 5: 379–386

De Witte T, Zwann F, Hermans J et al 1990 Allogeneic bone marrow transplantation for secondary leukaemia and myelodysplastic syndrome: a survey by the Leukaemia Working Party of the European Bone Marrow Transplant Group (EBMTG). British Journal of Haematology 74: 151–155

Eguchi M, Sakakibara H, Suda J et al 1989 Ultrastructural and ultracytochemical differences between transient myeloproliferative disorder and megakaryoblastic leukaemia in Down's syndrome. British Journal of Haematology 73: 315–332

Evans J P M, Czepulkowski B, Gibbons B, Swansbury G J, Chessells J M 1988 Childhood monosomy 7 revisited. British Journal of Haematology 69: 41–45

Freedman M H, Estrov Z, Chan H S L 1988 Juvenile chronic myelogenous leukemia. American Journal of Pediatric Hematology/Oncology 10: 261–267

Gale R P, Butturini A 1990 Ph-chromosome positive acute leukemias and acute phase CML: one or two diseases? Two. Leukaemia Research 14: 295–297

Ganesan T S, Rassool F, Guo A-P et al 1986 Rearrangement of the bcr gene in Philadelphia chromosome-negative chronic myeloid leukemia. Blood 68: 957–960

Goldman J M, Bortin M M, Champlin R E et al 1985 Bone-marrow transplantation for chronic myelogenous leukaemia. Lancet II: 1295

Gualtieri R J, Emanuel P D, Zuckerman K S et al 1989 Granulocyte-macrophage colony-stimulating factor is an endogenous regulator of cell proliferation in juvenile chronic myelogenous leukemia. Blood 74: 2360–2367

Hardisty R M, Speed D E, Till M 1964 Granulocytic leukaemia in childhood. British Journal of Haematology 10: 551–566

Herrod H G, Dow L W, Sullivan J L 1983 Persistent Epstein-Barr virus infection mimicking juvenile chronic myelogenous leukemia: immunologic and hematologic studies. Blood 61: 1098–1104

Hocking W G, Golde D W 1989 Polycythemia: evaluation and management. Blood Reviews 3: 59–65

Hows J M, Bradley B A 1990 The use of unrelated marrow donors for transplantation. British Journal of Haematology 76: 1–6

Inaba T, Hayashi Y, Hanada R, Nakashima M, Yamamoto K, Nishida T 1988 Childhood myelodysplastic syndromes with 11p15 translocation. Cancer Genetics and Cytogenetics 34: 41–46

Ingram L, Mott M G, Mann J R, Raafat F, Darbyshire P J, Morris Jones P H 1987 Second malignancies in children treated for non-Hodgkin's lymphoma and T-cell leukaemia with the UKCCSG regimens. British Journal of Cancer 55: 463–466

Jacobs A 1989 Oncogenes in the myelodysplastic syndrome. Blood Reviews 3: 105–109

Kaldor J M, Day N E, Clarke A et al 1990 Leukemia following Hodgkin's disease. New England Journal of Medicine 322: 7–13

Kaneko Y, Maseki N, Sakurai M et al 1989 Chromosome pattern in juvenile chronic myelogenous leukemia, myelodysplastic syndrome, and acute leukemia associated with neurofibromatosis. Leukemia 3: 36–41

Kastan M B, Strauss L C, Civin C I 1989 The role of hematopoietic growth factors and oncogenes in leukemogenesis. American Journal of Pediatric Hematology/Oncology 11: 249–267

Klingebiel T, Creutzig U, Dopfer R 1990 Bone marrow transplantation in comparison with conventional therapy in children with adult type chronic myelogenous leukemia. Bone Marrow Transplantation 5: 317–320

Le Beau M M, Albain K S, Larson R A et al 1986 Clinical and cytogenetic correlations in 63 patients with therapy-related myelodysplastic syndromes and acute non-lymphoblastic leukaemia: further evidence for characteristic abnormalities of chromosomes No 5 and No 7. Journal of Clinical Oncology 4: 325–345

Leiper A D, Stanhope R, Lau T et al 1987 The effect of total body irradiation and bone marrow transplantation during childhood and adolescence on growth and endocrine function. British Journal of Haematology 67: 419–426

Lilleyman J S, Harrison J F, Black J A 1977 Treatment of juvenile chronic myeloid leukemia with sequential subcutaneous cytarabine and oral mercaptopurine. Blood 49: 559–562

List A F, Garewal H S, Sandberg A A 1990 The myelodysplastic syndromes: biology and implications for management. Journal of Clinical Oncology 8: 1424–1441

McGlave P B, Beatty P, Ash R, Hows J M 1990 Therapy for chronic myelogenous leukemia with unrelated donor bone marrow transplantation: Results in 102 cases. Blood 75: 1728–1732

Michels S D, McKenna R W, Arthur D C, Brunning R D 1985 Therapy-related acute myeloid leukemia and myelodysplastic syndrome: a clinical and morphologic study of 65 cases. Blood 65: 1364–1372

Morris S W, Daniel L, Ahmed C M I, Elias A, Lebowitz P 1990 Relationship of bcr breakpoint to chronic phase duration, survival, and blast crisis lineage in chronic myelogenous leukemia patients presenting in early chronic phase. Blood 75: 2035–2041

Mufti G J, Stevens J R, Oscier D G, Hamblin T J, Machin D 1985 Myelodysplastic syndromes: a scouring system with prognostic significance. British Journal of Haematology 59: 425–433

Nix W L, Fernbach D J 1981 Myeloproliferative diseases in childhood. American Journal of Pediatric Hematology/Oncology 3: 397–407

Nowell P C, Hungerford D A 1960 A minute chromosome in human granulocytic leukemia. Science 132: 1497

Nowell P, Bergman G, Besa E, Wilmoth D, Emanuel B 1984 Progressive preleukemia with a chromosomally abnormal clone in a kindred with the Estren-Dameshek variant of Fanconi's anemia. Blood 64: 1135–1138

Paul B, Reid M M, Davison E V, Abela M, Hamilton P J 1987 Familial myelodysplasia: progressive disease associated with emergence of monosomy 7. British Journal of Haematology 65: 321–323

Pearson T C 1991 Primary thrombocythemia—diagnosis and management. British Journal of Haematology 78: 145–148

Pugh W C, Pearson M, Vardiman J W, Rowley J D 1985 Philadelphia chromosome-negative chronic meylogenous leukaemia: a morphological reassessment. British Journal of Haematology 60: 457–467

Pui C H, Behm F G, Raimondi S C et al 1989 Secondary acute myeloid leukemia in children treated for acute lymphoid leukemia. New England Journal of Medicine 321: 136–142

Randall D L, Reiquam C W, Githens J H, Robinson A 1965 Familial myeloproliferative disease. American Journal of Diseases in Children 110: 479–490

Rowley J D 1973 A new consistent chromosomal abnormality in chronic myelogenous leukemia identified by quinicrine fluorescence and Giemsa staining. Nature 243: 290–293

Sanders J E, Pritchard S, Mahoney P et al 1986 Growth and development following marrow transplantation for leukemia. Blood 68: 1129–1135

Sanders J E, Buckner C D, Thomas E D et al 1988 Allogeneic marrow transplantation for children with juvenile chronic myelogenous leukemia. Blood 71: 1144–1146

Schwartz C L, Cohen H J 1988 Preleukaemic syndromes and other syndromes predisposing to leukemia. Pediatric Clinics of North America 35: 853–871

Sieff C A, Malleson P 1980 Familial myelofibrosis. Archives of Disease in Childhood 55: 888–893

Sieff C A, Chessells J M, Harvey B A M, Pickthall V J, Lawler S D 1981 Monosomy 7 in childhood: a myeloproliferative disorder. British Journal of Haematology 49: 235–249

Smith K L, Johnson W 1974 Classification of chronic myelocytic leukemia in children. Cancer 34: 670–679

Talpaz M, Kantarjian H M, McCredie K, Trujillo J M, Keating M J, Gutterman J U 1986 Hematologic remission and cytogenetic improvement induced by recombinant human interferon alpha A in chronic myelogenous leukemia. New England Journal of Medicine 314: 1065–1069

Teasdale J M, Worth A J, Corey M J 1970 A missing group C chromosome in the bone marrow cells of three children with myeloproliferative disease. Cancer 25: 1468–1477

Tefferi A, Thibodeau S N, Solberg L A Jr 1990 Clonal studies in the myelodysplastic syndrome using X-linked restriction fragment length polymorphisms. Blood 75: 1770–1773

Third MIC Cooperative Study Group 1988 Recommendations for a morphologic, immunologic, and cytogenetic (MIC) working classification of the primary and therapy-related myelodysplastic disorders. A report of the workshop held in Scottsdale, Arizona, USA, on February 23–25 1987. Cancer Genetics and Cytogenetics 32: 1–10

Thomas E D, Clift R A 1989 Indications for marrow transplantation in chronic myelogenous leukemia. Blood 73: 861–864

Travis S F 1983 Fetal erythropoiesis in juvenile chronic myelocytic leukemia. Blood 62: 602–605

Tutschka P J, Copelan E A, Klein J P 1987 Bone marrow transplantation for leukemia following a new busulfan and cyclophosphamide regimen. Blood 70: 1382–1388

Urban C, Schwinger W, Slavc I et al 1990 Busulfan/cyclophosphamide plus bone marrow transplantation is not sufficient to eradicate the malignant clone in juvenile chronic myelogenous leukemia. Bone Marrow Transplantation 5: 353–356

Weatherall D J, Edwards J A, Donohoe W T A 1968 Haemoglobin and red cell enzyme changes in juvenile chronic myeloid leukaemia. British Medical Journal 1: 679–681

Wegelius R 1986 Preleukaemic states in children. Scandinavian Journal of Haematology 36: 133–139

Weinberg R S, Leibowitz D, Weinblatt M E, Kochen J, Alter B P 1990 Juvenile chronic myelogenous leukaemia: the only example of truly fetal (not fetal-like) erythropoiesis. British Journal of Haematology 76: 307–310

Weiss K, Stass S, Williams D et al 1987 Childhood monosomy 7 syndrome: clinical and in vitro studies. Leukemia 1: 97–104

Woods W G, Roloff J S, Lukens J N, Krivit W 1981 The occurrence of leukemia in patients with the Shwachman syndrome. Journal of Pediatrics 99: 425–428

Woods W G, Nesbit M E, Buckley J et al 1985 Correlation of chromosome abnormalities with patient characteristics, histologic subtype, and induction success in children with acute nonlymphocytic leukemia. Journal of Clinical Oncology 3: 3–11

4. Acute myeloid leukaemia

I. M. Hann

INTRODUCTION

It is always instructive to look back over the history of a medical subject before considering the current status of the art. Textbooks in the period immediately after the First World War noted that acute myeloid leukaemia (AML) was a disease occurring in adults and only very rarely in children, the chronic form of myeloid leukaemia being more usual. This latter assertion is, of course, untrue, but AML does in fact account for only one-fifth of childhood leukaemia and as a consequence most of what we have learnt has been gleaned from work performed in adults. Little of this mattered because during this period no effective treatment was available and the approach was largely nihilistic, with arsenic being the treatment of choice. By the late 1920s, a firmer differentiation of acute leukaemia from other blood disorders, such as aplastic anaemia and reactive changes, was possible because bone marrow examination became more widely practical; this technique remains the mainstay of diagnosis and management. However, despair was still the order of the day and chapters on the subject often had poetic headings such as that of Vaughan's: 'Can anyone tell me what it is? Can you, that wind your thoughts into a clue, to guide out others?' By the time of the Second World War, diagnosis was on a much firmer footing, and Dr Still was able to extol the benefits of supportive care, refinements of which have facilitated the development of effective therapy.

Very few patients with AML were cured until the 1970s, even then success rates reported in series of children such as those from Great Ormond Street in London were uniformly poor, at about 10%. The real breakthrough has occurred within the last 10 years, with the introduction of high-intensity chemotherapy and allogeneic bone marrow transplantation during first remission of the disease. Today, approximately one-third to one-half of all children with AML are cured of their primary disease. Excitement at this dramatic development has to be tempered by uncertainty as to the role of certain modalities of treatment, particularly very high-dose chemotherapy with autologous bone marrow rescue (usually called autologous bone marrow transplantation or ABMT). This chapter will attempt to look at the current state of knowledge as to the nature of AML, the types of treatment known to be effective and what we need to do to have a chance of advancing our capability of curing the disease.

THE BIOLOGICAL NATURE AND EPIDEMIOLOGY OF ACUTE MYELOID LEUKAEMIA

Our knowledge of the nature of AML and its causes is advancing very rapidly. Such research will hopefully lead to further advances in cure and prevention, but at the time of writing has contributed little to the cure of patients.

Epidemiology

Most of the studies which have looked at potential environmental causes of AML are of limited value because they are too small or have not adequately classified the leukaemia. Overall, AML accounts for 1.2% of all cancer deaths in the USA (US OHRST Report 1981). It accounts for approximately 10–12% of leukaemia in US and UK children under the age of 10 years with a doubling of this incidence in young adolescents. However, there is wide geographic variation, suggesting a potential genetic effect. Childhood AML predominates over ALL in several African countries and in Japan (Linet 1985), and there are apparent racial differences within the USA with a significant increasing incidence over time for black children in Baltimore (Gordis et al 1981). Suggestions that greater than expected numbers of cases occur amongst siblings and other relatives of children with AML have not yet been fully substantiated. However, certain chromosomal disorders, such as Down's syndrome (trisomy 21) and Klinefelter's syndrome, predispose to an increased risk of childhood AML. In Down's syndrome there is a preponderance of the megakaryoblastic subtype (French-American-British [FAB] type M7). Disorders characterized by increased susceptibility to chromosome breakage – for examples ataxia-telangiectasia, Bloom's syndrome and Fanconi's anaemia (Linet 1985) – also carry an increased risk of acute leukaemia. Twin studies suggest increased concordance for childhood leukaemia among monozygotic twins; this may result from a common exposure or single leukaemic transformation leading to malignancy in both children through the shared placental circulation (Hartley & Sainsbury 1981). A number of studies have appeared to link prenatal exposure of mothers to smoking, aspirin or antihistamines with childhood leukaemia but none have been proven. There is some evidence that paternal exposure to hydrocarbons and radiation may be of importance, but more careful prospective studies are urgently required. A number of case-control studies are being undertaken to investigate apparent increased risks of childhood leukaemia related to direct exposure to irradiation, high intensity electricity cables and infections. These studies may ultimately give us some insight into what is probably a multistep and multifactorial aetiological process.

Biology

Jacobsen and co-workers in 1984 and Fearon in 1986 have demonstrated that AML is a clonal disease – i.e. it is derived from a single clone of cells. This has been demonstrated in females heterozygous for X-linked enzyme markers and using DNA polymorphisms. The process whereby genetic change creates a leukaemic stem cell and causes it to 'freeze' at a particular stage of differentiation is not clearly understood. What can be demonstrated are well-defined clonal chromosomal abnormalities in a high proportion of cases of AML, and there are no significant differences between adults and children in this respect. This is one of the findings indicating that adult and childhood AML are biologically similar and should be treated along similar lines. The chromosomal findings will be dealt with in detail in a later section but those commonly seen include t(8;21), –7, t(15;17), inv16, 5q–, +8. No oncogenes have been clearly associated with these abnormalities but three of the haemopoietic growth factors (GM-CSF, M-CSF and interleukin-3) are located on chromosome 5(q20–q30) which also contains the locus for the M-CSF receptor which is identical to the oncogene c-fms. 5q– is present in therapy-related myelodysplasia and acute leukaemia (Nimer & Golde 1987). The G-CSF gene is located at 17(q11), close to the breakpoint t(15;17) seen in most acute promyelocytic leukaemia cases.

None of these observations tells us what the basic defect is leading to leukaemia, but recent interesting work has demonstrated that an autocrine network of self-stimulation of leukaemia cells producing G-CSF leads to autonomous growth of these cells. What remains unclear at present is the role of networks of interacting growth factors and inhibitory factors in this process. In fact, the lack of action of inhibitory substances such as T-cell derived growth factors may be crucial in the sustained and uncontrolled growth and failure of differentiation that occurs in leukaemia.

CLINICAL FEATURES AND DIAGNOSIS

The majority of children with AML present with features related to bone marrow failure. Anaemia produces lethargy, pallor, anorexia and headaches. Thrombocytopenia leads to purpura, petechiae, overt bleeding (often from the nose or gastrointestinal tract) and sometimes internal bleeding. The latter is usually intracranial and there is a strong association with high presenting white cell count and leukostasis. Rarely, bleeding occurs in other sites, such as the lung, also often associated with leukostasis and high white cell counts. Reduction in normal neutrophil numbers and function predisposes to infection and fever. Symptoms are often present for several days before presentation. Bone pain and irritability are also frequently seen at diagnosis.

The clinical findings in children with AML are often less dramatic than those seen in ALL, but those with the FAB M4 and M5 subtypes (see below) have more extramedullary disease, including skin and gum infiltration, and more CNS involvement (Chessells et al 1986). Other rare distinctive findings are myeloblastic chloromas; these are solid tumours found around the orbits, spinal cord or cranium. Testicular involvement is very rare, although meningeal involvement affects about one in six children with AML at diagnosis (Stevens et al 1990). Modest hepatomegaly and more striking splenomegaly are common, but generalized lymphadenopathy is unusual other than in monocytic cases (M4 and M5).

Morphological classification

The diagnosis of acute myeloid leukaemia still rests largely upon the examination of good quality smears of aspirated bone marrow. The two main exceptions to this rule are the rare cases where very high blood blast counts preclude the need, and the rare patients whose marrow cannot be aspirated. The latter occurs when there is very extensive marrow fibrosis, usually associated with acute megakaryoblastic leukaemia (FAB subtype M7). Myelofibrosis in children is a secondary reactive event associated with leukaemia, disseminated infections, myelodysplasias and other causes; it is probably rarely, if ever, a primary phenomenon and the various outmoded titles of 'acute myelofibrosis', 'idiopathic myelofibrosis', 'familial myelofibrosis', etc. are thus inappropriate. In the context of M7 AML, the diagnosis can usually be confirmed by immunological staining of bone marrow trephine preparations with anti-platelet antibodies such as CD51 or anti-factor VIII. Having said this, the majority of cases fall into convenient FAB groups based on morphology using simple Romanowsky stains together with Sudan black and combined esterases (Table 4.1):

M1 (Acute myeloid leukaemia undifferentiated)

These cases are difficult to distinguish from the macrolymphoblastic type of ALL (FAB L2). The blasts are usually devoid of Auer rods, and negative with the immunological marker terminal deoxynucleotidyl transferase (TdT). Granulation is not prominent and there is little if any differentiation. Some workers use the designation M0 for cases which appear even more difficult to distinguish from ALL but this is not very helpful.

M2 (Acute myeloid leukaemia with differentiation)

In contrast, the myeloid differentiation is obvious here, and Auer rods are usually present. When

Table 4.1 Summary of the quantitative bone marrow criteria proposed for the diagnosis of acute myeloid leukaemia subtypes

Bone marrow cells	Subtype[1]				
	M1	M2	M4	M5	M6
Blasts (%)					
All nucleated cells	–	> 30	> 30	–	< 30 or > 30
Nonerythroid cells	90 (I + II)[2]	> 30	> 30	> 80[3]	> 30
Erythroblasts, all nucleated cells (%)	–	< 50	< 50	–	> 50
Granulocytic components[4], nonerythroid cells (%)	< 10	> 10	> 20[5]	< 20	Variable
Monocytic component[6], nonerythroid cells (%)	< 10	< 20	> 20	> 80[3]	Variable

[1] Lysozyme estimations and cytochemical tests are required if the peripheral blood monocyte counts is 5×10^9/l or more but the marrow suggests M2, and if the marrow suggests M4 but the peripheral blood monocyte count is less than 5×10^9/l (see text).
[2] Blasts type I and II, as previously described (10).
[3] Monoblasts in M5a; and in M5b the predominant cells are promonocytes and monocytes.
[4] Promyelocytes, myelocytes, metamyelocytes and neutrophils.
[5] May include myeloblasts.
[6] Promonocytes and monocytes.
(Reproduced from Bennett et al 1985, with permission.)

looked at in AML overall, Auer rod positivity indicates a better prognosis, but this needs to be looked at along with other features in larger studies (Ritter et al 1989). Sudan black and chloroacetate esterase positivity are present.

M3 (Acute promyelocytic leukaemia)

Most of these cases are obvious, with extremely prominent granulation and multiple Auer rods ('faggots') with strong Sudan black positivity. In occasional cases, the granulation can be less prominent but the folded nuclei ('cottage-loaf' effect) indicate the diagnosis. Disseminated intravascular coagulation is often present and is probably initiated by proteolysis of fibrinogen.

M4 (Acute myelomonocytic leukaemia)

Monocytes, promonocytes, myeloblasts and other myeloid cells are intermixed, with cytochemical stains showing positivity for myeloid (Sudan black) and monocytic (nonspecific esterase) cells.

M5 (Acute monoblastic M5a and monocytic M5b)

This variety shows positivity with nonspecific esterase only, and has a minimal myeloid component. Half of the cases occur in children, below the age of 2 years. Patients often exhibit hyperleukocytosis and leukostasis due to the physical properties of monocytic cells which have great adhesiveness, lack of deformability and motility (Odom et al 1990). In addition to nonspecific esterase, acid phosphatase stains are strongly positive with a diffuse pattern.

M6 (Erythroleukaemia)

Nucleated red cells as well as primitive erythroblasts occur in the blood of some patients. The marrow shows a striking increase in megaloblastic erythroblasts with a minor population of myeloblasts in some cases. Some bizarre giant forms may be present. There are characteristic multiple globules of PAS positivity (Malkin & Freeman 1989).

M7 (Acute megakaryocytic leukaemia)

Properly classified only in the last 5 years, this disorder is associated with Down's syndrome,

younger age and osteosclerosis. The marrow is usually densely fibrotic and often impossible to aspirate. Blasts are positive, with anti-platelet glycoprotein, IIb/IIIa complex and other platelet markers. CD51 is amongst the best. The cells are often small and undistinguished, but cytoplasmic blebs are often prominent and bizarre megakaryocytes are sometimes seen along with big platelet fragments. They do not stain with Sudan black, but PAS and acid phosphatase are often positive in a localized pattern. The nonspecific esterase is strongly positive but alpha-naphthol butyrate esterase negative, distinguishing them from monocytes. Children with this disease can respond surprisingly well to therapy, but bone marrow recovery can be slow whilst the fibrosis is recovering.

Immunophenotyping

With the development of more and better characterised antibodies, surface and cytoplasmic immunological markers have come to play a major part in the diagnosis and management of AML. Now that more patients are surviving, it is also possible to look at correlates with prognostic outcome. A small proportion of AML cases, usually a few M1, some M6, and all M7 cases, are difficult to define without these markers. The undifferentiated cases can usually be distinguished from ALL by their lack of B- and T-cell markers and terminal deoxynucleotidyl transferase (TdT) negativity. The M6 erythroleukaemia cases are positive for markers detecting spectrin and glycophorin, and M7 by the platelet markers already mentioned. Studies performed mainly in adults have looked at various monoclonal antibodies (McAb) and established that: CD34 is expressed on progenitor cells, AML and 30% of ALL; CD15 stains AML cells with granulocytic differentiation and the normal granulocytic lineage from promyelocytes onwards; CD13 recognizes AML with granulocyte or monocyte differentiation; CD11c and CD14 recognize monocytes; and CD33 recognizes most AML cases. CD13 and CD33 are, however, present in rare cases of ALL in childhood and all of these tests must be interpreted with some caution.

Table 4.2 shows the correlations between FAB

Table 4.2 Correlations between FAB classification and surface antigen expression

	FAB subtype								
	M0	M1	M2	M3	M4	M5a	M5b	M6	M7
Total no. cases	7	18	21	19	27	25	25	5	1
No. cases expressing > 20% McAb positivity									
NHL 30.5*	6	10	11	1	18	12	6	4	0
CD13	5	12	18	13	19	16	15	3	1
CD14	1	5	5	6	14	12	20	4	1
CD15	5	13	19	18	22	14	14	4	1
CD33	0	6	7	3	7	12	15	4	1
CD34	6	11	11	5	19	13	7	3	0

*Recognizes a 180-kDa protein expressed on AML cells and normal marrow progenitors. Askew et al, Blood 67; 1098, 1985.
McAb = Monoclonal antibody
Table adapted from Campos et al, Br J Haematol 72: 161, 1989 with permission.

classification and surface antigen expression in a series of adult AML cases recently reported by Campos et al (1989). This shows a correlation of CD14 with monocytic subtypes, and that CD15 was mainly expressed in M2 and M3 types. CD34 and NHL 30.5 were expressed in particular on the undifferentiated and M1 cases.

This series was of interest because the patients were treated with the same intensive protocol and studied prospectively. Positivity for NHL 30.5 was associated with shorter survival, and CD15 positivity with longer survival, but duration of complete remission was not affected. Further studies along these lines are under way in various trials including the UK Medical Research Council Acute Myeloid Leukaemia Trial 10.

Recently, van der Schoot et al have described a McAb against myeloperoxidase (MPO). This substance is localized in the azurophilic granules of myeloid cells and synthesis occurs at an early stage of differentiation. It is therefore potentially specific for myeloid cells and this does indeed seem to have been demonstrated. 206 cases of AML were studied and the McAb was shown to have a higher diagnostic sensitivity and specificity for AML than the McAbs described above. It will now be studied in prospective trials.

Cytogenetics

There have been many studies of chromosomal abnormalities in children and adults with acute myeloid leukaemia. We are indebted to the St Jude's Group (Kalwinsky et al 1990) for clarifying the situation with a comprehensive study of 155 children treated between 1980 and 1987. Adequate banding was achieved in 120, and 20% were normal, 30% had miscellaneous clonal abnormalities, and 50% fell into known cytogenetic subgroups (Fig. 4.1). These were: inv(16)/del(16q) n=15, t(8;21) n=14, t(15;17) n=9, t(9;11) n=9, t(11;v)/del(11q) n=7, and -7/del(7q) n=6. The inv(16)/del (16q)-positive AML cases frequently had central nervous system (CNS) disease at diagnosis or initially relapsed in this site, indicating that more intensive CNS-directed therapy is required in these patients. There was no predilection for any FAB subtype in this group. The

DISTRIBUTION OF FAB SUBTYPES AMONG CYTOGENETIC SUBSETS OF CHILDHOOD AML

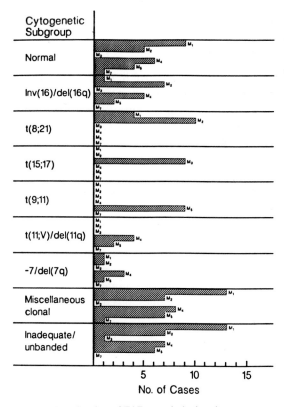

Fig. 4.1 Distribution of FAB morphologic subtypes among cytogenetically defined subsets of patients with de novo childhood AML. (Reproduced from: Kalwinsky et al 1990, with permission.)

infants with M5 disease and t(9;11) did significantly better than others within the M5 group. The other infants often had high white cell counts and frequent coagulation abnormalities and usually relapsed early during therapy; none survived past 16 months.

Children with monosomy 7 had resistant leukaemia and only 17% entered remission, indicating that they need different induction therapy. Those with t(15;17) had M3 disease and did relatively badly because of haemorrhagic deaths during remission induction therapy. Leukaemia-free survival is comparably good in this group, underlining the importance of supporting the patients through the initial few days of therapy.

PROGNOSTIC FACTORS

With improved survival from AML has come a natural desire to predict those patients who will do better or worse. Although it is still early days, it does look as though patients can be segregated into risk groups and so it is possible to begin to think about means of producing better results. The best examples of this include the need to improve CNS disease control in monocytic varieties and those with inv(16)/del(16q) chromosomal changes, and the prevention of early deaths from bleeding in children with promyelocytic leukaemia. However, care must be taken to avoid the danger (also present in trials of ALL stratified by 'risk group') of making premature assumptions about certain modalities of therapy (e.g. etoposide for monocytic variants or retinoids for promyelocytic leukaemia, or cranial irradiation where CNS disease is a problem) which then become accepted practice without proper randomized studies. We should continue to enter patients into randomized trials of intensive therapy without prejudice until therapeutic questions have been properly answered.

At present, there is broad agreement that the following are adverse prognostic factors: monosomy 7, previous myelodysplasia, blast crisis of chronic myeloid leukaemia, high white cell count, monocytic varieties, CNS disease at diagnosis, and longer time to achieve remission. Good prognostic factors are more difficult to define and more uncertain, but may include: the presence of

Auer rods, a high percentage Sudan black positivity, marrow eosinophilia and, of course, lack of all the bad risk features. (Swirsky et al 1986, Creutzig et al 1987, Grier et al 1987, Weinstein et al 1987). There is no real evidence that young age is of independent significance, but infants of course exhibit a higher incidence of the poor risk features, as previously described.

There are continuing attempts to predict response to drugs by in vitro tests, rather like microbiological testing of antibiotics against pathogens. Although this is unlikely to have wide clinical application in the near future, the results are beginning to look interesting and further work is at last underway (Dow et al 1986).

SUPPORTIVE CARE

Success with leukaemia treatment has paralleled improvements in supportive care in a similar way as the advances in surgery consequent upon modern anaesthesia. The subject is a large one and it is not the purpose of this text to produce a menu for management of intensive therapy any more than it is to produce detailed chemotherapy protocols. Treatment of children with AML is extremely tricky and depends most of all upon nurses and junior doctors with paediatric training, supported by the complex and expensive ancillary services provided within children's units.

Haemorrhage

The management of AML has been considerably easier since the more intensive use of blood products. While there are, of course, no randomized trials to prove this assertion, we rarely see haemorrhagic deaths nowadays and those that do occur are confined almost entirely to children with high white cell counts. It is likely that leukostasis in the brain and lungs (usually of monocytes/monoblasts) contributes significantly to the internal bleeding which occurs in these patients. It is thus important to reduce the blast count as quickly as possible using full-dose conventional therapy as soon as the diagnosis is established. This does run the risk of producing tumour lysis syndrome (see below) but this may occur whatever antileukaemic therapy is given and there is no evidence that a gradualist approach is any better.

Children with AML need to be very closely and regularly monitored, which includes blood counts and full coagulation screening. The usual approach is to keep the platelet count above $20 \times 10^9/l$ at all times, and probably higher when the child is febrile because there is then a higher risk of bleeding. It is sometimes necessary to replace blood products in line with *defined* coagulation abnormalities, although it is not essential to do so when the abnormality is mild or moderate and the patient is afebrile, not bleeding and does not have a very high white cell count.

Patients with promyelocytic leukaemia (M3) are also at risk of haemorrhage, although this disease is relatively rare in childhood. Unfortunately, proper controlled studies of various supportive measures have not been carried out. The balance of evidence is if anything in favour of using intensive blood product support without heparinization (Goldberg et al 1986). A tricky problem with heparin use is how one should monitor the dose in the face of already disordered coagulation. The best method is probably to keep the anti-Xa levels between 0.60 and 0.80 U/ml, although an alternative approach is to give a standard dose of 7.5 U/kg per hour by continuous i.v. infusion, rising to a maximum of 15 U/kg per hour depending on whether or not the fibrinogen level continues to decline. However, it should be pointed out that there is no real evidence that this approach works, and the incidence of life-threatening and fatal bleeding between trials which used and did not use heparin is remarkably similar, at about 20% (Cunningham et al 1988, Goldberg et al 1986). It would be of some interest to perform more trials in this area, but they would need to be multicentre and possibly multinational, and should also look at the efficacy of the new low molecular weight heparin compounds (Nieuwenhuis & Sixma 1985). In addition, the use of antifibrinolytic agents, such as tranexamic acid, should be investigated, because one small controlled randomized study (Avvisati et al 1989) showed beneficial effects of the drug over placebo. Trials of retinoids are in progress and look promising.

At present, the important points about managing M3 patients are that they should be very carefully monitored, treated with intensive blood product support and induced into a remission as

rapidly and as gently as possible, at which time the risk of bleeding will dramatically reduce. Retinoids (trans retinoic acid) may offer an alternative to conventional chemotherapy (Coco et al 1991).

Tumour lysis syndrome and other problems with high white blood cell counts

The problem of hyperuricaemia, hyperkalaemia, hyperphosphataemia and hypocalcaemia is much less common in AML than it is in acute lymphoblastic leukaemia (ALL) of childhood. In fact, it is confined to those patients with high counts, and this is almost entirely the patients in the M4 and M5 categories. There have been a number of attempts to produce menus for the avoidance and treatment of these problems, but the prevention of serious difficulties by the use of allopurinol (intravenous or oral) along with forced alkaline diuresis and supplemented by treatment of specific metabolic derangements as they arise is a highly skilled process. More than in any other field of paediatric oncology, tumour lysis syndrome highlights the need for specialist paediatric trained nurses and doctors who monitor progress by the minute and hour, including through the night. With such an approach, very few patients should die of this complication and each death should be regarded as a tragedy in an otherwise potentially curable child.

All children with AML are at risk of isolated hyperuricaemia which can lead to pre-renal failure, convulsions and other complications. They should thus all receive allopurinol 100 mg/m^2 three times a day, which can be given i.v. or by mouth. Higher doses are potentially dangerous and can lead to xanthine nephropathy.

Patients with high white blood cell (WBC) counts are more susceptible to bleeding (see above) and to the problems of leukostasis. This can present with cerebral dysfunction and lung dysfunction with chest X-ray changes as the most common manifestations. These problems were often fatal in the past and their avoidance has largely been achieved by avoidance of blood transfusion until the WBC falls significantly, by adequate hydration and, most importantly, by pressing on with full antileukaemic therapy. Lysis or removal of the leukaemic white cells is mandatory and the best way to do this is with active chemotherapy. Leukapheresis in children is difficult, dangerous and not very effective, and this author cannot think of a situation in which its use is justified.

Nutrition

In the past, most patients were marasmic within a few weeks of starting treatment for AML. The introduction of planned enteral and parenteral feeding has dramatically improved this situation, and in so doing has generally improved the child's condition, ability to recover more quickly from extremely intensive therapy and ability to ward off infection. In most modern centres, patients are encouraged to exercise as much as possible, and the combination of good nutrition with a more active approach to 'physiotherapy' has undoubtedly been of benefit. All patients with AML require that a right atrial indwelling silastic catheter be inserted before or very shortly after instituting therapy. In order to facilitate intravenous feeding, which is required eventually in the majority of patients, a dual or triple-lumen Broviac variety is probably preferable. Some patients manage without any special feeding measures and others will tolerate enteral feeding, but these are the exceptions.

Vomiting is a real problem with AML therapy and the various conventional antiemetics have not ablated this problem. However, the new serotonin antagonists such as ondansetron look more hopeful and are now undergoing clinical trials. The key to parenteral feeding is to anticipate the need for it rather than using it when marasmus and other problems have already arisen. The administration of intravenous feeding is very expensive in terms of money and manpower and requires the presence of clean air suites for preparation. Units which are not expert in managing this vital aspect of therapy should not undertake AML treatment.

Infection

In view of the size of the subject, the complexity of the problems and the apparently infinite numbers of organisms involved, this chapter will discuss only the most important and controversial forms of therapy and the organisms which commonly cause significant illness. The reader is referred to textbooks such as the excellent one by Rubin & Young (1987) for more details.

Children undergoing AML treatment are probably the highest risk group for serious infection that any paediatric haematologist/oncologist has to deal with. Thus, it would seem absolutely reasonable to direct the main effort at prevention. Unfortunately, very few of the measures which have been enthusiastically adopted are of any proven benefit. The reasons for this are twofold: firstly, very few properly conducted trials have been carried out; and secondly the measures generally have only one effect, which is to heighten anxiety and make medical and nursing staff feel better. The only approaches to infection control and treatment of proven value are as follows:

1. *High efficiency air filtration* reduces the risk of aspergillus infection and the other, much rarer, airborne organisms. Laminar flow isolation is of no proven value.

2. *Prophylactic acyclovir.* Patients seropositive for herpes simplex virus (HSV) can be protected against recrudescence following bone marrow transplantation (BMT) by prophylactic acyclovir orally 7 mg/kg 3 times a day or i.v. 5 mg/kg twice a day.

3. *Cotrimoxazole* 480 mg/m^2 twice daily, 3 times a week prevents *Pneumocystis carinii* pneumonia following BMT. Inhaled pentamidine may have the same effect but has not been properly tried out and there are indications that it may not suppress systemic infection elsewhere.

4. *Broad spectrum empirical antibiotics.* The best-tested and efficacious initial empirical antibiotic regimen for treating febrile neutropenic patients is an aminoglycoside and ureidopenicillin (Sage et al 1988) or an aminoglycoside and ceftazidime (EORTC 1987). AML patients are at very high risk of overwhelming infection, and broad-spectrum therapy must be instituted as a matter of urgency in the face of pyrexia and neutropenia. Many studies have shown that the highest risk group for a poor outcome of infection is that with persistent and profound ($< 0.1 \times 10^9$/l) granulocytopenia. The use of double beta-lactam combinations and monotherapy, and the use of newer agents such as imipenem are not justified until they have been subjected to large randomized trials in the highest risk patients. All the evidence is in favour of giving the antibiotic course for

about 5 days after temperature resolution, with a minimum course of 9 days for bacteraemias. Longer courses have been shown to be associated with an increasing risk of severe fungal infection.

5. *Persistent pyrexia of unknown origin.* Patients who are persistently pyrexial for 72–96 hours, persistently severely granulocytopenic, not responding to broad-spectrum antibiotics and with no organism found are the biggest challenge to cure. The EORTC trials have shown that this group of patients has a high mortality and high incidence of fungal infection found at post mortem. It has also been shown that patients in this situation treated with empirical amphotericin B at 72–96 hours do better than those who just have antibiotics fiddled about with. The toxic side-effects are usually easily dealt with by pretreatment with hydrocortisone and chlorpheniramine. This knowledge allows us to develop a planned progressive approach to therapy of infection, the author's version of which is shown in Figure 4.2.

An additional problem noted in recent years is the markedly increasing incidence of hepatosplenic candidiasis. Any patient developing hepatosplenomegaly and fever may have this infection or a viral infection due to CMV or HSV.

6. *Gut decontamination.* Gut sterilization of various types is of no proven value and is extremely unpalatable for children. Compliance is poor and psychological disturbance frequent. The *quinolone antibiotics* (e.g. ciprofloxacin/norfloxacin) preserve the anaerobic gut flora and selectively decontaminate. Preliminary studies in adults (see Hann 1988) are producing very encouraging results which suggest good compliance and a genuine reduction in Gram-negative bacteraemia. Unfortunately, these agents are not yet licensed for use in children because of possible toxicity to growing cartilage. Sterile diets are not of proven value, but a 'clean' diet is a justified approach.

7. *Renal tubular leak.* Patients receiving an aminoglycoside, particularly if given with a ureido-

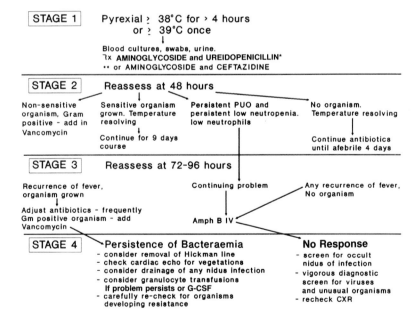

Fig. 4.2 A planned progressive approach to infection in severely neutropenic cancer patients.* If the patient has recently received a ureidopenicillin eg piperacillin we would usually start with an aminoglycoside and ceftazidine, especially if ureidopenicillin-resistant Gram-negative rods are present in stool cultures. **The choice of an initial regimen depends upon the local flora and fauna which *must* be carefully and continually monitored especially for aminoglycoside resistance. If this develops then amikacin will probably be the first choice. If ureidopenicillin resistance occurs then ceftazidine will be the first choice at the present time.

penicillin and amphotericin B, are very susceptible to renal tubular leaks of various salts. The most important of these is potassium and severe hypokalaemia may ensue. The problem can largely be abrogated by the use of the potassium-sparing diuretics amiloride or spironolactone. Potassium, calcium and magnesium supplements are also often required. The oto- and nephro-toxicity of the regimens used can be contained at a low level (Sage et al 1988) with very careful monitoring of aminoglycoside and vancomycin levels. There is little evidence that one aminoglycoside is better than another in this respect.

8. *Haemopoietic growth factors.* White cell transfusions are of extremely limited value in the management of infection. The dose which can be collected by leukapheresis of steroid-treated donors is too small to be of great benefit. Occasionally, a patient with persistent bacteraemia can perhaps be helped over by a prolonged course of daily or twice daily infusions. In future, it is likely that the recombinant growth factors, such as granulocyte-macrophage colony-stimulating factors (GM-CSF) or granulocyte colony stimulating factor (G-CSF), will fulfil this role by stimulating endogenous production of neutrophils if it can be shown that they do not at the same time stimulate the leukaemic blasts. Trials are under way in which these agents (sometimes in combination with interleukin-3 [IL-3] or other growth factors) are used from the outset of AML chemotherapy courses and prior to and throughout bone marrow transplantation (BMT) in order to shorten the duration of severe neutropenia to a more manageable length of time. It is likely that the introduction of these agents will alter our approach to therapy in the near future.

9. *Metronidazole* is used far too frequently in the management of AML and for very flimsy reasons and indications. The EORTC and other trials have repeatedly shown that anaerobic infections are very uncommon in such patients. To use it as an empirical agent is not justified especially when the indications are as vague as oral mucositis and diarrhoea. When loose stools occur a vigorous search for potentially treatable organisms (e.g. *Clostridium difficile*, campylobacter, isospora, cryptosporidium) is required and specific therapy given if required.

10. *Management of interstitial pneumonia.* One of the most awkward problems is still that of interstitial pneumonia. Diagnosis is difficult and potentially hazardous and there is a myriad of causative organisms. The author's approach is to give high-dose co-trimoxazole for up to 48 hours at the same time as instituting a vigorous search for usual and unusual organisms by culture of nasopharyngeal aspirates (NPA), blood and swabs and also by serology. In this way we hope to eventually detect a proportion of the most common organisms such as measles, *Pneumocystis carinii*, mycoplasma, legionella, cytomegalovirus and other respiratory viruses. A chest X-ray can be diagnostically helpful, demonstrating cavitating fungus balls in aspergillus infection, for example. However, in the author's experience its value often rests only in assessing response to therapy.

In patients who do not respond by 48 hours and in whom the various tests such as NPA for measles, IgM mycoplasma and blood cultures are negative, a bronchoalveolar lavage should be seriously considered and, if this did not give the answer, an open lung biopsy. However, in patients who remain fairly stable at this stage the author would probably favour the empirical addition of high-dose erythromycin before proceeding to a more interventionist approach. This is always a difficult decision because rapid deterioration can occur and it is always best to know what one is dealing with before the patient becomes too ill to tolerate diagnostic procedures. One problem frequently seen after BMT is cytomegalovirus (CMV) pneumonia, and the results of therapy have dramatically improved probably because of therapy with gancyclovir and high-dose CMV immunoglobulin.

Other supportive care

Much has been written about the psychosocial aspects of management in childhood leukaemia. The only way to obtain experience in this area is to be actively involved in the team management of a number of children over many years. As with all aspects of management of children with malignant disease, there really is no room for the type of individualism which has existed over the years. These children need to be managed in units which can provide *comprehensive* care and this aspect is a particularly important one. Ideally, the team of doctors and nurses should also include the following: dietitian, occupational therapist, liaison health visitor, play therapist, psychologist and physiotherapist. The majority should attend at least weekly ward rounds, and in most units they also constitute the nucleus of psychosocial 'rounds' and the 'continuing care team' which provides essential community liaison and, if appropriate, terminal care. This team of workers will also provide the contact with local 'shared care' hospitals and can provide a certain amount of treatment in the home including management of central venous catheters.

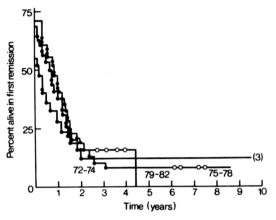

Fig. 4.3 Duration of first remission in three consecutive series of patients treated at the Hospital for Sick Children, London, 1972–1982. There was no improvement in survival (12% at 3 years) over the 10-year period studied.

TREATMENT REGIMENS

When one is called upon to review the treatment of AML in children, two things become apparent. Firstly, the dramatic improvement in therapy over the last 10 years, which outstrips that of any other advance in paediatric oncology. This is well illustrated when comparing current results of chemotherapy and BMT (see Fig. 4.6, p. 96) with a typical series for the period 1972–1982 in which the survival remained static at 12% at 3 years (Fig. 4.3). Secondly, despite the myriad possible regimens, modern published series produce remarkably similar results despite the use of different statistical methods for reporting events. The details of these trials are summarized in Table 4.3. The complete remission rates of studies carried out in the 1980s vary between 75% and 91%; this may be compared with the current United Kingdom

Medical Research Council AML Trial (MRC AML 10) which has a 90% rate for the first hundred patients entered to Spring 1990. The event-free survival rates vary between 20 and 52%, with the most recent studies hovering around 40%. There is no evidence that one regimen is better than any other, and assertions to the contrary are ridiculous in view of the small numbers entered into all the studies except USCCSG 251. The main questions still to be answered are as follows:

1. Can we reduce the high relapse rate associated with current regimens (about 40%) and deal with primary disease resistance (about 10%)?
2. Can we further reduce the deaths related to infection and haemorrhage (about 10%)?
3. Will very high dose chemotherapy with

Table 4.3 Results of recent therapeutic studies of AML in childhood (Adapted from: Lie S 1989, with permission.)

Study	BFM-78[1]	St Jude 80[2]	AIEOP 82043[3]	BFM-83[4]	VAPA[5]	Boston 80-035[6]	USCCSG 251[7]	UK[8]
Years entered	1978–82	1980–83	1982–86	1983–86	1976–80	1980–84	1979–83	1982–85
Total no. entered	151	87	133	143	61	64	508	66
Induction deaths	19	16	13	18	16	19	161	6
Resistant disease	13	6	13	21				
Complete response rate	80%	75%	80%	79%	74%	70%	68%	91%
Event-free survival excluding BMT	49%	20%	33%	52%	33%	29%	25%	42%

[1] Creutzig et al Am J Paed Hem/Onc 9: 324–30 1987
[2] Dahl et al Acute Leukaemias Springer 83–87 1987
[3] Amadori et al J Clin Oncol 5: 1356–1363 1987
[4] Creutzig et al 4th Int Symp on Acute leukaemia Rome 220 1987
[5] Weinstein et al Blood 62: 315–9 1983
[6] Weinstein et al Acute leukaemias Springer 88–92 1987
[7] Nesbit et al Proc Am Soc Clin Oncol 6: 163, 1987
[8] Marcus et al Acute Leukaemias Springer 346–351 1987

autologous bone marrow transplant rescue (ABMT) add anything to intensive chemotherapy?
4. Does allogeneic BMT add to the survival of patients following intensive chemotherapy?
5. Should certain phenotypes (e.g. M4 and M5 FAB subtypes) be treated in different ways, for instance with cranial radiotherapy?

I am afraid that we do not know the answers to these questions at the present time and this is the strongest possible reason to support the multi-centre randomized studies currently under way in some countries. The assertion, with minimal evidence, that certain therapies should be given to certain groups of patients is the best way to ensure that we never learn how best to treat them. Thus, the nontrialled introduction of retinoids for the treatment of M3 AML, and cranial radiotherapy and etoposide for monocytic variants is to be deprecated.

Chemotherapy

The basic idea behind the treatment schedules which have improved results in the last decade is dose intensity, although there are differences of emphasis, such that the BFM studies use a more sustained type of therapy unlike the usual pulsed therapy used elsewhere. The basic drugs have remained the same, with cytarabine and an anthracycline being the mainstay. Whether or not etoposide or thioguanine add anything to this type of induction regimen is uncertain, and randomized trials of their relative efficacy (e.g. ADE* versus DAT** in MRC AML 10) are under way. The cytarabine and anthracycline doses have been 'racked up' to the limit of tolerance which is determined by severe gut and infection-related toxicity. A multiplicity of dosage regimens have been used but the commonest current practice is to use cytarabine 100–200 mg/m² day for 7–10 days by continuous infusion, with daunorubicin 30–75 mg/m² given by i.v. bolus at the beginning, or end, or in 3 divided doses through the course. Other regimens such as MIDAC† and MACE+ have been used as remission induction courses, but there have been no large randomized trials of their use and no evidence that they are better or less

toxic than ADE/DAT. As stated above, about 90% of children will survive the first two courses of therapy and achieve a complete remission; 5% fall by the wayside because of toxic death, and 5% because of resistant disease. It is common practice to give two courses of the same or similar treatment in order to achieve remission, and three-quarters will do so after one course. The evidence that those patients who require to receive more than one course of chemotherapy in order to achieve remission do worse is scanty at present, but it seems likely that this will be shown to be the case. It has commonly been thought that children with Down's syndrome tolerate therapy less well and have more gut and infection-related toxicity. This is not true on the whole; they tolerate treatment quite well (Lie S 1989) but are at higher risk of developing M7, megakaryo-blastic leukaemia. In addition, recovery of blood counts in this particular group of patients is often delayed, presumably due to slow resolution of myelofibrosis.

Consolidation therapy consists of either chemotherapy or bone marrow transplantation. Allogeneic transplantation (see below) would usually be considered after at least one further course of chemotherapy following remission; the total is usually three followed by BMT. Those who advocate high-dose therapy with autologous bone marrow rescue (ABMT) are usually more nervous of the efficacy of this modality of therapy and advocate four courses followed by ABMT. The idea behind consolidation chemotherapy is to get rid of 'minimal residual disease'. The assumption (with some experimental proof) is that resistant clones of leukaemia cells exist amongst this residuum. For this reason, therapy should be intensive at this stage and consist of different drugs from those used at the beginning to minimize the chance of survival for these troublesome clones. It is at this stage that the MACE and MIDAC-like courses are given. To achieve maximum intensity, the drugs are given as soon as the counts rise so that the leukaemia does not get a 'breather'. The trend

---

*   ADE = cytosine Arabinoside, Daunorubicin, Etoposide
**DAT = Daunorubicin, cytosine Arabinoside, Thioguanine
†MIDAC = MItoxantrone, high Dose Arabinosyl Cytosine
+MACE = aMsAcrine, Cytarabine, Etoposide

has also been to ratchet up the doses of drugs in these consolidation courses; for example the present UK policy is to give four very intensive courses of chemotherapy which leads to an approximately 10% overall toxic death rate and about 15 weeks total stay in hospital during which the patients spend most of the time receiving intravenous nutrition, multitudes of antimicrobials and often some degree of intensive care. The drug regimens used in the current trial MRC AML 10 are given in outline in Figure 4.4. The chemotherapy questions being asked by this trial are:

1. Is etoposide superior to thioguanine in the induction regimen for toxicity and efficacy? Patients with M4 and M5 disease can of course be compared on both regimens.
2. Is this very high dose regimen tolerable?
3. How do remission induction and event-free survival rates compare with similar groups of patients being treated in other countries, bearing in mind that all patients are entered into this trial and all are analyzed with no exclusions?

The intention is to admit children and adults up to the age of 50 years into this trial in view of the probable lack of basic differences in the underlying nature of the disease. The aim is to randomize approximately 200 children and 800 adults in order to have a good chance of answering the chemotherapy questions above and the BMT questions discussed below. Two residual questions

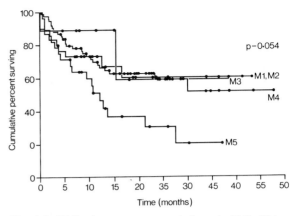

Fig. 4.5 FAB subtype as a prognostic factor in AML. This trial included adults and children and demonstrates that the only significant effect is a worse outcome for M5 patients, especially those with CNS disease at diagnosis. (Reproduced from Marcus et al 1987, with permission.)

are not being addressed; the role of maintenance chemotherapy and that of cranial irradiation. The trial of Marcus and others (Fig. 4.5) showed that the M5 FAB subtype was a risk factor for relapse especially when central nervous system (CNS) disease is present at diagnosis. However, in the author's view the very low failure rate in the CNS (7%, for example, in total in the BFM 1/82 trial) does not justify routine cranial radiotherapy in M5 cases, except when CNS disease is present at diagnosis and a BMT is not contemplated.

Maintenance (or, more properly, 'continuation') chemotherapy, is an unresolved issue. It is highly questionable that long-term sporadic treatment will add anything to modern short and very intensive treatment (Bloomfield 1985), and there have been no randomized studies to justify its use in children.

High-dose therapy with autologous marrow rescue (ABMT)

Like all other forms of transplantation, AMBT is best thought of as just another type of high-dose therapy. The marrow in ABMT just rescues the haemopoietic system from the intensity of treatment. In allogeneic BMT there is probably an additional anti-leukaemic affect, possibly mediated through cytotoxic T-cells and natural killer cells, which depends on transfusion of the bone

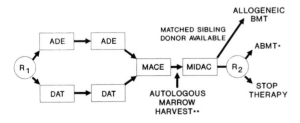

Fig. 4.4 Outline schema of UK MRC AML 10 Trial. *ABMT = High dose therapy with autologous marrow rescue. **Marrow harvest to be used for STOP patients who consequently relapse. RI = Randomization one. R2 = Randomization two. ADE = cytArabine, Daunorubicin, Etoposide. DAT = Daunorubicin, cytArabine, Thioguanine. MACE = aMsAcrine, Cytarabine, Etoposide. MIDAC = MItoxantrone, high Dose Arabinosyl Cytosine.

marrow graft. ABMT is usually a very well-tolerated procedure with a low risk of cytomegalo-virus (CMV) infection, and is comparable for tox-icity with an intensive course of chemotherapy. With the advent of therapeutic haemopoietic growth factors, it may even become possible to reduce the period in hospital to a few days, so long as such substances do not also have a stimulatory effect on the leukaemia. The current situation is that various studies have shown quite promising results for ABMT, but we will not know whether they are significantly better than current highly-intensive chemotherapy regimens until the results of trials such as MRC AML 10 and comparable US studies become available. What we *do* know is that current preparative therapy prior to ABMT is very toxic (see late-effects section). In order to try to reduce this problem, non-total body irradiation (TBI) regimens such as busulphan/cyclophosphamide have been tried out, but whether this approach will be less toxic or equally effective is as yet unknown. The type of questions that need to be answered are as follows:

1. Does AMBT add to the efficacy of very intensive chemotherapy?
2. Does allogeneic BMT add to the efficacy of very intensive chemotherapy and how does it compare with ABMT?
3. Can less toxic but similarly effective preparative regimens for BMT be designed? This is especially important in children below the age of 2 years for whom TBI is very toxic.
4. What are the late effects associated with each type of approach?

Questions 1, 2 and 4 are being asked in MRC AML 10 and other trials; question 3 will be addressed if and when question 1 or 2 is answered in the affirmative.

Allogeneic bone marrow transplantation (BMT)

Allogeneic BMT from matched sibling donors is widely regarded as the treatment of choice for childhood AML. However, it is very important to keep an open mind on this question, particularly in view of the severe toxic late effects of TBI, the

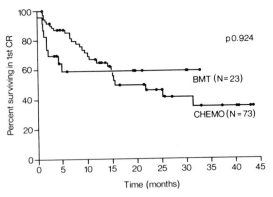

Fig. 4.6 Comparison of allogeneic BMT with chemotherapy in AML. A combined sequential series of children and adults. BMT was performed whenever a donor was available. The usual 'lozenge-shaped' effect on the survival curves is shown with a worse early survival in the BMT group almost entirely due to procedure-related mortality, mainly in adults, due to graft-versus-host disease. The ultimate results for BMT look better but are not significant due to the early 'fall-off'. The results include only those patients who went into remission, i.e. about 90% of children. (Adapted from: Marcus et al 1987, with permission.)

improving results of high-dose chemotherapy and the fact that only about one in three patients has a suitable donor.

The results of allogeneic BMT have usually been compared with chemotherapy in studies which have 'randomized' the patients to BMT depend-ing on the availability of a donor (Fig. 4.6). A number of important points can be drawn from this survival curve. Firstly, as with almost all publications, the results for BMT do not start at presentation. The longer the procedure is delayed the better the results will be because vulnerable patients will have fallen by the wayside through relapse, resistant disease and toxic deaths. The result is no better than 50% survival, which is not a great deal different from chemotherapy, although if the children had been separated out from the adults the results would have been better.

A more helpful idea of outcome can be obtained from single-institution studies, looking at all-comers and comparing the results of matched allogeneic BMT where it is available with chemotherapy where it is not (Fig. 4.7). It can then be seen that allogeneic BMT does appear to confer some advantage, but the difference is not great, largely because of the early procedure-related mortality of BMT. However, the results of transplantation are

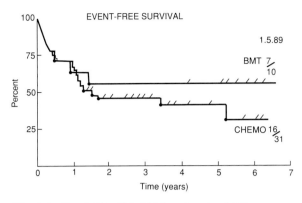

Fig. 4.7 Hospital for Sick Children, London AML treatment results 1983–1987. Patients received BMT in first remission if a donor was available, or alternatively intensive chemotherapy. There is no statistical difference but the transplant results plateau out at 53% EFS by one year. The chemotherapy survival curve continues to fall off.

improving dramatically now that cyclosporin A is being used with a short course of methotrexate to prevent graft-versus-host disease. We are also getting better at preventing CMV infections by the use of screened seronegative blood products, and at treating this and other infections, thus, we must await the results of current trials to see whether BMT remains the apparent treatment of choice for first remission AML where a histocompatible sibling donor is available.

The standard pre-transplant myeloablative therapy for allogeneic BMT is also high-dose cyclophosphamide and TBI (usually given in 6–8 fractions to a total dose of 12–14 Gy). However, efforts are being made to reduce the toxicity and retain the efficacy of these regimens by adding in other drugs such as high-dose cytarabine, and changing to a drugs-only regimen such as busulphan/cyclophosphamide. At present, there is insufficient evidence to justify a change from the cyclophosphamide/TBI regimen.

The use of matched unrelated donors is in its infancy but it may in the future offer hope where none presently exists for relapsed patients who do not have a matched sibling donor (Hann 1990).

LATE TOXIC EFFECTS OF THERAPY

Very little information exists on this aspect of management, largely because very few patients have lived long enough for the problem to be assessed. The time has now come for such studies. At present, it would appear that the risk of second malignancy is small, other than for those patients who have a pre-existing myelodysplastic disorder. There is no evidence about other toxicities of chemotherapy alone, although the author is concerned about persisting oto- and nephrotoxicity in his own patients who have been heavily treated with multiple long-sustained antimicrobial combinations. There is also a fear that the cardiac insult provided by these drugs may lead to significant adverse late effects.

Much is known about the late effects of allogeneic BMT with TBI (Hann 1990). It would seem that introduction of fractionated radiotherapy over several days has reduced immediate and late problems, particularly cataracts, but has not completely eradicated them. One important point is that it may take a number of years for the effects on growth and hormonal status to become manifest, so that careful long-term follow-up is essential. One-third of children treated with cyclophosphamide/TBI develop compensated hypothyroidism with elevated TSH and normal T4. About 8% develop overt hypothyroidism. The risk of thyroid malignancy has not been quantitated, but in one series two of 116 children developed a neoplasm 4 and 8 years after BMT. The level of adrenal abnormalities is unknown but gonadal dysfunction is more clearly defined. Two-thirds of prepubertal boys have delayed onset of secondary sexual characteristics and many require androgen therapy. Two-thirds of prepubertal girls experience delayed puberty and many require replacement therapy. Most of the post-pubertal boys and girls develop primary gonadal failure. All of the girls develop amenorrhoea; one-third recover but some may again develop ovarian failure thereafter. All of the post-pubertal boys studied have azoospermia. Two-thirds (at least) of patients develop growth hormone deficiency, and the response to recombinant growth hormone is still being evaluated. All of this, of course, argues for less toxic preparative regimens and this will be the next step if the current set of trials confirms the superiority of allogeneic BMT (and possibly ABMT) over the best current drug regimen.

REFERENCES

Askew D S, Eaves A C, Eaves C J, Takei F 1985 Restricted expression of a new acute myelogenous leukaemia-associated antigen (NHL-30.5) on normal hemopoietic progenitor cells. Blood 67: 1098–1102

Avvisati G, Tencate J W, Buller H R, Mandelli F 1989 Tranexamic acid for control of haemorrhage in acute promyelocytic leukaemia. Lancet 122–124

Bennett J M, Catovsky D, Daniel M-T et al 1985 Criteria for the diagnosis of acute leukaemia of megakaryocytic lineage (M7). Annals of Internal Medicine 460–462

Bloomfield C D 1985 Postremission therapy in AML. Journal of Clinical Oncology 3: 1570–1572

Campos L, Guyotat D, Archimbaud E et al 1989 Surface marker expression in adult acute myeloid leukaemia: correlations with initial characteristics, morphology and response to therapy. British Journal of Haematology 72: 161–166

Chessells J M, O'Callaghan U, Hardisty R M 1986 Acute myeloid leukaemia in childhood: clinical features and prognosis. British Journal of Haematology 63: 555–564

Coco F L, Avvisati G, Deverio D et al 1991 Molecular evaluation of response to all-trans retinoic acid therapy in patients with acure promyelocytic leukemia. Blood 77: 1657–1659

Creutzig U, Ritter J, Riehm H et al 1987 The childhood AML studies BFM 78 and 83: treatment results and risk factor analysis. Haematology and Blood Transfusion Springer 30: 71–75

Cunningham I, Gee T S, Reich L M et al 1988 Acute promyelocytic leukaemia: treatment results during a decade at Memorial Hospital. Blood 73: 1116–1122

Dow L W, Dahl G V, Kalwinsky D K et al 1986 Correlation of drug sensitivity in vitro with clinical responses in childhood AML. Blood 68: 400–405

EORTC International Antimicrobial Therapy Cooperative Group 1987 Ceftazidine combined with a short or long course of amikacin for empirical therapy of Gram-negative bacteraemia in cancer patients with granulocytopenia. New England Journal of Medicine 317: 1692–1698

Fearon E, Burke P, Schiffer C et al 1986 Differentiation of leukaemia cells to polymorphonuclear leukocytes in patients with AML. New England Journal of Medicine 315: 15–24

Goldberg M A, Ginsburg D, Mayer R J et al 1986 Is heparin administration necessary during induction chemotherapy for patients with acute promyelocytic leukaemia? Blood 69: 187–191

Gordis L, Szklo M, Thompson B et al 1981 An apparent increase in the incidence of AML in black children. Cancer 47: 2763–2768

Grier H, Gelber R D, Cammitta B M et al 1987 Prognostic factors in childhood AML. Journal of Clinical Oncology 5: 1026–1032

Hann I M 1988 Infections in immunosuppressed children. Current Opinion in Infectious Diseases 1: 607–609

Hann I M 1990 Bone marrow transplantation. Current Opinion in Paediatrics 2: 143–150

Hartley S E, Sainsbury C 1981 Acute leukaemia and the same chromosome abnormality in monozygote twins.

Human Genetics 58: 408–410

Jacobsen R J, Temple M J, Singer J W et al 1984 A clonal complete remission in a patient with AML originating in a multipotent stem cell. New England Journal of Medicine 310: 1513–1517

Lie S O 1989 Acute myelogenous leukaemia in children. European Journal of Paediatrics 148: 382–388

Linet M S 1985 The leukaemias: epidemiological aspects. In: Lilienfield A M (ed) Monographs in epedimology and biostatistics. OUP, New York, p 1–293

Malkin D, Freeman M H 1989 Childhood erythroleukaemia: review of clinical and biological features. American Journal of Pediatric Haematology and Oncology 11: 348–359

Marcus R E, Catovsky D, Prentice H G et al 1987 Intensive induction and consolidation chemotherapy for adults and children with AML. Joint AML Trial 1982–1985. Haematology and Blood Transfusion Vol 30: Acute Leukaemias. Springer, Berlin, p 346–351

Nieuwenhuis H K, Sixma J J 1985 Treatment of disseminated intravascular coagulation in APML with low molecular weight heparinoid Org 10172. Cancer 58: 761–764

Odom L F, Lampkin B C, Tannous R et al 1990 Acute monoblastic leukaemia – a review from the CCSG. Leukaemia Research 14: 1–10

Rees J K H, Gray R G, Swirsky D, Hayhoe F G S 1986 Principal results of the MRC 8th AML Trial. Lancet 1236–1241

Ritter J, Vormoor J, Creutzig U, Schellong G 1989 Prognostic significance of Auer rods in childhood acute myelogenous leukaemia: results of the studies AML-BFM-78 and 83. Medical Pediatric Oncology 17: 202–209

Rubin R H, Young L S 1987 Clinical approach to infection in the compromised host, 2nd ed. Plenum, New York

Sage R, Hann I, Prentice H G et al 1988 A randomised trial of empirical antibiotic therapy with one of four β-lactam antibiotics in combination with netilmicin in febrile neutropenic patients. Journal of Antimicrobial Chemotherapy 22: 237–247

Stevens R, Burnett A K, Goldman A H, Gray R G et al on behalf of the MRC Adult and Childhood Leukaemia Working Parties 1990 Medical Research Council's 10th AML Trial. British Journal of Haematology 74(suppl 1): 4

Swirsky D M, de Bastos M, Parish S E et al 1986 Features affecting outcome during remission induction of AML in 619 adult patients. British Journal of Haematology 64: 435–453

United States OHRST, National Centre for Health Statistics 1981 Vital Statistics of the US. Vol II Mortality, Part A. US Government Printing Office, Washington D C

Van der Schoot C E, Daams G M, Pinkster J et al 1990 Monoclonal antibodies against myeloperoxidase are valuable immunological reagents for the diagnosis of AML. British Journal of Haematology 74: 173–178

Verdeguer A, Fernandez J M, Esquembre C et al 1990 Hepatosplenic candidiasis in children with acute leukaemia. Cancer 65: 874–877

Weinstein H, Grier H, Gelber R, Cammitta B 1987 Postremission induction intensive sequential chemotherapy for children with AML – treatment results and prognostic factors. Haematological Blood Transfusion 30: 88–92

5. Nonmalignant disorders of granulocytes and monocytes

R. F. Stevens

INTRODUCTION

Neutrophils are the most important cellular constituents in the control of infection. When released from the bone marrow they circulate briefly, sometimes migrating along the vascular endothelium, before being attracted to foci of infection by chemotactic factors. There they ingest opsonized organisms and enclose the microbe within a vesicular phagosome into which they discharge their granule contents. Finally, they enzymatically reduce oxygen to reactive metabolites which aid in the killing of the organisms.

Bone marrow granulocyte development

Granulocyte-macrophage progenitor cells can be demonstrated in bone marrow, blood, spleen and cord blood. Granulocyte-macrophage colony-forming units, (CFU-GM) can give rise to mature granulocyte and macrophage populations from a common CFU-GM that morphologically resembles a primitive blast cell or lymphocyte. The CFU-GM population represents a continuation of cells with varying proliferative and cell cycle qualities leading to mixed marrow colonies that are heterogeneous in size.

Certain regulatory glycoproteins known as colony-stimulating factors (CSFs) influence the growth of granulocytes and monocytes in culture. CSFs are produced by a variety of tissues including endothelial cells, T-lymphocytes and mononuclear phagocytes. Several CSFs (e.g. GM-CSF, G-CSF, M-CSF) which are more selective in their stimulatory capacity have been isolated and cloned. G- and GM-CSF are now becoming available in therapeutic quantities as a result of recombinant DNA technology.

Table 5.1 illustrates the kinetics of mature neutrophil production. In the peripheral blood a relatively small number of neutrophils make up the circulating and marginating pools. In the marrow there is an immense cellular reserve made up of dividing and maturing cells.

The release of neutrophils from the marrow to the circulation is multifactorial. Neutrophil deformability, cell-releasing factor, blood flow through the marrow and localization of cells in relation to the vascular channels can all affect release of granulocytes into the blood stream.

NEUTROPENIA

Neutropenia is an absolute reduction in the number of circulating neutrophils. Normal values are age dependent (see Ch. 1). Classification of the neutropenias can be based on one of several approaches, including pathophysiology, kinetics, metabolism, function and the severity of the neutropenia. None of these classifications is ideal, but in this chapter emphasis will be given to the severity and variability of the neutropenia.

Symptoms are relatively uncommon with neutrophil counts above $1.0 \times 10^9/1$, but become increasingly severe as the count falls. A neutrophil

Table 5.1 Neutrophil production and kinetics

Compartment	Compartment size ($\times 10^9$ cells/kg)	Compartment transit time (hours)
Myeloblast	0.15	18
Promyelocyte	0.5	24
Myelocyte	2.0	104
Metamyelocyte	3.0	40
Segmented neutrophil	3.0	96
Peripheral neutrophil	0.7	10

count of 0.5–1.0 × 10⁹/1 can be considered as moderate, and one below 0.5 × 10⁹/1 as severe neutropenia. Within a particular neutrophil range there is considerable variation in infective symptoms both within a patient population and within a single individual.

Bacterial infections are the commonest problem associated with neutropenia. Fungal, viral and parasitic infections are relatively uncommon in isolated neutropenia as opposed to the severe pancytopenias associated with hypoplasia (as seen after intensive chemotherapy or marrow transplantation). Cellulitis, superficial and deep abscess formation, pneumonia and septicaemia are particularly associated with neutropenia. The typical inflammatory response may be much modified with a poor localization of infection and a tendency to rapid dissemination.

Profound and prolonged neutropenia

Reticular dysgenesis

This condition results from the failure of marrow progenitor cells which are committed to myeloid and lymphoid proliferation (de Vaal & Seynhaeve 1959). Affected infants are susceptible to fatal bacterial and viral infections because of severe neutropenia and lymphopenia. As well as a virtual absence of marrow myeloid precursors there is a total lack of lymphoid cells, both marrow- and thymic-derived. Lymph nodes show absent germinal follicles. Lymphocytes are also lacking from the tonsils, spleen and Peyer's patches. Red cell and platelet maturation is normal. No specific treatment is available other than bone marrow transplantation.

Neutropenia and lymphocyte abnormalities (See also Ch. 6)

The association between X-linked hypogammaglobulinaemia and neutropenia has been recognized for some time (Rosen et al 1968). Approximately one-third of males with X-linked agammaglobulinaemia have neutropenia at some stage during their illness. Absence of IgG and IgA with normal or raised IgM has also been reported in association with severe neutropenia. Bone marrow examination usually reveals a maturation arrest, with early myeloid precursors but little maturation beyond the myelocyte stage. Children usually have severe recurrent bacterial infections, hepatosplenomegaly and failure to thrive. Patients may die in early childhood and no specific treatment is available other than immunoglobulin replacement therapy or marrow transplantation.

The syndrome of T-cell lymphocytosis and neutropenia, where an acquired excess of suppressor T-cells is associated with a profound neutropenia, is occasionally seen in children though is more common in adults. The condition is not neoplastic, the cause if obscure and there is no effective therapy. Morbidity can be considerable (Murray & Lilleyman 1983).

Severe congenital neutropenia (Kostmann's syndrome)

This autosomal recessive condition was first described by Kostmann in 1956. The neutropenia is severe, with absolute counts usually below 0.2 × 10⁹/1 although the total white cell count may be normal because of the accompanying monocytosis and eosinophilia. Infective episodes usually begin shortly after birth and are frequently very severe. Bone marrow examination shows variable degrees of abnormality but there is usually normal myeloid maturation to the promyelocyte/myelocyte stage and a scarcity of more mature forms. Nevertheless, normal numbers of myeloid progenitor cells have been detected in many patients, and in vitro culture appears to progress beyond the myelocyte stage with the appearance of neutrophils (Parmley et al 1980). There is ultrastructural and cytochemical evidence of an intrinsic myeloid precursor cell defect, with defective primary granules, a reduced number of secondary granules and autologous ingestion of mature neutrophils.

The majority of patients used to die of severe infection although leukaemic transformation has also been reported (Gilman et al 1970). Antibiotics may help prolong life, but androgens, steroids or splenectomy have been of no proven benefit. Bone marrow transplantation has helped in some patients (Pahwa et al 1977), but may now have been superseded by successful therapy with G-CSF.

Variable neutropenia

Several syndromes have been described where neutropenia is associated with other phenotypic abnormalities. These include Shwachman's syndrome, cartilage hair hypoplasia, Fanconi's anaemia and dyskeratosis congenita. Although of variable severity, these conditions are not usually as devastating as Kostmann's syndrome or reticular dysgenesis.

Shwachman's syndrome

Shwachman's syndrome is a rare multi-organ disease of unknown cause which is probably transmitted as an autosomal recessive trait (Shwachman et al 1964). Its features include exocrine pancreatic insufficiency, growth retardation, metaphyseal dyschondroplasia, bone marrow hypoplasia, neutropenia, anaemia, thrombocytopenia and a raised level of fetal haemoglobin. Diarrhoea, weight loss, failure to thrive, eczema, otitis media and chest infections tend to occur in the neonatal period, whereas growth failure and dwarfism tend to become apparent in infancy and early childhood. Abnormal gait follows the metaphyseal chondroplasia. Other features include reduced thoracic gas volume and chest wall compliance, mild mental handicap, hypotonia, deafness, retinitis pigmentosa, diabetes mellitus, dental abnormalities, delayed puberty and renal tubular acidosis (Aggett et al 1980, Marra et al 1986).

The degree of neutropenia is variable, usually averaging between 0.2 and $0.5 \times 10^9/l$. The bone marrow is usually hypoplastic or may show myeloid maturation arrest (Aggett et al 1980).

If the neutropenia is not noted then the diagnosis may be mistaken for cystic fibrosis in the young, although the sweat test is normal. The malabsorption tends to diminish with time, although the pancreatic insufficiency persists and is probably the result of pancreatic fatty infiltration and acinar degeneration (Aggett et al 1980). Although the majority of patients are diagnosed before the age of 2 years, occasional cases have been described as presenting during the second decade (Hislop et al 1982).

Although the precise abnormality in Shwachman's syndrome is unknown, it has been postulated that the condition is the result of a cytoskeletal defect in neutrophils as reflected by an abnormal distribution of concanavalin A receptors (Rothbaum et al 1982). This does not, however, explain the non-neutrophil features of the condition. Aggett et al (1980) have speculated that the syndrome may be the result of a defect in microtubular and microfilament cellular elements, but this hypothesis awaits confirmation. The malabsorption of Shwachman's syndrome responds to oral pancreatic enzymes. Associated infections can be treated with antibiotics.

The disorder is a premalignant condition and secondary leukaemia is well described. Otherwise, the prognosis is probably better than that of cystic fibrosis, with most patients surviving to adulthood, given adequate supportive therapy.

Cartilage hair hypoplasia

This condition is characterized by short-limbed dwarfism, fine hair, frequent infections and a moderate neutropenia. Impaired cellular immunity together with more variable immunological abnormalities are found (McKusick et al 1965). Bone marrow transplantation has been used successfully to correct the condition (O'Reilly et al 1984).

Dyskeratosis congenita

This X-linked recessive condition is associated with dystrophic nails, leukoplasia and skin hyperpigmentation. Neutropenia is seen in approximately one-third of patients and is the result of marrow hypoplasia. The majority of patients reach adult life, and life-threatening infections are uncommon.

Fanconi's syndrome

This condition is dealt with in Chapter 2. Patients often show some degree of leukopenia, which is usually of mild or moderate severity initially but eventually becomes profound with the development of marrow aplasia. Infections are relatively uncommon prior to the development of severe marrow hypoplasia or acute leukaemia.

Chronic benign neutropenia

In the relatively common chronic benign neutropenia, the severity of illness and susceptibility to infection is closely related to the severity of the neutropenia. Except for the low neutrophil count, no other specific phenotypic features have been reported. The condition may be the result of a defect in committed myeloid progenitor cells (Greenberg et al 1980) or a diminished release of colony-stimulating activity by the marrow micro-environment.

The peripheral blood neutrophil count usually remains static over many years, but spontaneous remissions have been reported, usually in younger children (Dale et al 1979). The lack of associated dysmorphic or chromosomal features in chronic benign neutropenia may be connected with the lack of evidence for an increased incidence of secondary leukaemia. In the majority of patients no genetic pattern has been identified.

Bone marrow appearances are variable. Most frequently there are plentiful early myeloid forms but a marked reduction of mature segmented forms. This coincides with the presence of peripheral blood segmented ('band') forms but few mature neutrophils. Marrow myeloid progenitor cells are also very variable in number (Falk et al 1977).

Patients with chronic benign neutropenia have a relatively low risk of serious infections and hence should not be subjected to therapy with potential side-effects unless indicated. Therapy should be based on symptoms and not on the neutrophil count.

Myelokathexis

This is a form of neutropenia in which the granulocyte nuclei show marked morphological abnormalities, with filaments connecting the nuclear lobes and cytoplasmic vacuolation. Bone marrow cellularity is usually increased and shows numerous degenerating neutrophils which may be hypersegmented. The peripheral blood neutropenia is probably the result of increased marrow granulocyte destruction (Zuelzer 1970).

Metabolic neutropenia

Neutropenia has been associated with a variety of inherited metabolic disorders including propionic acidaemia, isovaleric acidaemia, methyl-

malonic acidaemia and hyperglycinaemia (Tanaka & Rosenberg 1983). The neutropenia may be the result of a direct inhibition of progenitor cell maturation.

Cyclical neutropenia

Cyclical neutropenia is an unusual disorder characterized by regular recurring episodes of severe neutropenia (peripheral neutrophil count less than $0.2 \times 10^9/1$) lasting usually 3–6 days and occurring approximately every 3 weeks. The condition was first reported by Leale in 1910. Since then, over 100 cases have been described.

When the patient is neutropenic, symptoms such as oral ulceration, stomatitis and pharyngitis are common. More serious localized and disseminated infections can occur, the severity of which is usually related to the degree of neutropenia, although it is not unusual for patients to be asymptomatic throughout periods of neutropenia. Patients frequently know when they have a fall in neutrophils because they experience anorexia and malaise and develop oral ulcers and white exudates over the tongue. As the neutrophil count recovers, the patient's wellbeing also improves. There is no evidence that affected individuals are especially prone to viral, fungal or parasitic infections. Although usually considered benign, up to 10% of patients have died of infectious complications (Lange 1983).

In many patients, mild chronic neutropenia (less than $2.0 \times 10^9/1$) is seen in addition to periods of severe neutropenia (Wright et al 1981). Monocytes, lymphocytes, eosinophils, platelets and reticulocytes are also seen to cycle. When a patient is at the neutrophil nadir, blood monocyte counts are elevated. Mild anaemia is common, particularly when there is severe infection, and is probably a nonspecific consequence of inflammation.

At the beginning of each period of neutropenia, the bone marrow shows a rapid increase in the number of promyelocytes and myelocytes followed by an increase in later forms (metamyelocytes and segmented forms). About 10 days after the beginning of the neutropenic period, the marrow shows a high percentage of mature neutrophils and fewer early myeloid precursors. Because of the cyclical changes in marrow lymphoid, erythroid and platelet precursors, the name 'periodic or cyclic haematopoiesis' has also been used (Guerry et al 1973).

Cyclic neutropenia should be suspected in patients with the typical pattern of regularly recurring symptoms. Total and differential white cell counts should be performed at least twice a week for 2 months to confirm the diagnosis. Greatest confusion occurs when differentiating cyclical neutropenia from chronic benign neutropenia, a more common diagnosis (Dale et al 1979). In both conditions, splenomegaly is usually absent, there is a monocytosis and the marrow shows a myeloid 'maturation arrest'. Although patients with chronic benign neutropenia may show fluctuating counts, they do not have the strict regularity of cyclical neutropenia, though it is probable that the conditions may in fact overlap to some extent. Families have been described with both cyclic and noncyclical members (Morley et al 1967).

Family studies have demonstrated an inherited pattern to cyclical neutropenia and/or symptoms highly suggestive of the condition in almost one-third of reported cases. The pattern of occurrence suggests an autosomal dominant mode of inheritance. In nearly all the familial cases, symptoms start in infancy or early childhood (Morley et al 1967). In other cases the onset appears to be spontaneous and the condition is diagnosed in both children and adults (Lange 1983). The collie dog shows the veterinary equivalent of cyclical neutropenia, where inheritance is autosomal recessive (Lund et al 1967).

Two lines of evidence suggest that cyclical neutropenia may occur by heterogeneous mechanisms. Firstly, it has been shown that some older patients with the disorder have a clonal proliferation of large granular lymphocytes (Loughran et al 1986), whereas children do not. It appears the cyclical neutropenia can be acquired late in life. Secondly, there are now reports of cyclical neutropenia responding to androgens and steroids (Rogers & Shuman 1982, Roozendaal et al 1981). In all cases these have been adult patients. There are reports of neutrophil cycling in association with leukaemia (Lensink et al 1986), but there are no reports of typical childhood-onset cyclical neutropenia evolving into malignancy. Based on these observations, Dale & Hammond (1988) proposed the classification shown in Table 5.2.

Several lines of evidence suggest that the primary defect in cyclical neutropenia is in the regulation of haemopoietic stem cells or progenitors committed to the neutrophil cell line. For example, in dogs, it has been shown that the disease can be transmitted and cured by marrow transplantation (Dale & Graw 1974). In man, the marked swings in marrow cell populations seen in serial bone marrows support this idea. The condition has also been transfered between humans by allogeneic marrow transplantation (Krance et al 1982).

At present, there are three suggested mechanisms for cyclical neutropenia (Dale & Hammond 1988):

1. A stem cell defect resulting in altered response to haemopoietic regulation.
2. A defect in humoral or cellular stem cell control.
3. A periodic accumulation of an inhibitor of stem cell proliferation.

Cell culture studies of blood and bone marrow indicate that stem cells, or at least the committed stem cells of the neutrophil series, have little if any defect in their proliferative capacity (Englehard et al 1983). At the present time it has not been substantiated whether specific colony-stimulating factors or interleukins fluctuate cyclically and, if so, whether they are a cause or effect of the disease. Recent studies suggest that there may be a basic defect in endogenous generation of colony-stimulating factors in some patients, which raises the possibility of treatment with recombinant growth factors (Dale & Hammond 1988). Although cyclical variations in potentially toxic nucleotides have been demonstrated in cyclical neutropenia, these mitotic inhibitors may be

Table 5.2 Classification of cyclical neutropenia

1. Childhood onset
   a. family history
   b. without large granular lymphocytes
2. Adult onset
   a. with large granular lymphocytes
   b. without large granular lymphocytes
3. Associated with haematological malignancy
4. Associated with other cyclical phenomena
5. Possible cyclical neutropenia (inadequate data)

(From: Dale & Hammond 1988)

secondary to recurrent inflammation and intense cyclical proliferation (Osborne et al 1985).

The management of patients with cyclical neutropenia requires an understanding of symptoms associated with neutropenic episodes and appropriate treatment of infections during periods of neutropenia. Good oral hygiene and dental care are extremely important. Fortunately, symptoms are often milder as patients become older. Prednisone, androgenic steroids and possibly plasmapheresis (von Schulthess et al 1983) can affect the disease but are not of practical value. Lithium therapy is of no benefit. Although bone marrow transplantation offers a definitive cure, the associated mortality and morbidity does not justify this treatment. Recombinant growth factors offer the possibility of disease modification and regulation and G-CSF looks particularly promising.

Disorders of neutrophil survival

Neonatal isoimmune neutropenia

This condition is analogous to isoimmune haemolytic disease and isoimmune thrombocytopenia in the neonate. It has been estimated to affect up to 3% of newborns (Verheugt et al 1979). Mothers are sensitized by the passage of fetal antigens across the placenta during gestation. IgG antineutrophil antibodies subsequently cross the placenta and destroy the infant's neutrophils. Despite the theoretically high incidence of this condition, less than 100 reported cases have been described (Curnutte & Boxer 1987). Affected infants tend to suffer from fever, skin infections (particularly *Staphylococcus aureus*), and respiratory and urinary infections. Septicaemia may also occur.

The bone marrow shows compensatory myeloid hyperplasia with a 'maturation arrest' and reduction in mature neutrophils. Erythroid precursors and megakaryocytes are normal. The peripheral blood shows severe neutropenia often with an associated monocytosis and eosinophilia.

Neutrophil antibodies may be found in the sera of child and mother. The antibody reacts against the neutrophils of the patient, father and possibly some siblings, but does not react against the mother's neutrophils. Minchinton (1984) has classified the neutrophil antigens as NA1, NA2, NB1 and NC1. Neutrophil counts usually return to normal by 2 months of age, associated with the decay of the maternal antibody.

Isoimmune neonatal neutropenia is best treated with appropriate antibiotics. Occasionally, in severe cases, plasma or whole blood exchange may have to be considered to remove the antibody. Transfusion of maternal neutrophils (which will lack the antigen) may be helpful in exceptional circumstances (Boxer 1981).

HLA antigens are also present on neutrophils and it might be expected that neonatal neutropenia could occur in the offspring of multiparous women with the transplacental transfer of maternal HLA antibodies (Payne 1964). This seldom happens, perhaps because HLA antigens are present on other tissues and the antibodies are rapidly absorbed so that insufficient remain to cause neutropenia.

Autoimmune neutropenia

Autoimmune neutropenia of infancy. This is an uncommon but well defined condition which has distinctive clinical features. After an initial asymptomatic period, infants develop recurrent mild infections. The majority of children present within the first year of life, and many patients have symptoms for several months before a blood count is performed. The neutrophil count is probably normal at birth. Neutropenia is usually severe (less than $0.5 \times 10^9/l$) and is often associated with an eosinophilia and monocytosis. Bone marrow examination shows myeloid hyperplasia but reduced or absent mature neutrophils ('maturation arrest'). The condition does not appear to be familial and is more common in girls.

The autoimmune nature of this disease can be established in more than 98% of patients by demonstrating neutrophil-bound and circulating antibodies in the patients and the absence of antibodies in maternal blood (Lalezari et al 1986). Antibodies can be demonstrated by direct and indirect immunofluorescence in over 80%, and by agglutination in approximately 75% of cases. Some antibodies can only be detected by one of these techniques. Neutrophil antibodies may be directed against neutrophil-specific antigens, whereas in other patients the antigen specificity remains undefined. Autoantibodies may be IgG, lgM, IgA or a mixture (Verheugt et al 1978). Late in the course of self-limiting disease, antibodies may become undetectable even though the patients are still neutropenic. This may present a diagnostic dilemma when patients are seen for the first time late in the disease.

Approximately half the children show abnormal circulating immune complexes but these are probably not the cause of the neutropenia but, rather, a secondary phenomenon. The exact mechanism of neutrophil destruction remains unclear. The autoantibodies opsonize neutrophils in vitro (Boxer et al 1975). Other suggested mechanisms for the neutropenia include intravascular lysis, antibody-dependent cell-mediated cytotoxicity and entrapment of agglutinated neutrophils in the microcapillaries (Lalezari 1985).

The disorder should be differentiated from other immunologically induced neutropenias which include:

1. isoimmune neonatal neutropenia.
2. transient neonatal neutropenia which occurs in infants born to mothers who have an immune neutropenia.
3. the rare infant neutropenia associated with autoimmune haemolytic anaemia and thrombocytopenia.

In general, patients with autoimmune neutropenia of infancy tolerate the disease well, and treatment should be based on antibiotics to control severe infective episodes. Systemic steroids may result in a temporary rise in the neutrophil count but carries the theoretical risk of disseminating infection. Temporary remission can be induced with high-dose intravenous immunoglobulin (Bussel 1983).

Acquired autoimmune neutropenias in older children are occasionally seen in

1. patients with no other obvious autoimmune phenomena
2. patients who have additional autoantibodies against platelets and/or red cells
3. in patients with associated multisystem disorders such as systemic lupus erythematosus, rheumatoid arthritis and chronic active hepatitis.

Morbidity can be considerable with bacterial and fungal infections (Fig. 5.1).

Felty's syndrome. This condition may also be associated with antineutrophil antibodies. It is characterized by rheumatoid arthritis, splenomegaly and leukopenia (Logue & Shimm 1980). Its exact nature is not understood. Neutrophil survival appears shortened, with increased release of marrow neutrophils and impaired myelopoiesis. This may result from antineutrophil antibodies, immune complexes or circulating inhibitory factors (Joyce et al 1980). It has also been suggested that the shortened neutrophil survival may be the result of impaired marrow release of neutrophils or increased neutrophil margination (Dancey & Brubaker 1979).

Autoimmune neutropenia has also been reported following bone marrow transplantation, both autologous and allogeneic (Minchinton & Waters 1985). A variety of mechanisms for the formation of autoantibodies have been postulated and include:

1. neutrophil sensitization to alloantigens common with engrafted progenitor cells as a result of sensitization by blood products
2. altered T-helper/suppressor cell ratios
3. abnormal neutrophil antigen expression secondary to in vitro stem cell damage
4. an altered immune state secondary to the underlying malignancy.

Infective neutropenia

In children, viral infections are a common cause of neutropenia. The commonest offending organ-

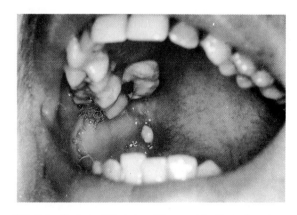

Fig. 5.1 Oral candidiasis in a 13-year-old with profound chronic autoimmune neutropenia. The condition has persisted for over 5 years with several life-threatening infections.

isms include respiratory syncytial virus, influenza, hepatitis (A and B), measles, varicella and rubella (Murdock & Smith 1972). The neutropenia usually corresponds to the period of viraemia and may result from increased neutrophil utilization following viral-induced tissue damage (MacGregor et al 1980). Transient neutropenia is also often seen in association with infectious mononucleosis and may be the result of neutrophil destruction by anti-neutrophil antibodies (Stevens et al 1979). Neutropenia has also been described in association with tuberculosis, brucellosis, typhoid and paratyphoid fevers, malaria and rickettsial infections (Murdock & Smith 1972). In most cases, the pathophysiology of the neutropenia remains obscure.

Septic neutropenia may be particularly profound and may be the result of severe marrow toxic changes affecting myelopoiesis (Christensen & Rothstein 1980). Bacteraemic neutropenia may also result from excessive destruction of neutrophils (Craddock et al 1979), and the neutropenia may be the result of complement activation and aggregation of neutrophils in the pulmonary vasculature contributing to the adult respiratory distress syndrome. Other possible mechanisms include neutrophil destruction following microbial phagocytosis.

Drug-associated neutropenia

The commonest cause of drug-induced neutropenia is that associated with treatment for malignancy. Outside that context, drug-induced neutropenia can be defined as a severe and selective reduction in the numbers of circulating neutrophils (less than $0.2 \times 10^9/1$) due to an idiosyncratic reaction to the offending drug. This also implies that drug-associated neutropenia is unpredictable in its frequency and distribution. The list of drugs which have been implicated in neutropenia is extensive (Young & Vincent 1980) but is summarized in Table 5.3.

In most cases, the pathogenesis in children is unknown. Girls are more often affected than boys. Three basic mechanisms are suggested:

1. increased sensitivity of myeloid progenitor cells to drugs
2. alterations in the immune response as a result of drug administration

3. differences in drug pharmacokinetics leading to toxic drug (or metabolite) levels in the marrow microenvironment.

It is probable that genetic factors also contribute.

An example of the first mechanism is given by the phenothiazines (Young & Vincent 1980). Such compounds may act as haptens, stimulating the formation of antibodies which then complex with the drug and cause myeloid progenitor suppression. Penicillin, thiouracil and gold can also cause neutropenia by this mechanism (Weitzman & Stossel 1978). An example of the second mechanism is given by quinidine, which can activate a cellular immune response, or by phenytoin which produces a humoral response, both of these suppress myelopoiesis (Young & Vincent 1980). The third mechanism, differences in the pharmacokinetics of drugs, is exemplified by sulphasalazine, where some patients who are slow acetylators show greater toxicity than those who are fast acetylators (Schröder & Evans 1972).

Bone marrow appearances in drug-induced neutropenia are very variable. Myeloid precursors may be normal, reduced or increased. Frequently there is a 'maturation arrest' with a reduction in mature forms. After withdrawal of the drug, there is an increase in early myeloid forms followed by a rapid expansion of all myeloid elements.

It is not usually practical or possible to predict the onset of neutropenia with serial blood counts. If neutropenia occurs, withdrawal of the offending drug is the most important therapeutic action. Antibiotics should be used to treat infective episodes. Corticosteroids and granulocyte transfusions are of little benefit. The duration of the neutropenia is very variable. Acute idiosyncratic reactions may last only a few days, whereas chronic episodes may persist for years. Immune-mediated neutropenia usually lasts for about 7 days.

Table 5.3   Drugs causing neutropenia

Antimicrobial agents – particularly penicillins and sulphonamides
Antirheumatics – particularly gold, phenylbutazone and penicillamine
Sedatives – including barbiturates and benzodiazepines
Antithyroid drugs
Phenothiazines
Antipyretics

Table 5.4 Investigation of the child with neutropenia

1. Full blood counts at least weekly to check for cyclical neutropenia and to confirm persistent absolute neutropenia.
2. Blood film examination for white cell morphology.
3. Leucocyte alkaline phosphatase and peroxidase reactions, to detect abnormal neutrophil granulation.
4. Quantitative immunoglobulins, to exclude hypogammaglobulinaemia.
5. Lymphocyte T and B subsets, to exclude reticular dysgenesis.
6. Complement levels, to exclude dysgammaglobinaemia.
7. HLA antibodies, to exclude association with neutropenia.★
8. Neutrophil antibodies, to exclude isoimmune and autoimmune neutropenia.★
9. Bone marrow examination, to exclude agranulocytosis, maturation arrest, dyserythropoiesis or megaloblastic change.
10. Bone marrow culture:
    a. Increased colonies with abnormal morphology suggests severe congenital neutropenia.
    b. Increased colonies with normal morphology suggests Shwachman syndrome or chronic benign neutropenia.
    c. Reduced colonies suggests immune neutropenia, chronic neutropenia or progenitor cell disorder.
11. Autoantibodies to exclude SLE or Felty's syndrome.
12. B_{12} and folate assays to exclude megaloblastic neutropenia.
13. Exocrine pancreatic function tests to exclude Shwachman's syndrome.
14. Sucrose lysis and Ham's test to exclude paroxysmal nocturnal haemoglobinuria.
15. Chromosomal analysis to exclude Fanconi's anaemia.
16. Skeletal survey to exclude cartilage hair syndrome, Fanconi's syndrome, Shwachman's syndrome, dyskeratosis congenita.
17. Rebuck skin window to exclude neutrophil chemotactic defect.
18. Plasma and urine amino acids to exclude organic acidaemia.
19. Neutrophil stimulation tests (see Table 5.5).

★ May be performed on the patient's mother in some cases

Evaluation of neutropenia

Particular attention should be focused on the frequency and duration of infective symptoms and any drugs or potentially toxic agents which may produce neutropenia. A family history may indicate other family members with repeated infections. Physical examination should concentrate on any evidence of superficial infection (e.g. skin and mucous membranes), hepatosplenomegaly, lymphadenopathy or any dysmorphic or phenotypic abnormality. Table 5.4 gives a basis for the investigation of a neutropenic child. This list should be considered only as a guide. In many cases, a large

Table 5.5 Neutrophil stimulation tests

1. Hydrocortisone stress test
   a. 5 mg/kg of hydrocortisone hemisuccinate intravenously and monitor neutrophil count hourly from 0 to 6 hours.
   b. A normal response is a rise in the absolute neutrophil count of $> 2.0 \times 10^9/l$.
   c. Cells are released into the circulating pool from the bone marrow.
   d. Abnormal results seen in chronic neutropenia, drug- or toxin-induced hypoplasia, infection-induced hypoplasia, ineffective myelopoiesis and increased peripheral neutrophil destruction.

2. Adrenalin stress test
   a. 0.03 ml/kg of 1:10,000 adrenaline subcutaneously and monitor neutrophil count at 0, 5, 10, 15 and 30 minutes.
   b. A normal response shows a doubling of the absolute neutrophil count within 20 minutes.
   c. Cells are mobilized from the marginating pool.

number of the tests may prove necessary. Table 5.5 indicates some neutrophil stimulation tests which may also occasionally be helpful.

NEUTROPHILIA

In adults, neutrophilia can be applied to patients with an absolute neutrophil count of greater than $7.5 \times 10^9/l$. This definition is too restrictive in children, as neutrophil counts are age-dependent (Ch. 1).

An increase in the number of circulating neutrophils results from an alteration in the normal steady state of neutrophil production, transit and migration, and destruction. Neutrophilia is usually the result of one of the following mechanisms (Cronkite 1979):

1. increased neutrophil mobilization from the marginating pools or bone marrow
2. prolonged neutrophil survival due to impaired transit into the tissues
3. expansion of the neutrophil circulating pool due to (a) increased progenitor cell proliferation, and (b) increased frequency of cell division of committed neutrophil precursors.

Acute neutrophilia

Neutrophils can be mobilized very rapidly, as indicated by the adrenaline stress test where they are released by the marginating cell pool in less than

20 minutes. It has been postulated that adrenaline stimulates receptors on endothelial cells, with the release of cyclic AMP, and reduces neutrophil adhesion. This mechanism is probably of particular importance when neutrophilia is associated with acute bacterial infection, stress, exercise and various toxic agents.

A slightly slower rise in neutrophil count occurs when cells are released from the bone marrow storage pool; this is demonstrated by the hydrocortisone stress test, where neutrophilia may not appear for a few hours. The response may also be mediated via endotoxins released by various microbial agents, or complement activation with the formation of C3e (Ghebrehiwet & Muller-Eberhard 1979). Corticosteroids may also reduce the passage of circulating neutrophils into the tissues, and congenital disorders of neutrophil motility, such as the congenital neutrophil actin dysfunction syndrome, may have a similar effect. The phenomenon may be reflected by an abnormal Rebuck skin window test (Crowley et al 1980).

Chronic neutrophilia

Chronic neutrophilia is usually the result of prolonged stimulation of neutrophil production resulting from increased marrow myeloid progenitor cell proliferation. The majority of reactions last a few days or weeks but some may persist for many months. Chronic neutrophilia may follow long-term corticosteroid therapy, long-standing inflammatory reactions, infections or chronic blood loss. Infections include less common organisms such as disseminated herpes and varicella, poliomyelitis and leptospira.

Chronic inflammatory conditions are frequently associated with neutrophilia, and include juvenile rheumatoid arthritis and Kawasaki's disease. Splenectomy or functional hyposplenism may result in neutrophilia due to reduced removal of neutrophils from the circulation. Other 'noninfectious' causes of neutrophilia include diabetic ketoacidosis, disseminated malignancy, haemolysis, severe burns, uraemia and postoperative states.

Leukaemoid reactions

'Leukaemoid reaction' is an overused term and

Table 5.6   Causes of leukaemoid reactions

Infections
    Bacterial (especially *Staph. aureus* and *Strep. pneumoniae*)
    Tuberculosis
    Brucellosis
    Toxoplasmosis
Marrow infiltrative disease (often with leucoerythroblastosis)
Systemic disease
    Acute glomerulonephritis
    Acute liver failure

is not pathognomonic of any disease process. It is usually applied to a chronic neutrophilia where there is a marked leucocytosis (usually in excess of $50 \times 10^9/1$). A usual feature is a 'shift to the left' of myeloid cells in the peripheral blood, including metamyelocytes, myelocytes, promyelocytes and occasional myeloblasts. The main causes are listed in Table 5.6. Leukaemoid reactions may be confused with leucoerythroblastic anaemias, where similar myeloid precursors may be seen, but the main differentiating feature is the coexistence of nucleated red cells in the peripheral blood, and the leucocyte count may not be raised.

Leukaemoid reactions and myeloproliferative disease

A transient leukaemoid reaction of the newborn may be seen in up to one-third of patients with Down's syndrome. The reaction usually regresses spontaneously within 12 months, but at its zenith may be indistinguishable from acute leukaemia. Bone marrow chromosomal changes may also be found. The reaction appears to arise from an intrinsic intracellular defect in the regulation of neutrophil proliferation and maturation within the bone marrow (Engel et al 1964). A true leukaemia may follow later in childhood in some cases.

A familial myeloproliferative disease resembling chronic myeloid leukaemia has also been described (Randall et al 1965). As well as neutrophilia and immature precursors in the peripheral blood, such patients are anaemic and have hepatosplenomegaly. Some of those described die in early life, whereas others improve with time.

The differentiation between a leukaemoid reaction and chronic granulocytic leukaemia is usually straightforward; the presence of massive splenomegaly, a low leucocyte alkaline phosphatase score and the Philadelphia chromosome indicate the latter condition. Juvenile chronic myeloid leukaemia (better known as subacute myelomonocytic leukaemia) is less likely to be confused, as thrombocytopenia is usually present and frequently there is a raised concentration of fetal haemoglobin.

Neonatal neutrophilia

When compared to those of adults, neutrophil counts are relatively high in the first few days of life, being in the range $8–15 \times 10^9/1$, but by 3 days of age they usually fall to between 1.5 and $5 \times 10^9/1$. This early physiological neutrophilia is often associated with a few myeloid precursors (promyelocytes and blast cells) in the peripheral blood, together with segmented forms. Persisting neutrophilia beyond the first few days of life requires explanation and may be associated with bacterial infection.

EOSINOPHILIA

Eosinophils are proportionately reduced in numbers during the neonatal period. They also exhibit a diurnal variation, being relatively higher during the evenings. Both of these features are of no clinical importance.

The causes of eosinophilia are legion but can be considered under the following headings: allergy, parasites, malignancy, drugs, skin disorders, gastrointestinal disorders, the hypereosinophilic syndrome, and a group of miscellaneous disorders.

Allergy

This is the commonest cause of eosinophilia in the western world. Acute allergic reactions may cause 'leukaemoid' eosinophilic responses with absolute eosinophil counts exceeding $20 \times 10^9/l$. Chronic allergic states are rarely associated with counts above $2 \times 10^9/l$. Over 75% of asthmatic children have eosinophil counts of $0.6 \times 10^9/l$. Other allergic disorders such as hay fever and acute urticaria are also associated with modest eosinophilia.

Parasites

Outside the western world, invasive parasitic in-fections are the commonest cause of eosinophilia. The helminths usually produce a more marked response than do protozoan infections (Teo et al 1985). The eosinophilia associated with parasitic infections is probably not due to a specific factor in the parasites, but to a granulomatous response of the tissues requiring the participation of intact parasites. Some organisms, such as *Giardia lamblia*, do not induce eosinophilia, probably because they do not enter the circulation but remain localized in the gastrointestinal tract. *Toxicara canis* may result in a marked systemic involvement with respiratory, retinal and central nervous system signs. Marked leucocytosis and eosinophilia may persist for years.

Malignant disease

Mild eosinophilia may be associated with Hodgkin's disease in about one-quarter of patients, although occasionally a very marked eosinophilia may be seen. Eosinophilia is also seen occasionally in association with non-Hodgkin's lymphoma, chronic myeloid leukaemia (often with basophilia), acute leukaemias (uncommon), malignant histiocytosis and brain tumours.

Drugs

Of the myriad of drugs causing raised eosinophil counts, many are preceded by the prefix 'anti-', such as antibiotics (penicillin, ampicillin, cephalosporins, nitrofurantoin), antituberculins (para-aminosalicylic acid), antiepileptics (phenytoin) and antihypertensives (hydralazine).

Skin disorders

A variety of skin diseases have been associated with eosinophilia, including atopic dermatitis, eczema, acute urticaria, toxic epidermal necrolysis and dermatitis herpetiformis.

Gastrointestinal disorders

Crohn's disease is often associated with modest eosinophilia, whereas in ulcerative colitis there may be large numbers of eosinophils infiltrating the bowel and relatively few in the peripheral blood.

Milk intolerance and gastrointestinal saccharide intolerance may be associated with a moderate eosinophilia. Chronic liver disease, in particular chronic hepatitis, may also produce a mild rise in circulating eosinophils.

The hypereosinophilic syndrome

In 1968, Hardy & Anderson drew attention to the fact that persistent hypereosinophilia of any type could be associated with a range of similar complications, and they grouped these together as the hypereosinophilic syndrome (Hardy & Anderson 1968). Cushid et al (1975) restricted the diagnosis to patients in whom no underlying cause for the hypereosinophilia could be shown.

In order to make the diagnosis, the following criteria have been suggested: a peripheral blood eosinophilia of more than $1.5 \times 10^9/1$ persisting for more than 6 months (or fatal in a shorter period), resulting in organ system dysfunction and in the absence of any obvious cause for the eosinophilia.

The term encompasses various syndromes including disseminated eosinophilic collagen disease and Loeffler's fibroplastic endocarditis with eosinophilia (Alfaham et al 1987). Some patients have hypereosinophilia with only lung involvement and angioedema. Others present with, or develop, severe cardiac or central nervous system complications. A third group have eosinophilic cytogenetic abnormalities and features of an eosinophilic leukaemic process (see below).

A cause for the condition remains to be identified, although it has been postulated that it may be autoimmune or neoplastic in nature (Fauci et al 1982). Although it is commonest between the ages of 20 and 50 years, the hypereosinophilic syndrome is well-recognized in children, although very rare below the age of 5 (Alfaham et al 1987).

Involvement of the cardiovascular system is the main cause of morbidity and mortality. In the heart, both ventricles are usually involved but the cardiac outflow tracts are spared. Mitral and tricuspid regurgitation are common, and endocardial thrombi give rise to embolic disease. Disease of small blood vessels with intimal thickening also occurs. Cases previously described as Loeffler's syndrome are probably hypereosinophilia with cardiac involvement. Other organs may be involved, as indicated by hepatosplenomegaly, pulmonary fibrosis, central nervous system damage, fever, weight loss and anaemia.

Eosinophilic leukaemia

Rickles & Miller (1972) suggest that the following criteria should be met for a diagnosis of eosinophilic leukaemia: pronounced and persistent eosinophilia associated with immature forms, either in the peripheral blood or bone marrow, more than 5% of bone marrow blasts, tissue infiltration by immature eosinophilic cells, and an acute history with anaemia, thrombocytopenia and increased infection.

Chromosomal abnormalities, abnormal leucocyte alkaline phosphatase activity, high serum B_{12} levels and an associated basophilia suggest leukaemic change and a poor prognosis due to eventual bone marrow failure, but it is more common for patients to succumb to cardiac damage secondary to endocardial and myocardial fibrosis.

The mainstay of treatment for the hypereosinophilic syndrome is corticosteroids. These have brought about a notable improvement in survival and prognosis. Hydroxyurea can be used in non-responders or to allow a reduction in steroid dosage. Vincristine has also been used in association with aggressive disease. Many patients are given anticoagulants. Treatment is given with the aim of reducing the leucocytosis and eosinophilia and alleviating organ dysfunction.

Miscellaneous causes

Most immune deficiency syndromes are associated with a mild eosinophilia. This is particularly noteworthy in the Wiskott–Aldrich syndrome, but may be due in part to the severe eczema associated with that condition. In children with hypogammaglobulinaemia, the presence of eosinophilia may be an indication of *Pneumocystis carinii* infection. Peritoneal and haemodialysis for chronic renal failure and congenital heart disease (with or without hyposplenism) have also been associated with a moderate eosinophilia (Beeson & Bass 1977), as has the thrombocytopenia/absent radius syndrome (see Ch. 6).

Two fungal conditions can produce a marked

eosinophilia – coccidioidomycosis and allergic bronchopulmonary aspergillosis.

BASOPHILIA

As basophils are the least common of the granulocytes, they are the most subject to counting error. A true basophilia is most commonly associated with hypersensitivity reactions to drugs or food substances or in association with acute urticaria.

Inflammatory and infective conditions such as ulcerative colitis, juvenile rheumatoid arthritis, renal failure, influenza, chicken pox and tuberculosis are also associated with a mild-to-moderate basophilia (May & Waddell 1984). Other conditions include Hodgkin's disease, cirrhosis, chronic haemolysis and post splenectomy.

Basophilia is particularly associated with adult-type (Philadelphia chromosome-positive) chronic myeloid leukaemia. The cells may appear abnormal both morphologically and ultrastructurally. Basophil counts may exceed 30% of the white cell population and may rise during the accelerated stage of the disease.

MONOCYTOSIS

The absolute monocyte count is age dependent, and during the first 2 weeks of life the level is greater than $1.0 \times 10^9/1$. Thereafter, the monocyte count rarely exceeds this figure or 10% of the total leucocyte count.

Monocytes are derived from bone marrow progenitor cells, but as there is no substantial bone marrow reserve pool, mature monocytes are released into the peripheral circulation several days earlier than neutrophils following an episode of myelosuppression. They are sometimes a useful harbinger of engraftment following allogeneic marrow transplantation.

Conditions associated with a monocytosis can be grouped into infections, malignant diseases, connective tissue disorders, granulomatous diseases and miscellaneous diseases (Table 5.7).

DISORDERS OF GRANULOCYTE FUNCTION

Functional granulocyte disorders usually produce signs and symptoms similar to those associated with neutropenia or low levels of complement and immunoglobulins. The possibility of a granulocyte dysfunction should be considered after these disorders have been excluded.

It is convenient to consider the various granulocyte disorders under the same headings as neutrophil function, namely: adherence and margination, chemotaxis, ingestion and recognition, degranulation, oxidative metabolism and oxidant scavenging.

Disorders of adherence and margination

Plasma membrane glycoprotein deficiency

Between the mid-1970s and early 1980s, several investigators reported over 20 patients with a previously unrecognized disorder associated with severe recurrent bacterial infections (see Todd & Freyer 1988 for review). The infections mainly affected soft tissues, the middle ear, produced pneumonitis or involved the oropharyngeal mucosa. Other more specific features included a persistent leucocytosis, gingivitis/periodontitis and delayed separation of the umbilical cord. The most striking physical finding was the failure of neutrophils to accumulate at foci of infection despite a peripheral blood neutrophilia. The defect was most dramatically demonstrated using the Rebuck skin window technique, where there was almost complete absence of neutrophils more than 4 hours after the skin abrasion.

In 1980, Crowley et al suggested a molecular basis for this striking defect. They showed that granulocytes from patients with the illness apparently lacked a series of membrane glycoproteins.

Table 5.7 Conditions associated with a reactive monocytosis

Infections	Connective tissue disorder
Infective endocarditis	Ulcerative colitis
Tuberculosis	Sarcoidosis
Brucellosis	Crohn's disease
Typhoid fever	Miscellaneous
Congenital syphilis	Post splenectomy
Leishmaniasis	
Malignant disease	
Myelodysplastic syndromes	
Myeloid leukaemias	
Hodgkin's disease	
Non-Hodgkin lymphomas	

This lack of membrane glycoproteins resulted in a defect of neutrophil adherence to surfaces, a necessary prerequisite for cells to migrate across tissues in response to chemotactic signals. Affected neutrophils also failed to recognize microorganisms coated with the complement fragment C3bi. Although the defective neutrophils degranulated and showed normal exudative burst activity if stimulated with soluble stimuli, they did not show these responses when triggered by complement C3bi binding.

Three glycoproteins have been identified which together are now known as the CD11/CD18 glycoprotein family (Todd & Freyer 1988). These are:

1. LFA-1 which is present on all leucocytes and which acts as an adhesion-promoting molecule facilitating lymphocyte cytotoxicity and lymphocyte-endothelial cell adhesion
2. Mo1 which is present on monocytes, neutrophils and NK cells and which is the receptor for C3bi facilitating polymorph aggregation, adhesion and chemotaxis
3. P150, 95 which is present on monocytes and neutrophils but the function of which is not well defined.

The name CD11/CD18 membrane glycoprotein deficiency has recently been given to the disorder which can be recognized by flow cytometric analysis using CD11/CD18-specific monoclonal reagents (Shaw 1987).

The syndrome is inherited in an autosomal recessive fashion, although X-linked inheritance has also been reported in at least one family (Crowley et al 1980). Prenatal diagnosis of the condition has recently been described using fetal leucocytes obtained by amniocentesis (Weisman et al 1987).

No specific treatment has been shown to be beneficial except possibly vitamin C in one case (Hayward et al 1979). Most bacterial infections are controlled with the appropriate antibiotics, and granulocyte transfusions have been used. Successful allogeneic bone marrow transplantation has also been carried out (Fischer et al 1983). Prophylactic therapy with trimethoprin–sulphamethoxazole may also be helpful (Abramson et al 1981).

Acquired neutrophil adherence disorders

Various drugs are known to affect the adhesion of neutrophils to surfaces and may result in a marked transient neutrophilia. Adrenaline and corticosteroids are probably the best examples, and these responses form part of the basis of the adrenaline and corticosteroid stimulation tests. Adrenalin causes the stimulation of cyclic AMP in the vascular endothelium which appears to reduce neutrophil adherence, and hence marginating neutrophils are released into the circulating pool (Bryant & Sutcliff 1974). Steroids may change neutrophil adherence by affecting arachidonic acid metabolism, impairing neutrophil fatty acid metabolism, or interfering with the binding of chemotactic molecules to cells (Oseas et al 1982, Hirata et al 1980).

Increased neutrophil aggregation has been reported with the use of granulocyte transfusions where these have been obtained by filtration rather than centrifugation, and with the use of amphotericin B, particularly when these two therapies are combined. Neutrophil aggregation can result in the formation of pulmonary aggregates causing respiratory insufficiency (Boxer et al 1981).

Complement activation, and the generation of C5a in particular, is an important trigger to the activation of neutrophils and increased adhesion. The reaction is probably mediated via membrane glycoproteins. Stimulating factors probably include bacterial sepsis, thermal injury, extensive tissue necrosis and possibly haemodialysis. Aggregated neutrophils may then result in the liberation of proteases, endothelial cell damage and, in the lungs, the development of the adult respiratory distress syndrome (Tate & Repine 1983).

Chemotactic disorders

Chemotaxis refers to the attractions of cells by chemical substances; it has been recognized since the turn of the century, when Metchnikoff appreciated the importance of phagocytes and their ability to recognize bacterial products (Metchnikoff 1905).

Normal chemotaxis is dependent upon an integrated chain of events. Firstly, chemotactic factors must be produced in order to create a 'chemotactic gradient'. Monocytes and neutrophils must then process their appropriate receptors to identify these factors and be able to identify the direction of the gradient. Neutrophils must then be able to adhere to the endothelial wall and other connective tissues, and migrate to the point of inflammation (margination) with the aid of cytoplasmic contractile proteins. Finally, the stimulating chemotactic factors must be inactivated once an adequate neutrophil/monocyte response has taken place.

Phagocytes (i.e. neutrophils and monocytes) are known to contain plasma membrane receptors for leucokines, bacterial products, complement and colony-stimulating factors (CSFs). Receptors are more densely concentrated on the cell's leading edge, and intracellular receptors for the complement factor CR3 (C3bi) have also been identified (Fearon & Collins 1983). Alcohols can increase phagocyte receptor affinity whereas amphotericin can produce the opposite effect (Snyderman & Pike 1984). Minute concentrations of GM-CSF can result in an initial rise and subsequent fall in receptor affinity (Weisbart et al 1985).

Neutrophils cannot swim; they crawl towards sites of inflammation. Chemotactic factors reduce the normal cellular negative charge and enhance endothelial adherence. Increased adhesion appears to involve the CD11/CD18 neutrophil glycoprotein complex as well as endotoxins and interleukins (Schleimer & Rutledge 1986). After surface attachment, neutrophils become more elongated, with the nucleus moving to the back of the cell with the granule-rich cytoplasm and the microtubular apparatus positioned between the nucleus and the front of the cell. Both the microtubule apparatus and actin polymerization changes play a critical role in cell orientation and locomotion (Brown & Gallin 1988).

Lymphokines are also important in chemotaxis. Gamma interferon stimulates monocyte chemotaxis (Sechler & Gallin 1987). Tumour necrosis factor causes increased adherence of neutrophils to endothelial cells and increased phagocytic capacity (Schleimer & Rutledge 1986).

Laboratory diagnosis

Most in vitro assays of chemotaxis measure the movement of neutrophils under agarose or through a cellulose nitrate filter (Boyden chamber). After a set period, the cells are fixed and stained and their patterns of movement analyzed. Migration under agarose is not as sensitive as through cellulose nitrate filters, and conditions such as the Chédiak-Higashi syndrome may be missed as the agarose method does not detect defects in deformability. The agarose method, however, requires fewer neutrophils and identification of individual cell types is easier.

Radioisotope assays of chemotaxis using ^{51}Cr–labelled neutrophils are available which are simple and, when used in the form of a multicell microassay, require small numbers of cells and minimal chemoattractant (Falk et al 1980).

In vivo assessment of neutrophil movement usually involves the Rebuck skin window or skin blister technique. The Rebuck assay is rather nonspecific, as it measures not only chemotaxis but also the ability of leucocytes to adhere to glass. Nevertheless, the technique provides a simple screening test for the integrity of the inflammatory response. The suction blister apparatus yields information of neutrophil locomotion and is particularly useful for studying large numbers of functional neutrophils and quantitation of the number and types of cells arriving at inflammatory exudates.

Clinical features

Several chemotactic disorders have specific and distinct clinical features. These include the Chédiak-Higashi syndrome, Job's syndrome, CR3-receptor deficiency and localized juvenile periodontitis. Other disorders may not be associated with such specific characteristics, but all are associated with increased susceptibility to a variety of infections, including sinusitis, gingivitis, pneumonia, bronchiectasis, otitis, dermatitis and other skin infections. Frequent and severe soft tissue abscesses are also commonly associated with chemotactic disorders, and recurrent or chronic fungal and bacterial infections can occur despite a peripheral blood leucocytosis. Pneumonia and lung abscesses are the most frequent fatal complication.

Infections and dermatitis may present in the neonatal period but thereafter may be periodic and unpredictable. *Staphylococcus aureus* is the commonest infecting organism, but Gram-negative bacilli, fungi, *Haemophilus influenzae* and *Staph. epidermidis* may also be troublesome. Streptococci and particularly *Strep. pneumoniae* are not associated with chemotactic disorders, being more common in children with hypogammaglobulinaemia.

It is important to remember that severe infections may be associated with minimal signs and symptoms, probably because of the delayed movement of leucocytes to the focus of infection. The infections tend to become indolent, with a high recurrence rate and poor antimicrobial response. Determined investigation and therapy is therefore required.

Cellular disorders

CR3 deficiency. CR3 (C3bi receptor) deficiency usually presents in infancy with delayed separation of the umbilicus. The children can exhibit poor wound healing, with recurrent bacterial and fungal infections and little or no pus formation. Mucositis and oral periodontal infections are particularly common, as are more serious osteomyelitis and pneumonia. *Pseudomonas* and *Staph. aureus* are the most common infecting organisms.

As well as defective chemotaxis, a deficiency of neutrophil CR3 can be demonstrated using fluorescent or peroxidase-labelled anti-CR3 antibodies.

The mode of inheritance is autosomal recessive. CR3 is related to the CD11/CD18 neutrophil glycoprotein complex, and the severity of the glycoprotein deficiency correlates with the clinical severity of the condition. CR3 is also important in neutrophil adherence to endothelial cells, and its expression can be increased by endotoxin, interleukin-l and tumour necrosis factor.

Chédiak–Higashi syndrome. This is a rare, recessively inherited abnormality characterized by partial oculocutaneous albinism, mental retardation, photophobia, peripheral neuropathy and recurrent infections, particularly oral and cutaneous. All cells containing lysosomal granules show giant forms which are the result of fusion of different granules (Fig. 5.2). The majority of patients enter a phase of accelerated morbidity, usually during their second decade, which is characterized by a stormy febrile course, pancytopenia and widespread lymphohistiocytic organ infiltrates. Those

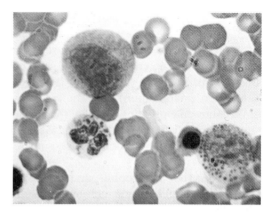

Fig. 5.2 Giant neutrophil inclusions seen in the Chédiak-Higashi syndrome. A myelocyte in the picture also shows abnormal giant granules.

patients who do not suffer an accelerated phase fall prey to recurrent serious infections, progressive peripheral neuropathy and, sometimes, CNS disease with cerebellar ataxia, cranial nerve palsies and raised intracranial pressure (Brown & Gallin 1988). The neurological effects may be the result of giant granule infiltration of cells in the CNS, particularly Schwann cells.

The haematological features of the Chédiak–Higashi syndrome are summarized in Table 5.8. The abnormal cytoplasmic granules form during myelopoiesis, and the majority of marrow progenitor stem cells are defective as judged by in vitro colony assays (Oliver & Essner 1985). This observation has led to the suggestion that the marrow stem cells are affected by the genetic defect (Barak et al 1986). The moderate neutropenia seen is the result of ineffective medullary myelopoiesis and recurrent infections are the result of neutropenia together with defective chemotaxis, degranulation and antibacterial activity (Root et al 1972).

It has been suggested that NK cells in the Chédiak-Higashi syndrome possess abnormal membrane and cytoplasmic structural components which are necessary for their function (Nair et al 1987). In addition, storage pool platelet defects have been described, resulting in prolonged bleeding times and haemorrhagic manifestations associated with normal platelet counts (Buchanan & Handin 1976).

Both Gram-positive and Gram-negative organisms are troublesome for children with the Chédiak-

Table 5.8 Laboratory features of the Chédiak-Higashi syndrome

Stable phase
Neutrophils
1. Giant azurophilic and specific granules
2. Neutropenia resulting from ineffective myelopoiesis
3. Reduced bacterial activity:
    a. impaired chemotaxis
    b. delayed degranulation
    c. reduced granule proteases

Monocytes/macrophages
1. Giant inclusion bodies
2. Impaired chemotaxis

Lymphocytes (NK cells) + platelets
1. Giant cytoplasmic granules
2. Absence of dense bodies
3. Platelet storage pool defect

Accelerated phase
1. Epstein-Barr infection
2. Diffuse polyclonal non-neoplastic lymphohistiocytic infiltrate
3. Histiocytic haemophagocytosis
4. Massive hepatosplenomegaly resulting in pancytopenia

Adapted from: Boxer & Smolen 1988

Higashi syndrome. Infections are often repeated and debilitating, with the skin and mucous membranes most often affected. *Staph. aureus* is the commonest organism.

Although the basic nature of the underlying abnormality is unknown, it is likely that anomalous neutrophil membrane function is an important factor in the functional defect (White & Clawson 1980). The neutrophils act as though unable to control membrane activation. They spontaneously aggregate molecules into caps, and show increased oxygen consumption, reduced surface adherence and impaired chemotactic responses (Oliver 1978). They also form giant neutrophil granules, changing the primary granules into large secondary lysosomes which have a reduced enzyme content (Kimball et al 1975). Despite normal ingestion, neutrophils kill microorganisms slowly due to the reduced and erratic delivery of diluted hydrolytic enzymes from the giant granules (Stossel et al 1972). An abnormal membrane fluidity has been demonstrated in neutrophils and red cells of patients (Ingraham et al 1981), and this concept may serve to link the abnormal motility, granule fusion, platelet abnormality and abnormal NK cell structure seen in the syndrome.

Management of the Chédiak-Higashi syndrome is based predominantly on the treatment of infec-

tious episodes. Prophylactic co-trimoxazole may be helpful, but acute infections should be treated aggressively. High doses of ascorbic acid have been found helpful in some, but not all, patients (Gallin et al 1979). Treatment for the accelerated phase has included vincristine, corticosteroids and antithymocyte globulin, but without obvious benefit (Nair et al 1987). Bone marrow transplantation has been successfully performed in a few patients (Fischer et al 1986).

Kartagener's syndrome. Patients with this disorder experience recurrent infections of the respiratory tract, middle ear and sinuses, and have associated situs inversus. Neutrophils exhibit defective locomotion and chemotaxis (Malech et al 1979).

Specific granule deficiency. This very rare disorder can be detected by blood film examination in patients who suffer from repeated infections (Boxer & Smolen 1988). Standard Romanowsky stains show agranular neutrophils, whereas peroxidase stain shows the primary granules to be intact. The absence of specific granules can be confirmed by immunochemical stains or demonstration of the absence of lactoferrin in either mature neutrophils or bone marrow precursors. There are also abnormalities of nuclear shape resembling the Pelger-Huet abnormality.

Individuals with specific granule deficiency are prone to recurrent bacterial and fungal infections of the skin and deep tissues (Gallin 1985) and a variety of abnormalities of neutrophil function. These include poor chemotaxis, failure of neutrophil disaggregation following stimulation and reduced recruitment of monocytes to sites of inflammation by neutrophils (Lomax et al 1989)

Recent work has also suggested that the absence of lactoferrin in the neutrophils is the result of an abnormality of lactoferrin gene expression which is limited to cells of the myeloid series (Lomax et al 1989). This would suggest that the lactoferrin lack in neutrophil-specific granule deficiency is a result of a failure of gene expression at the myelocyte/metamyelocyte stage of maturation.

Treatment is based on the prompt use of appropriate antibiotics with surgical drainage of abscesses. Morbidity and mortality may be less than those associated with phagocytic defects.

Localized juvenile periodontitis. This

condition usually affects older children and adolescents, and infection is usually localized to the mouth, with premature loss of teeth and periodontitis resulting in alveolar bone resorption (van Dyke 1985). There is a moderate defect of leucocyte chemotaxis as well as radiological evidence of periodontal bone loss.

Lazy leucocyte syndrome. Several miscellaneous disorders have been described in which there is abnormal neutrophil chemotaxis. The lazy leucocyte syndrome is characterized by recurrent dermatitis, otitis media, gingivitis, respiratory infections and congenital neutropenia (Miller et al 1971). Bone marrow examination shows normal myeloid precursors, but abnormal chemotaxis is demonstrable using the Rebuck skin window. The condition is relatively mild.

Humoral disorders

Hyper-immunoglobulin-E (HIE) syndrome (Job's syndrome). HIE syndrome is characterized by recurrent skin and sinopulmonary infections beginning in infancy or early childhood. Typical infective problems include the development of subcutaneous abscesses and chronic mucocutaneous candidiasis, usually involving the oesophagus, vagina and nails. Other problems include pneumonia, recurrent ear infections, dermatitis and chronic eczema. Chronic lung illnesses can be the most dangerous and debilitating, with bronchiectasis and fistula formation (Leung & Geha 1988). Patients frequently have characteristic facies with a broad nasal bridge and prominent jaw. The most commonly associated bacterial infections are *Staph. aureus* and *Haemophilus influenzae*.

HIE syndrome is extremely rare but should be considered in children and infants presenting with severe atopic dermatitis and recurrent staphylococcal skin infections. Most such patients will have other disorders, including primary skin complaints, hypogammaglobulinaemia, Wiskott-Aldrich syndrome or Di George's syndrome (Ch. 11). The diagnosis is based on the clinical history and the presence of an IgE level usually at least 10 times the age-related value (Donabedian & Gallin 1983).

The associated neutrophil chemotactic defect (Clark et al 1973) is present only intermittently.

Although immune complexes have been shown to inhibit neutrophil chemotaxis, serum from patients with HIE syndrome does not affect normal phagocyte function; however, their mononuclear cells have been shown to produce an inhibitor of leucocyte chemotaxis. Thus, the suggestion is that the neutrophils themselves are not abnormal, but that some sporadically produced factor causes the reversible chemotactic defect, a factor which does not appear to be plasma derived, but may be of monocytic origin, or may be an IgE-mediated histamine release (Hill et al 1976).

Treatment is much the same as for other leucocyte disorders and is based on effective use of antibiotics. Surgery may be necessary for abscess drainage. Other therapies that have been tried include ascorbic acid, cimetidine and levamisole. None has been shown to be of proven benefit, and a double-blind placebo-controlled trial actually demonstrated an increased incidence of infection in patients receiving levamisole. As patients with HIE syndrome have low levels of circulating antibody against bacterial antigens, a trial of intravenous immunoglobulin would appear logical, but no comparative study has been performed. There is anecdotal evidence that plasmapheresis may be beneficial for patients who fail to respond to antibiotics (Leung & Geha 1988).

Chemotactic inhibitors of the neutrophil response. Various clinical disorders have been described where the production of inhibitors interferes with the normal response of neutrophils to chemotactic factors. The mechanisms by which these inhibitors work are not known. Some immune complex diseases are associated with such chemotactic defects (Hanlon et al 1980). IgG-binding to neutrophils has been shown to inhibit locomotion. Similar effects have been seen in patients with IgA paraproteinaemias and solid tumours (mainly melanoma and breast cancer in adults).

Viral and bacterial products can also interfere with chemotaxis. Herpes simplex and influenza viruses can inhibit monocyte chemotaxis but this has not been shown with vaccinia, polio or retroviruses. Mouse CMV infection can reduce chemotaxis but this has not been demonstrated for human strains (Brown & Gallin 1988). HIV infection may have a direct effect on neutrophil chemotaxis, or an indirect effect via raised, inhibitory levels of IgA (Estevez et al 1986).

Neutrophils of donor origin in patients who have recently undergone bone marrow transplantation may show reduced chemotaxis particularly when associated with graft-versus-host disease (Clark et al 1976).

There are many other anecdotal reports of defective chemotaxis in association with systemic disease. These include alpha-mannosidase deficiency, myotonic dystrophy, alpha-1-antitrypsin deficiency, Pelger-Huet abnormality, cirrhosis and sarcoidosis (Brown & Gallin 1988).

Chemotactic factor phagocyte deactivation. Abnormal phagocyte chemotaxis has been observed in the Wiskott–Aldrich syndrome and appears to be the result of excessive production of lymphocyte-derived chemotactic factor (Ochs et al 1980). This finding goes together with the other features of this X-linked disorder (eczema, thrombocytopenia, abnormal cell-mediated immune responses and a deficiency of IgM production to polysaccharide antigens). Plasma from Wiskott patients inhibits the chemotaxis of normal leucocytes. It has been suggested that the excessive production of this chemotactic lymphokine leads to deactivation of chemotactic receptors.

DISORDERS OF OXIDATIVE METABOLISM

Chronic granulomatous disease

Chronic granulomatous disease (CGD) is an inherited disorder of neutrophil function in which phagocytes are unable to produce antimicrobial oxidant factors. Since the discovery of the disease nearly 25 years ago, (Holmes, Page & Good 1967) its increasing complexity has become apparent (Karnousky 1973).

Disease characteristics

The neutrophils from patients with CGD show normal chemotaxis, engulfment and degranulation, but have a reduced capacity to kill microorganisms (Babior & Crowley 1983). Affected neutrophils stimulated in vitro by appropriate particulate, or soluble stimuli fail to consume oxygen necessary for the production of superoxide, hydrogen peroxide and hydroxyl radicals. CGD can be suspected when there is evidence of absent or diminished oxidative metabolism of stimulated phagocytes. The diagnosis is confirmed when granulocytes are shown to be unable to kill ingested catalase-producing bacteria.

A variety of techniques are available to detect the defective oxidative metabolism. The reduction of the yellow dye, nitro blue tetrazolium (NBT) by superoxide to form an insoluble dark blue pigment which precipitates on normal activated neutrophils remains the standard and convenient way of demonstrating the defect (Baehner & Nathan 1968). The histochemical (slide) method is particularly useful because it allows assessment of individual cells and can also suggest the existence of a variant form of CGD (Meerhof & Roos 1986). It is also useful in diagnosing the carrier state, as a mixed population of NBT-positive and -negative cells are seen (Ochs & Igo 1973). Other tests of oxygen uptake, hydrogen peroxide and superoxide production are available, but usually only in specialist laboratories.

Classification

CGD has long been recognized as a heterogeneous disorder. The majority of patients are male and inherit the condition in an X-linked manner, but as long as 20 years ago females were observed with the condition where the inheritance appeared to be autosomal recessive (Baehner & Nathan 1968, Chandra et al 1969, Holmes et al 1970). Classification can therefore be made on the mode of inheritance, and also on whether or not the neutrophils contain cytochrome b_{558} (see below and Tables 5.9 and 5.10).

CGD occurs with a frequency of about one case

Table 5.9 The classification of CGD: 2. Neutrophil phenotypes

Type	Inheritance	Cytochrome b_{558}	Cytosol factor	Frequency (% of cases)
I	X-linked	Absent	Normal	65%
II	Autosomal recessive	Normal	Markedly reduced	30%
III	Autosomal recessive	Absent	Normal	Very rare
IV	X-linked	Normal	Normal	Exceedingly rare

Table 5.10 The classification of chronic granulomatous disease: 1. Inheritance

---

X-linked CGD
1. X-linked family distribution (i.e. male patients and female carriers)
2. NBT test on patient's mother and female carriers shows two cell populations
3. Gene probes may indicate an absent or defective CGD gene in the patient's DNA

Autosomal recessive CGD
1. Occurs in both male and female family members
2. NBT test normal in carriers
3. In some patients the cytosolic factor is missing (DNA probes for AR-CGD not yet available)

---

per million of the population, of which approximately two thirds are the X-linked variant (X-CGD), and one-third autosomal recessive (AR-CGD).

The molecular basis of CGD

The exposure of neutrophils and other phagocytes (eosinophils and monocytes) to certain stimuli results in the production of microbicidal oxidizing agents by the partial reduction of oxygen. This event is known as the 'respiratory burst' and results in the production of cellular superoxide (O_2^-), peroxide (H_2O_2), oxidizing radicals and a rise in glucose catabolism via the hexose monophosphate shunt. The key event in the respiratory burst is the activation of the enzyme responsible for O_2^- generation. This enzyme, the respiratory burst oxidase, catalyses the reduction of O_2 to O_2^- (Rossi & Zatti 1964) thus:

$$2\,O_2 + NADPH \longrightarrow 2\,O_2^- + NADP^+ + H^+$$

The reaction occurs when resting phagocytes are exposed to activating agents. In CGD patients activity of the oxidase is depressed.

O_2^--Forming activity

Attempts have been made to purify and characterize the active oxidase (Gabig et al 1978). It has been shown to require flavin adenine dinucleotide (FAD) and phospholipids for its activity. The most active of the purified preparations suggest that the oxidase is made up of three non-identical subunits (32 K, 48 K and 66 K) with the NADPH-binding site being on the 66K subunit (Umei et al 1986).

Cytochromes and CGD

In 1978 Segal and Jones (1978) identified a b-type cytochrome in human neutrophils. It is known as b_{558} (on the basis of spectroscopic measurement at 558mm) or b_{-245} (corresponding to an electron oxidation potential of -245 mV) (Segal 1988). Evidence strongly suggests that cytochrome b_{558} is connected with the respiratory burst and that it is missing from some patients with CGD (Ohno et al 1986). Most males with X-linked CGD have neutrophils which lack the cytochrome, whereas most (but not all) patients with the autosomal recessive type of CGD do not. What remains in doubt is the exact function of cytochrome b_{558}. It is believed that it may be the end component of an electron transport chain that carries electrons from NADPH to oxygen to form O_2^- (Cross et al 1985), but this hypothesis is not universally supported (Curnutte & Babior 1987). Cytochrome b_{558} may be made up of several components, in particular large and small subunits (Dinauer & Orkin 1988), with classic X-linked CGD being caused by a mutation in the large subunit of the cytochrome b heterodimer. Autosomal recessive CGD, on the other hand, is probably the result of an entirely different type of defect involving a cytosolic factor necessary for activation of the respiratory burst (see below).

The gene responsible for X-CGD has been localized to the X21 region of the X chromosome (Lomax et al 1989) and the X-CGD gene has been cloned.

The cytosolic factor

Most patients with the autosomal recessive type of CGD (the second-commonest type) have normal leucocyte levels of cytochrome b_{558}. Under normal circumstances, activation of the NADPH-dependent superoxide generating system of phagocytes can be achieved in a cell-free system, but this requires both cytosol and cell membranes (Curnutte et al 1988). It has been shown that cytochrome b_{558}-positive AR-CGD patients have a neutrophil cytosol defect, while X-CGD patients and cytochrome b_{558}-negative AR-CGD patients share a defect of neutrophil membranes (cytochrome b_{558} is an integral membrane protein). The cytosolic factor appears to be a 240K protein or proteins

Table 5.11 Clinical features suggestive of CGD

1. Recurrent lymphadenitis
2. Multiple site osteomyelitis
3. Family history of recurrent infections
4. Hepatic bacterial abscesses
5. Unusual catalase positive infections
6. Purulent, slowly healing skin lesions
7. Subcutaneous immunization related abscesses
8. Infantile rash of ears and nares
9. Ulcerative stomatitis
10. Persistent rhinitis
11. Conjunctivitis
12. Association of the above with chronic inflammatory bowel disease

(Curnutte et al 1987). Except for the fact that it requires magnesium in order to be active, little else is known about how it works.

From Table 5.9 it can be seen that a phenotypic classification of CGD can be based on the presence or absence of cytochrome b_{558} and cytosol factor. More important, however, especially for genetic counselling, is the establishment of the mode of transmission (Table 5.10).

Clinical features

Table 5.11 lists some of the clinical problems which should alert the clinician to the possibility of CGD. Infections tend to occur most often in the skin, lung and mucous membranes, all areas which act as surface environmental barriers (Fig. 5.3). Once organisms have penetrated those barriers, neutrophils play an important part in controlling infection. In CGD, the defect in microorganism killing results in a perpetuating cycle of phagocytosis, leucocyte rupture and re-engulfment of released organisms.

Lymphadenopathy and hepatomegaly occur in the majority of patients. Persistently discharging nodes are not uncommon. Hepatic abscesses also occur in over one-third of patients. Osteomyelitis is particularly common in the small bones of the feet and hands, and may be associated with recurrent foot furuncles or paronychia.

Multiple granulomata can develop in virtually any organ and are particularly common in the reticuloendothelial system. Such lesions can result in obstruction of the genito-urinary or gastrointestinal tracts. Granulomata formation in the antrum of the stomach can masquerade as pyloric stenosis, eosinophilic gastroenteritis or Crohn's disease. The mechanism of granuloma formation in CGD is unknown, but one possibility is that the delayed clearance of microorganisms leads to persistent inflammation because chemoattractants are not oxidized (Gallin & Buescher 1983).

Recurrent respiratory infections remain a particular source of morbidity (Fig. 5.4). The almost routine use of long-term prophylactic antibiotics has prolonged survival and decreased time in hospital, but has also been associated with an increase in late complications, such as chronic suppurative lung disease, progressive pulmonary fibrosis and

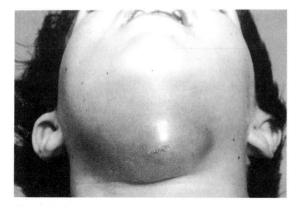

Fig. 5.3 Chronic granulomatous disease. Persisting submandibular soft tissue infection with incipient skin breakdown and chronic discharge.

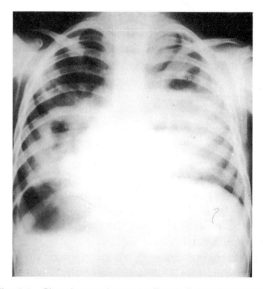

Fig. 5.4 Chronic granulomatous disease. Lung abcess and chronic inflammatory changes.

bronchiectasis. These secondary lung changes are not infrequently compounded by terminal *Aspergillus* fungal infections.

During acute infective episodes, patients usually have a neutrophil leucocytosis. The anaemia of chronic disorders may be a feature of chronic sepsis and may only improve with resolution of the infection. Care should be taken in transfusing red cells, as patients with X-linked CGD may be lacking in Kell blood group antigens (McLeod) and produce anti-Kell or anti-Cellano following red cell sensitization. Subsequent provision of compatible red cells becomes very difficult.

Management

Control of infection is the mainstay of management of CGD. Before the introduction of long-term prophylactic antibiotics, recurrent bacterial infections were much more frequent. Forrest et al (1988) reported that the use of trimethoprim/sulphamethoxazole (TMP-SMZ) lengthened the infection-free period in 19 patients from 3.7 to 10.7 months. Patients were affected less by dermatitis, osteomyelitis and hepatic abscesses. Although similar numbers of isolates of Gram-negative enteric organisms were cultured before and after prophylaxis, the incidence of staphylococcal infections in patients on prophylaxis was much reduced.

Many organisms are sensitive to TMP-SMZ prophylaxis, particularly *Enterobacteriaceae* and staphylococci. TMP-SMZ also exhibits good intercellular penetration and drug concentrations (Gmünder & Seger 1981).

Energetic supportive care also remains an important part of treatment for CGD. Cultures must be obtained as soon as infection is suspected, as unusual organisms may arise. Some abscesses will require surgical drainage either for diagnostic or therapeutic purposes or both. Nutritional support is often required, particularly if there is a gastric outlet obstruction. Corticosteroids may occasionally be helpful in gastrointestinal obstructive lesions (Chin et al 1987), but their use is not widely recommended.

Bone marrow transplantation remains the only known cure for CGD (Johnston 1983), but when and whether to transplant remain difficult decisions because of the variable nature of the disease.

Interferon

Recent in vitro studies using recombinant alpha-interferon have demonstrated increased respiratory burst activity of polymorphs and macrophages in the X-linked type I disease but not in the autosomal types II and III (Newburger & Ezekowitz 1988). Preliminary in vivo studies also showed complete or partial correction of the CGD defect in patients who had shown an in vitro response – interferon therefore offers some therapeutic potential in the treatment of patients with X-linked CGD, and is an example of pharmacological modulation of gene expression in human disease.

The potential for gene therapy

Theoretically, genes can be introduced into fetal cells, germ cells or specific somatic cells. Bone marrow provides a very suitable target tissue. Several methods are available for the introduction of genes into mammalian cells, and recent work has concentrated on the use of recombinant retrovirus vectors to effect gene transfer into bone marrow cells. Marrow cells are infected with a retrovirus gene vector and the gene transfer is quantitated by use of clonal assays, either in vitro agar culture or in vivo murine assays.

Several disorders of neutrophil function are potential candidates for gene transfer. These include CGD, myeloperoxidase deficiency, specific granule deficiency and leucocyte glycoprotein deficiency. The copy DNAs for both subunits of the CGD protein have been cloned (Dinauer et al 1987). The treatment of this and similar disorders, although rare, may provide useful models for gene therapy in the future.

Glucose-6-phosphate dehydrogenase (G6PD) deficiency

NADPH is the basic substrate for the respiratory burst reaction necessary for the formation of superoxide (O_2^-). It is produced by glucose-6-phosphate dehydrogenase (G6PD) and 6-phosphogluconate dehydrogenase (6PGD), the first two enzymes of the hexose monophosphate shunt. Absence of G6PD results in reduced availability of NADPH, reduced respiratory burst activity and a clinical picture similar to chronic granulomatous disease.

Similar microorganisms are involved (i.e. predominantly catalase-positive bacteria).

The gene for leucocyte G6PD deficiency is identical to that for the red cell enzyme, and patients have the associated haemolytic anaemia (Yoshida & Stamatoyannopoulos 1968), but unlike red cell G6PD deficiency, fewer than 10 patients with severe leucocyte G6PD deficiency have been described (Gray et al 1973). A possible explanation for this discrepancy in disease frequency is that neutrophils must have a severe (less than 5%) deficiency before neutrophil function is affected. Most cases of neutrophil dysfunction are found in Mediterranean G6PD deficiency, but even in this variant, clinically important leucocyte dysfunction is rare.

Myeloperoxidase deficiency

Myeloperoxidase (MPO) is a haem-containing enzyme found in primary neutrophil granules. It is essential for the formation of hypochlorite ions which react with free amine groups to form potent microbicidal agents. Although myeloperoxidase deficiency may affect up to 1 in 400 persons (Parry et al 1981), the clinical disorder is usually mild and is mainly expressed by *Candida albicans* infections in individuals with coexistent diabetes. When stimulated, neutrophils lacking myeloperoxidase show prolonged superoxide production, suggesting that peroxidase activity may play a role in normal termination of the respiratory burst (Nauseef et al 1983). Lengthening of the respiratory burst may partly compensate for absence of the myeloperoxidase–hydrogen peroxide reaction.

MPO deficiency is inherited as an autosomal recessive trait. With blood counters which incorporate automated white cell differential counters based on a peroxidase stain, patients with MPO deficiency may be incorrectly indicated to have an absolute neutropenia (Kitahara et al 1979). The disorder is diagnosed by demonstrating the absence of cytochemically stainable enzyme.

Recent cloning of cDNA for myeloperoxidase has indicated that in some patients the deficiency may result from derangement of post-translocational processing of an abnormal precursor peptide, and that the defect is probably on chromosome 17 (Lomax et al 1989). Weil et al (1988) have examined patients with acute promyelocytic leukaemia (M_3) which is associated with the chromosomal translocation t(15:17)(q22:q 11.2). In all cases studied, the myeloperoxidase gene was translocated from chromosome 17 to 15. The importance, if any, of the myeloperoxidase gene in development of this subtype of leukaemia remains to be determined.

Disorders of oxidant scavenging

Superoxides produced by the respiratory burst are very efficient at destroying microorganisms, but may diffuse into leucocyte cytoplasm resulting in serious cellular damage. Consequently, neutrophils are equipped with enzymes and antioxidants to remove these damaging oxygen derivatives from the cytoplasm (Babior & Crowley 1983) whilst not interfering with the normal microbicidal reactions within the phagolysosomes.

Superoxide is destroyed by the reaction:

$$O_2^- + O_2^- + 2\,H^+ \longrightarrow H_2O_2 + O_2$$

Hydrogen peroxide is then degraded into oxygen and water by cytoplasmic catalase or glutathione peroxidase and the glutathione reductase system.

Glutathione reductase maintains adequate amounts of reduced glutathione (GSH) by the reactions:

$$GSSG + NADPH + H^+ \longrightarrow 2\,GSH + NADP^+$$
$$\text{(glutathione reductase)}$$

Reduced glutathione then destroys hydrogen peroxide with the aid of glutathione peroxide:

$$H_2O_2 + 2\,GSH \longrightarrow 2H_2 + GSSG$$
$$\text{(glutathione peroxidase)}$$

Catalase deficiency

This very rare syndrome has not been associated with an increased incidence of infection. Ross et al (1980) reported two patients with reduced levels of both erythrocyte (less than 2% activity) and neutrophil (10–20%) catalase activity. They proposed that whilst affected neutrophils may be able to cope with endogenously generated hydrogen peroxide, they may exhibit reduced activity against exogenous superoxides.

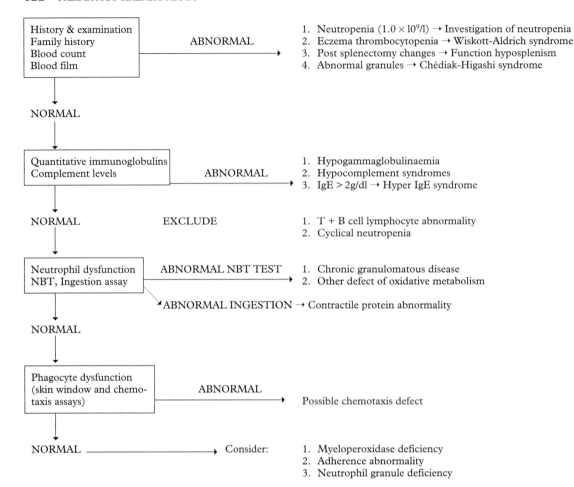

Fig. 5.5 Investigation of the child with recurrent infection

Glutathione reductase deficiency

One family has been reported in which three siblings of a consanguineous marriage showed marked neutrophil glutathione reductase deficiency (Loos et al 1976). The children had activity levels of 10–15% of normal, whereas both parents showed neutrophil glutathione reductase levels of 50%, suggesting that the defect was inherited as an autosomal recessive trait. As with G6PD, both red cell and neutrophil glutathione reductase are under the control of the same gene, and affected patients haemolyse when subjected to oxidative stress.

None of the affected patients showed signs of excessive infections, but their neutrophils showed a reduced respiratory burst because of an inadequate production of GSH. This suggests that only a brief respiratory burst is necessary for complete destruction of bacteria (Roos et al 1979).

Glutathione peroxidase deficiency

Deficiency of glutathione peroxidase has been described in three unrelated patients where the neutrophil enzyme level was approximately 25% of normal and red cell levels were undetectable (Holmes et al 1970, Matsuda et al 1970). All three had a clinical syndrome resembling chronic granulomatous disease. It is not clear how the severity of the illness relates to the modest reduction in neutrophil enzyme levels and it is possible that these patients may not represent a distinct clinical entity (Babior & Crowley 1983) or may in fact have had CGD (Whitin & Cohen 1988).

Glutathione peroxidase deficiency has also been seen in cases of dietary selenium deficiency (Baker & Cohen 1983).

Glutathione synthetase deficiency

Glutathione (GSH) is a tripeptide synthesized from glutamyl-cysteine by the enzyme glutamyl synthetase. Deficiency results in reduced levels of glutathione and a mild phagocytic defect. Several types of enzyme deficiency have been described which show autosomal recessive inheritance. Phagocytic abnormalities are only seen in those cases in which the glutathione synthetase deficiency is severe (Spielberg et al 1979). Patients usually also have a haemolytic anaemia (due to low erythrocyte enzyme levels) and a severe metabolic acidosis due to raised oxyproline levels (which cannot be metabolized to glutathione because of the synthetase deficiency).

Boxer et al (1979) suggested that increased sensitivity of neutrophils to oxidants resulting from glutathione synthetase deficiency could be corrected by administration of vitamin E, a powerful antioxidant.

INVESTIGATION OF THE CHILD WITH RECURRENT INFECTION

It is important to remember that neutrophils are only one component of the normal defence mechanisms against infection, and that many different phagocytic defects may present in a similar clinical fashion. The nature of the infecting organisms may be helpful, as in CGD, which is particularly associated with staphylococci and other catalase producers. Lymphopenia tends to result in fungal infections and pneumocystis.

Figure 5.5 attempts to lead the reader through the maze of clinical possibilities.

REFERENCES

Abramson J S, Mills E L, Sawyer M K et al 1981 Recurrent infections and delayed separation of the umbilical cord in an infant with abnormal phagocytic cell locomotion and oxidative response during particle phagocytosis. Journal of Paediatrics 99: 887–894

Alfaham M A, Fergusson S D, Shira B, Davies J 1987 The idiopathic hypereosinophilic syndrome. Archives of Disease in Childhood 62: 601–613

Aggett P J, Cavanagh N P, Matthew D J et al 1980 Shwachman's syndrome: a review of 21 cases. Archives of Disease in Childhood 55: 331–334

Babior B M, Crowley C A 1983 Chronic granulomatous disease and other disorders of oxidative killing by phagocytes. In: Stanbury J B, Wyngaarden J B, Frederickson D S et al (eds) The metabolic basis of inherited disease. McGraw Hill, New York p 1956

Baehner R L, Nathan D G 1968 Quantitative nitro blue tetrazolium test in chronic granulomatous disease. New England Journal of Medicine 278: 971–976

Baker S S, Cohen H J 1983 Altered oxidative metabolism in selenium-deficient rat granulocytes. Journal of Immunology 130: 2856–2860

Barak Y, Karov Y, Nir E et al 1986 The American Journal of Paediatric Hematology/Oncology 8(2): 128–133

Beeson P B, Bass D A 1977 The eosinophil. W B Saunders Co., Philadelphia

Boxer L A 1981 Immune neutropenias. Clinical and biological implications. American Journal of Pediatric Hematology Oncology 3: 89–96

Boxer L A, Greenberg M S, Boxer G J, Stossel T P 1975 Autoimmune neutropenia. New England Journal of Medicine 293: 748–753

Boxer L A, Oliver J M, Spielberg S P et al 1979 Protection of granulocytes by vitamin E in glutathione synthetase deficiency. New England Journal of Medicine 301: 901–905

Boxer L A, Oseas R S, Oliver J M et al 1981 Amphotericin B promotes leukocyte aggregation of nylon wool fibre treated polymorphonuclear leukocytes. Blood 58: 518–521

Boxer L A, Smolen J E 1988 Neutrophil granule constituents and their release in health and disease. Hematology/ Oncology Clinics of North America 2: 101–134

Brown C C, Gallin J I 1988 Chemotactic disorders Hematology/Oncology Clinics of North America 2: 61–79

Bryant R E, Sutcliff M C 1974 The effect of 3'5'-adenosine monophosphate on granulocyte adhesion. Journal of Clinical Investigation 54: 1241–1244

Buchanan G B, Handin R I 1976 Platelet function in the Chédiak Higashi syndrome. Blood 47: 941–945

Bussel J, Lalezari P, Hilgartner M et al 1983 Reversal of neutropenia with intravenous gammaglobulin in autoimmune neutropenia of infancy. Blood 62: 398–402

Chandra R K, Cope W A, Soothill J F 1969 Chronic granulomatous disease: evidence for an autosomal mode of inheritance. Lancet 2:71–74

Chin T W, Stiehm E R, Falloon J et al 1987 Corticosteroids in the treatment of obstructive lesions of chronic granulomatous disease. Journal of Pediatrics 111: 349–352

Christensen R D, Rothstein G 1980 Exhaustion of mature marrow neutrophils in neonates with sepsis. Journal of Pediatrics 96: 316–318

Clark R A, Johnson F L, Klebanoff S J et al 1976 Defective neutrophil chemotaxis in bone marrow transplant patients Journal of Clinical Investigation 58: 22–31

Clark R A, Root R, Kimball H et al 1973 Defective neutrophil chemotaxis and cellular immunity in a child with recurrent infections: Annals of Internal Medicine 78: 515–519

Craddock P R, Hammerschmidt D E, Moldow C F et al 1979 Granulocyte aggregation as a manifestation of membrane interactions with complement: possible role in leukocyte margination, microvascular occlusion, and endothelial damage. Seminars in Hematology 16: 140-147

Cronkite E P 1976 Kinetics of granulopoiesis. Clinical Haematology 8: 351–370

Cross A R, Parkinson J F, Jones O T G 1985 Mechanism of the superoxide-producing oxidase of neutrophils. Biochemical Journal 226–881–884

Crowley C A, Curnutte J T, Rosin R E et al 1980 An inherited abnormality of neutrophil adhesion: its genetic transmission and its association with a missing protein. New England Journal of Medicine 302: 1163–1168

Curnutte J T, Babior B M 1987 Chronic granulomatous disease. In: Harris H, Hirschorn K (eds) Advances in human genetics, vol 16. Plenum Publishing, New York p 229

Curnutte J T, Berkow R L, Roberts R L, Shurrin S B, Scott P J 1988 Chronic granulomatous disease due to a defect in the cytosolic factor required for NADPH oxidase activation. Journal of Clinical Investigation 81: 606–610

Curnutte J T, Boxer L A 1987 Disorders of granulopoiesis and granulocyte function. In: Nathan D G, Oski F A (eds) Haematology of infancy and childhood. Saunders, Philadelphia

Curnutte J T, Kuver R, Scott P J 1987 Activation of neutrophil NADPH oxidase in a cell-free serum: partial purification of components and characterisation of the activation process. Journal of Biological Chemistry 262: 5563–5569

Cushid M J, Dale D C, West B C, Wolf S M 1975 The hypereosinophilic syndrome: analysis of fourteen cases with review of the literature. Medicine (Baltimore) 54: 1–5

Dale D C, Hammond W P 1988 Cyclic neutropenia: a clinical review. Blood Reviews 2: 178–185

Dale D C, Guerry D, Werweka J R et al 1979 Chronic neutropenia. Medicine 58: 128–144

Dale D C, Graw R G 1974 Transplantation of allogeneic bone marrow in canine cyclic neutropenia. Science 183: 83–84

Dancey J T, Brubaker L H 1979 Neutrophil marrow profiles in patients with rheumatoid arthritis and neutropenia. British Journal of Haematology 43: 607–617

DeVaal O M, Seynhaeve V 1959 Reticular dysgenesis. Lancet 2: 1123–1125

Dinauer M C, Orkin S H, Brown R et al 1987 The glycoprotein encoded by the X-linked chronic granulomatous disease locus is a component of the neutrophil cytochrome b locus. Nature 327: 717–720

Dinauer M C, Orkin S H 1988 Chronic granulomatous disease: molecular genetics Hematology/Oncology Clinics of North America 2: 225–240

Donabedian H, Alling D W, Gallin J I 1982 Levamisole is inferior to placebo in the hyperimmunoglobulin E recurrent infection (Job's) syndrome, New England Journal of Medicine 307: 290–292

Donabedian H, Gallin J I 1982 Mononuclear cells from patients with the hyperimmunoglobulin E-recurrent infection syndrome produce an inhibitor of leukocyte chemotaxis. Journal of Clinical Investigation 69: 1155–1163

Donabedian H, Gallin J I 1983 The hyperimmunoglobulin E recurrent infection (Job's) syndrome. A review of the NIH experience and the literature. Medicine 62: 195–200

Engel R R, Hammond D, Eitzman D V et al 1964 Transient congenital leukaemia in seven children with mongolism.

Journal of Pediatrics 65: 303–305

Engelhard D, Landreth K S, Kapoor N et al 1983 Cycling of peripheral blood and marrow lymphocytes in cyclic neutropenia. Proclamation of the National Academy of Science USA 13: 5734–5738

Estevez M E, Ballart I J, Diez R A et al 1986 Early defect of phagocytic cell function in subjects at risk for acquired immune deficiency syndrome. Scandinavian Journal of Immunology 24: 215–221

Falk P M, Rich K, Feig S et al 1977 Evaluation of congenital neutropenic disorders by in vitro bone marrow culture. Pediatrics 59: 739–748

Fauci A S, Harley J B, Roberts W C et al 1982 The idiopathic hypereosinophilic syndrome: clinical, pathophysiologic and therapeutic considerations. Annals of Internal Medicine 97: 78–92

Fearon D T, Collins L A 1983 Increased expression of C3b receptors on polymorphonuclear leukocytes induced by chemotactic factors and by purification procedures. Journal of Immunology 130: 370–375

Fischer A, Griscelli C, Friedrick W et al 1986 Bone marrow transplantation for immunodeficiencies and osteopetrosis: European survey, 1968–85. Lancet 2: 1080–1084

Fischer A, Trung P H, Descamps–Latscha B et al 1983 Bone marrow transplantation for inborn errors of phagocytic cells associated with defective adherence, chemotaxis and oxidative response during opsonized particle phagocytosis. Lancet 2: 473–476

Forrest C B, Forehand J R, Axtell R A, Roberts R A, Johnson R B 1988 Hematology/Oncology Clinics of North America 2: 253–266.

Falk W, Goodwin R H, Leonard E J 1980 A 48-well micro chemotaxis assembly for rapid and accurate measurements of leukocyte migration. Journal of Immunological Methods 33: 239–247

Gabig T G, Kipnes R S, Babior B M 1978 Solubilisation of the O_2^- forming activity responsible for the respiratory burst in human neutrophils. Journal of Biological Chemistry 253: 6663–6665

Gallin J I 1985 Neutrophil-specific granule deficiency. Annual Reviews of Medicine 36: 263–274

Gallin J I, Buescher E S 1983 Abnormal regulation of inflammatory skin response in male patients with chronic granulomatous disease. Inflammation 7: 227–230

Gallin J I, Elin R J, Hubert R T et al 1979 Efficacy of ascorbic acid in Chédiak-Higashi syndrome. Studies in humans and mice. Blood 53: 226–234

Ghebrehiwet B, Müller-Eberhart H J 1979 C3e: an acidic fragment of human C3 with leukocytosis-inducing activity. Journal of Immunology 123: 616–621

Gilman P A, Jackson D P et al 1970 Congenital agranulocytosis: prolonged survival and terminal acute leukaemia. Blood 36: 576–579

Gmünder F K, Seger R A 1981 Chronic granulomatous disease: Mode of action of sulfamethoxazole/trimethoprin. Pediatric Research 15: 1533–1537

Gray G R, Stannatoyannopoulos G, Naiman S C et al 1973 Neutrophil dysfunction, chronic granulomatous disease, and non-spherocytic haemolytic anaemia caused by complete deficiency of glucose-6-phosphate dehydrogenase. Lancet 2: 530–534

Greenberg P L, Mara B, Steed S, Boxer L A 1980 The chronic idiopathic neutropenic syndrome: Correlation of clinical features with in vitro parameters of granulopoiesis. Blood 55: 915–921

Guerry D, Dale D C, Omine M, Perry S, Wolf S M 1973 Periodic hematopoiesis in human cyclic neutropenia. Journal of Clinical Investigation 52: 3220–3229

Hanlon S M, Panayi G S, Laurent R 1980 Defective polymorphonuclear leukocyte chemotaxis in rheumatoid arthritis associated with a serum inhibitor. Annals of Rheumatic Diseases 39: 68–74

Hardy W R, Anderson R E 1968 The hypereosinophilic syndrome. Annals of Internal Medicine 68: 1220–1229

Hayward A R, Harvey B A M, Leonard J et al 1979 Delayed separation of the umbilical cord, widespread infections, and defective neutrophil motility. Lancet 1: 1099–1101

Hill H R, Estensen R D, Hogan N A et al 1976 Severe staphylococcal disease associated with allergic manifestations, hyperimmunoglobulin E and defective neutrophil chemotaxis. Journal of Laboratory and Clinical Medicine 88: 796–806

Hirata F, Schiffman E, Venkata Subramanian et al 1980 A phospholipase A_2 inhibitory protein in rabbit neutrophils induced by glucocorticoids. Proceedings of the National Academy of Sciences USA 77: 2533–2536

Hislop W S, Hayes P C, Boyd E J S 1982 Late presentation of Shwachman's syndrome. Acta Paediatrica Scandinavia 71: 677–679

Holmes B, Page A R, Good R A 1967 Studies of the metabolic activity of leukocytes from patients with a genetic abnormality of phagocyte function. Journal of Clinical Investigation 46: 1422–1432

Holmes B, Park B H, Malawista S E et al 1970 Chronic granulomatous disease in females. A deficiency of leukocyte glutathione peroxidase. New England Journal of Medicine 283: 217–221

Ingraham L M, Burns C P, Hack R A et al 1981 Fluidity properties and lipid composition of erythrocyte membranes in Chédiak–Higashi syndrome. Journal of Cell Biology 89: 510–516

Johnston R B 1983 Management of patients with chronic granulomatous disease. In: Gallin J I, Fauci A S (eds) Advances in host defences mechanisms, vol 3. Chronic granulomatous disease. Raven Press New York, p 77

Joyce R A, Boggs D A, Chervenick P A, Lalezari P 1980 Neutrophil kinetics in Felty's syndrome. American Journal of Medicine 69: 695–702

Karnousky M L 1973 Chronic granulomatous disease – pieces of a cellular and molecular puzzle. Federation Proceedings 32: 1527–1533

Kimball H R, Ford G H, Wolff S M 1975 Lysosomal enzymes in normal and Chédiak-Higashi blood leukocytes. Journal of Laboratory and Clinical Medicine 86: 616–630

Kitahara M, Simonian Y, Eyre H J 1979 Neutrophil myeloperioxidase: A simple reproducible technique to determine activity. Journal of Laboratory and Clinical Medicine 93: 232–237

Kostmann R 1956 Infantile genetic agranulocytosis. A review with presentation of ten new cases. Acta Pediatrica Scandinavica 64: 362–366

Krance R A, Spruce W E, Forman S J et al 1982 Human cyclic neutropenia transferred in allogeneic bone marrow grafting. Blood 60: 1263-1266

Lalezari P 1985 Autoimmune neutropenia. In: Rose M R, Mac Kay I R (eds) The autoimmune disease Blackwell, Oxford p 523.

Lalezari P, Khorshidi M, Petrosova M 1986 Autoimmune neutropenia of infancy. Journal of Pediatrics 109: 764–767

Lange R D 1983 Cyclic hematopoiesis: human cyclic neutropenia. Experimental Hematology 11: 435–451

Leale M 1910 Recurrent furniculosis in an infant showing an unusual blood picture. Journal of The American Medical Association 54: 1845

Lensink D B, Barton A, Appelbaum F R, Hammond W P 1986 Cyclic neutropenia as a premalignant manifestation of acute lymphoblastic leukaemia. American Journal of Hematology 22: 9–16

Leung D Y, Geha R S 1988 Clinical and immunologic aspects of the hyperimmunoglobulin E syndrome. Hematology/Oncology Clinics of North America, 2: 81–100

Logue G L, Shimm D S 1980 Autoimmune granulocytopenia. Annual Reviews of Medicine 31: 191–200

Lomax K J, Malech H L, Gallin J I 1989 The molecular biology of selected phagocyte defects. Blood Reviews 3: 94–104

Loos H, Roos D, Weening R et al 1976 Familial deficiency of glutathione reductase in human blood cells. Blood 48: 53–62

Loughran T P, Clark E A, Price T H, Hammond W P 1986 Adult onset cyclic neutropenia is associated with increased large granular lymphocytes. Blood 68: 1082–1087

Lund J E, Pagett G A, Ott R L 1967 Cyclic neutropenia in grey collie dogs. Blood 29: 452–461

Malech H L, Englander L, Zakhinehb A 1979 Abnormal polymorphonuclear neutrophil function in Kartagener's syndrome. Clinical Research 27 (abstract 590A)

Matsuda I, Oka Y, Taniguchi N et al 1970 Leukocyte glutathione peroxidase deficiency in a male patient with chronic granulomatous disease. Journal of Pediatrics 88: 581–584

Marra G, Appiani A C, Romeo L et al 1986 Renal tubular acidosis in a case of Shwachman's syndrome. Acta Paediatrica Scandinavica 75: 682–684

May M E, Waddell C C 1984 Basophils in peripheral blood and bone marrow. A retrospective review. American Journal of Medicine 76: 509–511

Meerhof L J, Roos D 1986 Heterogeneity in chronic granulomatous disease detected with an improved nitroblue tetrazolium slide test. Journal of Leukocyte Biology 39: 699–711

Metchnikoff E 1905 Immunity in infective disease. Cambridge University Press, Cambridge

MacGregor R R, Friedman H M, Macarak E J et al 1980 Virus infection of endothelial cells increases granulocyte adherence. Journal of Clinical Investigation 65: 1469–1477

Miller M E, Oski F A, Harris M B 1971 'Lazy leukocyte' syndrome. A new disorder of neutrophil dysfunction. Lancet 1: 665–669

Minchinton R M 1984 The occurrence and significance of neutrophil antibodies. British Journal of Haematology 56: 521–524

Minchinton R M, Waters A H 1985 Autoimmune thrombocytopenia and neutropenia after bone marrow transplantation. Blood 3: 752–757

McKusick V A, Eldridge R, Hostetler J A et al 1965 Dwarfism in the Amish. Cartilage hair hypoplasia. Bulletin of the Johns Hopkins Hospital 116: 285–326

Morley A A, Carew J P, Baikie A G 1967 Familial cyclical neutropenia. British Journal of Haematology 13: 719–738

Murdoch R M, Smith C C 1972 Haematological aspects of systemic disease: infection. Clinical Hematology 1: 619–625

Murray J A, Lilleyman J S 1983 T cell lymphocytosis with

neutropenia. Archives of Disease in Childhood 58: 635–636

Nair M P, Gray R H, Boxer L A, Schwartz S 1987 Deficiency of inducible suppressor cell activity in the Chédiak-Higashi syndrome. American Journal of Hematology 26: 55–66

Nauseef W M, Metcalf J A, Root R K 1983 Role of myeloperoxidase in the respiratory burst of neutrophils. Blood 61: 483–492

Newburger P E, Ezekowitz R A 1988 Cellular and molecular effects of recombinant interferon gamma in chronic granulomatous disease. Haematology/Oncology Clinics of North America 2: 267–276

Ochs H D, Slichter S J, Harker L A et al 1980 The Wiskott-Aldrich syndrome: studies of lymphocytes, granulocytes and platelets. Blood 55: 243–252

Ochs H D, Igo R P 1973 The NBT slide test: a simple screening method for detecting chronic granulomatous disease and female carriers. Journal of Pediatrics 83: 77–82

Ohno Y, Buescher E S, Roberts R, Metcalf J A, Gallin J I 1986 Revaluation of cytochrome b and flavin adenine dinucleotide in neutrophils from patients with chronic granulomatous disease. Blood 67(4): 1132–1138

Oliver J M 1978 Cell biology of leukocyte abnormalities in membrane and cytoskeletal function in normal and defective cells. A review. American Journal of Pathology 93: 221–270

Oliver C, Essner E 1985 Formation of anomalous lysozomes in monocytes neutrophils and eosinophils from bone marrow of mice with Chédiak–Higashi syndrome. Laboratory Investigation 32: 17–21

O'Reilly R J, Bochstein J, Dinsmore R et al 1984 Marrow transplantation for congenital disorders. Seminars in Haematology 21: 188-221

Osborne W R A, Hammond W P, Dale D C 1985 Human cyclic haematopoiesis is associated with aberrant purine metabolism. Journal of Laboratory and Clinical Medicine 105: 403–409

Oseas R S, Allen J, Yang H H et al 1982 Mechanism of dexamethasone inhibition of chemotactic factor-induced granulocyte aggregation. Blood 59: 265–269

Pahwa R N, O'Reilly R J, Pahwa S et al 1977 Partial correction of neutrophil deficiency in congenital neutropenia following bone marrow transplantation (BMT). Experimental Haematology 5: 45–50

Parmley R T, Crist W M, Ragab A H et al 1980 Congenital dysgranulopoietic neutropenia: clinical, serologic, ultrastructural and in vitro proliferative characterisation. Blood 56: 465–450

Parry M F, Root R K, Metcalf J A et al 1981 Myeloperoxidase deficiency. Prevalence and clinical significance. Annals of Internal Medicine 95: 293–301

Payne R 1964 Neonatal neutropenia and leukoagglutinins. Pediatrics 33: 194–197

Randall D L, Reiquam C N, Githens J H et al 1965 Familial myeloproliferative disease. A new syndrome closely simulating myelogenous leukaemia in childhood. American Journal of Disease in Childhood. 110: 479–500

Rickles F R, Miller D R 1972 Eosinophilic leukemoid reaction; report of a case, its relationship to eosinophilic leukaemia and review of paediatric literature. Journal of Pediatrics 80: 418–428

Rodgers G M, Shuman M A 1982 Acquired cyclic neutropenia : successful treatment with prednisone. American Journal of Hematology 13: 83–89

Roos D, Weening R S, Wyss S R et al 1979 Protection of

phagocytic leukocytes by endogenous glutathione: studies in a family with glutathione reductase deficiency. Blood 53: 851–866

Roos D, Weening R S, Wyss S R et al 1980 Protection of human neutrophils by endogenous catalase. Journal of Clinical Investigation 65: 1515–1522

Root R K, Rosenthal A S, Balestra D K 1972 Abnormal bactericidal, metabolic and lysosomal functions of Chédiak-Higashi syndrome leukocytes. Journal of Investigation 51: 649–665

Roozendaal K J, Dicke K A, Boonzajer Flaes M L 1981 Effect of oxymetholone on human cyclic haematopoiesis. British Journal of Haematology 47: 185–193

Rosen F S, Craig J et al 1968 The dysgammaglobulinaemias and X—linked thymic hypoplasia. In: Bergsma D (ed) Immunologic deficiency diseases in man National Foundation – March of Dimes, New York p 67

Rossi F, Zatti M 1964 Biochemical aspects of phagocytosis in polymorphonuclear leukocytes. NADPH oxidation by the granules of resting and phagocytosing cells. Experientia 20: 21–23

Rothbaum R J, Williams D A, Daugherty C C 1982 Unusual surface distribution of concanavolin A reflects a cytoskeletal defect in neutrophils in Shwachman's syndrome. Lancet 2: 800–801

Schleimer R, Rutledge B 1986 Cultured human vascular endothelial cells acquire adhesiveness for neutrophils after stimulation with interleukin 1, endotoxin and tumour-promoting phorbol esters. Journal of Immunology 136: 649–654

Schröder H, Evans D A P 1972 Acetylator phenotype and adverse effects of sulphasalazine in healthy subjects. Gut 13: 278–284

Von Schulthess G K, Fehr J, Dahinden C 1983 Cyclic neutropenia: amplification of granulocyte oscillations by lithium and long term suppression of cycling by plasmapheresis. Blood 62: 320–326

Shwachman H, Diamond L K, Oski F A et al 1964 The syndrome of pancreatic insufficiency and bone marrow dysfunction. Journal of Pediatrics 65: 645–663

Sechler J, Gallin J I 1987. Recombinant gamma interferon is a chemoattractant for human monocytes. Federation Proceedings 46: (abstract 5523).

Segal A W 1988 Cytochrome b-245 and its involvement in the molecular pathology of chronic granulomatous disease. In Hematology/Oncology Clinics of North America 2(2): 213–223

Segal A W, Jones O T G 1978 Novel cytochrome b system in phagocytic vacuoles from human granulocytes. Nature 276: 515–517

Shaw S 1987 Characterization of human leukocyte differentiation antigens. Immunology Today 8: 1–10

Snyderman R, Pike M C 1984 Transductional mechanisms of chemoattractant receptors on leukocytes. In: Snyderman R. (ed) Regulation of leukocyte function. Plenum Press, New York, p 1

Spielberg S P, Boxer L A, Oliver J M et al 1979 Oxidative damage to neutrophils in glutathione synthetase deficiency. British Journal of Haematology 42: 215–225

Stevens D L, Everett E D, Boxer L A et al 1979 Infectious mononucleosis with severe neutropenia and opsonic antineutrophil activity. Southern Medical Journal 72: 519–521

Stossel T P, Root R K, Vaughan K, 1972 Phagocytosis in chronic granulomatous disease and the Chédiak–Higashi syndrome. New England Journal of Medicine 286: 120–123

Tanaka K, Rosenberg L E 1983 Disorders of branched chain amino acid and organic acid metabolism. In: Stanbury J B, Wyngaarden J B (eds) The metabolic basis of inherited disease, 5th edn. McGraw Hill, New York p 440

Tate R M, Repine J E 1983 Neutrophils and the adult respiratory distress syndrome. American Reviews of Respiratory Disease 128: 552–559

Teo C G, Singh M, Ting W C et al 1985 Evaluation of the common conditions associated with eosinophilia. Journal of Clinical Pathology 38: 305–308

Todd R F, Freyer D R 1988 The CD11/CD18 leukocyte glycoprotein deficiency. Hematology/Oncology Clinics of North America 2: 13–31

Umei T, Takeshige K, Minakami S 1986 NADPH binding component of neutrophil superoxide-generating oxidase. Journal of Biological Chemistry 261: 5229–5232

van Dyke T E 1985 Role of the neutrophil in oral disease : receptor deficiency in leukocytes from patients with juvenile periodonitis. Reviews of Infectious Disease 7: 419–425

Verheugt F W A, von dem Borne A E, van Noord–Bokhorst J C et al 1978 Autoimmune granulocytopenia: the detection of granulocyte autoantibodies with the immunofluorescent test. British Journal of Haematology 39: 339–350

Verheugt F W A, van Noord-Bokhurst J, von dem Borne A E et al 1979. A family with allo-immune neutropenia: group specific pathogenicity of maternal antibodies. Vox Sanguinis 36: 1–8

Weisbart R H, Golde D W, Clark S C et al 1985 Human granulocyte-macrophage colony stimulating factor is a neutrophil activator. Nature 314: 361–362

Weisman S J, Mahoney M J, Anderson D C et al 1987 Prenatal diagnosis of Mo1 (CDW 18) deficiency. Clinical Research 35: 435a

Weitzman S A, Stossal T P 1978 Drug-induced immunological neutropenia. Lancet 1: 1068–1072

Weil S C, Rosner G L, Reid M S et al 1988 Translocation and rearrangement of myeloperoxidase gene in acute promyelocytic leukaemia. Science 240: 790–792

White J G, Clawson C C 1980 The Chédiak–Higashi syndrome. The nature of the giant neutrophil granules and their interaction with cytoplasm and foreign particles. American Journal of Pathology 98: 151–196

Whitin J C, Cohen H J 1988 Disorders of respiratory burst termination. Hematology/Oncology Clinics of North America 2: 289–299

Wright D G, Dale D C, Fauci A S et al 1981 Human cyclic neutropenia: clinical review and long-term follow-up of patients. Medicine 60: 1–13

Yoshida A, Stamatoyannopoulos G 1968 Biochemical genetics of glucose-6-phosphate dehydrogenase variation. Annals of the New York Academy of Science. 155: 868–872

Young G A, Vincent P C 1980 Drug-induced agranulocytosis. Clinical Haematology 9: 438–504

Zuelzer W W 1970 Myelokathexis – new form of chronic granulocytopenia. New England Journal of Medicine 282: 231–236

6. Disorders of platelets. I Thrombocytopenia and thrombocytosis

J. S. Lilleyman

The disorders of platelets described in the next two chapters are divided on the basis of whether the problem is one of abnormal numbers or defective function. In circumstances where both occur simultaneously, the condition is cross-referenced and dealt with in the section where the most clinically important abnormality lies. This chapter deals with diseases in which the chief feature is a lack or excess of platelets.

PLATELET KINETICS

Platelets are produced from megakaryocytes by a unique method of cytoplasmic shedding in an exception to the universal process of mitosis. Exactly where this process primarily takes place is not entirely clear, and while most would presume the site to be the bone marrow, there are persuasive data to suggest that the lungs might be a major, if not exclusive, alternative, with megakaryocytes arriving there via the circulation (Slater et al 1983). Megakaryocytes themselves are produced in the marrow from committed progenitor cells under the influence of various cytokines, the most important of which is megakaryocyte colony-stimulating factor (meg-CSF). Platelet production from existing megakaryocytes is influenced by the ill-characterized humoral agent thrombopoietin which (unlike the otherwise analogous erythropoietin) induces cell maturation rather than clonal proliferation (Eldor et al 1989). In health its production depends on the existing platelet mass which in most circumstances correlates closely with the circulating count, but where it is produced is not known (Penington 1987). Recent data suggest it may be related to interleukin-6 (Ishibashi et al 1989).

Best estimates of the life span of platelets in health are in the range of 8–11 days (Stuart et al 1975), and the normal range for platelet counts is $150–400 \times 10^9/l$. These figures apply to all ages. From them it can be roughly deduced that a 27-kg, 9-year-old child will have a total circulating platelet mass of 500×10^9, 10% of which will be replaced every day.

In any given individual, the circulating platelet count is closely correlated with the existing platelet mass, but the two are not synonymous. Platelet mass is influenced by the volume of each platelet produced, the rate of production, and the rate of loss or consumption. Circulating platelet counts are influenced by the rate of production, the distribution of platelets within the body, and the rate of loss. It is possible for an individual with a normal count to have an abnormal mass and vice versa. Normal counts may mask underlying pathology where there is increased turnover which is compensated for by increased production, but abnormal counts always require explanation.

Thrombocytopenia is more often a physical sign than a clinical problem, and it is only with counts below $10–20 \times 10^9/l$ that haemorrhagic problems regularly occur. The relationship between the platelet count and the defect in primary phase haemostasis produced by a fall to subnormal values can best be assessed by some version of the template bleeding time. Exploring that relationship, Harker & Schlicter (1972) studied 136 patients in 8 groups with a variety of different causes of thrombocytopenia. Seventy had stable thrombocytopenia due to impaired platelet production, 11 had 'modest' thrombocytopenia due to hypersplenism (Gaucher's disease, cirrhosis, and lymphoma), 12 had immune-mediated thrombocytopenia, 10 had familial thrombocytopenia (4 families), 4 had the Wiskott-Aldrich syndrome, and 29 with other conditions had normal platelet counts. Comparing the patients with each other and a reference group of 100 normal adult volunteers, the authors found that in those with stable production-failure thrombocytopenia there was a linear relationship between a dropping platelet count and prolongation of bleeding time as the count fell below $100 \times 10^9/l$. Exceptions to this rule were seen in two groups of patients with counts below $50 \times 10^9/l$; those in the early stages of recovery from chemotherapy-induced myelosuppression, and those with immune-mediated thrombocytopenia (ITP) where the bleeding time was considerably shorter than would have been predicted from the platelet count alone.

Harker and Schlicter's observations are clinically important because they indicate that the risk of haemorrhage is not simply related to the platelet count, but to the underlying disease. Conditions where there is increased production of young cells appear to carry less risk than those where production has failed. Aplastic anaemia is more dangerous than ITP, and this should be taken into account when assessing the risk:benefit ratio of any proposed treatment.

If thrombocytopenia is more often a physical sign than a clinical problem, the same may be said with more conviction for thrombocytosis. The number of occasions when a high platelet count per se has justified therapy to reduce the risk of vasoocclusive disease in children is very small, and the discovery of a high count usually requires explanation rather than intervention.

What follows is a discussion of, firstly, disorders associated with a low platelet count, and secondly those where the count is high. Emphasis has been placed on conditions which are either severe, or common, or both.

THROMBOCYTOPENIA DUE TO SHORT PLATELET SURVIVAL: I IMMUNE-MEDIATED

The chief immune-mediated causes thrombocytopenia due to short platelet survival are listed in Table 6.1 and considered further below.

Table 6.1 Causes of childhood thrombocytopenia due primary to shortened platelet survival: I Immune mediated

Idiopathic thrombocytopenic purpura (ITP)
Neonatal isoimmune thrombocytopenia
Associated with infection
Drug-induced*
Associated with autoimmune disorders
Associated with malignant disease
Post transfusion purpura

* Can be immune- or non-immune-mediated

Idiopathic (immune) thrombocytopenic purpura

Childhood idiopathic (immune) thrombocytopenic purpura (ITP) is a generic name for immune-mediated thrombocytopenia unassociated with drugs or other evidence of disease. It is not a specific condition in the sense that it has an understood common cause or pathology, nor does it have a predictable prognosis.

Over the last 25 years, referral centre or population-based studies have been carried out in Canada (Choi & McClure 1967), Australia (Benham & Taft 1972, Lammi & Lovric 1973, Robb & Tiedeman 1990), Scandanavia (Cohn 1976), England (Walker & Walker 1984), the United States (Simons et al 1975, Lusher et al 1984) and Scotland (Hoyle et al 1986). Together, these reports describe some 2000 patients, which allow broad conclusions about the natural history of the syndrome to be drawn.

Incidence

Best estimates put the historical incidence of symptomatic ITP at around 4 per 100 000 children per year (Walker & Walker 1984), and there is no evidence that this has varied greatly across the world. There must be many subclinical cases, and with the widespread introduction of routine platelet counting some may be unearthed that would otherwise be missed. The incidence in future may therefore rise.

Childhood ITP can be broadly divided into the common 'acute' self-limiting type (accounting for 80–90%) and the less usual 'chronic' variety (accounting for 10–20%). The accepted definition for 'chronic' ITP is any case which persists for over 6 months. There may be a third very small category of 'recurrent' 'cyclical' or 'relapsing' ITP, but from a practical point of view this can be considered as a subvariety of the chronic type.

Although the distinction between acute and chronic types is always difficult to make prospectively, there are differences in the age and sex distribution and the mode of onset, and it is probable that the two are distinct disorders. This is supported by differences in serological findings (see below), as well as the clinical course, so for these reasons the two varieties will be considered separately.

Clinical features

Acute ITP. Acute ITP usually presents with sudden-onset bruising and purpura in an otherwise well child. This can be spectacular, with conjunctival and retinal haemorrhages in 3–4%, and up to 25% will have associated nosebleeds. A few will have haematuria (Lusher et al 1984). The spleen tip may be palpable in 5–8% (Lusher & Zuelzer 1966, Choi & McClure 1967); otherwise, there are no abnormal physical signs.

There may be a history of a preceding upper respiratory infection, but this is too common in children to be specific. Any age can be affected, but there is a distinct peak between the ages of 2 and 4 years, after which time the disease becomes progressively more rare throughout childhood (Lusher et al 1984, Hoyle et al 1986). It is equally common in boys and girls. A seasonal incidence has been noted with a bias towards winter and spring, supporting a possible viral aetiology and leading to the suggestion that acute ITP might be called 'postinfectious' (Lusher et al 1984).

Chronic ITP. In contrast, chronic ITP more often has an insidious onset, with a history stretching back over some weeks (Walker & Walker 1984). The incidence is constant throughout childhood without any peaks or troughs, and girls are affected twice as frequently as boys (Lusher & Zeulzer 1966, Hoyle et al 1986). There is usually no history of preceding infection and there is no suggestion of any seasonal trend in incidence. The physical signs are the same as those of acute ITP, and at presentation the two conditions cannot be distinguished clinically with any reliability. Chronic ITP in children is very similar to the disease seen more commonly in adults (McVerry 1985).

Pathology

Acute ITP. There is little doubt that acute childhood ITP is immune-mediated, though the precise mechanism has proved hard to define. It has been known for several years that some patients with the disease have increased amounts of platelet-bound IgG (Lightsey et al 1979), but it has been unclear whether this represents binding of true platelet-specific autoantibodies or antibodies complexed to microbial antigens interacting with platelet Fc-receptors (the innocent bystander mechanism). The latter seems to be the case in infection-associated immune thrombocytopenia where the pathogen is recognized (see below), and may also be true in virus infections where no organism is identified.

A recent study has suggested an alternative explanation, at least in some cases. Using an immunoblotting technique to probe for antibodies to specific platelet antigens, Winiarski found that 4 of 21 children had IgG antibodies to glycoproteins Ib, IIb or IIIa, but, more importantly, that 13 had IgM antibodies to these or smaller antigens (Winiarski 1989). The suggestion is made that acute-phase antiviral IgM antibodies might cross-react with platelet antigens, and that such antibodies could play a role analogous to that of IgG in chronic ITP, a hypothesis which would explain the transient nature of the acute syndrome and why IgG antibodies have been hard to find.

Chronic ITP. In contrast, direct evidence of IgG autoantibodies to platelet-specific antigens in the majority of studied cases of chronic ITP is now beyond dispute (Woods & McMillan 1984), and using the most sensitive techniques antibodies to membrane glycoproteins can be found in up to 75% of cases (McMillan et al 1987). The condition is thus directly analogous to autoimmune haemolytic anaemia. Despite this, serology is of little value as a routine test to distinguish between acute and chronic ITP, or to contribute positively to the diagnosis, partly because the techniques involved are sophisticated, but mostly because there are still many cases where no antibody can be identified. When reflecting recently on the clinical usefulness of platelet serology, Harrington concluded that it had 'improved the ease of diagnosis very little' and 'had virtually no value in the formulation of management' (Harrington 1987).

Diagnosis

Given that serology is not helpful, the diagnosis of ITP in children is essentially one of exclusion of other causes of thrombocytopenia. Conditions which are most likely to generate confusion are low platelet counts associated with specific infections, drugs or collagen disorders (see below), familial thrombocytopenias (see below), leukaemia and aplastic anaemia, and, occasionally, portal hypertension with hypersplenism.

On the basis of the blood count and the clinical picture, it must be admitted that there is seldom much doubt about the diagnosis in typical cases, and for this reason routine marrow examination for all patients (to exclude leukaemia or aplasia) has been considered unnecessary (McIntosh 1982, Halperin & Doyle 1988).

On the other hand, mistakes can arise, and over the last decade three patients with leukaemia referred to the author's centre were initially thought to have ITP. The fact that all, in retrospect, had features to indicate the true diagnosis does not alter the initial error. In a survey of 322 American paediatric haematologists, 74% said that they did routine marrows on all children with apparent ITP, and of that 74% over half had been wrong in their clinical diagnosis on at least one occasion (Dubansky & Oski 1986).

The other argument for performing a marrow is to avoid inappropriate treatment for the wrong disease if any therapy is planned. This is particularly important if steroids are to be given. Partial treatment of an unsuspected leukaemia could jeopardise the patient's chances of long survival (Revesz et al 1985).

Marrow appearances in ITP are in no way specific, and examination is only helpful in the exclusion of other conditions. Megakaryocytes are usually plentiful. More accurate quantitation is seldom possible or necessary.

Prognosis

The distinction between acute and chronic ITP is based entirely on whether the condition persists for over 6 months. The duration of thrombocytopenia (platelets $<50 \times 10^9$/l) for a demographically defined cohort of 55 unselected consecutive children is shown in Figure 6.1, which indicates that nine cases proved to be chronic but that only two were still thrombocytopenic at two years. This underlines the possibility of late remission, which can be spontaneous and arise as late as 5 to 19 years after diagnosis (Walker & Walker 1984).

Morbidity and mortality. Morbidity in ITP is minimal; usually, the parents are more upset than the child. Apart from the obvious stigmata of a defect in primary-phase haemostasis, major haemorrhage in the acute phase is rare. The possibility of CNS purpura (as opposed to frank intra-

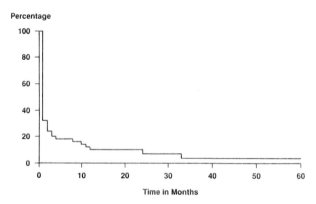

Fig. 6.1 Duration of thrombocytopenia (platelets $<50 \times 10^9$/l) in a demographically defined consective group of 55 children from the city of Sheffield from 1978–1990. Three had a splenectomy; the remainder received short-course steroids or no treatment.

cranial haemorrhage) causing brain dysfunction has been raised (Matoth et al 1971) but seems improbable in most cases.

Life-threatening intracranial haemorrhage is a very unusual event. Where it arises, some additional predisposing cause or alternative diagnosis should be considered. In the United Kingdom, data from three centres suggest the incidence to be less than 1% (3 of 380 patients), but the risk is probably cumulative the longer a child is thrombocytopenic (Lilleyman 1990). The problem is much more common in adults with ITP (Pizzuto & Ambriz 1984).

Mortality from ITP in children appears to have reduced over the years, but this has more to do with the recognition of serious diseases with which it used to be confused than a true improvement in prognosis (Lilleyman 1986). From studies published in the last 20 years (see above), the risk of death overall appears to be about 1 in 500.

Long-term sequelae. A 10-year follow-up on 171 ITP children was reassuring, in that none developed multisystem autoimmune disease or malignancy, nor had any evidence of immunodeficiency. Two of 33 women who had children several years after ITP had thrombocytopenic babies, despite the platelet count in one of the mothers being normal (Walker & Walker 1984).

Management

The management of ITP can conveniently be considered in two parts; the initial phase following diagnosis, and the subsequent chronic phase if the condition persists. Both are the subject of debate and individual practices and prejudices vary widely.

Following diagnosis. Most children with profound thrombocytopenia are admitted to hospital for diagnosis, though once ITP has been confirmed, unless some hospital-based therapy is planned, there is little reason to keep them there. The risks of serious bleeding in hospital are the same as the risks at home – very low. Confining children to bed or putting severe restrictions on their activities is of no proven benefit, and causes boredom in the patient and anxiety in the parents.

Therapy in the acute phase is the subject of some controversy. The three most widely considered options are steroids, intravenous high dose human pooled immunoglobulin (IVIG), or no treatment at all. Attempts at prospective trials have been fraught with difficulties, partly because of the rarity of ITP and the lack of centralization of care of patients with the condition, and partly because the morbidity and mortality is so low that the perceived benefits of therapy are hard to define other than by some arbitrary platelet count achieved after some arbitrary time.

Such randomized trials as there have been suggest that steroids are associated with slightly faster recovery of the platelet count when compared to no therapy (Sartorius 1984, Buchanan & Holtkamp 1984), and that IVIG may be superior to steroids by the same criteria (Imbach et al 1985). There is no evidence that either therapy affects mortality, nor could there be outside the context of a trial with thousands of patients. A single death among the 214 children in the three trials occurred in a child who received IVIG (Imbach et al 1985).

So far, the only trial comparing all three options in a single multicentre study has been carried out in Canada. Fifty three patients randomly allocated to no therapy, steroids or IVIG indicated that both steroids and IVIG were associated with fewer days of profound thrombocytopenia than no treatment, but did not differ significantly from each other (Blanchette 1990, personal communication).

On the basis of these studies it seems reasonable to opt for nothing or prednisolone, perhaps reserving therapy for patients who have the more spectacular physical signs. Low-dose regimens (0.25 mg/kg per day) appear to be as effective as conventional doses (1 mg/kg per day) in this context (Belluci et al 1988). The drug should be withdrawn after 3 weeks, irrespective of the platelet count, to avoid side-effects.

IVIG is expensive, and even though lower doses may be as effective as those originally suggested (Bussel & Hilgartner 1984), the material requires intravenous infusion and keeps the child in hospital. While the various preparations of IVIG appear to be microbiologically safe, at the time of writing rigorous studies showing them to be free of hepatitis C are lacking. The place of IVIG in the management of ITP is better reserved for the temporary relief of the chronic disease (see below).

Non-remitters. For the few children who do not remit within a few weeks, other therapies may be considered. Before any are tried, it is important to consider whether the child has any symptoms of the disease. If not, and if the platelet count is $> 20 \times 10^9/l$, it is unlikely that the cost, inconvenience or (most importantly) risk of any treatment is justified. Even if the platelet count is lower, it should be remembered that chronic profound thrombocytopenia is entirely compatible with normal activities and longevity (Walker & Walker 1984).

Despite this, there are a very few children who have real problems, such as menorrhagia, repeated distressing nosebleeds, unsightly bruises and purpura, which, together with the tiny but enlarging risk of intracranial bleeding (see above), prompt some sort of intervention. The alternatives are considered further below.

Splenectomy. Chronic ITP has been successfully treated by splenectomy for over 60 years (Williamson 1926), but the risks of the procedure have only been recognized for just over half that time (King & Schumacker 1952). Overwhelming sepsis may occur, and the risk persists for well over 10 years (Evans 1985). The mortality from infection after ITP splenectomy was estimated in 1973 to be 1.4% (Singer 1973). The true figure today may well be less than that, but the mortality of the treatment is probably of the same order or more than that of the disease.

The success rate of splenectomy seems to be around 65–75%. Of 380 British children with ITP seen in three centres over the last 25 years, 51 became chronic and had their spleens removed; one died postoperatively; two had late pneumococcal infections which they survived; but only 12 subsequently had persistent thrombocytopenia (Walker & Walker 1984, Hoyle et al 1986, Lilleyman 1988).

Despite the hazards, splenectomy still has its advocates (Harrington 1987) and may be justified in symptomatic children with profound thrombocytopenia of more than 12 months' duration where the diagnosis is not in doubt. Appropriate prophylaxis against infection should be given, probably for many years.

Alternatives to splenectomy. Alternatives used to be considered appropriate only for splenectomy

failures, but are increasingly being tried beforehand. The list of candidates is long and still growing. This underlines the fact that none fulfil the ideal of being universally effective and safe.

High-dose non-specific immunoglobulin. It is rarely possible to use intermittent IVIG to maintain a long-term remission in chronic ITP. True refractory cases usually require too much too often to make the treatment convenient or cost effective. The manoeuvre can be helpful as a temporary 'chemical' splenectomy to cover elective surgery or some other short-term problem.

Anti-D immunoglobulin. It was relatively recently noted that small doses of anti-D immunoglobulin injected into D-positive adults with chronic ITP caused their platelet counts to rise (Salama et al 1984). The same authors later extended their experience to include 10 children, and showed that giving 28–50 µg/kg for 1–4 consecutive days produced a rise of $> 50 \times 10^9/l$ on 26 of 45 occasions (Becker et al 1986). Whether this therapy has any advantages over IVIG in terms of efficacy or cost remains to be seen. It is certainly more convenient.

Pulse steroid therapy. High doses of prednisolone or methyl prednisolone can undoubtedly generate a satisfying temporary response in many children with chronic ITP (Menichelli et al 1984) but, as with IVIG, the effect is usually temporary. It is seldom possible to maintain a remission without steroid side-effects.

Vinca alkaloids. Unrelated to their cytotoxic effect, vinca alkaloids can generate a paradoxical reactive thrombocytosis in normal individuals, and this phenomenon has been exploited with some anecdotal success in childhood ITP (Manoharan 1986). The effect is usually short-lived, and repeated exposure may precipitate neuropathic side effects.

Danazol. Danazol is an impeded androgen which, through some ill-understood mechanism, can produce a rise in the platelet count in patients with chronic ITP (Ahn et al 1983). Results in children so far have not been particularly encouraging (Schaison et al 1985, Marwaha et al 1990), but further evaluation is needed.

Other treatments. A small group of patients with chronic ITP in an uncontrolled study showed an interesting pattern of response to interferon (Procter et al 1989), and an intriguing study using high doses of vitamin C has also recently appeared (Brox et al 1988) suggesting that this innocuous substance might also be useful. Both of these observations require confirmation, and experience in children has yet to be collected.

Cytotoxic immunosuppressives. No existing published reports offer much encouragement to use cytotoxic immunosuppressive therapy in children with ITP. The least toxic agent is azathioprine (Hilgartner et al 1970), a drug which still has advocates for its use in the adult disease (Quiquandon et al 1990). Cyclophosphamide has no place in the treatment of children. It is a potent leukaemogen and three adult ITP patients are described who developed a secondary leukaemia (Krause 1982).

Emergency treatment for life-threatening bleeding in ITP

The extremely rare but terrifying event of intracranial bleeding in ITP is by no means invariably fatal if treated promptly and aggressively (Woerner et al 1981). Craniotomy (if indicated) can be carried out at the same time as emergency splenectomy. The procedures can be covered by massive allogeneic platelet transfusions followed by IVIG and bolus doses of methyl prednisolone (in that order). Therapy during the postoperative phase can be dictated by clinical circumstances, but may include further platelets, IVIG and steroids. Using such a whole-hearted approach can reduce mortality to less than 50% with minimal disabling sequelae for the survivors (Lilleyman 1988).

Neonatal isoimmune thrombocytopenia

Babies are occasionally born thrombocytopenic due to transplacental passage of maternal antiplatelet antibodies. They fall into two groups: the first is affected by maternal antibodies produced as a result of direct sensitization to fetal platelet antigens, in a way analogous to haemolytic disease of the newborn (alloimmune neonatal thrombocytopenia, ANT); the second, much more common, is the result of maternal autoimmune thrombocytopenia (neonatal ITP). The presenting clinical features of these two groups are the same, but there are important differences between them in terms of management.

Alloimmune neonatal thrombocytopenia (ANT)

ANT is the product of fetomaternal incompatibility for platelet-specific antigens, most commonly Pl^{A1} (also known as Zw^a). Non-expression of this antigen is confined to less than 3% of the population (Mollison et al 1987a), so rare negative mothers have a high risk of having a positive child, and firstborns are frequently affected. Less commonly, other antigens may be involved. Successive infants tend to be equally or more severely affected, and the problem may arise in as many as 1 in 2000–3000 births (Blanchette et al 1986). It should be stressed, however, that not all pregnancies during or before which a mother has formed Pl^{A1} antibodies will result in the delivery of a thrombocytopenic infant, and only 6% of women with at-risk pregnancies (Pl^{A1}-negative mother, Pl^{A1}-positive fetus) will result in sensitization (Blanchette et al 1990).

In the absence of a history of a previously affected child, the condition can be suspected when a profoundly thrombocytopenic baby (who is otherwise well) is born to a mother with no history of ITP or autoimmune disease and who is not thrombocytopenic herself. The diagnosis can be confirmed by the demonstration of an IgG alloantibody in the mother's serum which reacts with the father's (and the infant's) platelets. If the mother is Pl^{A1}-positive, the chances of precisely identifying the offending antibody are not high. Anti-Pl^{A1} accounts for some 75–80% of cases, and in the remainder only some 10% will have demonstrable platelet-specific antibodies (Von dem Borne et al 1981), though recently in the largest serological study to date, Mueller-Eckhardt et al (1989) found another antibody – anti-Br^a – in 19% of babies with ANT.

Despite the fact that ANT is often a benign problem with a favourable outcome, there is still concern to avoid intracranial haemorrhage (ICH). The risk of this is far from negligible in severely affected babies, and may arise in over 10% (Mueller-Eckhardt et al 1989). If ICH occurs, residual neurological damage will ensue in up to 25%, and more than one baby in 10 will die

(Lancet Editorial 1989). For this reason, it has been common practice to avoid birth trauma, and deliver profoundly thrombocytopenic babies by caesarean section. However, as ICH can arise in utero during the third trimester, and even before (Herman et al 1986), attention more recently has been given to predicting those at greatest risk and attempting to alleviate the thrombocytopenia prior to delivery.

Two basic approaches have been tried. The first involves close monitoring of the fetal platelet count and giving intrauterine transfusions of washed irradiated maternal platelets during the later stages of pregnancy to those with very low platelet counts. This appears feasible and possibly successful (Kaplan et al 1988). Even more aggressive intervention has been advocated in the shape of weekly intrauterine platelet transfusions throughout the third trimester (Lancet Editorial 1989), but this would necessitate the use of unrelated platelet-pheresis donors, and could cause logistic problems.

The second approach is less invasive and revolves around maternal immunosuppression with high-dose intravenous immunoglobulin (IVIG). In a small study of seven at-risk pregnancies, where a previous child had been affected, Bussel et al (1988) found that the mothers had babies with higher platelet counts and less morbidity when given weekly IVIG (1 g/kg per week for 6–17 weeks prior to delivery). None of the treated babies had an ICH, compared to three of their earlier siblings. However, as with ITP, the response to this form of therapy appears to be variable between individuals.

It has to be concluded that, at present, the best prenatal management of ANT has not been established, though surveillance of babies at risk has improved due to the availability of fetal blood sampling. The postnatal management of affected thrombocytopenic babies is less difficult, and the low platelet count should spontaneously resolve in 2–3 weeks. Washed maternal platelets can be transfused if necessary, or compatible unrelated donor platelets – irradiated to avoid precipitating engraftment of viable lymphocytes – can be used. IVIG can also be given, but the effect is less predictable and less rapid. It has been thought helpful in at least 15 patients (Mueller-Eckhardt et al 1989) and may be the treatment of choice in an emergency when maternal or other compatible platelets are not easily available.

Neonatal ITP

The second group of thrombocytopenic newborns is that composed of babies born to mothers suffering from active or previous idiopathic immune thrombocytopenic purpura (ITP). Clinically similar to ANT (see above), the distinction is important because the treatment is different. Neonatal passive ITP cannot be treated by transfusing maternal platelets as these will be destroyed as rapidly as those already circulating.

It is difficult to predict which babies of mothers with ITP are likely to be affected. An attempt to do so by Cines et al (1982) concluded that there was no correlation between the platelet counts of mother and child, and that only 50% of babies born to mothers with active ITP would be thrombocytopenic. They also noted that five of 11 mothers in clinical remission from ITP at the time of delivery nonetheless produced thrombocytopenic children.

The only variable Cines et al could identify which (inversely) correlated with the infant's platelet count was the concentration of circulating free maternal anti-platelet antibody measured in an indirect radiolabelled antiglobulin test against normal random platelets. They suggested that this assay, or one similar, might be of predictive value and avoid the need for repeated fetal blood samples, but it should be stressed that the absence of such an antibody does not preclude the possibility that an infant might be affected. Two of 23 mothers in Cines et al's series had 'normal' antibody concentrations but their babies were thrombocytopenic.

The treatment of neonatal ITP revolves around estimating the risk to the fetus (direct platelet counting is perhaps the most reliable way), considering caesarean section for those with the lowest counts, and giving steroids to the mother for 10–14 days before delivery. Such steroid therapy has been found to be effective, in as much as babies born to steroid-treated mothers have, overall, significantly higher platelet counts than the offspring of untreated mothers, and antepartum prednisolone is thought to reduce the need for caesarean section (Karpatkin et al 1981). As steroids are not always effective (Scharfman et al 1982), a possible alternative is the use of IVIG, given either to the mother antepartum, or to the child postpartum. Both have been tried (Newland et al 1984). It is hard to define a consensus view on overall management of the problem (as in chronic ITP, see above) and individual circumstances demand individual consideration.

A point to note is that the mere discovery of a mild, symptomless thrombocytopenia in a pregnant woman should not necessarily be regarded as ITP and lead to invasive investigation of an unborn child. A recent survey of a large cohort of normal expectant mothers found that 8% of them were mildly thrombocytopenic (platelets $100–150 \times 10^9/l$), but that this had no effect on them or their babies, who had platelet counts similar to those of nonthrombocytopenic mothers. The cause of such thrombocytopenia is not clear (Burrows & Kelton 1988).

Immune thrombocytopenia associated with infections

Thrombocytopenia complicating some infections is known to be immune-mediated. In others, the mechanism is less clear, but where detailed studies have been possible, where shortened survival has been demonstrated or presumed, and where DIC has been excluded, the possibility of an immune mechanism has been suggested by the finding of increased amounts of platelet-adherent IgG in both bacterial (Kelton et al 1979) and viral infections (Feusner et al 1979). The distinction between some infection-associated immune thrombocytopenias, such as that seen with rubella or varicella, and acute ITP (see above) becomes semantic, but where a specific precipitating infection can be identified, it is easier to predict the clinical course.

Infectious mononucleosis

Thrombocytopenia has been recognized as a rare complication of infectious mononucleosis (IM) for many years (Radel & Schorr 1963). The incidence is hard to assess and depends on the definition of 'thrombocytopenia'. Carter found eight

of 57 unselected cases were associated with a platelet count of $<100 \times \times 10^9/l$ (Carter 1965), symptomatic thrombocytopenia is much more rare and probably arises in less than 0.05% of patients (Sharp 1969). There is no pre-existing pattern of symptoms or signs to suggest that one child is more likely to develop the problem than another, and those who do so mostly produce haemorrhagic signs in the second or third weeks of the disease. There is considerable circumstantial evidence that the thrombocytopenia is immune-mediated (Duncombe et al 1989).

The duration of the thrombocytopenia is variable, but seldom lasts more than 2 months, and very low counts usually last only a few days (Radel & Schorr 1963). One fatality has been recorded in a boy who had a spontaneous rupture of the spleen while profoundly thrombocytopenic (Radel & Schorr 1963), though splenic rupture, a well-known complication of IM in its own right, carries a 20% mortality irrespective of the platelet count. No intracranial haemorrhage has been reported in IM.

The thrombocytopenia of IM usually quickly disappears after the start of steroids, the conventional approach to therapy. Whether such treatment alters the morbidity of the condition in any clinically important way has not and probably will never be objectively assessed, but subjective impressions are that it might. Having said that, apart from the fatality referred to above, all 29 of Radel & Schorr's historical series recovered uneventfully and only nine had steroids. Occasional patients may *not* recover on steroids, and in two such young adults, high-dose intravenous immunoglobulin has been anecdotally successful (Duncombe et al 1989).

HIV-associated disease

An immune-mediated thrombocytopenia, clinically indistinguishable from subacute or chronic ITP, occurs in individuals infected with the human immunodeficiency virus (HIV) (Bellucci 1989, Karpatkin 1990). The complication is not rare and usually forms part of the aids related complex (ARC) syndrome. It can arise as an isolated problem in otherwise symptomless patients who are merely at the seropositive stage of their infection, and be the first marker of disease progression. Alternatively, it can appear for the first time in patients with AIDS. Experience in children has largely been confined to boys with haemophilia showing features similar to the adult patients described by Ratnoff et al (1983).

There are some serological differences between true chronic ITP and HIV thrombocytopenia in terms of anti-platelet antibodies and circulating immune complexes (Karpatkin 1990), but the clinical response to steroids, splenectomy or high-dose intravenous immunoglobulin appears to be similar (Beard & Savidge 1988). Anti-D immunoglobulin has also been tried with some success (Cattaneo et al 1989), and it has been claimed that antiviral therapy with azidothymidine (AZT) alleviates HIV-associated thrombocytopenia (Hymes et al 1988). Steroids should be used sparingly in HIV-infected children to avoid provoking opportunist infections.

The prognostic importance of thrombocytopenia in HIV infection, compared to generalized lymphadenopathy or other features of the ARC syndrome, is not clear.

Rubella

An acute self-limiting thrombocytopenia can follow clinically overt or silent rubella infection, and can be symptomatic and spectacular. Fatalities have been recorded (Morse et al 1966). The mechanism has been explored by Myllyla et al, who showed that such children have an antibody which causes platelet aggregation in vitro in the presence of rubella antigen, whereas convalescent serum from nonthrombocytopenic children does not (Myllyla et al 1969). The incidence is unknown but the problem is rare. The author has identified three unequivocal cases from a population of 1–200000 children in 15 years, but that is likely to be a falsely low figure, as examples following undiagnosed rubella would have been regarded as acute ITP in the absence of serial serological studies. The distinction is clinically unimportant as the management and outlook are the same.

Varicella

Apart and distinct from its rare association with the much more serious DIC and purpura fulminans (see below), varicella infection is also, and more commonly, accompanied by an acute ITP-like immune-mediated thrombocytopenia. The problem may arise during the viraemic phase or during the convalescent phase. Steroid therapy during the viraemic phase is theoretically risky and unnecessary. Most cases resolve within 2 weeks, though the later the onset the longer the problem may last (Lascari 1984a). Management, apart from the caution about steroids, is as for acute ITP.

Other specific virus infections

Acute and probably immune-mediated thrombocytopenia can complicate mumps (Graham et al 1974), measles or live measles vaccine (Bachand et al 1967). The problem is less common than with rubella or varicella (see above). In the case of measles, severe haemorrhagic symptoms ('black' measles) are more likely to be due to DIC than to simple immune thrombocytopenia (Lascari 1984a).

Congenital 'TORCH' infections

The 'TORCH' infections, toxoplasmosis, rubella, cytomegalovirus, and herpes simplex are a group of congenital infections (which should include congenital syphilis) having certain clinical features in common, one of which is thrombocytopenia. Affected newborns are ill, with jaundice, pallor, purpura and hepatosplenomegaly. Laboratory findings include haemolysis and a low platelet count, together with liver dysfunction and occasional abnormalities of coagulation (Oski & Naiman 1982a). From this, it is clear that the mechanism of the thrombocytopenia is complex and not necessarily immune-mediated, though it is quite possible that some immune mechanism contributes to the shortened platelet survival that is thought to occur.

Malaria

Thrombocytopenia frequently complicates malarial infections (outside the context of DIC in fulminating disease due to Plasmodium falciparum), and there are data to suggest that on some occasions this may be due to platelet-bound malarial antigen attracting antimalarial antibodies (Kelton et al 1983).

Drug-induced immune thrombocytonepia

Apart from the direct myelotoxic effect of anti-neoplastic drugs on platelet production (see below), in the past drugs have produced serious thrombocytopenia by causing direct non-immune-mediated aggregation of circulating platelets, as occurred with the antibiotic ristocetin and some early non-human clotting factor concentrates. These agents have now been withdrawn from use.

Mild thrombocytopenia of this type is still occasionally seen during the infusion of antilymphocyte (or antithymocyte) globulin (currently used as immunosuppressive therapy for aplastic anaemia graft-versus-host disease and transplant rejection episodes; (Champlin et al 1983)), and also occasionally arises in a few recipients of heparin (see below).

Much more commonly, drugs promote premature destruction of platelets by some immune-mediated mechanism. They do this in one of three currently understood ways:

1. by forming soluble drug–antibody immune complexes which attach themselves loosely to the surface of the platelet, fix complement and so lead to cell destruction
2. by attaching themselves firmly to the cell surface and acting as a hapten
3. by provoking the production of antibodies that cross-react with cell surface antigens thus creating a true autoimmune thrombocytopenia (Meischer & Graf 1980)

From a practical point of view, the distinction between the three mechanisms only becomes important in terms of how long the problem lasts after withdrawal of the offending agent, being slowest in the third.

The diagnosis of drug-induced immune-mediated thrombocytopenia is seldom easy. It rests on the exclusion of other causes of a low platelet count observed while the patient is taking the agent in question, and which resolves only after it is withdrawn. Direct *in-vitro* laboratory confirmation is seldom feasible, though demonstration of drug-dependent binding of IgG to

platelets can be attempted (Hackett et al 1982). The most likely source of confusion is the occurrence of ITP (see above) while a child is receiving innocent drugs for a coincidental reason.

The list of candidate drugs capable of causing immune-mediated thrombocytopenia is long (Meischer & Graf 1980), but in practice the majority of problems are due to only a few agents. Some important ones are shown in Table 6.2. Drugs are included there on the grounds that they are drugs commonly used in paediatrics which occasionally cause problems. On that basis, probably the single most important compound causing immune thrombocytopenia in children is sodium valproate, as it is frequently used. In a prospective study of 45 children, one-third had a measurable fall in their platelet count and one reached a nadir of $35 \times 10^9/l$ (Barr et al 1982). Bleeding problems have been described and appear to be due to a reduction in platelet numbers rather than drug-induced functional defects (Winfield et al 1976). Whether the thrombocytopenia is always or wholly immune-mediated is not clear. Defective platelet production through myelosuppression has been described (Ganick et al 1990).

Other frequently or increasingly used agents worthy of special mention are rifampicin (Blajchman et al 1970) and co-trimoxazole (Claas et al 1979). There are, of course, other drugs occasionally used in children which have been implicated as causes of thrombocytopenia. The classical examples of quinidine, quinine, gold, sulpha compounds and non-steroidal anti-inflammatory agents are well known (Meischer & Graf 1980) and there are many more. It should

Table 6.2 Commonly used paediatric drugs occasionally causing immune-mediated thrombocytopenia

Drug	Reference
Sodium Valproate	Barr et al 1982
Phenytoin	Weintraub et al 1962
Carbamazepine	Pearce & Ron 1968
Co-trimoxazole	Claas et al 1979
Rifampicin	Blajchman et al 1970
Acetozolamide	Bertino et al 1957
Cimetidine	Kelton et al 1981
Aspirin	Niewig et al 1963
Heparin*	Chong et al 1982

*Heparin can cause thrombocytopenia by a non-immune-mechanism also (see text)

be assumed that any drug is capable of producing an immune-mediated thrombocytopenia when a low platelet count occurs in any child for no other obvious reason. All should resolve within days or weeks after stopping the offending drug, with odd exceptions such as gold compounds. These produce thrombocytopenia of the type whereby true autoantibodies are stimulated (and which should not be confused with the irreversible aplastic anaemia also associated with their use), and which takes longer than that caused by other drugs to resolve after withdrawal of the drug because gold is very slowly excreted from the body (Kelton et al 1981).

Heparin-induced thrombocytopenia

Heparin is not nearly as frequently used in paediatrics as in adult medicine due to the much lower incidence of thromboembolic disease. It *is* used occasionally for conditions such as purpura fulminans (see below), and patients on intensive care invariably receive small amounts from indwelling catheters and arterial lines.

Low platelet counts can arise in as many as 5% of heparin recipients and may occur more frequently with bovine than porcine material (King & Kelton 1984). The thrombocytopenia produced by the drug is of two types: one is immediate, usually mild, and not immune mediated; the other is severe, arises after 8–10 days, and is associated with paradoxical arterial and venous thrombo-embolism (Chong et al 1982, Chong 1988). The second, much more serious, appears to be due to a heparin-dependent antibody which can activate platelet aggregation and cause major vascular occlusion. Though rare, and likely to be particularly so in children, this complication of heparin therapy is so devastating that all who use the drug should be aware of it. If necessary, it is possible to confirm the diagnosis of heparin-dependent thrombocytopenia using an in vitro test assessing the effect of patients' sera on the release of serotonin from normal platelets in the presence of heparin (Sheridan et al 1986).

Immune thrombocytopenia associated with autoimmune disorders

Immune cytopenias are not infrequently seen in

systemic lupus erythematosus (SLE), and chronic ITP-like thrombocytopenia was observed in 2–3% of a large number of adults attending a major SLE clinic (Miller et al 1983). The problem arises in children to the same extent as in adults and is occasionally a major cause of morbidity. It tends to be associated with the presence of the 'lupus anticoagulant', an antiphospholipid antibody inhibiting the formation of the phospholipid-dependent complexes in the coagulation cascade (Bellucci 1989).

The thrombocytopenia of SLE has much in common with chronic ITP (see above), though the serology may be different, with lupus-associated antiplatelet antibodies more commonly fixing complement (Dixon et al 1975). As might be anticipated, thrombocytopenic babies can be born to mothers with SLE (as they can to mothers with ITP, see above) if maternal anti-platelet antibodies cross the placenta.

Therapy for SLE-associated thrombocytopenia is as for chronic ITP, and the problem tends to respond to steroids along with other manifestations of the disease. There is evidence that splenectomy is less likely to be successful than in 'true' ITP (Hall et al 1985) and severe refractory cases are difficult to manage. The presence or otherwise of thrombocytopenia has no prognostic importance in terms of other manifestations and progress of the SLE (Miller et al 1983).

Immune thrombocytopenia has also been noted in mixed connective tissue disease, dermatomyositis and scleroderma (Richert-Boe 1987). It has been described complicating ulcerative colitis (Kocoshis et al 1979), and a clear association with autoimmune thyroid disease has been recorded (Marshall et al 1967). It has also been anecdotally reported complicating both myasthenia gravis (Anderson et al 1984) and sarcoidosis (Lawrence & Greenberg 1985) though it has rarely, if ever, been encountered associated with these two latter conditions in childhood.

Evans' syndrome

Some 1% of children with apparent ITP will have a preceding, coincident or succeeding autoimmune haemolytic anaemia, and the association between these two immune cytopenias has been called

Evans' syndrome (Evans et al 1951). Whether it is a distinct entity is not clear, but the condition tends to run a chronic or intermittent course. The disorder as it affects children has been well reviewed by Pui et al (1980) who make the point that it should be carefully distinguished from SLE and other connective tissue disorders. Neutropenia can accompany the disease and was noted in two of Evans' original series of eight. Other authors have seen it more frequently (Pui et al 1980).

Treatment is unsatisfactory. Temporary remissions can be gained with steroids, and splenectomy may help occasional patients, but no therapy is likely to produce a prolonged complete remission.

As an illustration of the syndrome, the author has seen a child who started with an immune haemolytic anaemia (warm type) at the age of 2 years, at which time his platelet count was normal. The problem resolved quickly on steroids, but briefly recurred at the age of 3. Shortly after his fourth birthday, he developed spectacular ITP. At that stage his haemoglobin was normal, but he had a reticulocytosis. There was a further relapse of the ITP just before his fifth birthday – on that occasion without a reticulocytosis – but 6 months later a further bout of haemolysis occurred. Since then both cytopenias have waxed and waned independently up to his present age of 10. Each episode has resolved on steroids and no more aggressive therapy has been necessary. His direct antiglobulin test has been negative in between attacks.

Immune thrombocytopenia associated with lymphomas

The association between immune thrombocytopenia and lymphomas is familiar to adult oncologists and has been well documented (Fink & Al-Mondhiry 1976). Excluding chronic lymphocytic leukaemia, the phenomenon is most often seen in Hodgkin's disease, and this is the context in which the disorder is most likely to be encountered in childhood. Hodgkin's disease can present as 'ITP' (Rudders et al 1972), can be preceded by it by many months (Fink & Al-Mondhiry 1976), or thrombocytopenia can arise later in the course of the disease. It can be the first sign of relapse (Hamilton & Dawson 1973), and occur in the presence or absence of the spleen (Fink & Al-

Mondhiry 1976). Increased amounts of platelet-associated IgG have been found in 39% of those with Hodgkin's disease, a variable which seems to correlate with disease activity, though very few become profoundly thrombocytopenic (Berkman et al 1984).

The association between immune thrombocytopenia and non-Hodgkin lymphomas in children is much rarer, and the problem has been described primarily in the more differentiated diseases seen in adults (Fink & Al-Mondhiry 1976).

Post transfusion purpura

Almost exclusively a disorder of women who have been pregnant, post-transfusion purpura is an ill-understood thrombocytopenia which occasionally arises in those previously sensitized to the ubiquitous platelet antigen P1^{A1} (also known as Zw^a, see alloimmune neonatal purpura, above). In some way the alloantibody such patients produce is responsible for the immune destruction of autologous platelets 2–14 days following the transfusion of red-cell-compatible whole blood, resulting in profound thrombocytopenia (Pegels et al 1981). High-dose IVIG may be useful therapy (Mueller-Eckhardt et al 1983). The condition has not affected children so far, but presumably could in any who were P1^{A1}-negative and who became sensitized.

THROMBOCYTOPENIA DUE TO SHORT PLATELET SURVIVAL: II NON-IMMUNE-MEDIATED

The chief non-immune-mediated causes of

Table 6.3 Causes of childhood thrombocytopenia due primarily to shortened platelet survival: II Non-immune-mediated

Disseminated intravascular coagulation (DIC)
Haemolytic uraemic syndrome (HUS)
Thrombotic thrombocytopenic purpura (TTP)
Haemangiomata (Kasabach-Merritt syndrome)
Cyanotic congenital heart disease (CCHD)
Liver disease
Drug-induced*
Perinatal aspiration syndromes
Neonatal undefined
Intravascular prosthetics
Photosensitivity

* Can be either immune- or non-immune-mediated

thrombocytopenia due to short platelet survival are listed in Table 6.3.

Disseminated intravascular coagulation

Disseminated intravascular coagulation (DIC) is a term which imprecisely defines the end result of a variety of serious physical or chemical insults to the intravascular milieu, and refers to activation of the whole or part of the coagulation cascade resulting in the generation of circulating thrombin. This causes the cleavage of fibrinogen and the aggregation of circulating platelets, and generates a severe secondary failure of haemostasis with paradoxical bleeding. Thrombocytopenia is a cardinal feature of DIC, and in children, particularly babies, once the condition has been recognized, the platelet count is a particularly useful indicator of its continued presence and progress. Most commonly, the condition is acute, severe, and found only in seriously ill patients, though occasionally a chronic low-grade consumption coagulopathy can arise with less spectacular laboratory findings in children who are not conspicuously ill. The disorder is described here as well as in Chapter 13, because thrombocytopenia is often the feature which indicates that a sick child has DIC.

Broadly, there are three aetiological groups. The first is triggered by chemically mediated damage to the vascular endothelium and occurs following exposure to bacterial toxins, acidosis, hypoxia, viraemia or immune complexes; this results in activation of the intrinsic coagulation system via factor XII. The second type is due to the physical disruption of tissues other than the vascular endothelium, and arises following trauma, cell lysis, hypoxia or hypothermia; it is mediated chiefly through the extrinsic pathway and activation of factor VII. The distinction between type 1 and type 2 may be somewhat artificial, as it is now felt that tissue thromboplastin expressed on the surface of endothelial cells or macrophages is the most important trigger procoagulant for all common intrinsic causes of DIC (Muller-Berghaus 1989).

The third group is a miscellaneous collection of rare disorders where there is direct activation of thrombin or factor X, or direct enzymatic degradation of fibrinogen, due to abnormal circulating

Table 6.4 Causes of acute disseminated intravascular coagulation in neonates*

1. Infections
    Septicaemia (Gram-
    positive or -negative)
    Viruses:
      congenital rubella
      congenital
      cytomegalovirus
      disseminated herpes
      simplex
      echovirus II
    Fungi
2. Deranged biochemistry
    Hypoxia
    Acidosis
	3. Tissue injury/cell
	    disruption
	    Hypothermia
	    Prolonged hypotension
	    Abruptio placentae
	    Severe maternal pre-
	    eclampsia/eclampsia
	    Dead twin
	    Severe birth asphyxia
	    Necrotizing enterocolitis
	    Intravascular haemolysis
	    Congenital malignant
	    disease
	4. Other causes
	    Homozygous protein C
	    deficiency
	    Hereditary fructose
	    intolerance

* See also Ch. 13

proteolytic enzymes such as snake venoms or the peculiar products of certain malignant cells. Some of the latter group are not, strictly speaking, DIC, and if they do not result in free circulating thrombin, thrombocytopenia may be absent. Platelets are not an important mediator for triggering DIC, and the thrombocytopenia it produces is a secondary phenomenon (Muller-Berghaus 1989).

Diagnosis

The diagnosis is usually not difficult, with gross derangement of the prothrombin, thrombin and partial thromboplastin times, together with profound thrombocytopenia. In the acute case, there is usually (but not invariably) a reduction in the circulating fibrinogen concentration, but there are seldom the striking red cell changes seen in the chronic syndrome unless the condition persists for some days. Fibrin/fibrinogen degradation products (FDP) are usually increased within 12 hours. Tests are now available to detect the D-dimers of crosslinked fibrin – the end product of thrombin activation – unlike earlier FDP assays which were nonspecific and cross-reacted with fibrinogen and fibrin monomers (Wilde et al 1989). Serial observations are necessary to make sense of a fluctuating clinical state, but the platelet count may be the easiest variable to monitor and provides a sensitive index of the progress of the condition.

Table 6.5 Causes of acute disseminated intravascular coagulation in older children*

1. Infections	3. Tissue or cell disruption
Septicaemias (Gram-positive or -negative)	Prolonged hypotension/shock
Haemorrhagic viruses	Hypothermia
Fulminating viral hepatitis	Trauma/crush injuries
Rickettsial diseases	Burns
Systemic fungal infections	Drowning
Falciparum malaria	Necrotizing enterocolitis
2. Deranged biochemistry	Malignant disease
Diabetic ketoacidosis	before therapy as part of disease process
Other acidosis	after therapy due to tumour lysis
Hypoxia/asphyxia	Status epilepticus
	Massive intravascular haemolysis
	Severe liver disease
	4. Other causes
	Snake venoms
	Haemorrhagic shock with encephalopathy**
	Reye's syndrome**

*See also Ch. 13
**The cause of DIC in these syndromes is unclear

Acute DIC

The causes of acute DIC are legion, but the more important ones arising in childhood are shown in Table 6.4 for neonates and Table 6.5 for other children. The distinction between the two groups is made because neonates, especially those born prematurely or small-for-dates, are particularly prone to develop DIC, due to the limited capacity of their reticuloendothelial systems to clear activated clotting factors from the circulation (Oski & Naiman 1982a). The frequency in one neonatal intensive care unit was noted to be around 5% of all patients admitted (Castle et al 1986). This, coupled with the different spectrum of diseases seen in the neonatal period, gives rise to a dissimilar incidence and variety of causes of DIC in newborns.

Of particular note as paediatric syndromes producing acute DIC are necrotizing enterocolitis (Hutter et al 1976) and the haemorrhagic shock with encephalopathy syndrome (Levin et al 1983).

Purpura fulminans. Although it has no single precipitating cause, this striking syndrome associated with acute DIC is recognizable due to the occurrence of widespread symmetrical peripheral gangrene chiefly involving fingers, toes, nose and ear lobes (Fig. 6.2). After 24–48 hours, fragmented red cells appear in the blood film, but the 'active phase', during which the condition progresses, usually lasts less than 3 days (Spicer & Rau 1976).

The incidence has two age peaks – childhood and old age. The condition has a high mortality if untreated (Chu & Blaisedell 1982), but with adequate supporting treatment (see below) this should now be less than 20%. Morbidity is still considerable, with loss of fingers or toes being a common consequence (Fig. 6.2).

The problem can follow meningococcal, pneumococcal or haemolytic streptococcal infections, or, rarely, varicella. Occasionally there is only a

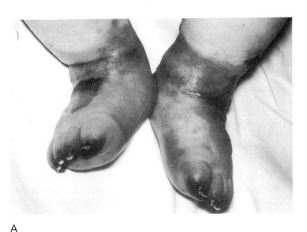

A

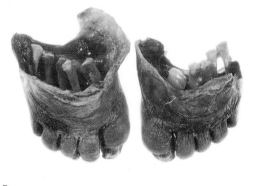

B

Fig. 6.2 Peripheral gangrene in purpura fulminans complicating pneumococcal septicaemia in an infant. **A.** Early stages. **B.** End result – amputation of non-vital tissue some weeks later. Otherwise the child made a full recovery.

vague history of preceding infection or no such history at all (Spicer & Rau 1976). A similar picture can arise in children on a recurrent basis, with homozygous deficiency of the naturally occurring anticoagulant protein C (Branson et al 1983; see Ch. 13).

Treatment of acute DIC

The treatment of acute DIC rests chiefly upon supportive measures and a vigorous attempt to remove the precipitating cause. After correction of hypovolaemia, consideration should be given to replacing clotting factors and platelets as these may hasten recovery and seldom make matters worse despite a theoretical 'fuel to the fire' risk.

More controversial is the use of heparin. In many cases it is probably unhelpful, but if the patient has evidence of continuing fibrin deposition, such as threatened peripheral gangrene, or venous thromboembolism, then active antithrombin therapy with heparin may be useful – as it appears to be in purpura fulminans (Spicer & Rau 1976). The route and dose of heparin are also the subject of debate, but in most instances a continuous intravenous infusion of 15 U/kg per hour has been advocated (Feinstein 1988).

Drugs blocking fibrinolysis should not be given in view of the risk of widespread fibrin deposition in the microcirculation. An exception to this rule may be the DIC seen in promyelocytic leukaemia which appears to be due to an acquired deficiency of alpha-2-antiplasmin, leading to proteolytic degradation of clotting factors rather than fibrin formation (Avvisati et al 1989).

Chronic DIC

The intravascular coagulation seen in chronic low-grade DIC is often, in fact, localized to one site in the body, as in the Kasabach-Merritt syndrome (see below), so perhaps should be called

Table 6.6 Causes of chronic low-grade intavascular coagulation in children

Giant cavernous haemangioma (Kasabach Merritt syndrome)
Other angiomas including:
  Chorangioma
  Diffuse angiomatosis
  Lymphangioma

LIC. The syndrome associated with mucin-secreting adenocarcinomas seen in adults does not arise in childhood, and low-grade DIC in paediatrics is essentially confined to that produced by giant haemangiomas (Table 6.6).

Kasabach–Merritt syndrome

Kasabach & Merritt first described and beautifully illustrated the association of bleeding and thrombocytopenia with giant haemangiomata in 1940. Shim, in a review of the problem in 1968, points out that the haemangiomata do not have to be large, and that low platelet counts have been seen with lesions as small as 5 cm. The site, too, is unimportant, as active examples have been described arising all over the body (Shim 1968). Occasionally, the lesions are occult, arising in the spleen, gut or lung.

The thrombocytopenia is associated with stigmata of a chronic consumption coagulopathy, and the consequent bleeding tendency can be severe. Schistocytes are usually seen on the patients' blood films. The proportion of haemangiomata that give rise to this syndrome is unknown, but may be larger than generally appreciated (Shim 1968). Unlike the approach to haemangiomata without thrombocytopenia, and although spontaneous regression can occur, treatment is considered necessary as the condition otherwise has a mortality of 21% (Shim 1968). Steroids may induce regression of the lesion in some cases; in others, low-dose radiotherapy may be justifiable (David et al 1983). Tranexamic acid has been used and thought helpful (Hanna & Bernstein 1989). Surgical resection is the treatment of choice but is often not possible.

Other angiomas

Chronic low-grade consumption coagulopathy and thrombocytopenia has occasionally been seen in other angiomas including chorangiomas (Bauer et al 1978), haemangiomatosis (Dadash-Zadeh et al 1976), and lymphangiomas (Dietz & Stuart 1977). The pathogenesis of the deranged haemostasis is presumably similar to that seen in the Kasabach-Merritt syndrome.

Haemolytic uraemic syndrome

First described by Gasser et al in 1955, the

haemolytic uraemic syndrome (HUS) is a hetero-geneous collection of disorders characterized by a combination of a microangiopathic haemolytic anaemia, thrombocytopenia, and renal failure. The thrombocytopenia is not associated with a consumption coagulopathy, and tests of coagulation are usually normal or only mildly deranged. The platelet count may be modestly or profoundly deduced. Platelet survival is shortened (Katz et al 1983), and platelet-aggregating activity has been found in the plasma of some affected children (Monnens et al 1985). The disease has occurred in epidemics during the summer months (Communicable Disease Surveillance Centre 1986), and usually has a prodromal illness of abdominal pain and bloody diarrhoea.

Evidence is accumulating to show that the epidemic form of HUS is frequently associated with an enteropathogenic *E. coli* producing an exotoxin called verotoxin. The precise mechanisms by which verotoxin causes the various features of the syndrome are still unknown, but the substance probably plays a major role in the pathogenesis of some cases. It may directly damage red cells, and normal plasma shows potent platelet-aggregating activity after incubation with it (Rose & Clark 1989, Rose et al 1985). A further contributory factor towards the thrombocytopenia of HUS might be the presence of abnormal factor VIII von Willebrand factor antigen (vWF:Ag) released by a direct cytopathic effect of verotoxin (or whatever) on the vascular endothelial cells (Rose et al 1984). The atypical vWF:Ag could cause platelet agglutination. Verotoxin is not the only cause of HUS, as it is not found in all cases, and some examples of what appears to be a very similar syndrome may be due to Shigella toxin (Raghupathy et al 1978), echovirus infection (O'Regan et al 1980) or even cytotoxic drugs (Weinblatt et al 1987).

Those mildly affected may present with anaemia or abdominal pain, and may recover without dialysis. Severely affected children may have other organ systems involved, including the brain and the myocardium, and may require dialysis for some weeks. The prognosis is variable, depending to some extent on age (younger children fare better), epidemiology and clinical prodrome. A few children die during the initial phase, and a few progress to chronic renal disease. Most eventually recover without sequelae. Trompeter et al, based on a series of 72 children, suggested that there are two basic subsets of children with HUS: One is commoner in toddlers, occurs in epidemics in the summer, and starts abruptly with explosive diarrhoea (the classical childhood syndrome); for them the outlook is good. The other variant, less well defined, occurs sporadically in older children, has a more insidious onset, more commonly involves systems outside the classical triad, and carries a worse prognosis for long-term renal function (Trompeter et al 1983). The second category may represent a heterogeneous group with a variety of noninfectious aetiologies.

Therapy, other than supportive measures for renal failure, anaemia and thrombocytopenia, is largely unsuccessful, though there are anecdotal reports of the use of heparin, antiplatelet drugs (aspirin and dipyridamole) and, more recently, infusions of prostacyclin (PGI$_2$), plasma exchange and alpha tocopherol (Powell et al 1984, Rose & Clark 1989). Platelet transfusions are seldom indicated except perhaps occasionally to cover the surgical insertion of dialysis catheters. As the mechanism producing the thrombocytopenia may be in vivo aggregation, there are theoretical grounds for keeping such transfusions to a minimum to avoid further microvascular thrombosis (see Thrombotic thrombocytopenic purpura (TTP) below).

In an older child with the insidious-onset sporadic type of HUS, if fever and neurological signs such as fits) are present, the distinction between HUS and TTP, (see below) becomes very difficult and may be semantic. The two conditions are distinguished purely on clinical grounds, and may represent different points on a common spectrum (Byrnes & Moake 1986).

Thrombotic thrombocytopenic purpura

Thrombotic thrombocytopenic purpura (TTP), also known as Moschcowitz's syndrome (after the first author to describe the disease in the early 1920s), is a syndrome of undetermined cause chiefly affecting young adults. It is characterized by a pentad of features which include: (a) thrombocytopenia, (b) microangiopathic haemolytic anaemia, (c) neurological disturbances, (d) renal failure and (e) fever. There is no evidence that the disorder observed occasionally in children differs from that encountered in adults (Sills 1984a). The classical pentad described above is the same as the classical triad for the haemolytic uraemic syndrome with the addition of two features – fever and neurological disturbances. It is probable that TTP and HUS (at least the sporadic type of the latter, see above) represent a similar pathological process with TTP being the more serious multisystem form of the disorder.

As with HUS, there is no evidence of DIC and the chief difference is the distribution of the disease process. The thrombocytopenia appears to be due to intravascular in vivo platelet aggregation due to a serum factor (platelet aggregating factor, PAF) (Berman & Finkelstein 1975) existing in sufferers. PAF can be neutralized by normal plasma, so it is not clear whether TTP patients lack an inhibitory substance or have an excess of a pro-aggregatory one. Some patients produce abnormal large multimers of von Willebrand factor (vWF) in the circulation which may induce the formation of platelet thrombi (Byrnes & Moake 1986). The clinical course of TTP is variable, but the disease is serious with a high mortality if untreated. Two-thirds of patients die within 3 months (Sills 1984a). The problem can wax and wane, with some patients pursuing a chronic relapsing course (Upshaw 1978).

There is no standard accepted therapy for TTP. Transfusions, plasmapheresis, steroids, immunosuppressives, antiplatelet drugs, prostacyclin, heparin, fibrinolytic agents and splenectomy have all been tried (Sills 1984b), and, with the exception of heparin, all have been anecdotally successful in some patients. Sills, in his detailed review, recommends a combination of plasma exchange with steroids as first line treatment, with the possible inclusion of vincristine if this is not successful. Byrnes & Moake suggest the simple rapid infusion of fresh frozen plasma (FFP), continuing at one plasma volume per day until the patient improves, and the use of plasmapheresis only if necessary for cardiovascular reasons (Byrnes & Moake 1986). The role of antiplatelet drugs is not clear, but the risk of haemorrhage may be justified in a non-responding patient. The use of long-term (6–12 months) aspirin and/or dipyridamole as 'maintenance' 'therapy once remission has been achieved

is logically attractive but of unproven benefit. During the acute phase, the use of platelet transfusions should be viewed with extreme caution, as some patients have had worsening neurological signs afterwards (Harkness et al 1981).

Despite the lack of a rationale for its application, splenectomy has been apparently successful in helping some patients. Its value may lie in the supportive transfusions given to cover the operation, and the good outcome overall may in part be due to patient selection. It may be worth considering as a last resort in an unresponsive individual (Sills 1984b). There is no established role for prosta-cyclin infusion (Byrnes & Moake 1986).

Cyanotic congenital heart disease

Some children with cyanotic congenital heart disease (CCHD) and secondary polycythaemia are prone to vasoocclusive disease, but paradoxically some become thrombocytopenic and may bleed excessively if subjected to corrective surgery. The cause of the thrombocytopenia is not well established, and there is debate about the presence or otherwise of DIC in such patients.

Wedemeyer et al (1972) studied 33 unselected children with CCHD, 12 of whom had a platelet count below $150 \times 10^9/l$, and four below $100 \times 10^9/l$. The severity of the thrombocytopenia was directly related to the haematocrit. All those over 70% had thrombocytopenia associated with a variety of abnormalities in clotting factor concentrations, though the authors concluded that none had DIC. Ihenacho et al (1973) studied 55 children with broadly similar results, but felt their findings *were* consistent with low-grade DIC, adding the observation that in 3 of 5 patients the platelet count rose after heparin therapy. A later study of autologous platelet survival in CCHD by Waldman et al (1975) found that those with the highest haematocrits had the shortest survival, but that short survival did not correlate with abnormal coagulation tests, and there was little evidence of DIC.

Naiman reviewed the problem without reaching a conclusion, though he pointed out the technical pitfalls of an uncorrected anticoagulant:plasma ratio in polycythaemic children when performing clotting factor assays. He recommended avoiding heparin therapy and suggested conservative management of the haemostatic defects by venesection and replacement by volume of fresh frozen plasma (Naiman 1970).

Liver disease

Acute and chronic liver disease can both be associated with disturbances of coagulation with or without thrombocytopenia. The mechanisms vary and the end results are complex. Coagulation factor deficiencies can be primary (decreased production through hepatocellular failure) or secondary due to some sort of consumption coagulopathy. There has been much debate about the presence or otherwise of 'true' DIC in liver disease (Bloom 1975), which has stemmed mostly from differing interpretations of the abnormalities seen, rather than different investigators obtaining different results. There is little doubt that fulminant hepatic failure can be associated with unequivocal DIC, but there is less certainty about whether grumbling low-grade DIC occurs in chronic liver disease. The topic is discussed more fully in Chapter 13.

The thrombocytopenia seen in liver disease is also complicated, being partly a consequence of congestive splenomegaly (see Hypersplenism, below), partly of shortened survival due to consumption, and (at least in adults with alcoholic liver disease) partly of decreased production due to ill-understood toxic myelosuppression. As the platelet count seems to fall with increasing age rather than being associated with any particular pattern of haemostatic disturbance, at least in biliary atresia, the major factor is probably hypersplenism (Yanofsky et al 1984). Therapy for the low platelet count *per se* is seldom required, abnormal bleeding usually arising from disturbances in coagulation, though occasionally replacement transfusion is warranted, particularly if platelet function as well as number is abnormal – as it may be (Ballard & Marcus 1976, Yanofsky et al 1984).

Perinatal aspiration syndromes

A particularly refractory form of persistent pulmonary hypertension seen in neonates can be distinguished from more responsive types by the presence of thrombocytopenia. The cause of the low platelet count is not certain, but it is possible that these children may inhale amniotic fluid, a powerful thromboplastin, which could cause thrombosis in the small vessels of the lung. Such an explanation would be compatible with the microthrombi seen in the pulmonary microcirculation at autopsy (Levin et al 1983).

Undefined neonatal thrombocytopenia

A large study of unselected consecutive neonates admitted to a regional intensive care unit indicated that 22% of them developed thrombocytopenia during the first week of life. An explanation for this could be found in only 80% of those affected: immune destruction accounted for around half, DIC for around 20% and exchange transfusion for around 10%. The remainder appeared to have short platelet survival with only very occasional patients showing evidence of underproduction (Castle et al 1986, Castle et al 1987). The reasons for the low platelet counts in such babies may not be fundamentally different from the rest, and the problem appears to be self-limiting. The thrombocytopenia tends to be less profound than in babies with recognizable causes.

Intravascular prosthetic devices

Umbilical catheters in neonates can generate thrombocytopenia – probably by promoting local thrombosis – though the mechanism is not clear (Nachman et al 1972). Otherwise, low platelet counts due to intravascular prosthetic devices are rarely seen in children. The shortened platelet survival demonstrable with some artificial heart valves and arterial repairs is usually compensated, so no thrombocytopenia arises (Burstein et al 1987). This is not so during prolonged extracorporeal cardiopulmonary bypass surgery, where consumptive thrombocytopenia is complicated by haemodilution and an acquired functional defect which compounds the haemostatic defect.

Phototherapy

Experimental data exist to indicate that photo-

Table 6.7 Causes of childhood thrombocytopenia due primarily to reduced production: I Congenital or inherited

---

1. Without megakaryocytes*:
   Thrombocytopenia/absent radius (TAR) syndrome
   Fanconi's anaemia
   Other amegakaryocytic thrombocytopenias
2. With megakaryocytes*:
   Wiskott Aldrich syndrome
   May-Hegglin anomaly
   Bernard-Soulier syndrome
   Epstein's syndrome
   Gray platelet syndrome
   Montreal syndrome
   Mediterranean thrombocytopenia
   Other hereditary thrombocytopenias
   Inherited megaloblastic anaemias
   Other metabolic disorders

---

*The classification into 'with' and 'without' megakaryocytes is not absolute but is clinically useful (see text).

therapy in neonates can increase platelet turnover with the occasional production of a mild and clinically unimportant thrombocytopenia if marrow compensation is inadequate (Maurer et al 1976).

THROMBOCYTOPENIA DUE TO IMPAIRED PLATELET PRODUCTION: I CONGENITAL

The chief congenital or inherited causes of thrombocytopenia due to impaired platelet production are listed in Table 6.7 and are considered further below.

The investigation of thrombocytopenia in small babies is always complicated by technical difficulties of adequate sampling, and this is particularly so when attempting to assess marrow megakaryocytes quantitatively. Ideally, that should be done by histological assessment of one or more marrow trephine biopsies, but such a technique is seldom possible in a thrombocytopenic neonate. Using cytological smears to decide whether megakaryocytes are present in normal, reduced, or increased numbers is often unreliable, but is nonetheless usually the basis for doing so in newborns. Consequently, to divide congenital production-failure thrombocytopenias into those 'with' and those 'without' megakaryocytes should be regarded as an imprecise science, though generally the distinction is clinically useful in a given case where megakaryocytes are easy or hard to find.

Type I: without megakaryocytes

Thrombocytopenia/absent radius (TAR) syndrome

Profound thrombocytopenia in association with forearm skeletal abnormalities – hypoplastic or absent radii – is a rare but well-recognized syndrome thought to be recessively inherited. The physical deformities are nearly always symmetrical (Fig. 6.3). The clinical features and pattern of inheritance are well reviewed by Hall (1987) who stresses the importance of distinguishing the syndrome from a Fanconi-type constitutional aplasia (see below) as the two disorders have very different outlooks. Severity of the thrombocytopenia is variable with some patients suffering considerable morbidity in the first year of life whilst others have few problems and may not be recognized until later in childhood. Morbidity lessens after the first year, and corrective orthopaedic surgery can often be carried out after that time without special precautions or replacement therapy. In symptomatic cases during the first 3–4 months of life, there is a risk of severe haemorrhage, often gastrointestinal,

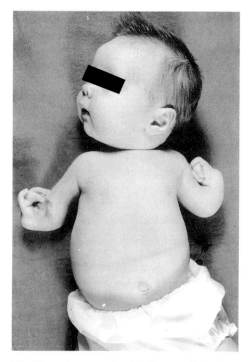

Fig. 6.3 Thrombocytopenia with absent radii (TAR) syndrome. Platelet count $30 \times 10^9/l$.

with a quoted mortality 20 years ago of 25% (Hall et al 1969), though it is likely that with the availability of platelet transfusions this figure will now be much less.

The marrow shows reduced or absent megakaryocytes, those present appearing small and dysplastic. Often, there is a background of apparent myeloid hyperplasia sometimes associated with a neonatal leukaemoid blood picture consisting of a neutrophilia peppered with myelocytes and metamyelocytes. The platelets are normal in size, and there is some evidence that their function may be slightly impaired by a storage pool defect (Sultan et al 1972), but this is not a constant finding (Armitage et al 1978).

Associated disorders include early failure to thrive and gastrointestinal bleeding due to cow's milk allergy (Whitfield & Barr 1976), and up to one-third may have heart defects. Congenital dislocated hips may be present, as may dysplasia of the jaw and clavicles.

There is no therapy known to correct the thrombocytopenia other than platelet transfusions; in particular, splenectomy is of no value. Transfusions should be given only when essential to minimize the risk of allosensitization.

Fanconi's anaemia

Fanconi described three brothers who had various congenital anomalies and pancytopenia in 1927. The term 'Fanconi's anaemia' has since come to describe a well-defined syndrome where a recessively inherited constitutional predisposition to develop irreversible pancytopenia declares itself usually in the middle years of childhood. Sufferers are often dysmorphic, short, and may have skeletal or genito-urinary abnormalities. Some are mentally handicapped. A cardinal feature of the disease is abnormal chromosome fragility, now best demonstrated as extreme sensitivity to in-vitro clastogens such as mitomycin-C. Exposure to this agent produces excessive chromatid breaks when compared to normal controls, and the lesion is consistently present from birth, before the pancytopenia and marrow hypoplasia evolve. Leukaemia (non-lymphoblastic) develops in some 10% of Fanconi patients and can occasionally be the presenting feature. For further details, see

Chapter 2 and the recent review by Gordon-Smith & Rutherford (1989).

Thrombocytopenia is usually the first haematological abnormality to appear and is often the reason the diagnosis is made. It is rarely present in the neonatal period and most commonly develops around the age of 6–7 years. Occasionally, the process may be delayed into adulthood. A lengthy asymptomatic prodrome of modest thrombocytopenia is usual and may last for a year or two before becoming symptomatic and being followed by neutropenia and anaemia. There is no effective long-term therapy other than bone marrow transplantation (Gluckman 1989), though androgens can produce a temporary response – in all cell lines – while a marrow donor is being sought. Recently, successful reconstitution of marrow cell lines has been achieved using umbilical cord blood from an HLA-identical sibling (Gluckman et al 1989).

Other amegakaryocytic thrombocytopenias

Over the years there has been a miscellany of anecdotes describing conditions which can be grouped under this broad heading. Some may merely be variants of the TAR syndrome, or have been described so infrequently that their existence as distinct diseases remains in doubt. They include: the multiple abnormalities and phocomelia associated with thrombocytopenia described by Cherstvoy et al (1980); the trisomy 18 syndrome including radial hypoplasia and thrombocytopenia described by Rabinowitz et al (1967); and the multiple malformations and neurological dysfunction described by Gardner et al (1983).

Sufficiently frequent reports have accumulated about a syndrome first described by O'Gorman Hughes in 1966 for it to be regarded as a separate entity. The disorder consists of congenital amegakaryocytic thrombocytopenia, unassociated with any other abnormalities, which evolves into aplastic anaemia in later childhood. That it may be a variant of Fanconi's anaemia is suggested by the similar evolution of pancytopenia (O'Gorman Hughes called it type III constitutional aplastic anaemia) and by the unpublished observation that in a case of the author's the chromosomes were more than normally fragile to the effect of clastogens to a degree rather less than that seen in the classical syndrome. The fragility observed was such that conventional tests could appear normal, which would make the finding compatible with earlier reports indicating children with this disease to be chromosomally unremarkable (Saunders & Freedman 1978). *In-vitro* culture studies would suggest the condition to be an intrinsic haemopoietic stem cell defect (Freedman & Estrov 1990).

Boys are affected more commonly than girls, and the condition has been described in siblings, giving rise to speculation that the condition may be sex-linked or recessively inherited. Less than 20 cases have been recorded so far (Freedman & Estrov 1990) with progression to aplasia occurring at any time from the neonatal period to later in childhood, though usually at the age of 3–4 years. At birth, the bone marrow is unremarkable save for the sparse distribution or absence of megakaryocytes. Platelet survival appears to be normal (Buchanan et al 1977), but there is early evidence of myelodysplasia with persistent elevation of the MCV (around 100 fl) and haemoglobin F concentration (between 5 and 10%, persisting well beyond 9 months of age). There is no known effective therapy though marrow transplantation would be a logical approach. The median survival from birth is 3 years (Alter 1987).

Type 2: with megakaryocytes

Wiskott-Aldrich syndrome

The triad of eczema, thrombocytopenia and immunodeficiency has been recognized for many years and was first described by Wiskott in 1937. It was later recognized as a sex-linked inherited disease by Aldrich et al in 1954. The condition is very rare, with an incidence of less than 1 in 1 000 000 per year. The immune deficiency is complex, involving both cellular and humoral immunity with absent or reduced isoagglutinins, increasing lymphopenia and failure to make antibodies to some antigens after appropriate challenge. This aspect of the syndrome is covered in Chapter 11. In addition to lymphocyte abnormalities, neutrophil and monocyte functional defects have also been described (Ochs et al 1980).

The thrombocytopenia of the Wiskott–Aldrich syndrome is variable but frequently profound and symptomatic (Fig. 6.4). Its mechanism is multi-

factorial and complex. The platelets are qualitatively abnormal in that they are small, about half the size of normal cells (mean platelet volume around 3–5 fl instead of 7–9 fl), and have ultra-structural abnormalities on electron microscopy (Grottum et al 1969). They have functional abnormalities indicated by storage pool defects, impaired aggregation in response to collagen and ADP, and reduced in-vitro adhesiveness (see Chapter 7 and Grottum et al 1969). Some, possibly many, patients have grossly elevated concentrations of platelet-bound IgG, and produce a large increase in their circulating count after splenectomy suggesting that there is an important immune-mediated element to the thrombocytopenia (Lum et al 1980). Platelet survival studies in the disorder have been attempted with ^{51}Cr-labelled autologous and allogeneic cells and with unlabelled allogeneic cells, and these give rise to the suggestion that short survival is invariable with autologous platelets, whereas allogeneic transfusions may survive normally (Grottum et al 1969, Krivit et al 1966) or be similarly short-lived (Ochs et al 1980).

Thus, the thrombocytopenia these patients suffer

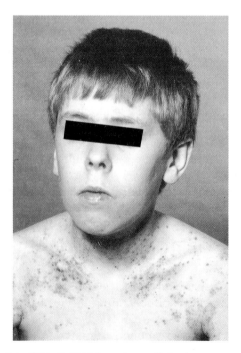

Fig. 6.4 Wiskott-Aldrich syndrome. Extensive purpura and haemorrhagic eczema.

is not just a failure of production of otherwise normal platelets. The immune-mediated component may be much more important than was initially realized, and despite the considerable hazard of splenectomy in patients who are already at abnormal risk of sepsis from encapsulated organisms such as *Streptococcus pneumoniae*, the operation may alleviate life-threatening thrombocytopenia-associated morbidity to the extent that the extra risk is justified (Lum et al 1980). High dose intravenous immunoglobulin may also be effective in temporarily pushing the platelet count up to satisfactory levels, with the added potential benefit of passive immunotherapy (Wodzinski & Lilleyman 1987), but in the author's limited experience steroids have not had any obvious effect on the platelet count in similar circumstances.

Other than splenectomy or immunoglobulin therapy, the only treatment which has proved effective in correcting the thrombocytopenia of Wiskott-Aldrich patients has been marrow transplantation (Parkman et al 1978). This, of course, corrects the other features of the syndrome as well, but it is interesting to note that in a patient in whom only a T-cell graft was established, the eczema was improved but the low platelet count persisted.

Carrier detection is not yet possible, but antenatal diagnosis by fetal platelet count and size may prove helpful (Holmberg et al 1983). The prognosis for sufferers has probably improved even if a marrow transplant is not possible, and many now survive to adulthood. The unlucky ones die of haemorrhage and/or infection.

May-Hegglin anomaly

Usually a curiosity rather than a clinical problem, the rare May-Hegglin anomaly, first described by May in 1909 and later again by Hegglin in 1945, consists of a mild thrombocytopenia associated with giant platelets and neutrophil inclusions. It is inherited as an autosomal dominant characteristic. One family has been described with an abnormality of chromosome 13 (Buchanan et al 1964), but the significance of that unconfirmed observation is not clear.

The neutrophil inclusions stain sky blue with Romanowsky stains, and on light microscopy are very similar in appearance to Döhle bodies seen in severe infections, but as they appear to be ultrastructurally distinct they should perhaps not be regarded as identical (Cawley and Hayhoe 1972). The platelets can be very large, more than 5 times normal size, with usually unremarkable morphology and ultrastructure though some examples contain giant granules (White & Gerrard 1976). Their survival and function are normal (Hamilton et al 1980). The thrombocytopenia per se is seldom profound enough to cause bleeding, and counts of $50-100 \times 10^9/l$ are not unusual. Occasional reports have described individuals with lower counts and clinical symptoms (Hegglin 1945, Oski et al 1962, Najean et al 1966). The condition is usually discovered fortuitously, and no treatment is effective or required.

Bernard-Soulier syndrome (see also Ch. 7)

First described by Bernard & Soulier in 1948, this recessively inherited disorder is characterized by a modest thrombocytopenia due to shortened platelet survival, but the most striking features are the abnormal platelet size, morphology and function. The condition produces a clinically important bleeding tendency.

Epstein's syndrome (see also Ch. 7)

Usually mild thrombocytopenia is found in this dominantly inherited disorder where large, functionally variable platelets produce a heterogeneous bleeding tendency. Other features of the syndrome are deafness and nephritis (Epstein et al 1972).

Gray platelet syndrome (see also Ch. 7)

So-called due to the hypogranularity seen on electron microscopy, this rare, dominantly inherited disorder produces a mild bleeding disorder and slightly reduced platelet count (Raccuglia 1971). The chief abnormalities are of platelet function.

Montreal syndrome (see also Ch. 7)

Chiefly characterized by abnormal platelet function, this dominantly inherited syndrome is also associated with large platelets which aggregate spontaneously, and a low platelet count.

Mediterranean thrombocytopenia

Slightly reduced platelet counts with large platelets, unassociated with a bleeding disorder, have been noted in individuals from the Mediterranean littoral when compared to North Europeans (Von Behrens 1975). Some 2% of such individuals have counts below $90 \times 10^9/l$, but the circulating platelet mass does not appear to be reduced in parallel.

Other hereditary thrombocytopenias

Described too infrequently, or without features sufficiently striking to warrant the status of a recognizable syndrome, there have been several kindreds reported with thrombocytopenia which is clearly familial. In some reported families, studies of platelet production, morphology and function have been much more detailed than in others. This makes it difficult to generalize about platelet and marrow appearances, or platelet survival and function. Also, because the reports have gradually accumulated over many years, some early papers describe families which today would perhaps be defined as established diseases.

Nonetheless, there are undoubtedly some well-documented families who have inherited thrombocytopenias which are not associated with a lack of megakaryocytes and which defy precise classification. They can be broadly divided into two groups: those where the inheritance pattern seems to be sex-linked, and those with an autosomal mode of transmission. All can potentially give rise to confusion with chronic ITP (see below) unless the familial nature of the disease is recognized.

Sex-linked. The sex-linked group may well include some variants of the Wiskott-Aldrich syndrome; this point has been made repeatedly (Vestermark & Vestermark 1964, Canales & Mauer 1967, Weiden & Blaese 1972, Murphy et al 1972), and has led these authors to suggest that such families have a partially expressed form of the syndrome. On the other hand, at least two kindreds have been described where the inheritance was apparently sex-linked but where there was no other feature to suggest any Wiskott-Aldrich association – one where there was an associated thalassaemia syndrome (Thompson et al 1977), and one where the family suffered mild thrombocytopenia but no eczema, infections or reduced

isoagglutinins (Chiaro et al 1972). Gutenberger et al (1970) described a family where sex-linked thrombocytopenia was associated with high serum IgA concentrations and glomerulonephritis, but concluded that it was not a variant of the Wiskott-Aldrich syndrome, chiefly because the sufferers showed no predisposition to infection, had no eczema, and suffered little other morbidity. Platelet size has been claimed to be useful in categorizing thrombocytopenias under such circumstances, as Wiskott platelets are usually small (Murphy et al 1972). It is not certain, though, that platelets in variants of the syndrome would necessarily be small, as platelet size can return to normal in those with the classical disease following splenectomy (Lum et al 1980), indicating that smallness is not irreversible or intrinsic.

Therapy in non-Wiskott sex-linked thrombocytopenia seldom appears to be necessary or successful. Splenectomy is particularly hazardous in such patients (Weiden & Blaese 1972), though the use of high-dose intravenous immunoglobulin has not been reported. It may be worth trying in severely affected individuals, for if any have a true Wiskott variant there may be an immune-mediated element to the thrombocytopenia as in the full-blown syndrome (see above). There is nothing to suggest that steroids are helpful.

Autosomal. The majority of 'miscellaneous' autosomal thrombocytopenias appear to be dominantly inherited. In some kindreds, there may be other nonhaematological abnormalities such as one recently reported with myopathy (Carrington et al 1989). Where platelet function has been assessed it has often been demonstrably abnormal, explaining a disproportionate bleeding tendency for a given platelet count (Cullum et al 1967, Kurstjens et al 1968, Sheth & Prankerd 1968, Danielsson et al 1980). Thrombopoiesis may be relatively ineffective, with increased numbers of megakaryocytes in the marrow, and platelet survival may be slightly reduced (Slichter & Harker 1978), or normal (Najean & Lecompte 1990). There is platelet anisocytosis with a tendency to larger cells than normal (Najean & Lecompte 1990).

Often confused with ITP, the conditions described have been essentially mild disorders, though mucosal bleeding, menorrhagia and dental extractions have caused problems. Occasional patients have had more serious morbidity (Kurtsjens et al 1968). The incidence and prevalence are hard to assess, but the problem may be more common than generally supposed (Najean & Lecompte 1990). No convincing claims for any effective therapy have been made, but treatment is seldom necessary except to cover a major haemostatic challenge. In that event, allogeneic platelet transfusion is the most logical approach, as the survival of such platelets is likely to be normal in unsensitized individuals (Murphy et al 1972).

One kindred observed by the author (unpublished) contained a father and three daughters (of a total of four), all of whom had a very mild bleeding disorder associated with longstanding platelet counts between 40 and $100 \times 10^9/1$. The proband, one of the daughters, presented at the age of 4 months and was thought initially to have ITP. She later developed 'common' lymphoblastic leukaemia at the age of 5, but completed therapy successfully, and continues 2 years later with a platelet count of $30\text{--}50 \times 10^9/1$. Her father, his sister, their mother, aunt and grandmother had all had primary thyrotoxicosis. The pattern of pathology in the family raises the possibility of an associated immune deficiency, and it is of interest to note that a child in the family described by Danielsson et al (1980) also developed leukaemia, as did four members of three families described by Najean & Lecompte (1990).

Inherited megaloblastic anaemias

Inherited childhood megaloblastic anaemias are discussed in Chapter 8 and have been well reviewed by Cooper (1976). Any are capable of producing a modest thrombocytopenia as part of the overall clinical picture, though low platelets are seldom the presenting or major feature.

Other metabolic disorders

Some organic acidaemias have thrombocytopenia and other cytopenias as part of their clinical picture (Rezvani & Auerbach, 1987). These include isovaleric acidaemia, proprionic acidaemia, and methylmalonic acidaemia – the latter being due to a variety of genetic defects most of which are not associated with megaloblastic anaemia (Cooper

Table 6.8 Causes of childhood thrombocytopenia due primarily to reduced production: II Acquired

Aplastic anaemia/myelosuppression
Idiopathic
Drug-induced
Toxin-induced
Radiation-induced
Hepatitis-associated
Marrow replacement
Leukaemia
Metastatic malignancy
Megaloblastic anaemias

1976). The mechanism producing the thrombocytopenia is not clear, though it may in part be consumptive due to acidosis (see DIC above). Such children are frequently also neutropenic, and fail to thrive due to vomiting and dehydration. Low platelet counts are usually the least of their problems.

THROMBOCYTOPENIA DUE TO IMPAIRED PLATELET PRODUCTION: II ACQUIRED

The chief acquired causes of thrombocytopenia due to impaired platelet production are listed in Table 6.8.

Aplastic anaemia

Aplastic anaemia is discussed in Chapter 2. Whether it is due to drugs, toxins, viruses, radiation or no known cause, thrombocytopenia is a cardinal feature of the disease, and in severe cases is frequently the direct cause of death. There is no specific therapy other than that for the primary disease (antilymphocyte globulin or marrow transplantation) or, temporarily, transfusion of random donor platelets. Such transfusions should be kept to a minimum if an allogeneic transplant is being considered, to avoid increasing the risks of graft rejection (Bacigalupo 1989).

Marrow replacement

Any extensive infiltration or replacement of bone marrow by malignant disease or fibrosis will generate secondary bone marrow failure, of which thrombocytopenia may be a prominent part. The leukaemias are described in Chapters 4 and 12, the myeloproliferative disorders and myelody-splasias in Chapter 3, and nonhaemic tumours which invade marrow in Chapter 15; they are not therefore discussed here.

Acquired megaloblastic anaemias

Megaloblastic anaemias due to any cause have a modest thrombocytopenia as part of the pancyto-penia they produce. Acquired varieties (see Ch. 8) are rare in children, compared to adults. The com-monest are: folate lack in premature neonates not given supplements, folate lack due to a generalized malabsorption syndrome, folate lack due to long-term anticonvulsants, and cobalamin deficiency secondary to chronic inflammatory bowel disease or following extensive gastrointestinal surgery. Other causes are very rare. Thrombocytopenia is seldom the main problem.

THROMBOCYTOPENIA DUE TO MALDISTRIBUTION, DILUTION, AND OTHER CAUSES

I: Maldistribution

The only recognized cause of thrombocytopenia due to maldistribution of a normal circulating platelet mass is splenic pooling in a large spleen (hypersplenism). The normal spleen harbours some 30% of the circulating platelets in dynamic equilibrium, and this proportion can be increased considerably in any circumstances where the spleen enlarges. It could be imagined that infiltra-tive diseases which replace splenic tissue, such as the storage disorders, might produce less splenic pooling than congestive splenomegaly due to por-tal hypertension, but there is little to suggest this, and it seems that any cause of splenic enlargement can have a broadly similar effect (Bowdler 1982).

The platelet count seldom falls below $50 \times 10^9/l$ due to hypersplenism alone, and so thrombocyto-penia itself is not a clinical problem. Patients with lower counts will have some additional reason. Impalpable spleens are not associated with hypersplenism (Burstein et al 1987).

II: Dilution: exchange and massive transfusion

A transfusion can be called 'massive' if a patient has a whole blood volume replacement within 24 hours. In paediatrics, this is most likely to arise in the context of an exchange transfusion in a sick neonate with hyperbilirubinaemia. Such in-fants may already be thrombocytopenic prior to exchange, but even if they are not, falls in plate-let counts to less than $100 \times 10^9/l$ can be expected in most patients with a few falling as low as $20 \times 10^9/l$. Full recovery to normal may take 7 days – longer if repeated exchanges are given (Oski & Naiman 1982b). At-risk children should have platelet supplements.

Massive replacement transfusion for surgery or trauma is less commonly encountered than in adults, and abnormal bleeding in such circum-stances depends upon whether there is already a bleeding tendency, such as DIC, due to widespread tissue damage. True dilutional thrombocytopenia due to simple replacement transfusion of stored blood is seldom a problem until two blood volumes have been transfused (Mollison et al 1987b). Difficulties can be avoided by giving adjuvant platelet transfusions.

III: Other causes

Spurious thrombocytopenia (in-vitro artefact)

Spurious thrombocytopenia can arise if there is a clot (even a small one) in the sample used for count-ing, and this is easily the most common cause. Much more rarely, platelet clumping can occur due to EDTA-dependent platelet agglutinins (Pegels et al 1982), when automated cell counters may recog-nize such clumps as leucocytes. Another rare pheno-menon is platelet satellitism, where platelets adhere to granulocytes in vitro and fail to be counted.

In paediatrics, the use of skin-puncture blood for platelet counting is satisfactory for clinical pur-poses provided care is taken over the technique of sample collection (Hinchliffe & Cassady 1987). In younger children, it may be more reliable than venous blood if the latter is only obtained after a lengthy struggle.

THROMBOCYTOSIS

Thrombocytosis, by definition, is an abnormally high platelet count. Conventionally, this is taken

Table 6.9   Incidence of thrombocytosis: Platelet counts ($\times 10^9$/l) at Sheffield Children's Hospital 1989–90

	All	>400	>500	>600	>700	>800	>900	>1000
Counts	12879	1322	567	285	122	88	36	16
%	100	10.3	4.4	2.2	0.9	0.7	0.3	0.1

Table 6.10   Conditions associated with thrombocytosis in children

Physiological	Primary
Premature infants	Essential thrombocythaemia
Secondary	Chronic granulocytic
Infection	leukaemia (adult type)
Malignant disease	Transient Down's
Chronic inflammation/	myeloproliferative
collagen disorders	Spurious
Iron lack	Cell fragments counting
Post splenectomy	as platelets
'Rebound' after	
thrombocytopenia	
Cerebral haemorrhage	
Vinca alkaloids	
Kawasaki's disease	
Infantile cortical	
hyperostosis	
Vitamin E deficiency	
Red cell aplasia	

to be one over 400×10^9/l, but at that threshold thrombocytosis is common, as has been appreciated since the widespread introduction of automated platelet counting of most routine laboratory samples (Heath & Pearson 1989). Of all platelet counts done over a 14-month period in the author's department, 10% were over 400×10^9/l, though only 0.1% exceeded 1000×10^9/l (Table 6.9)

Most high platelet counts in children are transient and secondary and in many instances are merely part of an acute phase response. Primary thrombocythaemia is extremely rare. The topic of childhood thrombocytosis was briefly reviewed several years ago (Addegio et al 1974), which indicated the wide variety of disorders with which it can be associated. The main groups of conditions where a high platelet count is likely to be encountered are shown in Table 6.10 and considered further below.

Thrombocytosis of prematurity

Low-birth-weight premature infants can have platelet counts in the range of $500–900 \times 10^9$/l during the first few months of life in the absence of any demonstrable pathology. In a recent study of 125 well babies born at less than 2000 g, 20% had counts over 500×10^9/l at 3 months of age, and in 3% the count was over 750×10^9/l (Lundstrom 1979). The count was independent of whether or not the children were receiving iron supplements. All were receiving supplements of vitamin E (see below).

Secondary thrombocytosis

Infection

In a prospective review of all children attending paediatric outpatients at the Yale-New Haven Hospital, Heath & Pearson (1989) noted that the 15 who had platelets in excess of 700×10^9/l all had a presumptive diagnosis of infection, and that the two with the highest counts were recovering from pyogenic abscesses. They found no clear suggestion that any specific infectious agent (bacterial or viral) was more likely to produce thrombocytosis than any other.

In a more specific study of a large group of children with *Haemophilus* meningitis, Thomas & O'Brien (1986) found counts over 500×10^9/l in 45% of them at some time during the course of the disease. They speculated that the thrombocytosis may be due to a rebound effect following thrombocytopenia associated with bacteraemia, and in support of this the child with pneumococcal-induced purpura fulminans depicted in Figure 6.2 subsequently developed a transient thrombocytosis with counts over 1000×10^9/l for several days during the recovery phase.

High platelet counts are also commonly found in patients with active pulmonary tuberculosis, and fluctuate in parallel with the activity of the disease. Such patients have increased thrombopoiesis-stimulating activity in their serum (Baynes et al 1987).

Malignant disease

High platelet counts can arise in children with cancer either due to the disease process itself, or as a 'rebound' phenomenon following a period of therapy-induced thrombocytopenia (see below).

Many neoplasms are associated with modest elevations in platelet counts, notably carcinomas (Levin & Conley 1964) but also lymphomas and even occasionally acute leukaemias (Lascari 1984b). Much higher values are seen in the adult-type of chronic granulocytic leukaemia, which can present with or evolve to a thrombocytosis well over $1000 \times 10^9/l$ (Mason et al 1974), though this is, of course, a primary myeloproliferative disorder and so akin to essential thrombocythaemia (see below).

Some patients with neuroblastomas show quite strikingly high platelet counts (Rao et al 1976), as do some with hepatoblastomas. There is evidence, at least in the latter group, that the thrombocytosis may be due to the tumour producing a thrombopoietin-like substance (Nickerson et al 1980). Langerhan's-cell histiocytoses, while probably not true neoplasms, can produce a thrombocytosis; this feature is secondary, occurs in the absence of marrow involvement, and may be amplified by the use of vinca alkaloids as single-agent therapy (Kamalakar et al 1977).

The thrombocytosis associated with childhood malignancy is seldom a clinical problem and is not associated with an increased tendency to vaso-occlusive disease. It requires no specific therapy.

Chronic inflammatory diseases

High platelet counts are found in most children with active juvenile rheumatoid arthritis (Calabro et al 1977), the majority with Crohn's disease (Dubois et al 1978), and many with ulcerative colitis (Morowitz et al 1968, Lake et al 1978). They are also seen in Wegener's granulomatosis (Fauci & Wolff 1973). In patients with chronic inflammatory bowel disorders it is difficult to be clear to what extent the thrombocytosis is due to the disease itself and to what extent chronic intermittent blood loss and iron deficiency complicate the picture. Occasional cases of immune thrombocytopenia have also occurred associated with inflammatory bowel disease (Kocoshis et al 1979).

Iron deficiency

Children with anaemia due to iron lack may have platelet counts that are low, normal or high, but as a group the mean values are significantly higher than iron-replete children and many will have counts over $600 \times 10^9/l$ (Gross et al 1964).

The reasons are not clear. Schloesser and colleagues showed that rats made iron-deficient after iron-free feeding developed a thrombocytosis which was corrected following iron replacement. They concluded that the presence of bleeding was not necessary for the stimulus to excess platelet production produced by iron lack (Schloesser et al 1965). In the series of 60 iron-deficient infants and toddlers reported by Gross et al (1964), 23 had some suggestion of gastrointestinal bleeding, but this did not correlate in any way with the presence or otherwise of thrombocytosis. Neither did the haemoglobin concentration, suggesting that iron deficiency probably has a direct thrombopoietic effect not mediated through erythropoietin.

In a review of the role of iron in the control of thrombopoiesis, Karpatkin et al (1974) concluded that both bleeding and iron lack were independently associated with thrombocytosis, but that the highest counts are likely to be seen in circumstances where chronic blood loss is being treated with iron supplements.

Irrespective of the initial value, the introduction of replacement therapy in iron-deficient children produces a transient rise in the platelet count followed by a return to normality over 4–5 weeks. The timing of the therapy-induced peak is in parallel with the reticulocyte response after parenteral iron (around 5 days), whereas after oral therapy the reticulocytes peak at 10 days but the platelets do not reach their zenith for 3 weeks (Gross et al 1964).

Postsplenectomy thrombocytosis

Modest thrombocytosis may follow fractures, parturition or any major surgery (Chesterman & Penington 1982). The most spectacular and long-lasting elevated counts are seen after removal of the spleen, where tissue trauma is less important than loss of the splenic platelet pool which contains up to one-third of the total body platelet mass.

In a review of 58 childhood splenectomies for

hereditary spherocytosis, Eraklis & Filler (1972) observed a rise from a preoperative mean of $322 \times 10^9/l$ to one of $1050 \times 10^9/l$ by the ninth postoperative day. This pattern is similar whatever the reason for the splenectomy, and the elevated count may persist for some months, though in most uncomplicated cases will settle to some 30% higher than the preoperative range within 3–8 weeks (Chesterman & Penington 1982). Morbidity associated with the thrombocytosis is minimal in children and no specific therapy is required.

Functional asplenia, as seen in children with sickle cell disease, can also produce a modest thrombocytosis of the type seen long after splenectomy (Kenny et al 1980).

'Rebound' thrombocytosis

Homeostatic control of the circulating platelet mass may go temporarily awry following a period of profound thrombocytopenia, resulting in an 'overshoot' and a short period where the platelet count is high (Ogston & Dawson 1969). Most commonly, this is seen following chemotherapeutic myelosuppression, but can occur following treatment of B_{12} or folate deficiency, or after an episode of consumption coagulopathy following severe infections (see above).

Cerebrovascular accidents

The few reports of thrombocytosis in association with cerebrovascular accidents in childhood do not make it clear whether the high platelet count is responsible for or reactive to the catastrophe, though both appear to be possible. In two infants with acute hemiplegia and thrombocytosis described by Huttenlocher & Smith (1968), the first patient had a rising platelet count following the event, whereas in the second a count of over $1000 \times 10^9/l$ preceded the problem by 3 weeks.

In a report from Sanyal et al (1966), two further babies, one comatose the other convulsing, both had a thrombocytosis on presentation. Only one had a lumbar puncture, which produced heavily bloodstained CSF, and again the platelet count subsequently rose. A 5-week infant reported by Lorber et al (1979) presented convulsing with bloodstained CSF, vitamin K deficiency and a

platelet count of $1154 \times 10^9/l$. The thrombocytosis in that instance was thought to be reactive, with the haemorrhage being precipitated by the bleeding tendency. In all five children the platelet count subsequently returned to normal, indicating that none had a primary thrombocytosis.

Vinca alkaloids

It has long been known that the cytotoxic alkaloids from *Vinca rosea* have the ability to induce a paradoxical thrombocytosis (Robertson & McCarthy 1969), an effect which has been used in the successful treatment of some cases of refractory ITP (see above). The phenomenon may be due to drug interference with feedback control of platelet production (Jackson & Edwards 1977).

Kawasaki's disease

Although thrombocytosis is associated with many infective and inflammatory conditions, there is a particularly noteworthy association with Kawasaki's disease (mucocutaneous lymph node syndrome). The platelet count typically rises to the 500–$1000 \times 10^9/l$ range during the second or third week of the illness.

First described in 1974 by Kawasaki et al, the disease is an acute febrile syndrome predominantly affecting infants and young children. The cause is unknown. The pathology is that of a systemic vasculitis with a predilection for the coronary arteries. The signs are fever, conjunctivitis, cervical lymphadenopathy, strawberry tongue, polymorphous macular erythema, and peeling of the fingers and toes. The acute phase lasts 1–3 weeks. The most serious complication is the development of coronary aneurysms in some 30% of patients (Novelli et al 1984).

The direct role of the platelet in the genesis of the vascular problems of Kawasaki's disease has been much debated, and aspirin is widely used as a primary therapy in the belief that it reduces the mortality, though the evidence that it reduces the incidence of coronary aneurysms is lacking (Corrigan 1986). The platelet count falls to normal values a few days after the end of the acute illness.

Infantile cortical hyperostosis (Caffey's disease)

A syndrome of unknown cause, infantile cortical hyperostosis usually presents within the first 3–4 months of life and consists of a relapsing febrile illness with marked swelling of soft tissues over the face and jaws associated with progressive cortical thickening of long bones and flat bones. During acute exacerbations, an associated thrombocytosis (over 500×10^9/l) may be present, and has been recorded in 50% of cases. Venous thrombosis has also been described (Pickering & Cuddigan 1969).

Vitamin E deficiency

Four of seven closely observed infants with haemolytic anaemia and vitamin E deficiency were noted by Ritchie et al (1968) to have platelet counts in excess of 500×10^9/l. Two corrected their platelet counts after replacement therapy over the subsequent 3 months, and two others, with counts of 400 and 350×10^9/l, showed a 30% fall (three were not tested). The reason for the thrombocytosis is not clear, and it should be emphasized that platelet counts in low-birth-weight infants can be high in the absence of pathology (see Thrombocytosis of prematurity, above).

Red cell hypoplasia

Red cell hypoplasia in childhood can be acquired, brief, and self-limiting (so-called transient erythroblastopenia of childhood, TEC) or congenital and chronic (Diamond–Blackfan anaemia). Both types can be associated with a high platelet count; some 34% of patients with TEC and 60% of children with Diamond–Blackfan anaemia may have counts over 450×10^9/l (Buchanan et al 1981, Alter 1987). The reason for this is not clear. Neither condition is associated with parvovirus infection, where the platelet count tends to be low (Wodzinski & Lilleyman 1989).

Primary thrombocytosis

Essential thrombocythaemia

Essential thrombocythaemia (ET), relatively common in adult practice, is extremely rare in children, with less than 15 cases ever having been described (Thieffry et al 1957, Ozer et al 1960, Spach et al 1963, Lumley 1971, Freedman et al 1973, Sceats & Baitlon 1980, Mitus et al 1990, Fernandez-Robles et al 1990). The disorder has arisen only in older children, with the youngest being 7 years old. It has been described in siblings (Fernandez-Robles et al 1990).

There appears to be little important difference between the adult and juvenile varieties of ET, with a similar constellation of symptoms (paradoxical bleeding and thrombosis, headaches, and myocardial and cerebral infarction) and signs (untreated platelet counts usually over 1000×10^9/l, often over 1500×10^9/l, together with megathrombocytes and splenomegaly).

The diagnosis is not usually difficult. It rests on the exclusion of other causes of grossly elevated platelet counts and distinguishing between ET and primary polycythaemia (PRV) or chronic granulocytic leukaemia (CGL). CGL can be recognized by the Philadelphia chromosome (or its molecular equivalent). PRV, with a modestly high haemoglobin, may be more difficult to distinguish, but the difference is perhaps academic–certainly from the therapeutic point of view.

Long survival appears to be the norm, mostly without treatment, though two patients have received busulphan (Lumley 1971, Sceats & Baitlon 1980). Morbidity, unlike that associated with secondary thrombocytosis, is not inconsiderable in some cases. Transient ischaemic attacks (or what sound like them) have been well described (Spach et al 1963), as has priapism (Sceats & Baitlon 1980). One 12-year-old, who was treated with radioactive phosphorous, subsequently developed acute myeloid leukaemia and died after 3 years (Ozer et al 1960). In retrospect, it is possible she had chronic granulocytic leukaemia from the outset, as the presenting white count was 19×10^9/l with 11% basophils.

Based on their experience of nine adolescents and young adults, Hoagland & Silverstein (1978) suggest that the management of young people with ET should differ from that of older patients, indicating that the disease is more benign and that aggressive therapy is not justified. Mitus et al, reporting on a larger group of young patients (of whom eight were less than 20 years), disagree, suggesting that morbidity is considerable and that active therapy should be considered at an early stage. What that therapy should be is unclear. It would certainly seem reasonable to hesitate to give known leukaemogens such as busulphan or ^{32}P, perhaps preferring alternative myelosuppressives and/or aspirin.

Other myeloproliferative disorders

Chronic granulocytic leukaemia – the adult variety – can present with a grossly elevated platelet count (see Malignant disease above and Mason et al 1974). The same phenomenon is also sometimes seen as part of the transient leukaemoid reaction occasionally encountered in the neonatal period of children with Down's syndrome (Miller et al 1967). Such children may develop true megakaryoblastic leukaemia later in childhood (Ch. 4).

Spurious thrombocytosis

Automated cell counters can recognize as platelets small fragments of larger cells, red or white, giving rise either to a spurious thrombocytosis, or, perhaps more commonly, and equally confusingly, to a normal count in the presence of true thrombocytopenia. Careful examination of the blood film should help to identify the problem (Hinchliffe & Cassady 1987).

REFERENCES

Addegio J E, Mentzer W C, Dallman P R 1974 Thrombocytosis in infants and children. Journal of Pediatrics 85: 805–807

Ahn Y S, Harrington W J, Simon S R, Mylvagnam R, Pall L M, So A G 1983 Danazol for the treatment of idiopathic thrombocytopenic purpura. New England Journal of Medicine 308: 1396–1399

Aldrich R A, Steinberg A G, Campbell D C 1954 Pedigree demonstrating a sex-linked recessive condition characterised by draining ears, eczematoid dermatitis and bloody diarrhea. Pediatrics 13: 133–139

Alter B P 1987 The bone marrow failure syndromes. In: Nathan D G, Oski F A (eds) Hematology of infancy and childhood, 3rd edn. W B Saunders, Philadelphia, p 159

Anderson M J, Woods V L, Tani P et al 1984 Antibodies to platelet glycoprotein IIb/IIIa and to the acetylcholine receptor in a patient with chronic idiopathic thrombocytopenic purpura and myasthenia gravis. Annals of Internal Medicine 100: 829–831

Armitage J O, Hoak J C, Elliott T E, Fry G L 1978 Syndrome of thrombocytopenia and absent radii: qualitatively normal platelets with remission following splenectomy. Scandanavian Journal of Haematology 20: 25–28

Avvisati G, Ten Cate J W, Buller H R, Mandelli F 1989 Tranexamic acid for control of haemorrhage in acute promyelocytic leukaemia. Lancet ii: 122–124

Bachand A J, Rubenstein J, Morrison A N 1967 Thrombocytopenic purpura following live measles vaccine. American Journal of Diseases in Children 113: 283–285

Bacigalupo A 1989 Treatment of severe aplastic anaemia. Balliere's Clinical Haematology 2: 19–35

Ballard H S, Marcus A J 1976 Platelet aggregation in portal cirrhosis. Archives of Internal Medicine 136: 316–319

Barr R D, Copeland S A, Stockwell M L, Morris N, Kelton J C 1982 Valproic acid and immune thrombocytopenia. Archives of Disease in Childhood 57: 681–684

Bauer C R, Fojaco R M, Bancalari E, Fernandez-Rocha L 1978 Microangiopathic hemolytic anemia and thrombocytopenia in a neonate associated with a large placental chorioangioma. Pediatrics 62: 574–577

Baynes R D, Bothwell T H, Flax H, McDonald T P 1987 Reactive thrombocytosis in pulmonary tuberculosis. Journal of Clinical Pathology 40: 676–679

Beard J, Savidge G F 1988 High-dose intravenous immunoglobulin and splenectomy for the treatment of HIV-related immune thrombocytopenia in patients with severe haemophilia. British Journal of Haematology 68: 303–306

Becker T, Kuenzlen E, Salama A et al 1986 Treatment of childhood idiopathic thrombocytopenic purpura (ITP) with Rhesus antibodies (anti-D). European Journal of Paediatrics 145: 166–169

Bellucci S 1989 Autoimmune thrombocytopenias. Balliere's Clinical Haematology 2: 695–718

Belluci S, Charpak C, Tobelem G 1988 Low doses v conventional doses of corticoids in immune thrombocytopenic purpura (ITP): results of a randomized clinical trial in 160 children, 223 adults. Blood 71: 1165–1169

Benham E S, Taft L I 1972 Idiopathic thrombocytopenic purpura in children: results of steroid therapy and splenectomy. Australian Paediatric Journal 18: 311–317

Berkman A W, Kickler T, Braine H 1984 Platelet-associated IgG in patients with lymphoma. Blood 63: 944–948

Berman N, Finkelstein J Z 1975 Thrombotic thrombocytopenic purpura in childhood. Scandanavian Journal of Haematology 14: 286–294

Bertino J R, Rodman T, Myerson R 1957 Thrombocytopenia and renal lesions associated with acetazoleamide (Diamox) therapy. Archives of Internal Medicine 99: 1006–1008

Blajchman M A, Lowry R C, Pettit J E, Stradling P 1970 Rifampicin-induced immune thrombocytopenia. British Medical Journal iii: 24–26

Blanchette V, Chen L, de Friedberg Z S, Hogan V A, Trudel E, Decary F 1990 Alloimmunization to the Pl a1 platelet antigen: results of a prospective study. British Journal of Haematology 74: 209–215

Blanchette V 1990 Personal communication

Blanchette V S, Peters M A, Pegg-Fiege K 1986 Alloimmune thrombocytopenia. Review from a neonatal intensive care unit. Current Studies in Hematology and Blood Transfusion 52: 87–96

Bloom A L 1975 Intravascular coagulation and the liver. British Journal of Haematology 30: 1–7

Bowdler A J 1982 The spleen in disorders of the blood. In:

Hardisty R M, Weatherall D J (eds) Blood and its disorders Blackwell, Oxford, p 751

Branson H E, Katz J, Marble R, Griffin J H 1983 Inherited protein C deficiency and coumarin-responsive chronic relapsing purpura fulminans in a newborn infant. Lancet ii: 1165–1168

Brox A G, Howson-Jan K, Fauser A A 1988 Treatment of idiopathic thrombocytopenic purpura with ascorbate. British Journal of Haematology 70: 341–344

Buchanan G R, Holtkamp C A 1984 Prednisone therapy for children with newly diagnosed idiopathic thrombocytopenic purpura – a randomised clinical trial. American Journal of Pediatric Hematology/Oncology 6: 355–361

Buchanan G R, Scher C S, Button L N, Nathan D G 1977 Use of homologous platelet survival in the differential diagnosis of chronic thrombocytopenia in childhood. Pediatrics 59: 49–54

Buchanan G R, Alter B P, Holtkamp C A, Walsh E G 1981 Platelet number and function in Diamond-Blackfan anaemia. Pediatrics 68: 238–241

Buchanan J G, Pearce L, Wetherley-Mein G 1964 The May Hegglin anomaly: a family report and chromosome study. British Journal of Haematology 10: 508–512

Burrows R F, Kelton J G 1988 Incidentally detected thrombocytopenia in healthy mothers and their infants. New England Journal of Medicine 319: 142–145

Burstein S A, McMillan R M, Harker L A 1987 Quantitative platelet disorders. In: Bloom A L, Thomas D P (eds) Haemostasis and thrombosis. Churchill Livingstone, Edinburgh, p 333

Bussel J B, Berkowitz R L, McFarland J G, Lynch L, Chitkara U 1988 Antenatal treatment of neonatal alloimmune thrombocytopenia. New England Journal of Medicine 319: 1374–1378

Bussel J B, Hilgartner M W 1984 The use and mechanism of action of intravenous immunoglobulin in the treatment of immune haematologic disease. British Journal of Haematology 56: 1–7

Byrnes J J, Moake J L 1986 Thrombotic thrombocytopenic purpura and the haemolytic uraemic syndrome: evolving concepts of pathogenesis and therapy. Clinics in Haematology 15: 413–442

Calabro J J, Staley H L, Burnstein S L, Leb L 1977 Laboratory findings in juvenile rheumatoid arthritis. Arthritis and Rheumatism 20(2): 268–9

Canales M L, Mauer A M 1967 Sex-linked hereditary thrombocytopenia as a variant of Wiskott-Aldrich syndrome. New England Journal of Medicine 277: 899–901

Carrington P A, Evans D I K, Cumming W J K, Mathon M 1989 Familial thrombocytopenia and myopathy. Clinical and Laboratory Haematology 11: 323–329

Carter R L 1965 Platelet levels in infectious mononucleosis. Blood 25: 817–829

Castle V, Andrew M, Kelton J, Giron D, Johnstone M, Carter C 1986 Frequency and mechanism of neonatal thrombocytopenia. Journal of Pediatrics 108: 749–755

Castle V, Coates G, Kelton J G, Andrew M 1987 111 In-Oxine platelet survivals in thrombocytopenic infants. Blood 70: 652–656

Cattaneo M, Gringeri A, Capitanio A M, Santagostino E, Mannucci P M 1989 Anti-D immunoglobulins for treatment of HIV related immune thrombocytopenic purpura. Blood 73: 357

Cawley J C, Hayhoe F G J 1972 The inclusions of the May-Hegglin anomaly and Dohle Bodies of infection: an ultrastructural comparison. British Journal of Haematology 22: 491–496

Champlin R, Ho W, Gale R P 1983 Antithymocyte globulin treatment in patients with aplastic anemia. New England Journal of Medicine 308: 113–118

Cherstvoy E, Lazjuk G, Lurie I, Ostrovskaya T, Shved I 1980 Syndrome of multiple congenital malformations including phocomelia, thrombocytopenia, encephalocele and urogenital abnormalities. Lancet ii: 485

Chesterman C N, Penington D G 1982 Platelet production and turnover: thrombocytopenia and thrombocytosis. In: Hardisty R M, Weatherall D J (eds) Blood and its disorders, 2nd edn. Blackwell, Oxford, p 971

Chiaro J J, Dharmkrong-at A, Bloom G E 1972 X-linked thrombocytopenic purpura. American Journal of Diseases in Children 123: 565–568

Choi S I, McClure P D 1967 Idiopathic thrombocytopenic purpura in childhood. Canadian Medical Association Journal 19: 562–568

Chong B H, Pitney W R, Castaldi P A 1982 Heparin induced thrombocytopenia: association of thrombotic complications with heparin-dependent IgG antibody that induces thromboxane synthesis and platelet aggregation. Lancet ii: 1246–1249

Chong B H 1988 Heparin-induced thrombocytopenia. Blood Reviews 2: 108–114

Chu D Z J, Blaisdell F W 1982 Purpura fulminans. American Journal of Surgery 143: 356–362

Cines D B, Dusak B, Tomaski A, Mennuti M 1982 Immune thrombocytopenic purpura and pregnancy. New England Journal of Medicine 306: 826–831

Claas F H J, van der Meer J W M, Langerak J 1979 Immunological effect of co-trimoxazole on platelets. British Medical Journal ii: 898–899

Cohn J 1976 Thrombocytopenia in childhood – an evaluation of 433 patients Scandanavian Journal of Haematology 16: 226–240

Communicable Disease Surveillance Centre 1986 British Paediatric Association/Communicable Disease Surveillance Centre surveillance of haemolytic uraemic syndrome 1983-4. British Medical Journal 292: 115–117

Cooper B A 1976 Megaloblastic anaemia and disorders affecting utilization of vitamin B_{12} and folate in childhood. Clinics in Haematology 5: 631–659

Corrigan J J 1986 Kawasaki disease and the plight of the platelet. American Journal of Diseases in Children 140: 1223–1224

Cullum C, Cooney D P, Schrier S L 1967 Familial thrombocytopenic thrombocytopathy. British Journal of Haematology 13: 147–159

Dadash-Zadeh M, Czapek E E, Schwartz A D 1976 Skeletal and splenic hemangiomatosis with consumption coagulopathy: response to splenectomy. Pediatrics 57: 803–806

Danielsson L, Jelf E, Lundkvist L 1980 A new family with inherited thrombocytopenia. Scandanavian Journal of Haematology 24: 427–429

David T J, Evans D I K, Stevens R F 1983 Haemangioma with thrombocytopenia (Kasabach-Merritt syndrome). Archives of Disease in Childhood 58: 1022–1023

Dietz W H, Stuart M J 1977 Splenic consumptive coagulopathy in a patient with disseminated lymphangiomatosis. Journal of Pediatrics 90: 421–423

Dixon R, Rosse W, Ebbert L 1975 Quantitative determination of antibody in idiopathic thrombocytopenic purpura. New England Journal of Medicine 292: 230–236

Dubansky A S, Oski F A 1986 Controversies in the management of acute idiopathic thrombocytopenic purpura; a survey of specialists. Pediatrics 77: 49–52

Dubois R S, Rosthchild J, Silverman A, Sabra A 1978 The pediatric corner; the varied manifestations of Crohn's disease in children and adolescents. American Journal of Gastroenterology 69: 203–211

Duncombe A S, Amos R J, Metcalfe P, Pearson T C 1989 Intravenous immunoglobulin therapy in thrombocytopenic infectious mononucleosis. Clinical and Laboratory Haematology 11: 11–15

Eldor A, Vlodavsky I, Deutch V, Levine R F 1989 Megakaryocyte function and dysfunction. Balliere's Clinical Haematology 2: 543–568

Epstein C J, Sahud M A, Piel C F et al 1972 Hereditary macrothrombocytopathia, nephritis and deafness. American Journal of Medicine 52: 299–310

Eraklis A J, Filler R M 1972 Splenectomy in childhood: a review of 1413 cases. Journal of Pediatric Surgery 7: 382–388

Evans D I K 1985 Postsplenectomy sepsis 10 years or more after operation. Journal of Clinical Pathology 38: 309–311

Evans R S, Takahashi K, Duane R T, Payne R, Lie C K 1951 Primary thrombocytopenic purpura and acquired hemolytic anemia: evidence for a common etiology. Archives of Internal Medicine 87: 48–65

Fauci A S, Wolff S M 1973 Wegener's granulomatosis; studies in 18 patients and a review of the literature. Medicine 52: 535–561

Feinstein D I 1988 Treatment of disseminated intravascular coagulation. Seminars in Thrombosis and Hemostasis 14: 351–362

Fernandez-Robles E, Vermylen C, Martiat P, Ninane J, Cornu G 1990 Familial essential thrombocythemia. Pediatric Hematology and Oncology 7: 373–376

Feusner J H, Slichter S J, Harker L A 1979 Mechanisms of thrombocytopenia in varicella. American Journal of Hematology 7: 255–264

Fink K, Al-Mondhiry H 1976 Idiopathic thrombocytopenic purpura in lymphoma. Cancer 37: 1999–2004

Freedman M H, Olivares R S, McClure P D, Weinstein L 1973 Primary thrombocythemia in a child. Journal of Pediatrics 83: 163–164

Freedman M H, Estrov Z 1990 Congenital amegakaryocytic thrombocytopenia : an intrinsic haemopoietic stem cell defect. American Journal of Pediatric Hematology/Oncology 12: 225–230

Ganick D J, Sunder T, Finley J L 1990 Severe hematologic toxicity of valproic acid: a report of four patients. American Journal of Pediatric Hematology/Oncology 12: 80–85

Gardner R J M, Morrison P S, Abbott G D 1983 A syndrome of congenital thrombocytopenia with multiple malformations and neurologic dysfunction. Journal of Pediatrics 102: 600–602

Gasser C, Gautier C, Steck A, Siebermann R E, Oechslin R 1955 Hamolytisch-uramische syndrome. Bilaterale neirenrindennekrosen bei akuten erwobenen hamolytischen anameen. Schweiz Medizinische Wochenschriff 85: 905–909

Gluckman E, Broxmeyer H E, Auerbach A D et al 1989 Hematopoietic reconstitution in a patient with Fanconi's anaemia by means of umbilical-cord blood from an HLA identical sibling. New England Journal of Medicine 321:1174–1178

Gluckman E 1989 Bone marrow transplantation for Fanconi's anaemia. Balliere's Clinical Haematology 2: 153–162

Gordon-Smith E C, Rutherford T R 1989 Fanconi anaemia – constitutional, familial aplastic anaemia. Balliere's Clinical Haematology 2: 139–152

Graham D Y, Brown C H, Benrey J, Butel J S 1974 Thrombocytopenia: a complication of mumps. Journal of the American Medical Association 227: 1162–1164

Gross S, Keefer V, Newman A J 1964 The platelets in iron deficiency anemia: 1. The response to oral and parenteral iron. Pediatrics 34: 315–323

Grottum K A, Hovig T H, Holmsen H, Abrahamsen A F, Jeremic M, Seip M 1969 Wiskott Aldrich syndrome: qualitative platelet defects and short platelet survival. British Journal of Haematology 17: 373–388

Gutenberger J, Trygstad C W, Stiehm E R et al 1970 Familial thrombocytopenia, elevated serum IgA levels and renal disease. American Journal of Medicine 49: 729–741

Hackett T, Kelton J G, Powers P 1982 Drug induced platelet destruction. Seminars in Thrombosis and Hemostasis 8: 116–137

Hall J G, Levin J, Kuhn J P, Ottenheimer E J, van Berkum K A P, McKusick V A 1969 Thrombocytopenia with absent radius (TAR). Medicine 48: 411–439

Hall J G 1987 Thrombocytopenia and absent radius (TAR) syndrome. Journal of Medical Genetics 24: 79–83

Hall S, McCormick J L, Griepp P R, Michet C J, McKenna C H 1985 Splenectomy does not cure the thrombocytopenia of systemic lupus erythematosus. Annals of Internal Medicine 102: 325–328

Halperin D S, Doyle J J 1988 Is bone marrow examination justified in idiopathic thrombocytopenic purpura? American Journal of Diseases in Children 142: 508–511

Hamilton P J, Dawson A 1973 Thrombocytopenic purpura as the sole manifestation of a recurrence of Hodgkin's disease. Journal of Clinical Pathology 26: 70–72

Hamilton R W, Shaikh B S, Ottie J N, Storch A E, Saleem A, White J G 1980 Platelet function, ultrastructure, and survival in the May Hegglin anomaly. American Journal of Clinical Pathology 74: 663–668

Hanna B D, Bernstein M 1989 Tranexamic acid in the treatment of Kasabach-Merritt syndrome in infants. American Journal of Pediatric Hematology and Oncology 11: 191–195

Harker L A, Slichter S J 1972 The bleeding time as a screening test for evaluation of platelet function. New England Journal of Medicine 287: 155–159

Harkness D R, Byrnes J J, Lian E C-Y et al 1981 Hazard of platelet transfusion in thrombotic thrombocytopenic purpura. Journal of the American Medical Association 246: 1931–1933

Harrington W J 1987 Are platelet-antibody tests worthwhile? New England Journal of Medicine 316: 211–212

Heath H W, Pearson H A 1989 Thrombocytosis in pediatric outpatients. Journal of Pediatrics 114:805–807

Hegglin V R 1945 Gleichzeitige konstitutionelle Veranderungen an Neutrophilen und Thrombozyten. Helvetica Medica Acta 4: 439–440

Herman J H, Jumbelic M I, Ancona R J, Kickler T S 1986 In utero cerebral hemorrhage in alloimmune thrombocytopenia. American Journal of Pediatric Hematology/Oncology 8: 312–317

Hilgartner M W, Lanzkowsky P, Smith C H 1970 The use of azathioprine in refractory idiopathic thrombocytopenic purpura in children. Acta Paediatrica Scandanavica 59: 409–415

Hinchliffe R F, Cassady G 1987 Basic laboratory techniques. In: Hinchliffe R F, Lilleyman J S (eds) Practical Paediatric Haematology. Wiley, Chichester, p 17

Hoagland H C, Silverstein M N 1978 Primary thrombocythemia in the young patient. Mayo Clinic Proceedings 53: 578–580

Holmberg L, Gustavii B, Jonsson A 1983 A prenatal study of fetal platelet count and size with application to fetus at risk for Wiskott-Aldrich syndrome. Journal of Pediatrics 102: 773–776

Hoyle C, Darbyshire P, Eden O B 1986 Idiopathic thrombocytopenia in childhood: Edinburgh experience 1962–82. Scottish Medical Journal 31:174–179

Huttenlocher P R, Smith D B 1968 Acute infantile hemiplegia associated with thrombocytosis. Developmental Medicine and Child Neurology 10: 621–625

Hutter J J, Hathaway W E, Wayne E R 1976 Hematologic abnormalities in severe neonatal necrotizing enterocolitis. Journal of Pediatrics 88: 1026–1031

Hymes K B, Greene J B, Karpatkin S 1988 The effect of azidothymidine on HIV-related thrombocytopenia. New England Journal of Medicine 318: 516–517

Ihenacho H N C, Breeze G R, Fletcher D J, Stuart J 1973 Consumption coagulopathy in congenital heart disease. Lancet i: 231–234

Imbach P, Berchtold W, Wagner H P et al 1985 Intravenous immunoglobulin versus oral corticosteroids in acute immune thrombocytopenic purpura in childhood. Lancet ii: 464–468

Ishibashi T, Kimura H, Shikama Y et al 1989 Interleukin-6 is a potent thrombopoietic factor in vivo in mice. Blood 74: 1241–1244

Jackson C W, Edwards C C 1977 Evidence that stimulation of megakaryocytopoiesis by low dose vincristine results from an effect on platelets. British Journal of Haematology 36: 97–105

Kamalakar P, Humbert J R, Fitzpatrick J E 1977 Thrombocytosis in histiocytosis X. Pediatric Research 11: 473 (abs)

Kaplan C, Daffos F, Forestier F et al 1988 Management of alloimmune thrombocytopenia: antenatal diagnosis and in-utero transfusion of maternal platelets. Blood 72: 340–343

Karpatkin M, Porges R F, Karpatkin S 1981 Platelet counts in infants of women with autoimmune thrombocytopenia. New England Journal of Medicine 305: 936–939

Karpatkin S 1990 HIV-1-related thrombocytopenia. Balliere's Clinical Haematology 3: 115–138

Karpatkin S, Garg S K, Freedman M L 1974 Role of iron as a regulator of thrombopoiesis. American Journal of Medicine 57: 521–525

Kasabach H H, Merritt K K 1940 Capillary hemangioma with extensive purpura. American Journal of Diseases in Children 59: 1063–1070

Katz J, Krawitz S, Sacks P V et al 1973 Platelet, erythrocyte and fibrinogen kinetics in the hemolytic uremic syndrome of infancy. Journal of Pediatrics 83: 739–748

Kawasaki T, Kosaki F, Okawa S, Shigematsu I, Yanagawa H 1974 A new infantile acute febrile mucocutaneous lymph node syndrome prevailing in Japan. Pediatrics 54: 271–276

Kelton J G, Meltzer D, Moore J et al 1981 Drug-induced thrombocytopenia is associated with increased binding of IgG to platelets both in vivo and in vitro. Blood 58: 524–529

Kelton J G, Keystone J, Moore J et al 1983 Immune-mediated thrombocytopenia of malaria. Journal of Clinical Investigation 71: 832–836

Kelton J G, Neame P B, Gauldie J, Hirsh J 1979 Elevated platelet-associated IgG In the thrombocytopenia of septicaemia. New England Journal of Medicine 300: 760–764

Kenny M W, George A J, Stuart J 1980 Platelet hyperactivity in sickle cell disease: a consequence of hyposplenism. Journal of Clinical Pathology 33: 622–625

King D J, Kelton J G 1984 Heparin-associated thrombocytopenia. Annals of Internal Medicine 100: 535–540

King H, Schumacker 1952 Spenic studies. 1. Susceptibility to infection after splenectomy performed in infancy. Annals of Surgery 136: 239–242

Kocoshis S A, Gartner J C, Gaffney P C, Gryboski J D 1979 Thrombocytopenia in ulcerative colitis. Journal of Pediatrics 95: 83–84

Krause J R 1982 Chronic idiopathic thrombocytopenic purpura (ITP). Development of acute non-lymphocytic leukemia subsequent to treatment with cyclophosphamide. Medical and Pediatric Oncology 10: 61–65

Krivit W, Yunis E, White J G 1966 Platelet survival studies in Aldrich syndrome. Pediatrics 37: 339–341

Kurstjens R, Bolt C, Vossen M, Haanen C 1968 Familial thrombopathic thrombocytopenia. British Journal of Haematology 15: 305–317

Lake A M, Stauffer J Q, Stuart M J 1978 Hemostatic alterations in inflammatory bowel disease: response to therapy. American Journal of Digestive Diseases 23: 897–902

Lammi A T, Lovric V A 1973 Idiopathic thrombocytopenic purpura: an epidemiologic study. Journal of Pediatrics 83: 31–36

Lancet editorial (anon) 1989 Management of alloimmune neonatal thrombocytopenia. Lancet i: 137–138

Lascari A D 1984a Viral infections. In: Lascari A D (ed) Hematologic manifestations of childhood diseases. Thieme-Stratton, New York, p 41

Lascari A D 1984b Malignant diseases. In: Lascari A D (ed) Hematologic manifestations of childhood diseases. Thieme-Stratton, New York, p 335

Lawrence H J, Greenberg B R 1985 Autoimmune thrombocytopenia in sarcoid. American Journal of Medicine 79: 761–764

Levin D L, Weinberg A G, Perkin R M 1983 Pulmonary microthrombi syndrome in newborn infants with unresponsive persistent pulmonary hypertension. Journal of Pediatrics 102: 299–303

Levin J, Conley C L 1964 Thrombocytosis associated with malignant disease. Archives of Internal Medicine 114: 497–500

Levin M, Hjelm M, Kay J D S et al 1983 Haemorrhagic shock and encephalopathy: a new syndrome with a high mortality in young children. Lancet ii: 64–67

Lightsey A L, Koenig H M, McMillan R, Stone J R 1979 Platelet associated immunoglobulin G in childhood idiopathic thrombocytopenic purpura. Journal of Pediatrics 94: 201–204

Lilleyman J S 1986 Changing perspectives in idiopathic thrombocytopenic purpura. In: Meadow R (ed) Recent

Advances In Paediatrics 8. Churchill Livingstone, Edinburgh, p 239

Lilleyman J S 1988 The management of chronic idiopathic thrombocytopenic purpura (ITP) in children. In: Del Principe D, Menichelli A, Rossi P, Guazzini S (eds) State of the art in idiopathic thrombocytopenic purpura (ITP) of childhood. Immuno, Pisa, p 75

Lilleyman J S 1990 Chronic idiopathic thrombocytopenic purpura: the pediatrician's dilemma. Pediatric Hematology and Oncology 7: 115–118

Lorber J, Lilleyman J S, Peile E B 1979 Acute infantile thrombocytosis and vitamin K deficiency associated with intracranial haemorrhage. Archives of Disease in Childhood 54: 471–472

Lum L G, Tubergen D G, Corash L, Blaese R M 1980 Splenectomy in the management of the thrombocytopenia of the Wiskott-Aldrich syndrome. New England Journal of Medicine 302: 892–896

Lumley S E 1971 Essential thrombocythaemia in childhood. Proceedings of the Royal Society of Medicine 64: 6–7

Lundstrom U 1979 Thrombocytosis in low birthweight infants: a physiological phenomenon in infancy. Archives of Diseases in Childhood 54: 715–717

Lusher J M, Emami A, Ravindranath Y, Warrier A I 1984 Idiopathic thrombocytopenic purpura in children. The case for management without corticosteroids. American Journal of Pediatric Hematology/Oncology 6: 149–157

Lusher J M, Zuelzer M D 1966 Idiopathic thrombocytopenic purpura in childhood. Journal of Pediatrics 68: 971–979

Manoharan A 1986 Vincristine by infusion for childhood acute immune thrombocytopenia. Lancet i: 317

Marshall J S, Weisberger A S, Levy R P, Breckenridge R T 1967 Co-existent idiopathic thrombocytopenic purpura and hyperthyroidism. Annals of Internal Medicine 67: 411–414

Marwaha R K, Singh R P, Garewal G, Marwaha H, Prakash D, Sarode R 1990 Danazol therapy in immune thrombocytopenic purpura. Pediatric Hematology and Oncology 7: 193–198

Mason J E, de Vita V T, Canellos G P 1974 Thrombocytosis in chronic granulocytic leukemia: incidence and clinical significance. Blood 44: 483–487

Matoth Y, Zaizov R, Frankel J J 1971 Minimal cerebral dysfunction in children with chronic thrombocytopenia. Pediatrics 47: 698–706

Maurer H M, Fratkin M, McWilliams N B et al 1976 Effects of phototherapy on platelet counts in low-birthweight infants and on platelet production and life span in rabbits. Pediatrics 57: 506–512

May R 1909 Leukocyteneinschlusse. Deutsches Archiv fur Klinishe Medizin 96: 1–6

McIntosh N 1982 Is bone marrow investigation required in isolated childhood thrombocytopenia? Lancet i: 956

McMillan R, Tani P, Millard F, Berchtold P, Renshaw L, Woods V L 1987 Platelet-associated and plasma anti-glycoprotein autoantibodies in chronic ITP. Blood 70: 1040–1045

McVerry B A 1985 Management of idiopathic thrombocytopenic purpura in adults. British Journal of Haematology 59: 203–208

Meischer P A, Graf J 1980 Drug-induced thrombocytopenia. Clinics in Haematology 9: 505–519

Menichelli A, Del Principe D, Rezza E 1984 Chronic idiopathic thrombocytopenia treated with pulse methylprednisolone therapy. Archives of Disease in Childhood 59: 777–779

Miller J M, Sherrill J G, Hathaway W E 1967 Thrombocythemia in the myeloproliferative disorder of Down's syndrome. Pediatrics 40: 847–850

Miller M H, Urowitz M B, Gladman D D 1983 The significance of thrombocytopenia in systemic lupus erythematosus. Arthritis and Rheumatism 26: 1181–1186

Mitus A J, Barbui T, Shulman L N et al 1990 Hemostatic complications in young patients with essential thrombocythemia. American Journal of Medicine 88: 371–375

Mollison P L, Engelfriet C P, Contreras M 1987a Antigens on leucocytes, platelets and serum proteins. In: Blood transfusion in clinical medicine. Blackwell, Oxford, p 688

Mollison P L, Engelfriet C P, Contreras M 1987b Transfusion in oligaemia. In: Blood transfusion in clinical medicine. Blackwell, Oxford, p 41

Monnens L, van de Meer W, Langenhuysen C, van Munster P, van Oustrom C 1985 Platelet aggregating factor in the epidemic form of haemolytic-uraemic syndrome of childhood. Clinical Nephrology 24: 135–117

Morowitz D A, Allen L W, Kirsner J B 1968 Thrombocytosis in chronic inflammatory bowel disease. Annals of Internal Medicine 68: 1013–1021

Morse E E, Zinkham W H, Jackson D P 1966 Thrombocytopenic purpura following rubella infection in children and adults. Archives of Internal Medicine 117: 573–579

Mueller-Eckhardt C, Kiefel V, Grubert A et al 1989 348 cases of suspected neonatal alloimmune thrombocytopenia. Lancet i: 363–366

Mueller-Eckhardt C, Kuenzlen E, Thilo-Korner D, Pralle H 1983 High-dose intravenous immunoglobulin for post-transfusion purpura. New England Journal of Medicine 308: 287

Muller-Berghaus G 1989 Pathophysiologic and biochemical events in disseminated intravascular coagulation: dysregulation of procoagulant and anticoagulant pathways. Seminars in Thrombosis and Hemostasis 15: 58–87

Murphy S, Oski F A, Naiman J L, Lusch C J, Goldberg S, Gardner F H 1972 Platelet size and kinetics in hereditary and acquired thrombocytopenia. New England Journal of Medicine 286: 499–504

Myllyla G, Vaheri A, Vesikari T, Penttinen K 1969 Interaction between human blood platelets viruses and antibodies. IV Post rubella thrombocytopenic purpura and platelet aggregation by rubella antigen-antibody interaction. Clinical and Experimental Immunology 4: 323–332

Nachman R L, Thomas M, Patel D, Gottbrath E 1972 Thrombocytopenia as evidence of local thrombus: the umbilical arterial catheter. Pediatrics 50: 825–826

Naiman J L 1970 Clotting and bleeding in cyanotic congenital heart disease. Journal of Pediatrics 76: 333–335

Najean Y, Schaison G, Binet J L, Dresch C, Bernard J 1966 Le syndrome de May-Hegglin. Presse Medicale 74: 1649–1652

Najean Y, Lecompte T 1990 Genetic thrombocytopenia with autosomal dominant transmission: a review of 54 cases. British Journal of Haematology 74: 203–208

Newland A C, Boots M A, Patterson K G 1984 Intravenous IgG for autoimmune thrombocytopenia in pregnancy. New England Journal of Medicine 310: 261–262

Nickerson H J, Silberman T L, McDonald T P 1980 Hepatoblastoma, thrombocytosis, and increased thrombopoietin. Cancer 45: 315–317

Niewig H O, Bouma H G, DeVries K, Janz A 1963 Haematological side effects of some antirheumatic drugs. Annals of the Rheumatic Diseases 22: 440–443

Novelli V M, Galbraith A, Robinson P J, Smallhorn J F, Marshall W C 1984 Cardiovascular abnormalities in Kawasaki disease. Archives of Disease in Childhood 59: 405–409

O'Gorman Hughes D W 1966 The varied pattern of aplastic anaemia in childhood. Australian Paediatric Journal 2: 228–236

O'Regan S, Chesney R W, Kaplan B S 1980 Red cell membrane phospholipid abnormalities in the haemolytic uraemic syndrome. Clinical Nephrology 15: 14-17

Ochs H D, Slichter S J, Harker L A, Von Behrens E, Clark R A, Wedgwood R J 1980 The Wiskott-Aldrich syndrome: studies of lymphocytes, granulocytes, and platelets. Blood 55: 243–262

Ogston D, Dawson A A 1969 Thrombocytosis following thrombocytopenia in man. Postgraduate Medical Journal 45: 754–756

Oski F A, Naiman J L, Allen D M, Diamond L K 1962 Leukocytic inclusions – Dohle bodies – associated with platelet abnormality (the May Hegglin anomaly). Report of a family and review of the literature. Blood 20: 657–667

Oski F A, Naiman J L 1982a Blood coagulation and its disorders in the newborn. In: Oski F A, Naiman J L (eds) Hematologic problems in the newborn. W B Saunders, Philadelphia, p 137

Oski F A, Naiman J L 1982b Disorders of the platelets. In: Oski F A, Naiman J L (eds) Hematologic problems in the newborn. W B Saunders, Philadelphia, p 175

Ozer F L, Truax W E, Miesch D C, Levin W C 1960 Primary hemorrhagic thrombocythemia. American Journal of Medicine 28: 807–823

Parkman R, Rappeport J, Geha R et al 1978 Complete correction of the Wiskott-Aldrich syndrome by allogeneic bone-marrow transplantation. New England Journal of Medicine 298: 921–927

Pearce J, Ron M A 1968 Thrombocytopenia after carbamazepine. Lancet ii: 223

Pegels J G, Bruynes E C E, Englefriet C P, von dem Borne A E G K 1981 Post-transfusion purpura: a serological and immunochemical study. British Journal of Haematology 49: 521–530

Pegels J G, Bruynes E C, Engelfriet C P, von dem Borne A E G K 1982 Pseudothrombocytopenia: an immunologic study on platelet antibodies dependent on ethylene diamine tetra-acetate. Blood 59: 157–161

Penington D G 1987 Thrombopoiesis. In: Bloom A L, Thomas D P (eds) Haemostasis and thrombosis. Churchill Livingstone, Edinburgh, p 1

Pickering D, Cuddigan B 1969 Infantile cortical hyperostosis associated with thrombocythaemia. Lancet ii: 464–465

Pizzuto J, Ambriz R 1984 Therapeutic experience on 934 adults with idiopathic thrombocytopenic purpura: multicentre trial of the co-operative Latin American group on hemostasis and thrombosis. Blood 64: 1179–1183

Powell H R, McCredie D A, Taylor C M, Burke J R, Walker R G 1984 Vitamin E treatment of haemolytic uraemic syndrome. Archives of Disease in Childhood 59: 401–404

Proctor S J, Jackson G, Carey P et al 1989 Improvement of platelet counts in steroid-unresponsive idiopathic immune thrombocytopenic purpura after short-course therapy with recombinant alpha2b interferon. Blood 74: 1894–1897

Pui C-H, Wilimas J, Wang W 1980 Evans' syndrome in children. Journal of Pediatrics 97: 754–758

Quiquandon I, Fenaux P, Caulier M T, Pagniez D 1990 Re-evaluation of the role of azathioprine in the treatment of adult chronic idiopathic thrombocytopenic purpura: a report of 53 cases. British Journal of Haematology 74: 223–228

Rabinowitz J G, Moseley J E, Mitty H A, Hirschhorn K 1967 Trisomy 18, esophageal atresia, anomalies of the radius and congenital hypoplastic thrombocytopenia. Radiology 89: 488–491

Raccuglia G 1971 Gray platelet syndrome: a variety of qualitative platelet disorder. American Journal of Medicine 51: 818–828

Radel E G, Schorr J B 1963 Thrombocytopenic purpura with infectious mononucleosis. Journal of Pediatrics 63: 46–60

Raghupathy P, Date A, Shastry J C M, Sudarsanam A, Jadhav M 1978 Haemolytic-uraemic syndrome complicating shigella dysentery in south Indian children. British Medical Journal 1: 1518–1521

Rao S P, Falter M L, Brown A K 1976 Thrombocytosis in neuroblastoma. Journal of Pediatrics 89: 682

Ratnoff O D, Menitove J E, Aster R H, Lederman M M 1983 Coincident classic hemophilia and 'idiopathic' thrombocytopenic purpura in patients under treatment with concentrates of antihemophilic factor (factor VIII). New England Journal of Medicine 308: 439–442

Revesz T, Kardos G, Kajtar P, Schuler D 1985 The adverse effect of prolonged prednisolone treatment in children with acute lymphoblastic leukemia. Cancer 55: 1637–1640

Rezvani I, Auerbach V H 1987 Defects in metabolism of amino acids. In: Behrman R E, Vaughan V C, Nelson W E (eds) Nelson textbook of pediatrics, 13th ed. W B Saunders, Philadelphia, p 280

Richert-Boe K E 1987 Hematologic complications of rheumatic disease. Hematology/Oncology Clinics 1: 301–320

Ritchie J H, Fish M B, McMasters V, Grossman M 1968 Edema and hemolytic anaemia in premature infants; a vitamin E deficiency syndrome. New England Journal of Medicine 279: 1185–1190

Robb L G, Tiedeman K 1990 Idiopathic thrombocytopenic purpura: predictions of chronic disease. Archives of Disease in Childhood 65: 502–506

Robertson J H, McCarthy G M 1969 Periwinkle alkaloids and the platelet count. Lancet ii: 353–355

Rose P E, Clark A J B 1989 Haematology of the haemolytic uraemic syndrome. Blood Reviews 3: 136–140

Rose P E, Armour J A, Williams C E, Hill F G H 1985 Verotoxin and neuraminidase induced platelet aggregating activity in plasma: their possible role in the pathogenesis of the haemolytic uraemic syndrome. Journal of Clinical Pathology 38: 438–441

Rose P E, Enayat S M, Sunderland R, Short P E, Williams C E, Hill F G H 1984 Abnormalities of factor VIII related protein multimers in the haemolytic uraemic syndrome. Archives of Disease in Childhood 59: 1135–1140

Rudders R A, Aisenberg A C, Schiller A L 1972 Hodgkin's disease presenting as 'idiopathic' thrombocytopenic purpura. Cancer 30: 220–230

Salama A, Kiefel V, Amberg R, Mueller-Eckhardt C 1984 Treatment of autoimmune thrombocytopenic purpura with Rhesus antibodies (anti Rho[d]). Blut 49: 29–35

Sanyal S K, Yules R B, Eidelman A I, Talner N S 1966 Thrombocytosis, central nervous system disease, and myocardial infarction pattern in infancy. Pediatrics

38: 629–636

Sartorius J A 1984 Steroid treatment of idiopathic thrombocytopenic purpura in children. American Journal of Pediatric Hematology/Oncology 6:165–169

Saunders E F, Freedman M H 1978 Constitutional aplastic anaemia: defective haemopoietic stem cell growth in vitro. British Journal of Haematology 40: 277–287

Sceats D J, Baitlon D 1980 Primary thrombocythaemia in a child. Clinics in Pediatrics 19: 298–300

Schaison G, Olive D, Fermand J P, Munck P 1985 Treatment of idiopathic thrombocytopenic purpura (ITP) in children with danazol. European Journal of Pediatrics 144:103 (abstr)

Scharfman W B, Babcock R B, Raugh A E 1982 Steroid administration in pregnant women with autoimmune thrombocytopenia. New England Journal of Medicine 306: 745

Schloesser L L, Kip M A, Wenzel F J 1965 Thrombocytosis in iron deficiency anaemia. Journal of Laboratory and Clinical Medicine 66: 107–114

Sharp A A 1969 Platelets, bleeding and haemostasis in infectious mononucleosis In: Carter R L, Penman H G (eds) Infectious mononucleosis. Blackwell, Oxford, p 99

Sheridan D, Carter C, Kelton J G 1986 A diagnostic test for heparin-induced thrombocytopenia. Blood 67: 27–30

Sheth N K, Prankerd T A J 1968 Inherited thrombocytopenia with thrombasthenia. Journal of Clinical Pathology 21: 154–156

Shim W K T 1968 Hemangiomas of infancy complicated by thrombocytopenia. American Journal of Surgery 116: 896–906

Sills R H 1984a Thrombotic thrombocytopenic purpura. 1. Pathophysiology and clinical manifestations. American Journal of Pediatric Hematology/Oncology 6: 425–430

Sills R H 1984b Thrombotic thrombocytopenic purpura: II. Principles of therapy and guidelines for management. American Journal of Pediatric Hematology/Oncology 6: 431–439

Simons S M, Main C A, Yaish H M, Rutzky J 1975 Idiopathic thrombocytopenic purpura in children. Journal of Paediatrics 87: 16–22

Singer D B 1973 Postsplenectomy sepsis. Perspectives in Pediatric Pathology 1: 285–311

Slater D N, Trowbridge E A, Martin J F 1983 The megakaryocyte in thrombocytopenia. A microscope study which supports the theory that platelets are produced in the pulmonary circulation. Thrombosis Research 31: 163–176

Slichter S J, Harker L A 1978 Thrombocytopenia: mechanisms and management of defects in platelet production. Clinical Haematology 7: 523–539

Spach M S, Howell D A, Harris J S 1963 Myocardial infarction and multiple thromboses in a child with primary thrombocytosis. Pediatrics 31: 268–276

Spicer T E, Rau J M 1976 Purpura fulminans. American Journal of Medicine 61: 566–571

Stuart M J, Murphy S, Oski F A 1975 A simple nonradioisotopic technic for the determination of platelet life-span. New England Journal of Medicine 292: 1310–1313

Sultan Y, Scrobohaci M L, Rendu F, Caen J P 1972 Abnormal platelet function, population, and survival time in a boy with congenital absent radii and thrombocytopenia. Lancet ii: 653

Thieffry S, Buhot S, Aicardi J 1957 Une observation de thrombocythemie essentielle. Sang 28: 264–266

Thomas G A, O'Brien R T 1986 Thrombocytosis in children with Haemophilus influenzae meningitis. Clinical Pediatrics 25: 610–611

Thompson A R, Wood W G, Stamatoyannopoulos G 1977 X-linked syndrome of platelet dysfunction, thrombocytopenia, and imbalanced globin chain synthesis with haemolysis. Blood 50: 303–316

Trompeter R S, Schwartz R, Chantler C et al 1983 Haemolytic-uraemic syndrome: an analysis of prognostic features. Archives of Disease in Childhood 58: 101–105

Upshaw J D 1978 Congenital deficiency of a factor in normal plasma that reverses microangiopathic hemolysis and thrombocytopenia. New England Journal of Medicine 298: 1350–1352

Vestermark B, Vestermark S 1964 Familial sex-linked thrombocytopenia. Acta Paediatrica Scandanavica 53: 365–370

von Behrens W 1975 Mediterranean macrothrombocytopenia. Blood 46: 199–208

von dem Borne A E G K, van Leeuwen E F, von Riesz L E, van Boxtel C J, Engelfriet C P 1981 Neonatal alloimmune thrombocytopenia: detection and characterization of the responsible antibodies by the platelet immunofluorescence test. Blood 57: 649–656

Waldman J D, Czapek E E, Paul M H, Schwartz A D, Levin D L, Schindler S 1975 Shortened platelet survival in cyanotic heart disease. Journal of Pediatrics 87: 77–79

Walker R W, Walker W 1984 Idiopathic thrombocytopenia, initial illness and long term follow up. Archives of Disease in Childhood 59: 316–322

Wedemeyer A L, Edson R, Krivit W 1972 Coagulation in cyanotic congenital heart disease. American Journal of Diseases in Children 124: 656–660

Weiden P L, Blaese R M 1972 Hereditary thrombocytopenia: relation to Wiskott-Aldrich syndrome with special reference to splenectomy. Journal of Pediatrics 80: 226–234

Weinblatt M E, Kahn E, Scimeca P G, Kochen J A 1987 Hemolytic uremic syndrome associated with cisplatin therapy. American Journal of Pediatric Hematology and Oncology 9: 295–298

Weintraub R M, Pechet L, Alexander B 1962 Rapid diagnosis of drug-induced thrombocytopenic purpura. Journal of the American Medical Association 180: 528–532

White J G, Gerrard J M 1976 Ultrastructural features of abnormal blood platelets. American Journal of Pathology 83: 590–632

Whitfield M F, Barr D G D 1976 Cows' milk allergy in the syndrome of thrombocytopenia with absent radius. Archives of Disease in Childhood 51: 337–343

Wilde J T, Kitchen S, Kinsey S, Greaves M, Preston F E 1989 Plasma D-dimer levels and their relationship to serum fibrinogen/fibrin degradation products in hypercoagulable states. British Journal of Haematology 71: 65–70

Williamson B 1926 Recent advances in the diagnosis and treatment of purpura haemorrhagica. Archives of Disease in Childhood 1: 39–50

Winfield D A, Benton P, Espir M L, Arthur L J H 1976 Sodium valproate and thrombocytopenia. British Medical Journal ii: 981

Winiarski J 1989 IgG and IgM antibodies to platelet membranes glycoprotein antigens in childhood idiopathic thrombocytopenic purpura. British Journal of Haematology 73: 88–92

Wiskott A 1937 Familiarer, angeborener Morbus Werlhofii? Monatsschr Kinderheilkd 68: 212–216

Wodzinski M, Lilleyman J S 1987 High-dose immunoglobulin therapy of Wiskott-Aldrich syndrome. Pediatric Hematology and Oncology 4: 345–348

Wodzinski M A, Lilleyman J S 1989 Transient erythroblastopenia of childhood due to human parvovirus B19 infection. British Journal of Haematology 73: 127–128

Woerner S J, Abildgaard C F, French B N 1981 Intracranial hemorrhage in children with idiopathic thrombocytopenic purpura. Pediatrics 67: 453–460

Woods V L, McMillan R 1984 Platelet autoantigens in chronic ITP. British Journal of Haematology 57: 1–4

Yanofsky R A, Jackson V G, Lilly J R, Stellin G 1984 The multiple coagulopathies of biliary atresia. American Journal of Hematology 16: 171–180

7. Disorders of platelets. II Functional abnormalities

Roger M. Hardisty

Bleeding disorders may result from defects of many different aspects of platelet function, even when the platelet count is normal. Functional defects may also accompany thrombocytopenia and aggravate the severity of the bleeding tendency which results. The most clearly characterized are the inherited disorders, which usually present clinically in infancy or childhood. Despite their rarity, these conditions are important for the extensive information which their study has provided concerning the physiology of the haemostatic mechanism and the relative clinical significance of its component parts. Platelet function may also be disturbed in a wide range of acquired diseases involving patients of all ages, or by a variety of drugs, but in most of these instances the pathogenetic mechanisms involved are much less clearly defined.

HAEMOSTATIC FUNCTIONS OF PLATELETS

The characteristic clinical diagnostic features of a platelet disorder, whether quantitative or functional, are a long bleeding time and spontaneous purpuric lesions; these show that the platelets are essential not only for the arrest of haemorrhage after injury to small vessels, but also for the maintenance of integrity of apparently uninjured vessels. The platelets do indeed play a central role in both these aspects of the haemostatic process. Originating as anucleate fragments of megakaryocyte cytoplasm, enveloped by a highly organized unit membrane, they circulate in the form of smooth discs. When the endothelial lining of the vessel wall is breached, bringing platelets into contact with subendothelium or deeper layers of the vessel wall, they rapidly adhere to these tissues, spread over their surface, undergo morphological

changes with the formation of pseudopodia, and aggregate together to form a haemostatic plug. These processes, which begin within seconds of injury, involve: the interaction of platelet membrane components with adhesive proteins in the vessel wall and the plasma; the secretion from the platelet of many active principles which themselves contribute to aggregation, vasoconstriction and vessel wall repair; and the activation of blood coagulation on the platelet surface. Defects of any of these steps in platelet plug formation can lead to haemostatic failure, while, in certain circumstances, increased platelet reactivity may contribute to a thrombotic tendency.

Platelet ultrastructure

The ultrastructural features of the unstimulated

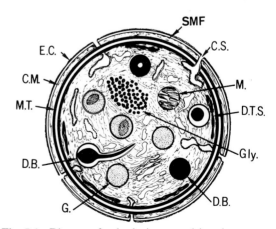

Fig. 7.1 Diagram of a platelet in equatorial section. EC = external coat; CM = cell surface membrane; SMF = submembranous microfilaments; MT = microtubules; DTS = dense tubular system; CS = surface-connected canalicular system; G = α-granule; DB = dense body; M = mitochondrion; Gly = glycogen granules. (Courtesy of Dr James G White)

167

Table 7.1 Platelet membrane glycoproteins

Glycoprotein	10^3 copies per platelet	Receptors	Alloantigens	Deficiency state
Ia	2–4	} Collagen	Br^a	
IIa	5–10			Single patient
		} Fibronectin, laminin		
Ic	3–6			
Ib } IX	25–30	vWF, thrombin, fibronectin?	Pl^{E1}, Ko^a	Bernard-Soulier syndrome
IIb } IIIa	40–50	{ Fibrinogen, vWF, fibronectin, vitronectin	Bak^a (Lek^a) } { Pl^{A1} (Zw^a) Pen^a }	Glanzmann's thrombasthenia
IV V		Collagen, thrombospondin Thrombin, C1$_q$	Nak^a	

discoid platelet are shown diagrammatically in Figure 7.1. The *plasma membrane* consists of a lipid bilayer, partially or completely penetrated by many glycoprotein (GP) molecules. These carry receptors for many different agonists and for adhesive proteins as well as specific alloantigenic sites, and are linked to elements of the platelet cytoskeleton. Several of them have been extensively characterized and have been shown to play key roles in the haemostatic process (Table 7.1), particularly as receptors for collagen, for adhesive proteins in the vessel wall, and for fibrinogen and von Willebrand factor, which are essential for the processes of aggregation and adhesion.

The most abundant glycoproteins are GPIIb and IIIa (Fig. 7.2), which form a heterodimer complex which carries receptors for fibrinogen, von Willebrand factor and fibronectin, and is therefore of crucial importance in haemostasis and thrombosis (see below). The GPIIb-IIIa complex (Phillips et al 1988) is a member of the superfamily of adhesion receptors known as *integrins* (Hynes 1987): these are heterodimers, present on many cell types, and consisting of an α subunit noncovalently linked to one of a restricted number of β subunits. They are transmembrane proteins, providing binding sites for adhesive proteins on their extracellular domains and attachment to cytoskeletal elements on their cytoplasmic domains. The platelet GPIa-IIa and Ic-IIa complexes are also integrins, providing binding sites for collagen and fibronectin respectively, and having identical

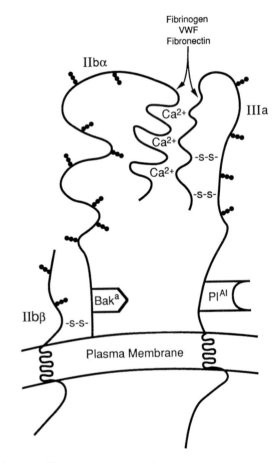

Fig. 7.2 The glycoprotein IIb-IIIa complex. The relative position of the Bak^a and Pl^{A1} alloantigens and approximate binding sites for adhesive proteins are shown.

structures to the VLA-2 and VLA-5 proteins of lymphocytes (Pischel et al 1988). Glycoprotein Ib (Wicki & Clemetson 1985; Fig. 7.3) carries receptors for von Willebrand factor and thrombin, and plays an essential part in platelet–vessel wall interaction (see below). It is closely associated in the membrane with GPIX and V, and its cytoplasmic domain is linked through actin-binding protein to actin, but this complex does not have the characteristic physicochemical features of an integrin.

Closely subjacent to the plasma membrane, in the equatorial plane, runs the circumferential band of *microtubules* which maintains the discoid shape of the resting platelet and disassembles on stimulation with aggregating agents. The *surface-connected canalicular system* (SCCS) consists of invaginations of the plasma membrane, through which granule contents are chiefly discharged during the secretory process, and the *dense tubular system* or

smooth endoplasmic reticulum is the chief site of thromboxane synthesis and of the sequestration and release of calcium ions for the control of intracellular calcium-dependent processes.

Other organelles within the platelet include mitochondria, glycogen granules, lysosomes, peroxisomes and two other specific types of storage organelle: the *dense osmiophilic granules* and *α-granules* (Table 7.2). The dense bodies contain the storage pool of adenine nucleotides and 5-hydroxytryptamine (5HT, serotonin), and the α-granules contain many different proteins; some of these (platelet factor 4, β-thromboglobulin, platelet-derived growth factor) are synthesized in the megakaryocyte and are specific to the platelet, while others, including coagulation proteins, are also found in other cell types and/or in the plasma. The contents of these granules are secreted by exocytosis in response to many stimuli, following the fusion of their membranes with the plasma

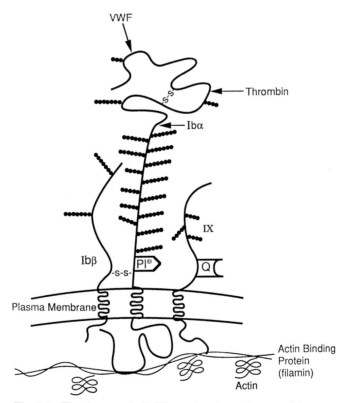

Fig. 7.3 The glycoprotein Ib-IX complex. Approximate positions are shown for von Willebrand factor and thrombin binding sites, and for the Pl^El alloantigen and the antigenic site (Q) for quinine/quinidine-dependent antibodies.

Table 7.2 Platelet storage organelles and their contents

Dense granules:	ATP, ADP
	5HT
	Ca^{2+}
α-granules	Platelet factor 4
	β-thromboglobulin
	Platelet-derived growth factor
	Von Willebrand factor
	Fibrinogen
	Factor V
	HMW kininogen
	Thrombospondin
	Fibronectin
	Plasminogen
	Plasminogen activator inhibitor I
	$α_2$-antiplasmin
	$α_2$-macroglobulin
	$α_1$-antitrypsin
	Histidine-rich glycoprotein
	Albumin

membrane. This process can be recognized by the appearance of specific granule contents in the plasma or by the identification of glycoproteins specific to the granule membranes on the outer surface of the platelet.

Haemostatic processes

Adhesion

The adhesion of platelets to subendothelium involves interactions between platelet membrane glycoproteins, elements of the vessel wall including collagen, and adhesive proteins including von Willebrand factor (vWF) and fibronectin. The relative importance of the various interactions involved varies with the conditions of flow (Turitto & Baumgartner 1979). Thus, at high shear rates, such as those that obtain in the microvasculature, the initial attachment of platelets to subendothelium is mediated chiefly through the binding of vWF (conformationally modified by its prior binding to the subendothelium; Bolhuis et al 1981) to glycoprotein Ib (Weiss et al 1974, Coller et al 1983). Under these conditions, however, vWF will also bind to GPIIb-IIIa, as also does the vWF secreted from the α-granules, and this interaction probably contributes to the subsequent spreading of the platelets on the subendothelial surface as well as to thrombus formation (Weiss et al 1986, Sakariassen et al 1986). At low shear rates similar to those on the venous side of the

circulation, GPIb and IIb-IIIa are still involved, but the role of vWF is less important, other adhesive proteins including fibronectin also being concerned in the adhesion reaction.

Aggregation

Adhesion to collagen, and many other stimuli, lead to a further series of reactions in the platelets, including a change of shape from discoid to spherical with the formation of many small pseudopodia, secretion of the contents of dense bodies and α-granules and the formation of aggregates. Aggregation in response to collagen is chiefly dependent on the secretion of active principles, including ADP and thromboxane A_2 from the platelets themselves, but aggregation in the absence of significant secretion can be studied in vitro in response to ADP and various other agonists. However induced, platelet aggregation is dependent on the binding of fibrinogen to specific receptors on the glycoprotein IIb-IIIa complex. These receptors are not available for fibrinogen binding on the surface of unstimulated platelets, but become expressed when the platelets are stimulated by an aggregating agent (Bennett & Vilaire 1979, Marguerie et al 1979). The nature of the signal transmitted from the receptor for the aggregating agent to GPIIb-IIIa is not known, but the binding of fibrinogen, unlike that of vWF to GPIb, is calcium-dependent, and involves at least two arg-gly-asp sequences on the Aα chain and a C-terminal peptide on the γ chain of fibrinogen. GPIIb-IIIa also binds arg-gly-asp sequences in vWF and fibronectin, but these adhesive proteins play no important physiological role in platelet aggregation, since fibrinogen is present at much higher molar concentration in plasma.

Secretion

Binding of many agonists to their receptors on the platelet membrane not only leads to expression of fibrinogen receptors, and so to aggregation, but sets in train a series of signal transduction mechanisms (Fig. 7.4). Agonist-receptor interaction leads via the activation of guanine nucleotide-binding proteins (G proteins) to the hydrolysis of phosphatidyl inositides in the platelet membrane by

PLATELET ACTIVATION

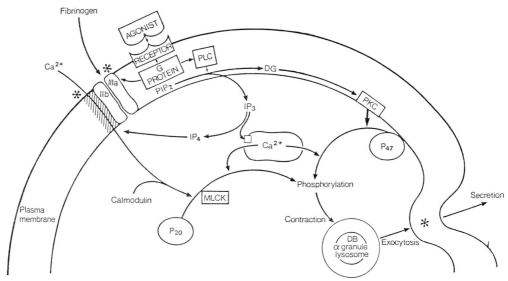

Fig. 7.4 Signal transduction mechanisms in the platelet. PIP_2 = phosphatidylinositol 4,5-bisphosphate; IP_3 = inositol 1, 4, 5-trisphosphate; IP_4 = inositol 1, 3, 4, 5-tetrakisphosphate; DG = diacylglycerol; PLC = phospholipase C; PKC = protein kinase C; MLCK = myosin light chain kinase; DB = dense body.

phospholipase C. The inositol trisphosphate thus produced promotes the mobilization of Ca^{2+} from its intracellular storage sites (chiefly the dense tubular system) and the influx of Ca^{2+} from the extracellular environment, while diacylglycerol activates protein kinase C (PKC). Amongst the intracellular reactions for which raised cytosolic Ca^{2+} is required, is the phosphorylation of myosin light chain (P20), while PKC brings about the phosphorylation of the 47 kD contractile protein (P47). The reactions together induce contraction and secretion, through which granule contents are secreted by a process of exocytosis. These processes are also regulated by cyclic AMP, the production of which by adenylate cyclase is also under the control of G proteins. Raised cAMP concentrations lower cytosolic free Ca^{2+} levels and inhibit aggregation and secretion. Meanwhile, arachidonic acid liberated from membrane phospholipids is converted to cyclic endoperoxides and thromboxane A_2 (Fig. 7.5), which themselves bind to specific receptors on secretion, and stimulate further activation of these pathways, as do ADP and 5HT secreted from the dense bodies.

Platelet procoagulant activity

Amongst the contents of platelet α-granules are several coagulation proteins – fibrinogen, factor V and high-molecular-weight kininogen – as well as a number of proteinase inhibitors; all of these may therefore reach high local concentrations when secreted from the platelets at sites of vascular injury. Probably the most important contribution of the platelets to blood coagulation, however, is in providing an active surface for the interaction of clotting factors. Much the most active phospholipid in this regard is phosphatidylserine. In the unstimulated platelet, most of this is situated in the inner leaflet of the membrane, but on stimulation by collagen and thrombin, a redistribution of the phospholipids in the bilayer occurs, resulting in translocation of phosphatidylserine to the outer leaflet (Bevers et al 1983). This greatly increases the ability of the platelets to enhance the activation of factor X and the conversion of prothrombin to thrombin, by providing binding sites for factors VIIIa-IXa and Va-Xa complexes respectively (Rosing et al 1985b). It is these activities of the platelets which were formerly loosely described as platelet factor 3.

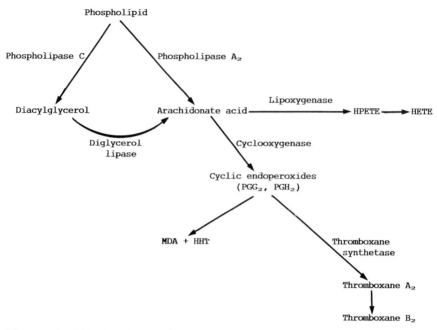

Fig. 7.5 Arachidonic acid metabolism in platelets. HPETE = 12-hydroperoxy-eicosatetraenoic acid; HETE = 12-hydroxy-eicosatetraenoic acid; MDA = malonyldialdehyde; HHT = 12-hydroxy-heptadecatrienoic acid.

Platelet function in the fetus and newborn infant

Prolonged bleeding from puncture wounds has been noted in fetuses at about 20 weeks' gestation (Bleyer et al 1971), and studies of the platelets of a small number of fetuses at about this stage of development have shown profoundly defective aggregation, relative to adult platelets, in response to adrenaline and collagen, and a lesser defect in response to ADP (Pandolfi et al 1972). Although healthy newborn infants have normal bleeding times (Feusner 1980) and do not suffer from a bleeding tendency, their platelets have been shown to be functionally defective compared with adult platelets in a number of respects. They aggregate less well in response to various agonists, including ADP, collagen and thrombin, but the aggregation defect is most marked in response to adrenaline (Mull & Hathaway 1970, Corby & Zuck 1976), apparently because newborn platelets lack α-adrenergic receptors (Corby & O'Barr 1981, Jones et al 1985). There is also evidence of impaired secretion of dense-body contents by newborn platelets, in response to various agonists (Whaun 1973), but no general agreement about

the reason for this. Corby & Zuck (1976) observed a minor decrease in both the metabolic and storage pools of adenine nucleotides, but no clear evidence of storage-pool deficiency, while Whaun (1980) found normal total nucleotides but concluded from their labelling pattern with ^{3}H-adenine that the storage pool was deficient. In view of the difficulty in obtaining clean cord blood samples, it is possible that some of these findings may have reflected in-vitro artefacts. Suarez et al (1988), however, found significantly raised plasma levels of the α-granule proteins platelet factor 4 and β-thromboglobulin in normal cord blood taken directly into a platelet inhibitory cocktail, suggesting that some degree of activation of the platelets had taken place in vivo.

Neonatal platelets appear to generate thromboxane A_2 and other arachidonic acid metabolites at least as effectively as do adult platelets (Stuart 1978, Stuart et al 1984, Kääpä et al 1984), and show enhanced release of arachidonate from membrane phospholipids on stimulation by thrombin (Stuart & Allen 1982). No significant differences from adult platelets have been observed in respect of platelet membrane glycoproteins or alloanti-

Table 7.3 Inherited disorders of platelet function

Defects of the platelet membrane
  Glanzmann's thrombasthenia
  Bernard-Soulier syndrome
  Platelet-type von Willebrand's disease
  Glycoprotein Ia deficiency
  Scott syndrome

Deficiency of storage organelles
  Dense-body deficiency
  Storage pool disease
  Hermansky-Pudlak syndrome
  Chediak-Higashi syndrome
  Wiskott-Aldrich syndrome
  Thrombocytopenia with absent radii
  α-granule deficiency
  Grey platelet syndrome
  Combined dense-body and α-granule deficiency

Defects of thromboxane generation
  Impaired liberation of arachidonic acid
  Cyclooxygenase deficiency
  Thromboxane synthetase deficiency

Defects of response to weak agonists
  Defective response to thromboxane A_2 and ionophores
  Defective response to adrenaline

Miscellaneous disorders of uncertain pathogenesis
  Giant platelet syndromes
  Montreal platelet syndrome
  May-Hegglin anomaly
  Epstein's syndrome, Fechtner syndrome, etc.
  Other disorders with normal platelet size

gens in fetuses at 18–26 weeks' gestation (Gruel et al 1986), and neonatal platelets have been found to have an essentially normal ultrastructure and an enhanced response to ristocetin (Ts'ao et al 1976).

Such functional differences as have been observed between newborn and adult platelets are evidently of little clinical significance, since they do not of themselves cause an enhanced tendency to bleed. They may, however, lead to an increased susceptibility to additional haemostatic stresses, such as the maternal ingestion of aspirin prior to delivery (Bleyer & Breckenridge 1970, Stuart et al 1982).

INHERITED DISORDERS OF PLATELET FUNCTION

These disorders are most conveniently classified (Table 7.3) according to the site and nature of the genetically determined defect:

1. abnormalities affecting plasma membrane glycoproteins or phospholipids, and resulting in impairment of adhesion, aggregation or procoagulant activity of the platelets
2. deficiency of specific intracellular organelles
3. defects of the mechanisms involved in secretion of granule contents.

A miscellaneous group of hereditary defects remains less well characterized with respect to their pathogenesis.

Plasma membrane disorders

Glanzmann's thrombasthenia

Glanzmann (1918) gave the first description of a hereditary disorder of platelet function, characterized by a long bleeding time and impaired clot retraction in the presence of a normal platelet count; he named it 'hereditary haemorrhagic thrombasthenia'. Nearly half a century later, the development of methods for measuring platelet aggregation led to the redefinition of Glanzmann's thrombasthenia (GT) as an autosomal recessive disorder of which the salient feature is a complete failure of the platelets to aggregate in response to ADP, collagen, thrombin or other agonists (Hardisty et all 1964, Caen et al 1966, Zucker et al 1966). Subsequent investigations have shown that this functional abnormality is due to a deficiency or molecular defect of the glycoprotein IIb-IIIa complex in the plasma membrane of the platelet (Nurden & Caen 1974, Phillips & Agin 1977, George et al 1984), resulting in a failure of the platelets to bind fibrinogen – an essential step in the aggregation process (Bennett & Vilaire 1979, Mustard et al 1979, Peerschke et al 1980).

Clinical features. Glanzmann's thrombasthenia is a rare disorder, with some 300 cases having been reported world-wide, although it may be more common in the Middle East. It cannot be distinguished on clinical grounds alone from other congenital platelet disorders or severe von Willebrand's disease. It commonly presents in infancy or early childhood with multiple bruises following minimal or unrecognized trauma, or with crops of petechiae or ecchymoses. Epistaxes are common, and may be difficult to control with local measures, and gingival haemorrhage is a frequent result of the shedding of deciduous teeth, or even tooth brushing. Large muscle haematomata and haemarthroses seldom occur, but menor-rhagia may present a serious hazard in pubertal girls. Serious accidental and surgical trauma will be life-threatening and will certainly call for intensive replacement therapy with platelet concentrates. In the absence of major trauma, the overall severity may appear to diminish as years of discretion are attained. Although the failure of platelet aggregation in vitro is always virtually complete, the clinical severity varies widely between patients and correlates poorly with the nature and degree of the molecular abnormality (George et al 1990).

Laboratory diagnosis. The essential diagnostic features are a normal platelet count and morphology and a greatly prolonged bleeding time, associated with a complete failure of platelet aggregation in response to ADP at any concentration. The aggregation defect is also seen in response to adrenaline, collagen, thrombin and, indeed, to all other aggregating agents which ultimately depend on fibrinogen binding to the platelet for their effect. These include arachidonic acid, thromboxane A_2 and its synthetic analogues, calcium ionophores and platelet activating factor (PAF-acether). Agglutination occurs normally, however, in response to ristocetin or bovine von Willebrand factor (vWF), which act through the binding of vWF to platelet glycoprotein Ib.

Having demonstrated the aggregation defect, the diagnosis can be confirmed – and in the case of unusual variants, extended – by measuring the amounts of GPIIb and IIIa in the platelet surface membrane. The methods available for this include one- and two-dimensional polyacrylamide gel electrophoresis, crossed immunoelectrophoresis using specific antibodies, and binding assays or flow cytometry with monoclonal antibodies to the constituent glycoproteins. The last of these has the advantage of being simply performed on very small volumes of whole blood (Montgomery et al 1983, Jennings et al 1986), making it particularly appropriate for prenatal diagnosis (see below) or for the investigation of small children. Fibrinogen binding can also be measured by flow cytometry on microlitre volumes of whole blood (Warkentin et al 1990), and this method can be useful for primary diagnosis of GT if insufficient blood can be obtained for platelet aggregation studies.

Clot retraction, platelet fibrinogen and platelet factor 3 availability are all defective in GT, but contribute no more to the diagnosis when the defective aggregation or fibrinogen binding has been demonstrated. Thrombasthenic platelets secrete their granule contents normally in response to strong agonists such as thrombin or high concentrations of collagen, but not in response to ADP or adrenaline, which depend on aggregation for their secretory effect.

Biochemical heterogeneity. Although, by definition, all patients with GT have a virtually complete failure of platelet aggregation, the underlying biochemical abnormality may vary from one kindred to another. Caen (1972) was the first to draw attention to a functional heterogeneity between cases, and proposed classifying GT into types I and II: type I patients, who were clinically more severely affected, had absent clot retraction and greatly reduced platelet fibrinogen, while in the rarer type II, clot retraction and platelet fibrinogen were only slightly diminished, though aggregation was equally defective. Since the discovery of the GPIIb-IIIa deficiency in typical severe (type I) GT, a variety of quantitative and qualitative abnormalities of the glycoprotein complex have been observed. Nurden et al (1985) found that two patients with type II GT by the old criteria had about 15% of the normal amount of GPIIb-IIIa on their platelets, while six out of seven type I patients had small residual amounts of GPIIb and/or IIIa, only one patient's platelets being completely deficient in both components. That such differences are genetically determined is strongly suggested by the observations of Coller et al (1987) on GT patients in Israel: they found that patients of Iraqi-Jewish origin had no demonstrable major GPIIIa band on immunoblots of their solubilized platelets, while Arab patients' platelets had clearly detectable amounts of this protein. Subsequent work (Newman et al 1990) has shown that the mutation in Arab patients resides in the GPIIb α-chain gene, and that in Iraqi-Jewish patients in the GPIIIa gene.

In addition to this heterogeneity amongst severely GPIIb-IIIa-deficient patients, a few cases have been reported in which the glycoproteins are present in normal or near-normal total amount, but are functionally defective. Ginsberg et al (1986) studied a patient from Guam with near-normal amounts of GPIIb-IIIa but greatly defective fibrinogen binding, which they presumed to be due to abnormal surface orientation of GPIIb. Nurden et al (1987) found that the quantitatively normal GPIIb-IIIa complex of their patient was abnormally sensitive to dissociation by EDTA and failed to bind fibrinogen; the patient described by Fournier et al (1989) appears to have a similar defect. The GPIIb-IIIa of the patient studied by Tanoue et al (1987) was normally dissociable but abnormally glycosylated. Jung et al (1988) found that their patient had 20% normal GPIIb, together with 35% of abnormal GPIIb of different molecular weight. It may be hoped that further study of the molecular defects in these patients' platelets will eventually lead to a coherent classification of the various forms of Glanzmann's thrombasthenia.

Molecular genetics. Both glycoproteins IIb and IIIa have now been cloned and their genes localized to the long arm of chromosome 17 (Bray et al 1987, Rosa et al 1988). Although human umbilical vein endothelial cells also synthesize GPIIb-IIIa (Newman et al 1986, Leeksma et al 1986), this is evidently under separate genetic control from that synthesized in the megakaryocyte, since endothelial cells from the umbilical cord of an infant with GT were found to express the complex normally (Giltay et al 1987). Russell et al (1988) found no major insertions or deletions of the GPIIb or IIIa genes of Israeli GT patients, and concluded that the condition must be due either to a small change in the nucleotide sequence of the coding region or a defect in the regulatory region of one or both genes. The subsequent work of Newman et al (1990) indicates small deletions in both Arab and Iraqi-Jewish patients, involving respectively 18 base pairs in the GPIIb α-chain gene, and 11 base pairs in the GPIIIa gene. Both these gene defects result in defective GPIIb-IIIa complex formation and thus in fibrinogen receptor deficiency. Study of GT patients from other ethnic groups may well reveal different molecular defects.

Detection of heterozygotes. Heterozygotes for GT usually have no significant bleeding symptoms, and no demonstrable defect of platelet aggregation. Characteristically, however, their platelets express about half the normal number of GPIIb-

IIIa complexes in the plasma membrane, and have a corresponding partial defect of fibrinogen binding. This provides a means of carrier detection, using a variety of methods for quantitative GPIIb-IIIa determination (Kunicki et al 1981, Stormorken et al 1982, Coller et al 1986, Jennings et al 1986) or fibrinogen binding (Warkentin et al 1990). Coller et al (1986) found good agreement between the results of monoclonal antibody binding, polyacrylamide gel electrophoresis and electroimmunoassay methods in a large series of obligatory carriers, who had about 60% of normal GPIIb-IIIa by all three methods.

Prenatal diagnosis. Now that the genes for GPIIb and IIIa have been localized to chromosome 17, it may be hoped that molecular probes will be constructed to allow the diagnosis of GT by chorionic villus sampling. For the present, however, prenatal diagnosis has to be carried out on fetal blood samples. Seligsohn et al (1985) measured GPIIb-IIIa in such samples by a monoclonal antibody binding assay, and Kaplan et al (1985) used the somewhat less direct method of Pl[A1] typing. These methods are applicable to families with the classical form of the disease, characterized by GPIIb-IIIa deficiency, and can even detect the heterozygous state in utero (Wautier et al 1987), but cannot be used for the prenatal diagnosis of GT variants with molecular defects of the GP complex. In such cases, prenatal diagnosis must rest on the demonstration of a defect of aggregation (Champeix et al 1988) or fibrinogen binding; micromethods for the latter (Warkentin et al 1990) are particularly appropriate.

The experience of Seligsohn et al (1988) shows that fetal sampling for the prenatal diagnosis of GT carries a high risk to the affected fetus of death from continuing haemorrhage. This underlines the importance of detailed counselling of the parents before the procedure is undertaken: it is clearly contraindicated if the parents wish the pregnancy to continue even if the fetus is affected.

Treatment. The only available curative treatment for GT is bone marrow transplantation, which has been successfully performed in one 4-year-old boy (Bellucci et al 1985). The risks of this procedure, however, are such as to confine its use to cases in which severe bleeding cannot be adequately controlled by more conservative measures. Gene therapy remains a more distant prospect in this, as in other, serious genetic disorders. Meanwhile, the management of GT consists of the avoidance of trauma and of drugs, such as aspirin, which may further interfere with platelet function, and the treatment of major bleeding episodes by platelet transfusion. Minor bleeding from accessible sites, such as deciduous tooth sockets, can usually be controlled by local measures, though epistaxis may continue despite packing, and require platelet transfusion in addition. The use of antifibrinolytic agents, such as tranexamic acid, may help to control bleeding after dental extractions, but has no other place in treatment. Good dental care is obviously essential if gum bleeding is to be minimized and tooth extraction avoided. Menorrhagia is likely to be a problem from the time of the first period, and may require hormonal therapy for its control: prepubertal counselling is important in this regard.

The chief limiting factor in the replacement therapy of GT is the risk of development of platelet antibodies. These may be directed against one or more of the platelet-specific alloantigens expressed on the GPIIb-IIIa complex (Pl[A1], Bak[a], Pen[a]) but probably arise more commonly against HLA determinants. For this reason, HLA-matched platelets, preferably from a single donor, should be used whenever possible.

Bernard–Soulier syndrome

Bernard & Soulier (1948) described a severe hereditary bleeding disorder characterized by a long bleeding time, moderate thrombocytopenia with giant and morphologically abnormal platelets, normal clot retraction but defective prothrombin consumption. Subsequent investigation of similar cases showed that their platelets aggregated normally with ADP, adrenaline and collagen (Howard et al 1973, Caen et al 1976) but were not agglutinated by bovine von Willebrand factor (Bithell et al 1972), or ristocetin (Howard et al 1973, Caen & Levy-Toledano 1973). In contrast to von Willebrand's disease, in which the defective response to ristocetin is due to deficiency of the plasma von Willebrand factor (vWF), in the Bernard-Soulier syndrome (BSS) it is the platelet membrane which is defective, lacking receptors for vWF.

Gröttum & Solum (1969) had previously postulated a membrane abnormality in BSS platelets, which they found to have a reduced sialic acid content, and this was confirmed by Nurden & Caen (1975), who demonstrated a specific deficiency of the sialic acid-rich glycoprotein I complex in the platelet membrane. This deficiency now appears to involve three closely associated membrane glycoproteins, designated GPIb, GPIX and GPV (Clemetson et al 1982, Berndt et al 1983b), the first two of which are associated as a heterodimer complex (Du et al 1987). This complex carries a receptor for vWF which is induced in vitro by ristocetin and which binds in vivo to vWF which has undergone a conformational change as a result of its prior binding to the vascular subendothelium (Sakariassen et al 1979). This platelet–vWF–subendothelium interaction is an essential step in the initial adhesion of platelets to damaged blood vessels, particularly at the shear rates which obtain in small arteries and capillaries, and it is the failure of this initial step in platelet plug formation which accounts for the bleeding tendency of the Bernard-Soulier syndrome (Weiss et al 1974, 1978).

The thrombocytopenia of BSS is chiefly due to a shortened platelet lifespan, which is probably an end result of the deficiency of the sialic-acid-rich glycoprotein. Other abnormalities which have been described include disordered phospholipid organization in the platelet membrane (Perret et al 1983), a failure of the platelets to bind and activate factor XI on stimulation by collagen (Walsh et al 1975), and a high basal prothrombinase activity in unstimulated platelets (Bevers et al 1986). The partial defect of thrombin binding and aggregation reported by Jamieson & Okumura (1978) suggested that the GPIb-IX complex carries a thrombin receptor, and this has subsequently been confirmed, and shown to be distinct from the vWF receptor (Takamatsu et al 1986, Yamamoto et al 1986). The binding site for quinine/quinidine drug-dependent antibodies has also been shown to be lacking on BSS platelets (Kunicki et al 1978); it has been localized within the membrane-associated region of the GPIb-IX complex (Berndt et al 1985), and more specifically to GPV (Stricker

& Shuman 1986). The Pl[E1] alloantigen is also lacking in BSS platelets, and has been localized to the α subunit of GPIb (Furihata et al 1988). The abnormally deformable membrane of BSS platelets (White et al 1984) is evidently also related to the GPIb-IX deficiency, since this complex plays an important part in linking the plasma membrane to the cytoskeleton of the platelet (Fox 1985).

Clinical features. The Bernard-Soulier syndrome is an extremely rare autosomal recessive disorder; only some 20–30 published cases meet the full diagnostic criteria. It is clinically indistinguishable from Glanzmann's thrombasthenia (see above) and, like it, usually presents early in life with multiple bruises and ecchymoses, and bleeding from mucous membranes and superficial grazes and cuts. Several children have died from uncontrollable bleeding, and the original patient of Bernard & Soulier, who presented with epistaxis and anal haemorrhage at the age of 15 days, had numerous bleeding episodes during his first 7 years, after which haemorrhage occurred less frequently and usually after injury; he died at the age of 28 from a cerebral haemorrhage following a bar-room brawl (Bernard 1983).

Laboratory diagnosis. The platelet count in BSS is usually only moderately reduced (commonly $50–100 \times 10^9/1$), but the bleeding time is very prolonged. The giant platelets may not be recognized as such by electronic cell counters, leading to spuriously low counts, but their presence in the blood film will suggest the diagnosis. It is difficult to prepare platelet-rich plasma for aggregation and other tests, since the large dense platelets tend to sediment with the red and white cells. The failure to agglutinate in response to ristocetin (even in the presence of normal plasma or vWF), together with the normal or even increased aggregation response to ADP, collagen and other agonists, and the demonstration of normal vWF in the patient's plasma, further establishes the diagnosis, which can be confirmed by demonstrating the deficiency of GPIb-IX complex in the platelet membrane. As for GPIIb-IIIa in thrombasthenia, this can be achieved by biochemical methods or by the use of specific monoclonal antibodies.

Molecular genetics. Of the three closely associated glycoproteins which are deficient in BSS, only the gene for the α subunit of GPIb has so far

been cloned; it is localized to the short arm of chromosome 17 (Wenger et al 1988, 1989). Nothing is yet known of the precise molecular defect(s) responsible for BSS; Drouin et al (1988), however, found residual amounts (10–47%) of GPIb, but an almost complete absence of GPIX, in the platelets of eight BSS patients from two unrelated families. Eight asymptomatic heterozygotes showed a double band pattern for GPIb and about half-normal levels of GPIb β chain and GPIX. The authors concluded that BSS was heterogeneous, and probably not due to gene deletions.

Detection of heterozygotes and prenatal diagnosis. George et al (1981) studied two families with BSS and found that the heterozygous parents, who were asymptomatic, had normal bleeding times, platelet counts and ristocetin-induced agglutination; three of them, however, had abnormally large platelets, with reduced GPIb and decreased sensitivity to a quinidine-dependent antibody. Quantitation of the GPIb-IX complex in small volumes of whole blood by means of monoclonal antibodies and flow cytometry provides the most suitable method for detecting heterozygotes and for antenatal diagnosis, but insufficient families have been studied to establish quantitative criteria. It is to be expected that prenatal blood sampling will carry a high risk to the affected fetus, as in the case of Glanzmann's thrombasthenia (see above).

Treatment. The general principles of treatment are the same as for Glanzmann's thrombasthenia: avoidance of injury and potentially harmful drugs, careful local haemostatic measures, platelet transfusions (preferably HLA-matched) for major bleeding episodes and hormonal control of menorrhagia if necessary. Treatment as for other thrombocytopenic conditions, such as steroids, intravenous immunoglobulin and splenectomy, are contraindicated, underlining the need for accurate diagnosis. Bone-marrow transplantation is a theoretical possibility for intractable cases, but has not yet been attempted in this condition.

Platelet-type von Willebrand's disease

An autosomal dominant bleeding disorder characterized by mild thrombocytopenia, a deficiency of the higher molecular weight forms of vWF in the plasma, and increased ristocetin-induced platelet agglutination, was described under this name by Miller & Castella (1982) and as 'pseudo-von Willebrand's disease' by Weiss et al (1982). The platelet vWF has a normal multimeric structure, and the essential abnormality appears to be an enhanced avidity of the platelet membrane — presumably GPIb-IX — for high-molecular-weight vWF multimers, which are selectively bound to the platelets from the plasma. Although this is in a sense the functional opposite of the Bernard-Soulier syndrome, no increase in GPIb-IX has been observed in the platelets of these patients. Takahashi et al (1984), however, studied four patients and found a structural abnormality of GPIb, which migrated as two distinct bands on polyacrylamide gel electrophoresis.

Most of the reported cases have had moderately prolonged bleeding times and a degree of thrombocytopenia, perhaps due to platelet aggregation in vivo, and some have had an increased platelet volume. Ristocetin-induced platelet agglutination is increased, and, indeed, the patient's platelets are agglutinated by the addition of normal plasma or vWF in the absence of ristocetin. The distinction from vWD type IIb depends on the demonstration of increased ristocetin-induced binding of normal vWF to the patient's platelets. Treatment with DDAVP is contraindicated in both these conditions, since the large vWF multimers released into the plasma are quickly bound to the platelets and aggravate their in-vivo aggregation. Platelet concentrates would seem to be the replacement therapy of choice in platelet-type von Willebrand's disease.

Glycoprotein Ia deficiency

Nieuwenhuis et al (1985) reported the case of a young woman who had suffered from easy bruising and menorrhagia since her teens, with a constantly prolonged bleeding time, whose platelets failed to respond by aggregation, secretion or thromboxane synthesis to collagen (though they responded normally to other agonists), or to adhere to purified type I or type III collagen or subendothelial microfibrils. They found that her platelet membranes were deficient in glycoprotein Ia, which is now known to form a heterodimer complex with GPIIa

(Pischel et al 1988), which complex carries a specific binding site for collagen. Although no similar abnormality could be found in the platelets of this patient's parents, sister or son, the defect seems likely to have been genetically determined.

Scott syndrome

Weiss et al (1979a) reported the case of a woman who had suffered from a moderately severe bleeding disorder since her teens, and whose only demonstrable abnormality was a defect of platelet procoagulant activity. The bleeding time was consistently normal, as were platelet aggregation and secretion. The abnormality appeared to consist of a failure to express binding sites for factors Va and Xa on the platelet membrane (Miletich et al 1979), as a result of a defect in the mechanism by which phosphatidyl serine becomes exposed on the outer leaflet of the membrane on activation of the platelets (Rosing et al 1985a). There was no family history, nor any detectable defect in the patient's parents' platelets, so that the hereditary nature of the defect remains in doubt. This patient remains unique, and her defect has been named after her. Her bleeding symptoms resembled those of a plasma coagulation disorder rather than a platelet defect, but surgical haemostasis was achieved by means of platelet transfusion.

Intracellular disorders

All the conditions considered under this heading (Table 7.3) result in a failure of secretion of granule contents on stimulation of the platelets. They may be divided into those in which the dense bodies and/or α-granules themselves are deficient or defective and those in which these storage organelles are normally present but the secretory mechanisms are at fault. The latter group comprises defects of thromboxane generation and of the other signal transduction mechanisms leading to secretion and aggregation. Disorders of platelet secretion may result from acquired diseases and drugs (see below), but the present account refers only to hereditable disorders. Most of these usually result in relatively mild bleeding states, less severe than the membrane disorders described above, and clinical presentation and diagnosis are therefore often delayed until later in childhood or even until adult life. Common presenting symptoms include easy bruising and somewhat prolonged bleeding from superficial cuts, epistaxes and menorrhagia. Apart from the risks of excessive haemorrhage following major surgical or accidental trauma, most patients are not seriously incommoded by their disorder.

Dense-body deficiency (storage pool deficiency)

Clinical associations. Deficiency of the dense osmiophilic granules, which normally contain the storage pool of adenine nucleotides and the serotonin (5-hydroxytryptamine, 5HT) of the platelets, has been observed in a number of families as an isolated defect, transmitted as an autosomal dominant trait (Weiss et al 1969, Maurer et al 1971, Ingerman et al 1978). In two such families, Weiss et al (1979b) found an associated partial deficiency of α-granules. Dense-body deficiency has also been demonstrated in association with other abnormalities of the platelets and other tissues in a number of hereditary bleeding disorders.

Hermansky-Pudlak syndrome. This is an autosomal recessive disorder characterized by the triad of tyrosinase-positive oculocutaneous albinism, a lifelong mild-to-moderate bleeding tendency and the presence of ceroid-like pigment in cells of the reticuloendothelial system (Hermansky & Pudlak 1959). The pigment was first observed in bone-marrow macrophages, but may also be deposited in the lungs and intestine – when it leads to pulmonary fibrosis and inflammatory bowel disease (Davies & Tuddenham, 1976, Garay et al 1979) – as well as in the buccal mucosa and urinary bladder. The bleeding tendency is primarily attributable to the deficiency of platelet dense bodies (White et al 1971, Hardisty et al 1972, Maurer et al 1972), though defects of phospholipase activation have also been observed (Rendu et al 1978, Weiss & Lages 1981). Heterozygotes are clinically unaffected, and their platelets have been found to contain normal amounts of adenine nucleotides and to aggregate normally. Gerritsen et al (1977), however, found that heterozygotes in a large Dutch family had platelet 5HT contents intermediate between homozygotes and normal controls.

Chediak-Higashi syndrome, an autosomal recessive disorder of lysosome formation in neutrophils and other cells, is more fully described in Chapter 5. Thrombocytopenia is common and is the chief cause of the bleeding tendency, but dense-body deficiency is also characteristic (Buchanan & Handin 1976, Boxer et al 1977, Rendu et al 1983, Apitz-Castro et al 1985). Like the neutrophils, the platelets also contain large abnormal granules (White 1978, Parmley et al 1979).

Wiskott-Aldrich syndrome. This X-borne recessive disorder is fully described in Chapter 11, and the thrombocytopenia, which is the chief cause of the bleeding tendency, is discussed in Chapter 6. It is mentioned here because the platelets have been shown to be structurally and functionally defective as well as deficient in number. They are smaller than normal (Murphy et al 1972, Ochs et al 1980) and deficient in dense bodies (Gröttum et al 1969) and have also been found to have defects of mitochondrial ATP synthesis (Akkerman et al 1982), and sometimes of membrane glycoproteins (Parkman et al 1981), though this is evidently not a constant feature (Pidard et al 1988).

Thrombocytopenia with absent radii (TAR syndrome). While the haemorrhagic tendency of this congenital disorder (Ch. 6) is fully explained by the thrombocytopenia, storage pool deficiency has also been observed (Day & Holmsen 1972).

Laboratory diagnosis. The bleeding time is usually moderately prolonged, and the aggregation pattern commonly reflects the defect of secretion, though it will not clearly distinguish dense-body deficiency from other secretory disorders. The typical features are normal primary aggregation in response to ADP and adrenaline, but without a second wave, and a marked defect of aggregation and ATP secretion in response to collagen. A normal response to arachidonic acid will serve to exclude a defect of thromboxane generation (Ingerman et al 1978, Minkes et al 1979). Nieuwenhuis et al (1987), however, found a typical aggregation pattern in only one-third of over 100 patients with storage pool deficiency (SPD), basing this diagnosis on a reduction of total platelet ADP and 5HT. These are indeed the hallmarks of SPD, together with the demonstration of the defect of secretion of these dense-body contents and of the dense-body deficiency by electron microscopy (White et al 1971, Witkop et al 1987) or by fluorescence microscopy of mepacrine-treated platelets (Rendu et al 1978). Israels et al (1990) also showed that SPD could be diagnosed in the absence of a demonstrable aggregation defect, on the basis of decreased ATP secretion and a diminished number of dense bodies.

Alpha-granule deficiency (Grey platelet syndrome)

Unlike dense-body deficiency, a pure deficiency of α-granules occurs in only a single hereditary disorder, described by Raccuglia (1971) as the grey platelet syndrome, from the appearance of the agranular platelets on a stained blood film. This extremely rare hereditary platelet disorder, which shows autosomal dominant heredity in some reported families (Kurstjens et al 1968, Libanska et al 1975), is sometimes surprisingly mild clinically, considering the profound nature of the structural and biochemical platelet defect. Epistaxes, menorrhagia and prolonged bleeding after serious injury are the commonest symptoms.

Diagnosis. The bleeding time is usually moderately prolonged, and unlike most other defects of platelet function, the first diagnostic clue comes from examination of the blood film, which reveals the characteristic grey agranular platelets. The platelet count is usually slightly below normal and the mean platelet volume increased. The α-granule deficiency can be confirmed by electron microscopy and by assay of the proteins normally contained in the α-granules; grey platelets have been shown to be profoundly deficient in β-thromboglobulin (βTG), platelet factor 4 (PF4), thrombospondin, platelet-derived growth factor (PDGF), fibrinogen, fibronectin, von Willebrand factor (vWF) and factor V (Gerrard et al 1980a, Levy-Toledano et al 1981, Nurden et al 1982, Berndt et al 1983a, Baruch et al 1987, Srivastava et al 1987). The defect is one of packaging within the organelles rather than of protein synthesis, as shown by normal or even slightly raised levels of βTG and PF4 in the plasma, and by the presence of fibrinogen and vWF in small granules within the platelets and megakaryocytes of patients with the grey platelet syndrome, which are thought to be precursors of α-granules in normal platelets (Cramer et al 1985). Grey platelets also contain normal amounts of an α-granule membrane protein, and redistribute it to the cell surface on thrombin stimulation (Rosa et al 1987). The defect in packaging of proteins evidently leads to their premature release from the megakaryocyte; the occurrence of myelofibrosis in some of these patients may result from leakage of PDGF and of PF4, which is an inhibitor of collagenase (Breton-Gorius et al 1981, Drouet et al 1981).

Other organelles – dense bodies, lysosomes and peroxisomes – are normally present in grey platelets (White 1979, Gerrard et al 1980a, Breton-Gorius et al 1981), but there is a partial defect of aggregation and dense-body secretion, particularly in response to thrombin and collagen. This appears to be due to a defect of phosphoinositide metabolism and cytosolic calcium transport (Rendu et al 1987, Srivastava et al 1987); its relation to the α-granule deficiency remains unexplained.

The grey platelet syndrome has not yet been diagnosed prenatally, but Wautier & Gruel (1989) were able to exclude the condition in the 19-week fetus of a woman with the grey platelet syndrome by demonstrating normal platelet βTG content and ultrastucture.

Defects of thromboxane generation

Aspirin ingestion is the commonest cause of defective thromboxane generation, and other drugs and even foods may have a similar effect. In a few cases, however, such abnormalities appear to have been congenital in origin, and some have shown a familial incidence. The characteristic laboratory features are an absence of the second wave of aggregation in response to ADP or adrenaline, and severe impairment of aggregation and dense-body secretion in response to collagen, despite evidence of normal platelet nucleotides and 5HT.

Impaired liberation of arachidonic acid

Rao et al (1984) studied three patients with a lifelong bleeding history, and the asymptomatic father of one of them; all had defective platelet aggregation in response to ADP, adrenaline and collagen, but a normal response to arachidonic acid and normal platelet ATP and ADP content. Liberation of ^{3}H-arachidonic acid from labelled platelet membrane phospholipids in response to thrombin was severely impaired, suggesting a deficiency or defect of activation of phospholipase A_2 or C. The possibility that such an abnormality might result from a defect of calcium mobilization appeared unlikely, since myosin light chain phosphory-lation, another calcium-dependent mechanism, occurred normally.

Impaired liberation of arachidonic acid has also been reported in several patients with storage pool deficiency (Rendu et al 1978, Minkes et al 1979, Weiss & Lages 1981), and in a patient with inherited thrombocytopenia and giant platelets (Greaves et al 1987).

Cyclooxygenase deficiency

It is to naturally-occurring deficiency of platelet cyclooxygenase that the term 'aspirin-like defect' ought properly to be confined. The distinction from the drug-induced defect may be somewhat easier to achieve in children than in adults, de-pending as it does on exclusion of drug ingestion and a lifelong history of bleeding symptoms. The best evidence that the defect is genetically deter-mined will be its demonstration in other family members; most of the reported cases have had negative family histories, but Horellou et al (1983) observed the defect in a mother and two of her children, suggesting autosomal dominant inherit-ance. This family was unusual in the severity of the bleeding symptoms, which included haemarthroses.

The characteristic laboratory findings, in addi-tion to those described above, are defective aggrega-tion and secretion in response to arachidonic acid, but a normal response to exogenous PGG_2, throm-boxane A_2 or their synthetic analogues (Malmsten et al 1975, Lagarde et al 1978, Pareti et al 1980). In some patients (Roth & Machuga 1982), normal levels of cyclooxygenase have been found by radio-immunoassay, suggesting a functional defect of the enzyme rather than an absolute deficiency.

Most patients with congenital cyclooxygenase deficiency suffer no more severe bleeding symp-toms than subjects on regular aspirin therapy. This may be because PGI_2 generation in vascular endothelial cells is also impaired, as shown by Pareti et al (1980) in their patient.

Thromboxane synthetase deficiency

Mestel et al (1980) and Defreyn et al (1981) have both described families in which a moderately severe lifelong bleeding tendency was shown to be due to a defect of thromboxane formation from arachidonic acid or from cyclic endoperoxides. The condition can be distinguished from cyclo-oxygenase deficiency by the failure of the platelets to aggregate in response to the cyclic endo-peroxides PGG_2 and PGH_2, or their synthetic analogues, as well as to arachidonic acid. The pa-tient of Mestel et al (1980) was a 3-year-old girl whose father and two siblings were similarly but less severely affected, suggesting an autosomal recessive mode of inheritance. In the family re-ported by Defreyn et al (1981), the degree of the defect appeared to be similar in a young woman and her father and daughter, making dominant inheritance more likely.

Defects of response to weak agonists

A miscellaneous group of lifelong bleeding ten-dencies have been found to be associated with defects of platelet secretion due neither to defi-ciency of organelles nor to defects of thromboxane synthesis. These defects are often observed only in response to 'weak' agonists, including ADP, adrena-line and low concentrations of collagen, which induce secretion only as a result of aggregation. Lages & Weiss (1988a) found that the initial rate of aggregation, as well as secretion, was impaired in eight such patients, and coined the designation 'weak agonist response defects' (WARD) for this heterogeneous group of disorders.

Defective response to thromboxane A_2 and ionophores

The weak agonist response defects include a number of patients whose platelets fail to respond to exogenous thromboxane A_2 or endoperoxide analogues, though they generate thromboxanes normally. These are themselves heterogeneous, as judged chiefly by the different responses of their platelets to calcium ionophores, suggesting vari-ous possible pathogenetic mechanisms: a throm-boxane receptor defect (Wu et al 1981), an ab-normality of intracellular calcium mobilization (Lages et al 1981), subsequently shown to be associated with a defect of phosphatidyl inositol metabolism (Lages & Weiss 1988b), or a defect of a calcium-dependent step in signal transduction (Hardisty et al 1983, Machin et al 1983).

The patient of Hardisty et al (1983) had the Silver-Russell form of dwarfism, but this condition has not otherwise been associated with a bleeding tendency. Easy bruising is, however, a common feature of the hereditary neuropsychiatric syndrome known as the attention deficit disorder (ADD), and Koike et al (1984) have found a defect of aggregation and secretion in 12 such patients in response to the ionophore A23187, showing that this condition falls into this general group of platelet disorders.

Defective response to adrenaline

The aggregatory response of normal platelets to adrenaline is notably variable (O'Brien 1964), and Scrutton et al (1981) and Gaxiola et al (1984) have shown that decreased responsiveness may be inherited without conferring any haemostatic failure. It can therefore be argued that tests of adrenaline-induced aggregation are best avoided in the investigation of bleeding disorders, or at least discounted in the absence of other demonstrable abnormalities. Stormorken et al (1983), however, reported a 16-year-old boy who had had frequent bleeding episodes since early childhood and whose platelets completely failed to aggregate in response to adrenaline. Like the haemostatically normal subjects studied by Scrutton et al (1981), his platelets had normal α_2-adrenergic receptors. The exact nature of the defect was not explained.

Management of intracellular platelet disorders

These disorders are usually of only mild or moderate clinical severity, and interfere little with everyday life. Excessive bleeding is likely to result from serious trauma, however, and may require replacement therapy as well as local haemostatic measures, though Mielke et al (1981) were able to reduce the bleeding time and surgical blood loss in a miscellaneous series of patients with platelet disorders by a short pre- and postoperative course of prednisone. Platelet transfusions have been used successfully in many such cases, but cryo-

precipitate (Gerritsen et al 1978) and DDAVP (Kobrinsky et al 1984, Schulman et al 1987) have, somewhat surprisingly, also been found to shorten the bleeding time and control surgical bleeding in patients with storage pool deficiency and other defects of secretion. Pfueller et al (1987) showed that DDAVP also shortened the bleeding time of a patient with the grey platelet syndrome, despite undetectable platelet vWF, suggesting that DDAVP does not exert its haemostatic effect in this group of disorders through stimulation of the secretion of platelet vWF; its mode of action remains to be explained.

Miscellaneous hereditary disorders

A number of other hereditary defects of platelet function have been described, whether as part of well-defined clinical syndromes or as isolated platelet abnormalities, which do not fall into any of the categories discussed above. Several of them are characterized by the presence of giant platelets, and therefore need to be distinguished from the Bernard-Soulier syndrome in particular.

Giant platelet syndromes

Montreal platelet syndrome. First described by Lacombe & d'Angelo (1963), this syndrome has subsequently been studied in detail by Milton & Frojmovic (1979) and Milton et al (1984). It is an autosomal dominant form of thrombocytopenia with giant platelets, normal ristocetin-induced agglutination as well as normal platelet aggregation responses to ADP and other agonists, but reduced sensitivity to thrombin, and an increased tendency to spontaneous aggregation. Glycoprotein Ib was normal in the platelets of two out of three patients examined, and no abnormality of platelet ultrastructure was found except for the presence of giant granules.

May-Hegglin anomaly (Ch. 6). This is an autosomal dominant trait comprising the presence of giant platelets and pseudo-Döhle bodies in the neutrophils. About one-third of patients have had some degree of thrombocytopenia, and an increase in giant platelet granules has been seen, but there is no significant disorder of platelet function (Hamilton et al, 1980). The condition is mentioned here only to distinguish it from other giant platelet syndromes.

Epstein's syndrome is an autosomal dominant trait in which mild thrombocytopenia with giant platelets is associated with Alport's syndrome of nephritis and nerve deafness. Minor defects of platelet function have been reported in most reported cases (Epstein et al 1972, Bernheim et al 1976, Clare et al 1979), but the bleeding tendency is probably chiefly attributable to the thrombocytopenia. A variant of this condition has been described under the name of *Fechtner syndrome* (Peterson et al 1985): eight out of 17 members of four generations of a family had various combinations of nephritis, deafness, congenital cataracts, giant platelets and leucocyte inclusions. The inclusions resembled those of the May-Hegglin anomaly on stained blood films, but could be distinguished from them by electron microscopy. Apart from a partial defect of thromboxane synthesis from arachidonic acid, no significant abnormality of platelet function was observed.

Other examples of familial thrombocytopenia with giant platelets, with or without demonstrable defects of platelet function, have been described by various authors (see also Chapter 6). Greaves et al (1987) studied a family in which congenital thrombocytopenia was dominantly inherited and associated with gross abnormalities of platelet ultrastructure, impaired arachidonic acid mobilization from membrane phospholipids and defective aggregation in response to ADP, adrenaline and collagen. Several affected members of this family had required transfusion for serious bleeding episodes during childhood. Stewart et al (1987) reported the case of a 13-year-old girl in whom thrombocytopenia and giant platelets were associated with stomatocytosis and pseudo-homozygous type II hypercholesterolaemia; platelet adhesion was reported to be slightly reduced, but aggregation was normal.

Other disorders with normal platelet size

Dowton et al (1985) described a large family of which 22 members suffered from an autosomal dominant bleeding disorder of moderate severity, usually presenting during their first decade, with mild-to-moderate thrombocytopenia, a long bleed-

ing time and normal platelet survival. Several of the affected members had defective aggregation in response to ADP, adrenaline and collagen. One patient also had congenital neuroblastoma, successfully treated but followed at the age of 7 by acute monocytic leukaemia, and five other family members, four of whom had the bleeding tendency, developed haematological neoplasms between the ages of 10 and 62.

Biochemical and/or functional abnormalities of the platelets have been described in Down's syndrome (Lott et al 1972, McCoy & Snedden 1984), adenosine deaminase deficiency (Ch. 11) and idiopathic scoliosis (Yarom et al 1980), but none of these conditions are associated with abnormal bleeding. Various platelet abnormalities have been reported in hereditary disorders of connective tissue, including Ehlers-Danlos and Marfan's syndromes and osteogenesis imperfecta, but the bleeding tendency in these conditions is more likely to result from the abnormality of the connective tissue itself. In Ehlers-Danlos syndrome, for example, skin collagen has been shown to be defective in aggregating normal platelets (Karaca et al 1972), and the aggregation defect in one family could be corrected by purified fibronectin (Furcht et al 1979). It is notable that the bleeding tendency is most severe in type IV Ehlers-Danlos syndrome, in which type III collagen, the most potent in activating the platelets, is deficient (Pope et al 1975).

Defective platelet aggregation has also been described in Bartter's syndrome (Stoff et al 1980), but is unassociated with a long bleeding time or a bleeding tendency, and is due to a plasma factor, the probable consequence of the metabolic disturbance (Solomon et al 1982).

The diagnostic approach to inherited platelet disorders

A lifelong history of 'easy bruising', prolonged bleeding after superficial injuries, or even apparently spontaneous bleeding from mucosal surfaces or into the skin, suggests the diagnosis either of a hereditary platelet disorder or of von Willebrand's disease. In the investigation of such a patient, the first clues to a more specific diagnosis may come from the family history or the association of the bleeding symptoms with other clinical features

Table 7.4 Diagnosis of inherited disorders of platelet function

Disorder	Inheritance	Platelet count	Platelet size	Platelet aggregation				Confirmatory findings	Associated abnormalities
				ADP	Collagen	Arachidonate	Ristocetin		
Glanzmann's thrombasthenia	Autosomal recessive	N	N	O	O	O	(1)★	GPIIb-IIIa deficiency	
Bernard-Soulier syndrome	Autosomal recessive	↓	↑	N	N	N	O	GPIb-IX deficiency	
Glycoprotein Ia deficiency		N	N	N	O	N		GPIa deficiency	
Idiopathic storage pool deficiency	Autosomal dominant	N	N or ↓	(1)★	↓	N	(1)★	Dense-body deficiency	
Hermansky-Pudlak syndrome	Autosomal recessive	N	N	(1)★	↓	N		Deficiency & failure of secretion of ATP, ADP, 5HT	Tyrosinase-positive albinism Pigmented macrophages in marrow
Wiskott-Aldrich syndrome	X-borne recessive	↓	↓	(1)★	↓				Eczema Recurrent infections
Chediak-Higashi syndrome	Autosomal recessive	N or ↓	N	(1)★	↓				Partial albinism Recurrent bacterial infections Abnormal neutrophil granules
Grey platelet syndrome	Autosomal dominant	↓	↑	N	N or ↓	N	N	α-granule deficiency	Myelofibrosis
Cyclo-oxygenase deficiency Thromboxane synthetase deficiency	?	N	N	(1)★	O	O	N	Defective TXB$_2$ synthesis	

★(1) = first-phase aggregation only

typical of particular conditions (Table 7.4); the Bernard-Soulier and grey platelet syndromes may first reveal themselves by the abnormal platelet morphology on the stained blood film, but a long bleeding time is the characteristic hallmark of this whole group of disorders. The combination of a long bleeding time with a normal (or perhaps moderately reduced) platelet count will indicate the need for platelet function tests, as may a strongly suggestive clinical history even in the presence of a normal bleeding time. Von Willebrand's disease can be excluded by appropriate investigations (see Ch. 13), and most of the recognized platelet abnormalities can be provisionally identified in the first instance by means of tests of aggregation and secretion in response to ADP, collagen, arachidonic acid and ristocetin, supplemented where necessary by determination of platelet size (Table 7.4).

These tests of aggregation should, however, be regarded as screening rather than as final diagnostic procedures; normal aggregation patterns are seen, for example, in a proportion of cases of storage pool deficiency (p. 179).

Confirmation of the diagnosis of thrombasthenia, the Bernard-Soulier syndrome or other membrane glycoprotein disorders requires biochemical tests for the glycoproteins or binding assays with specific monoclonal antibodies. Defects of aggregation in response to collagen and/or arachidonate call for a distinction to be made between deficiency of storage organelles, defective thromboxane synthesis and failure of response to thromboxane A$_2$. The relevant tests for dense-body deficiency are uptake and secretion of 5HT, content and secretion of adenine nucleotides and enumeration of dense bodies by fluorescence microscopy of

Table 7.5   Causes of acquired platelet dysfunction in childhood

Renal failure

Myeloproliferative disorders and myelodysplasia

Liver disease

Chronic hypoglycaemia
  Glycogen storage disease type I
  Fructose 1,6-diphosphatase deficiency

Acquired storage pool deficiency
  Autoimmune disease
  Disseminated intravascular coagulation
  Haemolytic uraemic syndrome, thrombotic
    thrombocytopenic purpura
  Severe burns
  Cardiopulmonary bypass, extracorporeal circulations
  Valvular heart disease

Antibodies against platelet membrane glycoproteins

Drugs (Table 7.6)

mepacrine-treated platelets or by electron microscopy; α-granule deficiency is identified by electron microscopy and by assay of β-thromboglobulin, PF4 or other α-granule constituents (Table 7.2). The final analysis of other secretory defects may require measurement of thromboxane B_2 production in response to collagen, arachidonate and endoperoxide analogues, and of phosphatidylinositol hydrolysis and Ca^{2+} mobilization in response to various stimuli.

ACQUIRED DISORDERS OF PLATELET FUNCTION

Abnormalities of platelet function occur in a wide range of conditions, often in association with other haemostatic defects including both thrombocytopenia and disorders of blood coagulation, so that it may be difficult to assess the relative importance of several observed abnormalities in the pathogenesis of the bleeding tendency. In most of these disorders, the nature of the platelet abnormality is much less clear cut than in the genetic disorders of platelet function, and a predominantly clinical rather than a pathogenetic classification is appropriate (Table 7.5). Many drugs may also interfere with platelet function, and these are listed in Table 7.6.

Enhanced platelet activity has been recorded in a number of conditions characterized by a thrombotic tendency. Although it is by no means always clear whether the observed changes in platelet behaviour are of primary pathogenetic significance, or merely secondary to other prothrombotic influences, a list of such conditions which may occur in childhood is given in Table 7.7, and some of them will be briefly discussed.

Conditions associated with defective platelet function

Renal failure

Coagulation defects and thrombocytopenia may both occur in patients in renal failure, but defective platelet function is evidently the chief cause of abnormal bleeding. This commonly presents as purpura, epistaxis or bleeding from the gums, though serious internal haemorrhage may also occur, and renal biopsy or surgical procedures present a special hazard. The pathogenesis of bleeding in renal failure, and its clinical management, have been reviewed by Remuzzi (1988). The bleeding time is typically prolonged, and abnormalities have been reported in a variety of platelet function tests, including adhesion to glass (Salzman & Neri 1966) and subendothelium (Castillo et al 1986), aggregation (Castaldi et al 1966, di Minno et al 1985) and platelet factor 3 activation (Horowitz et al 1967). These abnormalities can be at least partially corrected by haemodialysis or peritoneal dialysis (Stewart & Castaldi 1967, Remuzzi et al 1978a), but no general agreement has been reached on the identity of the dialysable component responsible for these effects on the platelets: urea (Eknoyan et al 1969), guanidinosuccinic acid (Horowitz et al 1970), phenolic acids (Rabiner & Molinas 1970) and uraemic middle molecules (Bazilinski et al 1985) have all been incriminated. Remuzzi and his colleagues (1978b, 1982, 1983) have described various defects of arachidonate metabolism in uraemic patients, leading to impaired generation of both thromboxane A_2 and prostacyclin, but Deckmyn et al (1983) observed increased prostacyclin production in children in chronic renal failure. Remuzzi et al (1981) have also shown that parathyroid hormone inhibits platelet aggregation and secretion in vitro, and suggested that the raised concentrations found in uraemic plasma might contribute towards the bleeding tendency in this way. Docci et al (1986), however, found no correlation between secondary hyperparathyroidism and bleeding in uraemic patients.

Apart from dialysis, uraemic bleeding has been treated successfully with cryoprecipitate (Janson et al 1980) and DDAVP (Mannucci et al 1983). The most effective therapeutic measure, however, is correction of the haematocrit, whether by red-cell transfusions (Livio et al 1982, Fernandez et al 1985) or by administration of human recombinant erythropoietin (Moia et al 1987, van Geet et al 1989). The beneficial effect on haemostasis of correcting the anaemia in uraemic patients remains to be fully explained: the mechanical effect of red cells in influencing flow conditions so as to promote interaction of platelets with the vessel wall (Turitto & Baumgartner 1975) is probably part of the explanation. Conjugated oestrogens have also been shown to correct the bleeding time of uraemic patients (Liu et al 1984, Livio et al 1986); the effect lasts for several days, though again the mechanism is not understood.

Myeloproliferative disorders and myelodysplasia

Both haemorrhagic symptoms and arterial thromboses are common in adults with this group of disorders, and both may occur in the same patient. The commonest bleeding symptoms are large superficial ecchymoses, epistaxes and haemorrhage from the gastrointestinal tract; thrombosis usually involves either the cerebral arteries or the peripheral arteries of the limbs. The platelet defects which have been described are not specifically associated with any one of the adult myeloproliferative disorders; similar defects have been observed in essential thrombocythaemia, polycythaemia vera, chronic granulocytic leukaemia and myelofibrosis. All these conditions are very rare in childhood, particularly the first two, but may also be associated with functional platelet disorders when they do occur in this age group. Bleeding in the juvenile form of chronic myeloid leukaemia (CML) typically results from thrombocytopenia, however, which is a usual presenting feature. Structural platelet abnormalities are commonly seen in the myeloproliferative disorders, and amongst the disturbances of platelet function which have been described are: defects of

aggregation, particularly in response to adrenaline (Schafer 1984); storage pool deficiency (Gerrard et al 1978, Rendu et al 1979, Russell et al 1981, Malpass et al 1984); defects of arachidonate metabolism (Okuma & Uchino 1979; Jubelirer et al 1980, Schafer 1982) and of platelet coagulant activities (Walsh et al 1977, Semeraro et al 1979); resistance to the action of the anti-aggregatory prostaglandin D_2 (Cooper et al 1978); and various abnormalities of the membrane glycoproteins (Clezardin et al 1985).

Michelson (1987) studied four children with juvenile (Ph[1]-negative) CML and two with Ph[1]-positive adult CML, all of whom (in contrast to age-matched controls and adults with Ph[1]-positive CML) showed two subpopulations of platelets, positive and negative respectively for both glycoproteins Ib and IIb-IIIa. Berndt et al (1988) described the case of a 9-year-old girl with a myelodysplastic syndrome characterized by monosomy 7, thrombocytopenia and giant platelets, who had had a bleeding tendency since the age of 5. She was also found to have two populations of platelets, the majority being large and deficient in the glycoprotein Ib-IX complex, as in the Bernard-Soulier syndrome, and the minority normal.

Some of the platelet abnormalities which have been observed would be expected to lead to abnormal bleeding and others to predispose to thrombotic episodes, but in practice the laboratory findings have usually been found to correlate poorly with the clinical course of the disease. When thrombocythaemia occurs in childhood, there is seldom any need for specific management of bleeding or thrombosis as such, and the treatment is that of the underlying disorder. Restoration of the platelet count to normal will usually correct any haemostatic abnormality which may exist.

Acute leukaemias and preleukaemic states

Bleeding in the acute leukaemias is usually the result of thrombocytopenia, but platelet dysfunction may also contribute, particularly in the myeloid leukaemias. Defects of aggregation and secretion have been described by several authors, and attributed variously to storage pool deficiency and defects of secretory mechanisms (Cowan et al 1975), impaired thromboxane production (Woodcock et al 1984), and a deficiency of thrombin binding sites on the platelet membrane (Ganguly et al 1978). Fäldt et al (1987) showed that myeloid leukaemia cells of various FAB types, like HL60 cells, but not normal polymorphs, secreted a low molecular weight inhibitor of platelet aggregation on incubation in vitro.

Bleeding in patients with preleukaemic states, including those with normal platelet counts, has also been attributed to defective platelet aggregation (Russell et al 1979, Stuart & Lewis 1982).

Liver disease

The haemostatic failure of liver disease results chiefly from defective synthesis of clotting factors, but low-grade intravascular coagulation and increased fibrinolysis may also occur. Defective platelet aggregation may be another contributory factor; the early suggestion (Thomas, 1972) that this might be due to the presence of FDP has not withstood critical examination (Solum et al 1973, Ballard & Marcus 1976), but acquired storage pool deficiency (see below) remains a likely mechanism. Defects of thromboxane synthesis (Laffi et al 1986) and membrane glycoproteins (Ordinas et al 1978) have also been reported. Although patients with liver disease usually have normal or raised levels of vWF, DDAVP has been found to shorten the prolonged bleeding time (Mannucci et al 1986), as well as improving the results of coagulation tests (Agnelli et al 1983).

Chronic hypoglycaemia

Patients with glycogen storage disease type I (glucose 6-phosphatase deficiency) and fructose 1,6-diphosphatase deficiency typically suffer from a mild bleeding tendency and have long bleeding times. The defect of platelet aggregation and adenine nucleotide secretion, to which the haemostatic failure appears to be due (Czapek et al 1973, Corby et al 1974), can be corrected by intravenous glucose administration; it appears that the chronic hypoglycaemia of these conditions leads to a failure of nucleotide synthesis within the platelets, affecting both the storage and the metabolic pool (Hutton et al 1976).

Acquired storage-pool deficiency

Many different stimuli can induce the secretion from platelets of their dense-body and α-granule contents, and if this occurs on a large scale in the circulation it may result in haemostatic failure due to the functional inadequacy of the depleted platelets, possibly combined with local thrombus formation at the site of platelet damage. A variety of conditions in which the platelets are subjected to either immune-mediated or mechanical damage (Table 7.4) may lead to abnormal bleeding and/or thrombosis in this way. The term 'acquired storage pool deficiency' derives from the original observations of depleted granule contents (Zahavi & Marder 1974, Khurana et al 1980, Hourdille et al 1981) or raised concentrations of platelet-specific proteins in the plasma (Harker et al 1980), but these methods are likely to be superseded by the detection of activated platelets by means of specific monoclonal antibodies (George et al 1986, Abrams et al 1990). Many of these disorders are likely also to result in thrombocytopenia, but the functional may precede the quantitative platelet defect. The activation of platelets during cardiopulmonary bypass can be largely prevented by infusion of prostacyclin (Longmore et al 1979, Malpass et al 1981), with correction of the bleeding time.

Antibodies against membrane glycoproteins

Many patients with immune thrombocytopenic purpura (ITP) have autoantibodies directed against determinants on GPIIb-IIIa or GPIb (Ch. 6). In a number of instances, such antibodies have been detected in patients with acquired bleeding disorders and long bleeding times, but normal platelet counts, resulting in functional defects resembling those of Glanzmann's thrombasthenia (Greaves et al 1983, Niessner et al 1986, Balduini et al 1987) and Bernard-Soulier syndrome (Stricker et al 1985) respectively. Vermylen & Blockmans (1989) reported a similar case in which the autoantibody was directed against GPIa and resulted in a specific failure of the platelets to aggregate in response to collagen. Of this group of five patients, one had Hodgkin's disease, one an unspecified lymphoproliferative disease and one myasthenia gravis and a thymoma; the other two had had chronic ITP, but the antibody-induced functional defect persisted after recovery of the platelet count. The patients of Stricker et al (1985) and Vermylen & Blockmans (1989) responded to repeated plasma exchange, and steroid therapy had a more lasting beneficial effect in two of the cases, but none in a third.

Platelet dysfunction due to drugs (Table 7.6)

Apart from the deliberate use of platelet inhibitory drugs as antithrombotic agents, bleeding may occasionally result from interference with platelet function as a side-effect of drugs used for other purposes. The following account is confined to this latter group.

Non-steroidal anti-inflammatory drugs. Aspirin ingestion is the commonest cause of platelet dysfunction, and may occasionally precipitate gastrointestinal or other haemorrhage, particularly in susceptible individuals. It should be forbidden in patients with known bleeding disorders. Aspirin inhibits the formation of cyclic endoperoxides and thromboxane A_2 by irreversible acetylation of cyclooxygenase (Vane 1971, Roth et al 1975); this results in a moderate prolongation of the bleeding time, absence of the second wave of aggregation with ADP and a failure of aggregation and secretion in response to collagen and arachidonic acid. These effects last throughout the lifespan of the platelet – hence the importance of ensuring abstention from aspirin for at least 10 days before platelet function testing

Table 7.6 Drugs that may cause bleeding through interference with platelet function

Acetylsalicylic acid

Other non-steroidal anti-inflammatory drugs
    Indomethacin
    Phenylbutazone
    Sulphinpyrazone

Antibiotics
    Penicillins
    Cephalosporins

Dextrans
Heparin
Sodium valproate
Intravascular radiographic contrast agents

for diagnostic purposes. Other non-steroidal anti-inflammatory drugs, including indomethacin, phenylbutazone and sulphinpyrazone, have a similar but less prolonged effect.

Antibiotics. Many of the β-lactam antibiotics, particularly the penicillins, are capable of causing a bleeding tendency by interfering with platelet function. This side-effect, which may persist for up to 12 days after withdrawal of the drug (Brown et al 1974), is seen only with high dosage regimes; patients in renal failure are at particular risk, since high drug concentrations resulting from impaired clearance may coexist with other haemostatic defects, and thrombocytopenic bleeding in patients on chemotherapy for malignant disease may be exacerbated by penicillin-induced platelet dysfunction (Fass et al 1987). Both penicillins and cephalosporins have been shown to inhibit platelet adhesion, aggregation and secretion in vitro, probably by coating the platelet surface and interfering with the binding of agonists to their receptors (Cazenave et al 1977, Shattil et al 1980).

Dextrans. Dextrans, particularly those of high molecular weight, have complex effects on the haemostatic mechanism. These include prolongation of the bleeding time and defects of platelet aggregation and secretion (Weiss 1967). The effects, which are dose-related, reach a maximum 4–8 hours after the end of the infusion, and Evans & Gordon (1974) have suggested that they may be due to refractoriness of the platelets following transient aggregation by the dextran itself.

Heparin. Heparins have been found to inhibit platelet function in certain experimental systems, possibly by inducing a refractory state following partial activation (Zucker 1977), and these effects might theoretically contribute towards the bleeding tendency of heparin overdosage. Heparin fractions of low molecular weight and high antithrombin affinity are the least likely to interfere with platelet function (Salzman et al 1980).

Other drugs. Amongst drugs used in paediatric practice which have occasionally been found to cause bleeding symptoms through an effect on platelet function are the anticonvulsant sodium valproate (Richardson et al 1976, Monnet et al 1979) and intravascular radiographic contrast media (Parvez et al 1984, Verdirame et al 1984).

Sodium valproate may also cause thrombocytopenia and minor coagulation abnormalities. Various other classes of drugs, including antihistamines, phenothiazines, tricyclic antidepressants, frusemide, daunorubicin, and both local and general anaesthetics, have been shown to inhibit platelet function in vitro, but do not significantly impair haemostasis at pharmacological doses. It is possible, however, that they may aggravate the bleeding tendency of patients with pre-existing haemostatic defects. Corby & Schulman (1971) found that the platelets of newborn infants were more susceptible than those of their mothers to the effects of promethazine and aspirin taken before delivery.

Blue fluorescent light, as used in the phototherapy of neonatal hyperbilirubinaemia, has been shown to damage platelets in vitro, depleting them of adenine nucleotides and glycogen (Mauer et al 1976), and a fall in platelet count has sometimes been observed during such treatment.

While foodstuffs do not inhibit platelet function to the extent of causing a bleeding tendency, they may do so sufficiently to interfere with the results of laboratory tests. Onions, garlic, ginger and the chinese black tree fungus, Mo-er, have all been incriminated, and should probably be avoided before diagnostic platelet function tests are performed.

Conditions associated with increased platelet activity (Table 7.7)

Diabetes mellitus

Diabetes mellitus is well known to be associated with vascular disease and thrombotic events at all ages, manifested by retinopathy, peripheral neuropathy, renal vascular disease, and an increased risk of cerebral and myocardial infarction. While raised levels of coagulation factors have

Table 7.7 Conditions associated with increased platelet activity

Diabetes mellitus
Nephrotic syndrome
Kawasaki's disease
Hyperlipoproteinaemia
Homocystinuria
Renal allograft rejection

been observed, as well as decreased fibrinolysis, the chief pathogenetic mechanism appears to concern platelet reactivity. Amongst the abnormalities which have been described are 'spontaneous' aggregation in vivo and in vitro, increased responsiveness to aggregating agents, and increased in vivo secretion of α-granule proteins (Kwaan et al 1972, Colwell et al 1976, Preston et al 1978). These are probably largely attributable to the increased production of thromboxane A_2 in platelets of diabetics, combined with reduced synthesis of prostacyclin by endothelial cells (Butkus et al 1980, Gerrard et al 1980b, Haluschka et al 1981). An increased sensitivity of the platelet thromboxane receptor has also been reported in patients with diabetic retinopathy (Collier et al 1986).

The platelet abnormalities appear early in the course of the disease, even in childhood diabetes (Kobbah et al 1985), sometimes pre-dating symptoms, and are not fully corrected by glycaemic control (Jackson et al 1984, Collier et al 1987). They have also been seen in infants born to mothers with inadequately controlled diabetes (Stuart et al 1979, 1985); such infants are known to have an increased incidence of thrombosis (Oppenheimer & Esterly 1965).

Nephrotic syndrome

Thrombosis is a common and serious complication of the nephrotic syndrome in childhood, as in later life, and platelet hyperaggregability appears to be an important factor in its pathogenesis (Bang et al 1973). The platelets' hyper-responsiveness to arachidonic acid, in terms of both aggregation and thromboxane production, is proportional to the degree of depletion of serum albumin and can be reversed by the addition of albumin in vitro or in vivo. This suggests that the hypoalbuminaemia is largely responsible for the functional platelet abnormality, probably as a result of decreased binding of arachidonic acid, which thus becomes available in excess for thromboxane synthesis (Yoshida & Aoki 1978, Remuzzi et al 1979, Jackson et al 1982). Bennett & Cameron (1987) found that ristocetin-induced agglutination was also increased in nephrotic patients, and was not correlated with hyper-responsiveness to arachidonate or with serum albumin. It was correlated, however, with the raised plasma vWF concentrations which are also found in these patients. While the correction of the thrombotic tendency must rely chiefly on the management of the renal disorder and the consequent correction of the plasma protein changes, the use of low-dose aspirin as an inhibitor of the excessive thromboxane production would also seem appropriate.

Kawasaki's disease

In this acute febrile vasculitis of infants and young children (Kawasaki et al 1974), involvement of the coronary arteries occurs in some 20% of cases, and coronary aneurysm formation and thrombosis are important causes of sudden death. Burns et al (1984) observed raised factor VIII and fibrinogen concentrations and raised platelet counts during the first 3 weeks of the illness, together with depletion of fibrinolytic activity; however, raised plasma β-thromboglobulin levels were observed only in children who developed aneurysms, suggesting increased in-vivo platelet activation specifically in this group. Yamada et al (1978) found heightened in-vitro aggregability of the platelets for as long as 9 months after the onset of the disease, which could be suppressed by aspirin treatment, and Hidaka et al (1983) showed increased thromboxane generation from arachidonate in vitro.

Aspirin probably has a place in the treatment of Kawasaki's disease, for its antiplatelet as well as its anti-inflammatory effects, but high-dose intravenous gamma globulin appears to offer the best means of reducing the incidence of coronary arterial disease (Newburger et al 1986).

Hyperlipoproteinaemia

Hyperlipidaemia is well known to predispose to atherosclerosis and thrombotic disease, but the relationship between plasma lipids and platelet function remains a matter for debate. Tremoli et al (1984) studied a large group of patients with type II hyperlipoproteinaemia aged from 11 years upwards, and found enhanced sensitivity of their platelets to aggregation by ADP, adrenaline and collagen, and increased production of thromboxane B_2 from endogenous arachidonic acid on stimulation with collagen. These abnormalities were not correlated with plasma cholesterol levels, but may have resulted from an increased cholesterol: phospholipid ratio in the platelet membrane.

Homocystinuria

The commonest cause of homocystinuria, cystathionine-B-synthase deficiency, is associated with a high incidence of thromboembolic disease, which is a major cause of death, sometimes even in the first decade of life. The most likely explanation of this is endothelial cell injury induced by the homocystine in plasma, leading to platelet-mediated intimal proliferation, as in the genesis of other atherosclerotic lesions (Harker et al 1974, 1976). There is no clear evidence for a primary effect of the plasma homocystine on platelet function, though both homocystine and homocysteine have been shown to increase thromboxane production in vitro (Graeber et al 1982). The use of dipyridamole and aspirin has been recommended as platelet inhibitors in this condition, and this would seem appropriate whether the primary injury is inflicted on the platelets themselves or the vascular endothelium.

REFERENCES

Abrams C S, Ellison N, Budzynski A Z, Shattil S J 1990 Direct detection of activated platelets and platelet-derived microparticles in humans. Blood 75: 128–138

Agnelli G, Berrettini M, De Cunto M, Nenci G G 1983 Desmopressin-induced improvement of abnormal coagulation in chronic liver disease. Lancet i: 645(letter)

Akkerman J W N, Van Brederode W, Gorter G, Zegers B J M, Kuis W 1982 The Wiskott-Aldrich syndrome: studies on a possible defect in mitochondrial ATP resynthesis in platelets. British Journal of Haematology 51: 561–568

Apitz-Castro R, Cruz M R, Ledezma E et al 1985 The storage pool deficiency in platelets from humans with the Chediak-Higashi syndrome: study of six patients. British Journal of Haematology 59: 471–483

Balduini C L, Grignani G, Sinigaglia F et al 1987 Severe platelet dysfunction in a patient with autoantibodies against membrane glycoproteins IIb-IIIa. Haemostasis 17: 98–104

Ballard H S, Marcus A J 1976 Platelet aggregation in portal cirrhosis. Archives of Internal Medicine 136: 316–319

Bang N U, Trygstad C W, Schroeder J E, Heindenreich R O, Csiscko B M 1973 Enhanced platelet function in glomerular renal disease. Journal of Laboratory and

Clinical Medicine 81: 651–655

Baruch D, Lindhout T, Dupuy E, Caen J P 1987 Thrombin-induced platelet factor Va formation in patients with a gray platelet syndrome. Thrombosis and Haemostasis 58: 768–771

Bazilinski N, Shaykh M, Dunea G et al 1985 Inhibition of platelet function by uremic middle molecules. Nephron 40: 423–428

Bellucci S, Devergie A, Gluckman E et al 1985 Complete correction of Glanzmann's thrombasthenia by allogeneic bone-marrow transplantation. British Journal of Haematology 59: 635–641

Bennett A, Cameron J S 1987 Platelet hyperaggregability in the nephrotic syndrome which is not dependent on arachidonic acid metabolism or on plasma albumin concentration. Clinical Nephrology 27: 182–188

Bennett S, Vilaire G 1979 Exposure of platelet fibrinogen receptors by ADP and epinephrine. Journal of Clinical Investigation 64: 1393–1401

Bernard J 1983 History of congenital hemorrhagic thrombocytopathic dystrophy. Blood Cells 9: 179–193

Bernard J, Soulier J P 1948 Sur une nouvelle variété de dystrophie thrombocytaire hémorrhagipare congenitale. Semaine des Hôpitaux, Paris 24: 3217–3223

Berndt M C, Castaldi P A, Gordon S, Halley H, MacPherson V J 1983a Morphological and biochemical confirmation of gray platelet syndrome in two siblings. Australian and New Zealand Journal of Medicine 13: 387–390

Berndt M C, Gregory C, Chong B H, Zola H, Castaldi P A 1983b Additional glycoprotein defects in Bernard-Soulier's syndrome: confirmation of genetic basis by parental analysis. Blood 62: 800–807

Berndt M C, Chong B H, Bull H A, Zola H, Castaldi P A 1985 Molecular characterization of quinine/quinidine drug-dependent antibody platelet interaction using monoclonal antibodies. Blood 66: 1292–1301

Berndt M C, Kabral A, Grimsley P, Watson N, Robertson T I, Bradstock K F 1988 An acquired Bernard-Soulier-like platelet defect associated with juvenile myelodysplastic syndrome. British Journal of Haematology 68: 97–101

Bernheim J, Dechavanne M, Bryon P A et al 1976 Thrombocytopenia, macrothrombocytopathia, nephritis and deafness. American Journal of Medicine 61: 145–150

Bevers E M, Comfurius P, Zwaal R F A 1983 Changes in membrane phospholipid distribution during platelet activation. Biochimica Biophysica Acta 736: 57–66

Bevers E M, Comfurius P, Nieuwenhuis H K et al 1986 Platelet prothrombin converting activity in hereditary disorders of platelet function. British Journal of Haematology 63: 335–345

Bithell T C, Parekh S J, Strong R R 1972 Platelet function in the Bernard-Soulier syndrome. Annals of the New York Academy of Sciences 201: 145–160

Bleyer W A, Breckenridge R T 1970 Studies on the detection of adverse drug reactions in the newborn. II The effects of prenatal aspirin on newborn hemostasis. Journal of the American Medical Association 213: 2049–2053

Bleyer W A, Hakami N, Shepard T H 1971 The development of hemostasis in the human fetus and newborn infant. Journal of Pediatrics 79: 838–853

Bolhuis P A, Sakariassen K S, Sander H J, Bouma B N, Sixma J J 1981 Binding of factor VIII-von Willebrand factor to human arterial subendothelium precedes increased platelet adherence and enhances platelet spreading. Journal of Laboratory and Clinical Medicine

97: 568–576

Boxer G J, Holmsen H, Robkin L, Bang N U, Boxer L A, Baehner R L 1977 Abnormal platelet function in Chediak-Higashi syndrome. British Journal of Haematology 35: 521–533

Bray P F, Rosa J P, Johnson G I et al 1987 Platelet glycoprotein IIb. Chromosomal localization and tissue expression. Journal of Clinical Investigation 80: 1812–1817

Breton-Gorius J, Vainchenker W, Nurden A, Levy-Toledano S, Caen J 1981 Defective α-granule production in megakaryocytes from gray platelet syndrome. Ultrastructural studies of bone marrow cells and megakaryocytes growing in culture from blood precursors. American Journal of Pathology 102: 10–19

Brown C H, Natelson E A, Bradshaw M W, Williams T W, Alfrey C P 1974 The hemostatic defect produced by carbenicillin. New England Journal of Medicine 291: 265–270

Buchanan G R, Handin R I 1976 Platelet function in the Chediak-Higashi Syndrome. Blood 47: 941–948

Burns J C, Glode M P, Clarke S H, Wiggins J, Hathaway W E 1984 Coagulopathy and platelet activation in Kawasaki syndrome: identification of patients at high risk for development of coronary artery aneurysms. Journal of Pediatrics 105: 206–211

Butkus A, Skrinska V A, Schumacher O P 1980 Thromboxane production and platelet aggregation in diabetic subjects with clinical complications. Thrombosis Research 19: 211–223

Caen J 1972 Glanzmann thrombasthenia. Clinics in Hematology 1: 383–392

Caen J P, Levy-Toledano S 1973 Interaction between platelets and von Willebrand factor provides a new scheme for primary haemostasis. Nature New Biology 244: 159–160

Caen J P, Castaldi P A, Leclerc J C et al 1966 Congenital bleeding disorders with long bleeding time and normal platelet count. I. Glanzmann's thrombasthenia (report of 15 patients). American Journal of Medicine 41: 4–26

Caen J P, Nurden A T, Jeanneau C et al 1976 Bernard-Soulier syndrome – a new platelet glycoprotein abnormality. Its relationship with platelet adhesion to subendothelium and with the factor VIII von Willebrand protein. Journal of Laboratory and Clinical Medicine 87: 586–596

Castaldi P A, Rozenberg M C, Stewart J H 1966 The bleeding disorder of uraemia. Lancet 2: 66–69

Castillo R, Lozano T, Escolar G, Revert L, Lopez J, Ordinas A 1986 Defective platelet adhesion on vessel subendothelium in uremic patients. Blood 68: 337–342

Cazenave J P, Guccione M A, Packham M A, Mustard J F 1977 Effects of cephalothin and penicillin G on platelet function in vitro. British Journal of Haematology 35: 135–152

Champeix P, Forestier F, Daffos F, Kaplan C 1988 Prenatal diagnosis of a molecular variant of Glanzmann's thrombasthenia. Current Studies in Hematology and Blood Transfusion 55: 180–183

Clare N M, Montiel M M, Lifshitz M D, Bannayan G A 1979 Alport's syndrome associated with macrothrombopathic thrombocytopenia. American Journal of Clinical Pathology 72: 111–117

Clemetson K J, McGregor J L, James E, Dechavanne M, Lüscher E F 1982 Characterization of the platelet membrane glycoprotein abnormalities in Bernard-Soulier syndrome and comparison with normal by surface-labelling techniques and high-resolution two-dimensional gel electrophoresis. Journal of Clinical Investigation 70: 304–311

Clezardin P, McGregor J L, Dechavanne M, Clemetson K J 1985 Platelet membrane glycoprotein abnormalities in patients with myeloproliferative disorders and secondary thrombocytosis. British Journal of Haematology 60: 331–344

Coller B S, Seligsohn U, Little P A 1987 Type I Glanzmann thrombasthenia patients from the Iraqi-Jewish and Arab populations in Israel can be differentiated by platelet glycoprotein IIIa immunoblot analysis. Blood 69: 1696–1703

Coller B S, Peerschke E I, Scudder L E, Sullivan C A 1983 Studies with a murine monoclonal antibody that abolishes ristocetin-induced binding of von Willebrand factor to platelets: additional evidence in support of GPIb as a platelet receptor for von Willebrand factor. Blood 61: 99–110

Coller B S, Seligsohn U, Zivelin A, Zwang E, Lusky A, Modan M 1986 Immunologic and biochemical characterization of homozygous and heterozygous Glanzmann thrombasthenia in the Iraqi-Jewish and Arab populations of Israel: comparison of techniques for carrier detection. British Journal of Haematology 62: 723–735

Collier A, Tymkewycz, Matthews D M, Jones R L, Clarke B F 1987 Changes in some aspects of platelet function with improvement of glycaemic control over 6 months. Diabetes Research 5: 79–82

Collier A, Tymkewycz P, Armstrong R, Young R J, Jones R L, Clarke B F 1986 Increased platelet thromboxane receptor sensitivity in diabetic patients with proliferative retinopathy. Diabetologia 29: 471–474

Colwell J A, Halushka P V, Sarji K, Levine J, Sagel J, Nair R M G 1976 Altered platelet function in diabetes mellitus. Diabetes 25: 826–831

Cooper B, Schafer A I, Puchalsky D, Handin R I 1978 Platelet resistance to prostaglandin D2 in patients with myeloproliferative disorders. Blood 52: 618–626

Corby D G, Schulman I 1971 The effects of antenatal drug administration on aggregation of platelets of newborn infants. Journal of Pediatrics 79: 307–313

Corby G, Zuck T F 1976 Newborn platelet dysfunction: a storage pool and release defect. Thrombosis and Haemostasis 36: 200–207

Corby D G, O'Barr T P 1981 Decreased α-adrenergic receptors in newborn platelets: cause of abnormal response to epinephrine. Developmental Pharmacology and Therapeutics 2: 215–225

Corby D G, Putnam C W, Greene H L 1974 Impaired platelet function in glucose-6-phoshatase deficiency. Journal of Pediatrics 85: 71–76

Cowan D H, Graham R C, Baunach 1975 The platelet defect in leukemia, platelet ultrastructure, adhesive nucleotide metabolism and the release reaction. Journal of Clinical Investigation 56: 188–200

Cramer E M, Vainchenker W, Vinci G, Guichard J, Breton-Gorius J 1985 Gray platelet syndrome: immunoelectron microscopic localization of fibrinogen and von Willebrand factor in platelets and megakaryocytes. Blood 66: 1309–1316

Czapek E E, Deykin D, Salzman E W 1973 Platelet dysfunction in glycogen storage disease type I. Blood 41: 235–247

Davies B, Tuddenham E G D 1976 Familial pulmonary fibrosis associated with oculocutaneous albinism and platelet function defect. Quarterly Journal of Medicine 45: 219–232

Day H J, Holmsen H 1972 Platelet adenine nucleotide 'storage pool deficiency' in thrombocytopenic absent radii syndrome. Journal of the American Medical Association 221: 1053–1054

Deckmyn H, Proesmans W, Vermylen J 1983 Prostacyclin production by whole blood from children: impairment in the hemolytic uremic syndrome and excessive formation in chronic renal failure. Thrombosis Research 30: 13–18

Defreyn G, Machin S J, Carreras L O, Dauden M V, Chamone D A F, Vermylen J 1981 Familial bleeding tendency with partial platelet thromboxane synthetase deficiency: variation of cyclic endoperoxide metabolism. British Journal of Haematology 49: 29–41

Di Minno G, Martinez J, McKean M R et al 1985 Platelet dysfunction in uremia. Multifaceted defect partially corrected by dialysis. American Journal of Medicine 79: 552–559

Docci D, Turci F, Delvecchio C et al 1986 Lack of evidence for the role of secondary hyperparathyroidism in the pathogenesis of uremic thrombocytopathy. Nephron 43: 28–32

Dowton S B, Beardsley D, Jamison D, Blattner S, Li F P 1985 Studies of a familial platelet disorder. Blood 65: 557–563

Drouet L, Praloran V, Cywiner-Golenzer C et al 1981 Déficit congénital en α-granules plaquettaires et fibrose réticulinique médullaire. Hypothèse physiopathogénique. Nouvelle Revue Française d'Hématologie 23: 95–100

Drouin J, McGregor J L, Parmentier S, Izaguirre C A, Clemetson K J 1988 Residual amounts of glycoprotein Ib concomitant with near-absence of glycoprotein IX in platelets of Bernard-Soulier patients. Blood 72: 1086–1088

Du X, Beutler L, Ruan C, Castaldi P A, Berndt M C 1987 Glycoprotein Ib and glycoprotein IX are fully complexed in the intact platelet membrane. Blood 69: 1524–1527

Eknoyan G, Wacksman S J, Glueck H I, Will J J 1969 Platelet function in renal failure. New England Journal of Medicine 280: 677–681

Epstein C J, Sahud M A, Piel C F et al 1972 Hereditary macrothrombocytopathia, nephritis and deafness. American Journal of Medicine 52: 299–310

Evans R J, Gordon J L 1974 Mechanisms of the antithrombotic action of dextran. New England Journal of Medicine 290: 748 (letter)

Fäldt R, Ankerst J, Zoukas E 1987 Inhibition of platelet aggregation by myeloid leukaemic cells demonstrated in vitro. British Journal of Haematology 66: 529–534

Fass R J, Copelan E A, Brandt J T, Moeschberger M L, Ashton J J 1987 Platelet-mediated bleeding caused by broad-spectrum penicillins. Journal of Infectious Diseases 155: 1242–1248

Fernandez F, Goudable C, Sie P et al 1985 Low haematocrit and prolonged bleeding time in uraemic patients: effect of red cell transfusions. British Journal of Haematology 59: 139–148

Feusner J H 1980 Normal and abnormal bleeding times in neonates and young children utilizing a fully standardized template technique. American Journal of Pathology 74: 73–77

Fournier D J, Kabral A, Castaldi P A, Berndt M C 1989 A

variant of Glanzmann's thrombasthenia characterized by abnormal glycoprotein IIb/IIIa complex formation. Thrombosis and Haemostasis 62: 977–983

Fox J E B 1985 Linkage of a membrane skeleton to integral membrane glycoproteins in human platelets. Identification of one of the glycoproteins as GPIb. Journal of Clinical Investigation 76: 1673–1683

Furcht L T, Wendelschafer-Crabb G, Mosher D F, Arneson M, Hammerschmidt D, Woodbridge P 1979 The role of fibronectin in normal platelet aggregation and demonstration of an inherited disease with defective platelet aggregation correctable with normal fibronectin. Journal of Cell Biology 83: 61a

Furihata K, Hunter J, Aster R H, Koewing G R, Shulman N R, Kunicki T J 1988 Human anti-P1E1 antibody recognises epitopes associated with the alpha subunit of platelet glycoprotein Ib. British Journal of Haematology 68: 103–110

Ganguly P, Sutherland S B, Bradford H R 1978 Defective binding of thrombin to platelets in myeloid leukaemia. British Journal of Haematology 39: 599–605

Garay S M, Gardella J E, Fazzini E P, Goldring R M 1979 Hermansky-Pudlak syndrome: pulmonary manifestations of a ceroid storage disorder. American Journal of Medicine 66: 737–747

Gaxiola B, Friedl W, Propping P 1984 Epinephrine-induced platelet aggregation. A twin study. Clinical Genetics 26: 543–548

George J N, Nurden A T, Phillips D R 1984 Molecular defects in interactions of platelets with the vessel wall. New England Journal of Medicine 311: 1084–1098

George J N, Caen J P, Nurden A T 1990 Glanzmann's thrombasthenia: the spectrum of clinical disease. Blood 75: 1383–1395

George J N, Reimann T A, Moake J L et al 1981 Bernard-Soulier disease: a study of four patients and their parents. British Journal of Haematology 48: 459–467

George J N, Pickett E B, Saucerman S et al 1986 Platelet surface glycoproteins. Studies on resting and activated platelets and platelet membrane microparticles in normal subjects and observations in patients during adult respiratory distress syndrome and cardiac surgery. Journal of Clinical Investigation 78: 340–348

Gerrard J M, Stoddard S F, Shapiro R S et al 1978 Platelet storage pool deficiency and prostaglandin synthesis in chronic granulocytic leukaemia. British Journal of Haematology 40: 597–607

Gerrard J M, Philips D R, Rao G H R et al 1980a Biochemical studies of two patients with the gray platelet syndrome. Selective deficiency of platelet alpha granules. Journal of Clinical Investigation 66: 102–109

Gerrard J M, Stuart M J, Rao G H R et al 1980b Alterations in the balance of prostaglandin and thromboxane synthesis in diabetes. Journal of Laboratory and Clinical Medicine 95: 950–958

Gerritsen S W, Akkerman J W N, Sixma J J 1978 Correction of the bleeding time in patients wih storage pool deficiency by infusion of cryoprecipitate. British Journal of Haematology 40: 153–160

Gerritsen S M, Akkerman J W N, Nijmeijer B, Sixma J J, Witkop C J, White J 1977 The Hermansky-Pudlak syndrome: evidence for a lowered 5-hydroxytryptamine content in platelets of heterozygotes. Scandinavian Journal of Haematology 18: 249–256

Giltay J C, Leeksma O C, Breederveld C, Van Mourik J A

1987 Normal synthesis and expression of endothelial IIb/IIIa in Glanzmann's thrombasthenia. Blood 69: 809–812

Ginsberg M H, Lightsey A, Kunicki T J, Kaufmann G, Marguerie G, Plow E F 1986 Divalent cation regulation of the surface orientation of platelet membrane glycoprotein IIb. Correlation with fibrinogen binding function and definition of a novel variant of Glanzmann's thrombasthenia. Journal of Clinical Investigation 78: 1103–1111

Glanzmann E 1918 Hereditäre hämorrhagische Thrombasthenie. Ein Beitrag zur Pathologie der Blutplättchen. Jahrbuch der Kinderheilkunde 88: 1–42

Graeber J E, Slott J H, Ulane R E, Schulman J D, Stuart M J 1982 Effect of homocysteine and homocystine on platelet and vascular arachidonic acid metabolism. Pediatric Research 16: 490–493

Greaves M, Pickering C, Porter N R, Magee J M, Preston F E 1983 Acquired Glanzmann's thrombasthenia. Blood 61: 209 (letter)

Greaves M, Pickering C, Martin J, Cartwright I, Preston F E 1987 A new familial 'giant platelet syndrome' with structural, metabolic and functional abnormalities of platelets due to a primary megakaryocyte defect. British Journal of Haematology 65: 429–435

Gröttum K A, Solum N O 1969 Congenital thrombocytopenia with giant platelets: a defect in the platelet membrane. British Journal of Haematology 16: 277–290

Gröttum K A, Hovig T, Holmsen H, Abrahamsen A F, Jeremic M, Seip M 1969 Wiskott-Aldrich syndrome: quantitative platelet defects and short platelet survival. British Journal of Haematology 17: 373–388

Gruel Y, Boizard B, Daffos F, Forestier F, Caen J, Wautier J L 1986 Determination of platelet antigens and glycoproteins in the human fetus. Blood 68: 488–492

Haluschka P V, Mayfield R, Wohltmann H J et al 1981 Increased platelet arachidonic acid metabolism in diabetes mellitus. Diabetes 30 (suppl. 2): 44–48

Hamilton R W, Shaikh B S, Ottie J N, Storch A E, Saleem A, White J G 1980 Platelet function, ultrastucture and survival in the May-Hegglin anomaly. American Journal of Clinical Pathology 74: 663–668

Hardisty R M, Dormandy K M, Hutton R A 1964 Thrombasthenia: studies on three cases. British Journal of Haematology 10: 371–387

Hardisty R M, Mills D C B, Ketsa-Ard K 1972 The platelet defect associated with albinism. British Journal of Haematology 23: 679–692

Hardisty R M, Machin S J, Nokes T J C, Rink T J, Smith S W 1983 A new congenital defect of platelet secretion: impaired responsiveness of the platelets to cytoplasmic free calcium. British Journal of Haematology 53: 543–557

Harker L A, Slichter S J, Scott C R, Ross R 1974 Homocystinemia. Vascular injury and arterial thrombosis. New England Journal of Medicine 291: 537–543

Harker L A, Ross R, Slichter S J, Scott C R 1976 Homocystine-induced arteriosclerosis. The role of endothelial cell injury and platelet response in its genesis. Journal of Clinical Investigation 58: 731–741

Harker L A, Malpass T W, Branson H E, Hessel E A II, Slichter S J 1980 Mechanism of abnormal bleeding in patients undergoing cardiopulmonary bypass: acquired transient platelet dysfunction associated with selective α-granule release. Blood 56: 824–834

Hermansky F, Pudlak P 1959 Albinism associated with

hemorrhagic diathesis and unusual pigmented reticular cells in the bone marrow: report of two cases with histochemical studies. Blood 14: 162–169

Hidaka T, Nakano M, Ueta T, Komatsu Y, Yamamoto M 1983 Increased synthesis of thromboxane A_2 by platelets from patients with Kawasaki disease. Journal of Pediatrics 102: 94–96

Horellou M H, Lecompte T, Lecrubier C et al 1983 Familial and constitutional bleeding disorder due to platelet cyclo-oxygenase deficiency. American Journal of Hematology 14: 1–9

Horowitz H I, Cohen B D, Martinez P, Papayoanou M F 1967 Defective ADP-induced platelet factor 3 activation in uremia. Blood 30: 331–340

Horowitz H I, Stein I M, Cohen B D, White J G 1970 Further studies on the platelet inhibitory effect of guanidinosuccinic acid: its role in uremic bleeding. American Journal of Medicine 49: 336–345

Hourdillé P, Bernard P, Belloc F, Pradet A, Sanchez R, Boisseau M R 1981 Platelet abnormalities in thermal injury. Study of platelet-dense bodies stained with mepacrine. Haemostasis 10: 141–152

Howard M A, Hutton R A, Hardisty R M 1973 Hereditary giant platelet syndrome: a disorder of a new aspect of platelet function. British Medical Journal 2: 586–588

Hutton R A, Macnab A J, Rivers R P A 1976 Defect of platelet function associated with chronic hypoglycaemia. Archives of Disease in Childhood 51: 49–55

Hynes R O 1987 Integrins: a family of cell surface receptors. Cell 48: 549–554

Ingerman C M, Smith J B, Shapiro S, Sedar A, Silver M J 1978 Hereditary abnormality of platelet aggregation attributable to nucleotide storage pool deficiency. Blood 52: 332–344

Israels S J, McNicol A, Robertson C, Gerrard J M 1990 Platelet storage pool deficiency: diagnosis in patients with prolonged bleeding times and normal platelet aggregation. British Journal of Haematology 75: 118–121

Jackson C A, Greaves M, Patterson A D, Brown C B, Preston F E 1982 Relationship between platelet aggregation, thromboxane synthesis and albumin concentration in nephrotic syndrome. British Journal of Haematology 52: 69–77

Jackson C A, Greaves M, Boulton A J M, Ward J D, Preston F E 1984 Near-normal glycaemic control does not correct abnormal platelet reactivity in diabetes mellitus. Clinical Science 67: 551–555

Jamieson G A, Okumura T 1978 Reduced thrombin binding and aggregation in Bernard- Soulier platelets. Journal of Clinical Investigation 61: 861–864

Janson P A, Jubelirer S J, Weinstein M J, Deykin D 1980 Treatment of the bleeding tendency in uremia with cryoprecipitate. New England Journal of Medicine 303:1318–1322

Jennings L K, Ashmun R A, Wang W C, Dockter M E 1986 Analysis of human platelet glycoproteins IIb-IIIa in Glanzmann's thrombasthenia whole blood by flow cytometry. Blood 68: 173–179

Jones C R, McCabe R, Hamilton C A, Reid J L 1985 Maternal and fetal platelet responses and adrenoceptor binding characteristics. Thrombosis and Haemostasis 53: 95–98

Jubelirer S J, Russell F, Vaillancourt R, Deykin D 1980 Platelet arachidonic acid metabolism and platelet function in ten patients with chronic myelogenous leukemia. Blood

56: 728–731

Jung S M, Yoshida N, Aoki N, Tanoue K, Yamazaki H, Moroi M 1988 Thrombasthenia with an abnormal platelet membrane glycoprotein IIb of different molecular weight. Blood 71: 915–922

Kääpä P, Viinikka L, Ylikorkala O 1984 Thromboxane B_2 production by fetal and neonatal platelets: effects of idiopathic respiratory distress syndrome and birth asphyxia. Pediatric Research 18: 756–758

Kaplan C, Patereau C, Reznikoff-Etievant M F, Muller J Y, Dumez Y, Kesseler A 1985 Antenatal Pl[A1] typing and detection of GPIIb-IIIa complex. British Journal of Haematology 60: 586–588

Karaca M, Cronberg L, Nilsson I M 1972 Abnormal platelet-collagen reaction in Ehlers-Danlos syndrome. Scandinavian Journal of Haematology 9: 465–469

Kawasaki T, Kosaki F, Okawa S, Shigematsu I, Yanagawa H 1974 A new infantile acute febrile mucocutaneous lymph node syndrome (MLNS) prevailing in Japan. Pediatrics 54: 271–276

Khurana M S, Lian E C Y, Harkness D R 1980 'Storage pool disease' of platelets: association with multiple congenital cavernous hemangiomas. Journal of the American Medical Association 244: 169–171

Kobbah M, Ewald U, Tuvemo T 1985 Platelet aggregation during the first year of diabetes in childhood. Acta Paediatrica Scandinavica (suppl.) 320: 50–55

Kobrinsky N L, Israels E D, Gerrard J M et al 1984 Shortening of bleeding time by 1-deamino-8-D-arginine vasopressin in various bleeding disorders. Lancet i: 1145–1148

Koike K, Rao A K, Holmsen H, Mueller P S 1984 Platelet secretion defect in patients with the attention deficit disorder and easy bruising. Blood 63: 427–433

Kunicki T J, Johnson M M, Aster R H 1978 Absence of the platelet receptor for drug-dependent antibodies in the Bernard-Soulier syndrome. Journal of Clinical Investigation 62: 716–719

Kunicki T J, Pidard D, Cazenave J P, Nurden A T, Caen J 1981 Inheritance of the human alloantigen Pl[A1] in type I Glanzmann's thrombasthenia. Journal of Clinical Investigation 62: 717–724

Kurstjens R, Bolt C, Vossen M, Haanen C 1968 Familial thrombopathic thrombocytopenia. British Journal of Haematology 15: 305–317

Kwaan H C, Colwell J A, Cruz S, Suwanwela N, Dobbie J G 1972 Increased platelet aggregation in diabetes mellitus. Journal of Laboratory and Clinical Medicine 80: 236–246

Lacombe M, D'Angelo G 1963 Etudes sur une thrombopathie familiale. Nouvelle Revue Française d'Hématologie 3: 611–614

Laffi G, La Villa G, Pinzani M et al 1986 Altered renal and platelet arachidonic acid metabolism in cirrhosis. Gastroenterology 90: 274–282

Lagarde M, Bryon P A, Vargaftig B B, Dechavanne M 1978 Impairment of platelet thromboxane A_2 generation and of the platelet release reaction in two patients with congenital deficiency of platelet cyclo-oxygenase. British Journal of Haematology 38: 251–266

Lages B, Weiss H J 1988a Heterogeneous defects of platelet secretion and responses to weak agonists in patients with bleeding disorders. British Journal of Haematology 68: 53–62

Lages B, Weiss H J 1988b Impairment of phosphatidylinositol metabolism in a patient with a bleeding disorder associated with defects of initial platelet responses. Thrombosis and Haemostasis 59: 175–179

Lages B, Malmsten C, Weiss H J, Samuelsson B 1981 Impaired platelet response to thromboxane A_2 and defective calcium mobilization in a patient with a bleeding disorder. Blood 57: 545–552

Leeksma O C, Zandbergen-Spaargaren J, Giltay J C, Van Mourik J A 1986 Cultured human endothelial cells synthesise a plasma membrane protein complex immunologically related to the platelet glycoprotein IIb/IIIa complex. Blood 67: 1176–1180

Levy-Toledano S, Caen J P, Breton-Gorius J et al 1981 Gray platelet syndrome: α-granule deficiency. Its influence on platelet function. Journal of Laboratory and Clinical Medicine 98: 831–848

Libanska J, Falcão L, Gautier A et al 1975 Thrombocytopénie thrombocytopathique hypogranulaire héréditaire. Nouvelle Revue Française d'Hématologie 15: 165–182

Liu Y, Kosfeld R E, Marcum S G 1984 Treatment of uraemic bleeding with conjugated oestrogen. Lancet ii: 887–890

Livio M, Gotti E, Marchesi D, Mecca G, Remuzzi G, De Gaetano G 1982 Uraemic bleeding: role of anaemia and beneficial effect of red cell transfusions. Lancet ii: 1013–1015

Livio M, Mannucci P M, Vigano G et al 1986 Conjugated estrogens for the management of bleeding associated with renal failure. New England Journal of Medicine 315: 731–735

Longmore D S, Bennett G, Gueirra D et al 1979 Prostacyclin: a solution to some problems of extracorporeal circulation. Lancet i: 1002–1005

Lott I T, Chase T N, Murphy D L 1972 Down's syndrome: transport, storage and metabolism of serotonin in blood platelets. Pediatric Research 6: 730–735

McCoy E E, Snedden J M 1984 Decreased calcium content and $^{45}Ca^{2+}$ uptake in Down's syndrome blood platelets. Pediatric Research 18: 914–916

Machin S J, Keenan J P, McVerry B A 1983 Defective platelet aggregation to the calcium ionophore A23187 in a patient with a lifelong bleeding disorder. Journal of Clinical Pathology 36: 1140–1144

Malmsten C, Hamberg M, Svensson J, Samuelsson B 1975 Physiological role of an endoperoxide in human platelets: hemostatic defect due to platelet cyclo-oxygenase deficiency. Proceedings of the National Academy of Sciences of the USA 72: 1446–1450

Malpass T W, Hanson S R, Savage B, Hessel E A II, Harker L A 1981 Prevention of acquired transient defect in platelet plug formation by infused prostacyclin. Blood 57: 736–740

Malpass T W, Savage B, Hanson S R, Slichter S J, Harker L A 1984 Correlation between prolonged bleeding time and depletion of platelet dense granule ADP in patients with myelodysplastic and myeloproliferative disorders. Journal of Laboratory and Clinical Medicine 103: 894–904

Mannucci P M, Remuzzi G, Pusineri F et al 1983 Deamino-8-D-arginine vasopressin shortens the bleeding time in uremia. New England Journal of Medicine 308: 8–12

Mannucci P M, Vicente V, Vianello L et al 1986 Controlled trial of desmopressin in liver cirrhosis and other conditions associated with a prolonged bleeding time. Blood 67: 1148–1153

Marguerie G A, Plow E F, Edgington T S 1979 Human platelets possess an inducible and saturable receptor specific for fibrinogen. Journal of Biological Chemistry 254: 5357–5363

Maurer H M, Still W J S, Caul J 1971 Familial bleeding tendency associated with microcytic platelets and impaired release of platelet adenosine diphosphate. Journal of Pediatrics 78: 86–94

Maurer H M, Haggins J C, Still W J S 1976 Platelet injury during phototherapy. American Journal of Hematology 1: 89–96

Maurer H M, Wolff J A, Buckingham S, Spielvogel A R 1972 'Impotent' platelets in albinos with prolonged bleeding times. Blood 39: 490–499

Mestel F, Oetliker O, Beck E, Felix R, Imbach P, Wagner H P 1980 Severe bleeding associated with defective thromboxane synthetase. Lancet i: 157 (letter)

Michelson A D 1987 Flow cytometric analysis of platelet surface glycoproteins: phenotypically distinct subpopulations of platelets in children with chronic myeloid leukemia. Journal of Laboratory and Clinical Medicine 110: 346–354

Mielke C H Jr, Levine P H, Zucker S 1981 Preoperative prednisone therapy in platelet function disorders. Thrombosis Research 21: 655–662

Miletich J P, Kane W H, Hofmann S L, Stanford N, Majerus P W 1979 Deficiency of factor Xa-factor Va binding sites on the platelets of a patient with a bleeding disorder. Blood 54: 1015–1022

Miller J L, Castella A 1982 Platelet-type von Willebrand's disease: characterization of a new bleeding disorder. Blood 60: 790–794

Milton J G, Frojmovic M M 1979 Shape-changing agents produce abnormally large platelets in a hereditary 'giant platelets syndrome' (MPS). Journal of Laboratory and Clinical Medicine 93: 154–161

Milton J G, Frojmovic M M, Tang S S, White J G 1984 Spontaneous platelet aggregation in a hereditary giant platelet syndrome (MPS). American Journal of Pathology 114: 336–345

Minkes M S, Joist J H, Needleman P 1979 Arachidonic acid-induced platelet aggregation independent of ADP-release in a patient with a bleeding disorder due to platelet storage pool disease. Thrombosis Research 15: 169–179

Moia M, Vizzotto L, Cattanes M et al 1987 Improvement of the haemostatic defect in uraemia after treatment with recombinant human erythropoietin. Lancet ii: 1227–1229

Monnet P, David M, Philippe N et al 1979 Altérations de l'hémostase lors des traitements au dipropylacetate de sodium (Depakine) (R). Pédiatrie 34: 603–620

Montgomery R R, Kunicki T J, Taves C, Pidard D, Corcoran M 1983 Diagnosis of Bernard-Soulier syndrome and Glanzmann's thrombasthenia with a monoclonal assay on whole blood. Journal of Clinical Investigation 71: 385–389

Mull M M, Hathaway W E 1970 Altered platelet function in newborns. Pediatric Research 4: 229–237

Murphy S, Oski F A, Naiman L, Lusch C J, Goldberg S, Gardner F H 1972 Platelet size and kinetics in hereditary and acquired thrombocytopenia. New England Journal of Medicine 286: 499–504

Mustard J F, Kinlough-Rathbone R L, Packham M A, Perry D, Harfenist E J, Pai K R M 1979 Comparison of fibrinogen association with normal and thrombasthenic platelets on exposure to ADP or chymotrypsin. Blood 54: 987–993

Newburger J W, Takahashi M, Burns J C et al 1986 The

treatment of Kawasaki syndrome with intravenous gamma globulin. New England Journal of Medicine 315: 341–347

Newman P J, Kawai Y, Montgomery R R, Kunicki T J 1986 Synthesis by cultured human umbilical vein endothelial cells of two proteins structurally and immunologically related to platelet membrane glycoproteins IIb and IIIa. Journal of Cell Biology 103: 81–86

Newman P J, Seligsohn U, Lyman S, Poncz M, Coller B S 1990 The molecular genetic basis of Glanzmann thrombasthenia in the Iraqi-Jewish and Arab populations in Israel. Clinical Research 38: 467a

Niessner H, Clemetson K J, Panzer S, Mueller-Eckhardt C, Santoso S, Bettelheim P 1986 Acquired thrombasthenia due to GPIIb/IIIa-specific platelet autoantibodies. Blood 68: 571–576

Nieuwenhuis H K, Akkerman J W N, Sixma J J 1987 Patients with a prolonged bleeding time and normal aggregation tests may have storage pool deficiency: studies on one hundred and six patients. Blood 70: 620–623

Nieuwenhuis H K, Akkerman J W N, Houdijk W P M, Sixma J J 1985 Human blood platelets showing no reponse to collagen fail to express surface glycoprotein Ia. Nature 318: 470–472

Nurden A T, Caen J P 1974 An abnormal platelet glycoprotein pattern in three cases of Glanzmann's thrombasthenia. British Journal of Haematology 28: 253–260

Nurden A T, Caen J P 1975 Specific roles for platelet surface glycoproteins in platelet function. Nature 253: 720–722

Nurden A T, Didry D, Kiefer N, McEver R P 1985 Residual amounts of glycoproteins IIb and IIIa may be present in the platelets of most patients with Glanzmann's thrombasthenia. Blood 65: 1021–1024

Nurden A T, Kunicki T J, Dupuis D, Soria C, Caen J P 1982 Specific protein and glycoprotein deficiencies in platelets isolated from two patients with the gray platelet syndrome. Blood 59: 709–718

Nurden A T, Rosa J P, Fournier D et al 1987 A variant of Glanzmann's thrombasthenia with abnormal glycoprotein IIb-IIIa complexes in the platelet membrane. Journal of Clinical Investigation 79: 962–969

O'Brien J R 1964 Variability in the aggregation of human platelets by adrenaline. Nature 202: 1188–1190

Ochs H D, Slichter S J, Harker L A, von Behrens W E, Clark R A, Wedgwood R J 1980 The Wiskott-Aldrich syndrome: studies of lymphocytes, granulocytes, and platelets. Blood 55: 243–252

Okuma M, Uchino H 1979 Altered arachidonate metabolism by platelets in patients with myeloproliferative disorders. Blood 54: 1258–1271

Oppenheimer E H, Esterly J R 1965 Thrombosis in the newborn: comparison between infants of diabetic and nondiabetic mothers. Journal of Pediatrics. 67: 549–556

Ordinas A, Maragall S, Castillo R, Nurden A T 1978 A glycoprotein I defect in platelets in three patients with severe cirrhosis of the liver. Thrombosis Research 13: 297–302

Pandolfi M, Åstedt B, Cronberg L, Nilsson I M 1972 Failure of fetal platelets to aggregate in reponse to adrenaline and collagen. Proceedings of the Society for Experimental Biology and Medicine 141: 1081–1083

Pareti F I, Mannucci P M, D'Angelo A, Smith J B, Sautebin L, Galli G 1980 Congenital deficiency of thromboxane and prostacyclin. Lancet i: 898–901

Parkman R, Remold-O'Donnell E, Kenney D M, Perrine S, Rosen F S 1981 Surface protein abnormalities in lymphocytes and platelets from patients with Wiskott-Aldrich syndrome. Lancet ii: 1387–1389

Parmley R T, Poon M S, Crist W M, Malluh A 1979 Giant platelet granules in a child with the Chediak-Higashi syndrome. American Journal of Hematology 6: 51–60

Parvez Z, Moncada R, Fareed J, Messmore H L 1984 Antiplatelet action of intravascular contrast media. Implications in diagnostic procedures. Investigative Radiology 19: 208–211

Peerschke E I, Zucker M B, Grant R A, Egan J J, Johnson M M 1980 correlation between fibrinogen binding to human platelets and platelet aggregability. Blood 55: 841–847

Perret B, Levy-Toledano S, Plantavid M et al 1983 Abnormal phospholipid organization in Bernard-Soulier platelets. Thrombosis Research 31: 529–537

Peterson L A, Rao K V, Crosson J T, White J G 1985 Fechtner syndrome – a variant of Alport's syndrome with leukocyte inclusions and macrothrombocytopenia. Blood 65: 397–406

Pfueller S L, Howard M A, White J G, Menon C, Berry E W 1987 Shortening of bleeding time by 1-deamino-8-arginine vasopressin (DDAVP) in the absence of platelet von Willebrand factor in gray platelet syndrome. Thrombosis and Haemostasis 58: 1060–1063

Phillips D R, Agin P P 1977 Platelet membrane defects in Glanzmann's thrombasthenia. Evidence for decreased amounts of two major glycoproteins. Journal of Clinical Investigation 60: 535–545

Phillips D R, Charo I F, Parise L V, Fitzgerald L A 1988 The platelet membrane glycoprotein IIb-IIIa complex. Blood 71: 831–843

Pidard D, Didry D, Le Deist F et al 1988 Analysis of the membrane glycoproteins of platelets in the Wiskott-Aldrich syndrome. British Journal of Haematology 69: 529–535

Pischel K D, Bluestein H G, Woods V L 1988 Platelet glycoproteins Ia, Ic and IIa are physicochemically indistinguishable from the very late activation antigens adhesion-related proteins of lymphocytes and other cell types. Journal of Clinical Investigation 81: 505–513

Pope F M, Martin G R, Lichtenstein J R et al 1975 Patients with Ehlers-Danlos syndrome type IV lack type III collagen. Proceedings of the National Academy of Sciences of the USA 72: 1314–1316

Preston F E, Ward J D, Marcola B H, Porter N R, Timperley W R, O'Malley B C 1978 Elevated beta-thromboglobulin levels and circulating platelet aggregates in diabetic microangiopathy. Lancet i: 238–240

Rabiner S F, Molinas F 1970 The role of phenol and phenolic acids on the thrombocytopathy and defective platelet aggregation of patients with renal failure. American Journal of Medicine 49: 346–351

Raccuglia G 1971 Gray platelet syndrome. A variety of qualitative platelet disorder. American Journal of Medicine 51: 818–828

Rao A K, Koike K, Willis J et al 1984 Platelet secretion defect associated with impaired liberation of arachidonic acid and normal myosin light chain phosphorylation. Blood 64: 914–921

Remuzzi G 1988 Bleeding in renal failure. Lancet i: 1205–1208

Remuzzi G, Livio M, Marchiaro G, Mecca G, De Gaetano G 1978a Bleeding in renal failure: altered platelet function in chronic uraemia only partially corrected by haemodialysis.

Nephron 22: 347–353

Remuzzi G, Marchesi D, Livio M et al 1978b Altered platelet and vascular prostaglandin generation in patients with renal failure and prolonged bleeding times. Thrombosis Research 13: 1007–1015

Remuzzi G, Mecca G, Marchesi D et al 1979 Platelet hyperaggregability and the nephrotic syndrome. Thrombosis Research 15: 345–354

Remuzzi G, Benigni A, Dodesini P et al 1981 Parathyroid hormone inhibits human platelet function. Lancet ii: 1321–1323

Remuzzi G, Benigni A, Dodesini P et al 1982 Platelet function in patients on maintenance hemodialysis: depressed or enhanced? Clinical Nephrology 17: 60–63

Remuzzi G, Benigni A, Dodesini P et al 1983 Reduced platelet thromboxane formation in uremia. Evidence for a functional cyclooxygenase defect. Journal of Clinical Investigation 71: 762–768

Rendu F, Lebret M, Nurden A, Caen J P 1979 Detection of an acquired platelet storage pool disease in three patients with a myeloproliferative disorder. Thrombosis and Haemostasis 42: 794–796

Rendu F, Breton-Gorius J, Trugnan G et al 1978 Studies on a new variant of the Hermansky-Pudlak syndrome: qualitative, ultrastructural and functional abnormalities of the platelet-dense bodies associated with a phospholipase A defect. American Journal of Haematology 4: 387–399

Rendu F, Breton-Gorius J, Lebret M et al 1983 Evidence that abnormal platelet functions in human Chediak-Higashi syndrome are the result of a lack of dense bodies. American Journal of Pathology 111: 307–314

Rendu F, Marche P, Hovig T et al 1987 Abnormal phosphoinositide metabolism and protein phosphorylation in platelets from a patient with the gray platelet syndrome. British Journal of Haematology 67: 199–206

Richardson S G N, Fletcher D J, Jeavons P M, Stuart J 1976 Sodium valproate and platelet function. British Medical Journal 1: 221–222

Rosa J P, George J N, Bainton D F, Nurden A T, Caen J P, McEver R P 1987 Gray platelet syndrome. Demonstration of alpha granule membranes that can fuse with the cell surface. Journal of Clinical Investigation 80: 1138–1146

Rosa J P, Bray P F, Gayet O et al 1988 Cloning of glycoprotein IIIa cDNA from human erythroleukemia cells and localization of the gene to chromosome 17. Blood 72: 593–600

Rosing J, Bevers E M, Comfurius P et al 1985a Impaired factor X- and prothrombin activation associated with decreased phospholipid exposure in platelets from a patient with a bleeding disorder. Blood 65: 1557–1561

Rosing J, van Rijn J L M L, Bevers E M, van Dieijen G, Comfurius P, Zwaal R F A 1985b The role of activated human platelets in prothrombin and factor X activation. Blood 65: 319–332

Roth G J, Machuga R 1982 Radioimmune assay of human platelet prostaglandin synthetase. Journal of Laboratory and Clinical Medicine 99: 187–196

Roth G J, Stanford N, Majerus P W 1975 Acetylation of prostaglandin synthetase by aspirin. Proceedings of the National Academy of Sciences of the USA 72: 3073–3076

Russell M E, Seligsohn U, Coller B S, Ginsberg M H, Skoglund P, Quertermous T 1988 Structural integrity of the glycoprotein IIb and IIIa genes in Glanzmann thrombasthenia patients from Israel. Blood 72: 1833–1836

Russell N H, Keenan J P, Bellingham A J 1979 Thrombocytopathy in preleukaemia; association with a defect of thromboxane A2 activity. British Journal of Haematology 41: 417–425

Russell N H, Salmon J, Keenan J P, Bellingham A J 1981 Platelet adenine nucleotides and arachidonic acid metabolism in the myeloprolifetative disorders. Thrombosis Research 22: 389–307

Sakariassen K S, Bolhuis P A, Sixma J J 1979 Human blood platelet adhesion to artery subendothelium is mediated by factor VIII-von Willebrand factor bound to the subendothelium. Nature 279: 636–638

Sakariassen K S, Nievelstein P F E M, Coller B S, Sixma J J 1986 The role of platelet membrane glycoproteins Ib and IIb-IIIa in platelet adherence in human artery subendothelium. British Journal of Haematology 63: 681–691

Salzman E W, Neri L J 1966 Adhesion of blood platelets in uremia. Thrombosis et Diathesis Haemorrhagica 15: 84–92

Salzman E W, Rosenberg R D, Smith M H, Lindon J N, Favreau L 1980 Effect of heparin and heparin fractions on platelet aggregation. Journal of Clinical Investigation 65: 64–73

Schafer A I 1982 Deficiency of platelet lipoxygenase activity in myeloproliferative disorders. New England Journal of Medicine 306: 381–386

Schafer A I 1984 Bleeding and thrombosis in the myeloproliferative disorders. Blood 64: 1–12

Schulman S, Johnsson H, Egberg N, Blombäck M 1987 DDAVP-induced correction of prolonged bleeding time in patients with congenital platelet function defects. Thrombosis Research 45: 165–174

Scrutton M C, Clare K A, Hutton R A, Bruckdorfer K R 1981 Depressed responsiveness to adrenaline in platelets from apparently normal human donors: a familial trait. British Journal of Haematology 49: 303–314

Seligsohn U, Mibashan R S, Rodeck C H, Nicolaides K H, Millar D S, Coller B S 1985 Prenatal diagnosis of Glanzmann's thrombasthenia. Lancet ii: 1419 (letter)

Seligsohn U, Mibashan R S, Rodeck C H et al 1988 Prevention program of type I Glanzmann's thrombasthenia in Israel: prenatal diagnosis. Current Studies in Hematology and Blood Transfusion 55: 174–179

Semeraro N, Cortellazzo S, Colucci M, Barbui T 1979 A hitherto undescribed defect of platelet coagulant activity in polycythaemia vera and essential thrombocythaemia. Thrombosis Research 16: 795–802

Shattil S J, Bennett J S, McDonough M, Turnbull J 1980 Carbenicillin and penicillin G inhibit platelet function in vitro by impairing the interaction of agonists with the platelet surface. Journal of Clinical Investigation 65: 329–337

Solomon L R, Bobinski H, Astley P, Goldby F S, Mallick N P 1982 Bartter's syndrome – observations on the pathophysiology. Quarterly Journal of Medicine 51: 251–270

Solum N O, Rigollot C, Budzynski A Z, Marder V J 1973 A quantitative evaluation of the inhibition of platelet aggregation by low molecular weight degradation products of fibrinogen. British Journal of Haematology 24: 419–434

Srivastava P C, Powling M J, Nokes T J C, Patrick A D, Dawes J, Hardisty R M 1987 Grey platelet syndrome: studies on platelet alpha-granules, lysosomes and defective response to thrombin. British Journal of Haematology

65: 441–446

Stewart G W, O'Brien H, Morris S A, Owen J S, Lloyd J K, Ames J A L 1987 Stomatocytosis, abnormal platelets and pseudo-homozygous hypercholesterolaemia. European Journal of Haematology 38: 376–380

Stewart J H, Castaldi P A 1967 Uraemic bleeding: a reversible platelet defect corrected by dialysis. Quarterly Journal of Medicine 36: 409–423

Stoff J S, Stemerman M, Steer M, Salzman E, Brown R S 1980 A defect in platelet aggregation in Bartter's syndrome. American Journal of Medicine 68: 171–180

Stormorken H, Gogstad G, Solum N O, Pande H 1982 Diagnosis of heterozygotes in Glanzmann's thrombasthenia. Thrombosis and Haemostasis 48: 217–221

Stormorken H, Gogstad G, Solum N O 1983 A new bleeding disorder: lack of platelet aggregatory response to adrenalin and lack of secondary aggregation to ADP and platelet activating factor (PAF). Thrombosis Research 29: 391–402

Stricker R B, Shuman M A 1986 Quinidine purpura: evidence that glycoprotein V is a target platelet antigen. Blood 67: 1377–1381

Stricker R B, Wong D, Saks S R, Corash L, Shuman M A 1985 Acquired Bernard-Soulier syndrome. Evidence for the role of a 210 000 molecular weight protein in the interaction of platelets with von Willebrand factor. Journal of Clinical Investigation 76: 1274–1278

Stuart J J, Lewis J C 1982 Platelet aggregation and electron microscopic studies of platelets in preleukemia. Archives of Pathology and Laboratory Medicine 106: 458–461

Stuart M J 1978 The neonatal platelet: evaluation of platelet malonyl dialdehyde formation as an indicator of prostaglandin synthesis. British Journal of Haematology 39: 83–90

Stuart M J, Allen J B 1982 Arachidonic acid metabolism in the neonatal platelet. Pediatrics 69: 714–718

Stuart M J, Gross S J, Elrad H, Graeber J E 1982 Effects of acetysalicylic-acid ingestion on maternal and neonatal hemostasis. New England Journal of Medicine 307: 909–912

Stuart M J, Duss E J, Clark D A, Walenga R W 1984 Differences in thromboxane production between neonatal and adult platelets in response to arachidonic acid and epinephrine. Pediatric Research 18: 823–826

Stuart M J, Sunderji S G, Walenga R W, Setty B N Y 1985 Abnormalities in vascular arachidonic acid metabolism in the infant of the diabetic mother. British Medical Journal 290: 1700–1702

Stuart M J, Elrad H, Graeber J E, Hakanson D O, Sunderji S G, Barvinchak M K 1979 Increased synthesis of platelet malonyldialdehyde and platelet hyperfunction in infants of mothers with diabetes mellitus. Journal of Laboratory and Clinical Medicine 94: 12–26

Suarez C R, Gonzalez J, Menendez C, Fareed J, Fresco R, Walenga J 1988 Neonatal and maternal platelets: activation at time of birth. American Journal of Hematology 29: 18–21

Takahashi H, Handa M, Watanabe K et al 1984 Further characterization of platelet-type von Willebrand's disease in Japan. Blood 64: 1254–1262

Takamatsu J, Horne III M K, Gralnick H R 1986 Identification of the thrombin receptor on human platelets by chemical crosslinking. Journal of Clinical Investigation 77: 362–368

Tanoue K, Hasegawa S, Yamaguchi A, Yamamoto N,

Yamazaki H 1987 A new variant of thrombasthenia with abnormally glycosylated GPIIb/IIIa. Thrombosis Research 47: 323–333

Thomas D P 1972 Abnormalities of platelet aggregation in patients with alcoholic cirrhosis. Annals of the New York Academy of Sciences 201: 243–250

Tremoli E, Maderna P, Colli S, Morazzoni G, Sirtori M, Sirtori C R 1984 Increased platelet sensitivity and thromboxane B2 formation in type-II hyperlipoproteinaemic patients. European Journal of Clinical Investigation 14: 329–333

Ts'ao C, Green D, Schultz K 1976 Function and ultrastructure of platelets of neonates: enhanced ristocetin aggregation of neonatal platelets. British Journal of Haematology 32: 225–233

Turitto V T, Baumgartner H R 1975 Platelet interaction with subendothelium in a perfusion system. Physical role of red blood cells. Microvascular Research 9: 335–344

Turitto V T, Baumgartner H R 1979 Platelet interaction with subendothelium in flowing rabbit blood – effect of blood sheer rate. Microvascular Research 17: 38–54

Vane J R 1971 Inhibition of prostaglandin synthesis as a mechanism of action for aspirin-like drugs. Nature New Biology 231: 232–235

Van Geet C, Hauglustaine D, Verresen L, Vanrusselt M, Vermylen J 1989 Haemostatic effects of recombinant human erythropoietin in chronic haemodialysis patients. Thrombosis and Haemostasis 61: 117–121

Verdirame J D, Davis J W, Phillips P E 1984 The effects of radiographic contrast agents on bleeding time and platelet aggregation. Clinical Cardiology 7: 31–34

Vermylen J, Blockmans D 1989 Acquired disorders of platelet function. Baillière's Clinical Haematology 2: 729–748

Walsh P N, Murphy S, Barry W E 1977 The role of platelets in the pathogenesis of thrombosis and hemorrhage in patients with thrombocytosis. Thrombosis and Haemostasis 38: 1085–1096

Walsh P N, Mills D C B, Pareti F et al 1975 Hereditary giant platelet syndrome: absence of collagen-induced coagulant activity and deficiency of factor XI binding to platelets. British Journal of Haematology 29: 639–655

Warkentin T E, Powling M J, Hardisty R M 1990 Measurement of fibrinogen binding to platelets in whole blood by flow cytometry: a micromethod for the detection of platelet activation. British Journal of Haematology 76: 387–394

Wautier J L, Gruel Y 1989 Prenatal diagnosis of platelet disorders. Baillière's Clinical Haematology 2: 569–583

Wautier J L, Gruel Y, Boizard B, Caen J P, Daffos F, Forestier F 1987 Antenatal diagnosis of thrombopathy. Thrombosis and Haemostasis 58: 401 (abstract)

Weiss H J 1967 The effect of clinical dextran on platelet aggregation, adhesion, and ADP release in man: in vivo and in vitro studies. Journal of Laboratory and Clinical Medicine 69: 37–46

Weiss H J, Lages B 1981 Platelet malondialdehyde production and aggregation responses induced by arachidonate, prostaglandin-G$_2$, collagen and epinephrine in 12 patients with storage pool deficiency. Blood 58: 27–33

Weiss H J, Turitto V T, Baumgartner H R 1978 Effect of shear rate on platelet interaction with subendothelium in citrated and native blood. I. Shear rate-dependent decrease of adhesion in von Willebrand's disease and the Bernard-Soulier syndrome. Journal of Laboratory and Clinical

Medicine 92: 750–764

Weiss H J, Turitto V T, Baumgartner H R 1986 Platelet adhesion and thrombus formation on subendothelium in platelets deficient in glycoproteins IIb-IIIa, Ib and storage granules. Blood 67: 322–330

Weiss H J, Vicic W J, Lages B A, Rogers J 1979a Isolated deficiency of platelet procoagulant activity. American Journal of Medicine 67: 206–213

Weiss H J, Witte L D, Kaplan K L et al 1979b Heterogeneity in storage pool deficiency: studies on granule-bound substances in 18 patients including variants deficient in α-granules, platelet factor 4, β-thromboglobulin and platelet-derived growth factor. Blood 54: 1296–1319

Weiss H J, Chervenick P A, Zalusky R, Factor A 1969 A familial defect in platelet function associated with impaired release of adenosine diphosphate. New England Journal of Medicine 281: 1264–1270

Weiss H J, Tschopp T B, Baumgartner H R, Sussman I I, Johnson M M, Egan J J 1974 Decreased adhesion of giant (Bernard-Soulier) platelets to subendothelium. Further implications on the role of the von Willebrand factor in hemostasis. American Journal of Medicine 57: 920–925

Weiss H J, Meyer D, Rabinowitz R et al 1982 Pseudo-von Willebrand's disease. An intrinsic platelet defect with aggregation by unmodified human factor VIII/von Willebrand factor and enhanced absorption of its high-molecular-weight multimers. New England Journal of Medicine 306: 326–333

Wenger R H, Kieffer N, Wicki A N, Clemetson K J 1988 Structure of the human blood platelet membrane glycoprotein Ibα gene. Biochemical and Biophysical Research Communications 156: 389–395

Wenger R H, Wicki A N, Kieffer N, Adolph S, Hameister H, Clemetson K J 1989 The 5' flanking region and chromosomal localization of the gene encoding human platelet membrane glycoprotein Ibα. Gene 85: 517–524

Whaun J M 1973 The platelet of the normal infant: 5-hydroxytryptamine uptake and release. Thrombosis et Diathesis Haemorrhagica 30: 327–333

Whaun J M 1980 The platelet of the newborn infant – adenine nucleotide metabolism and release. Thrombosis and Haemostasis 43: 99–103

White J G 1978 Platelet microtubules and giant granules in the Chediak-Higashi syndrome. American Journal of Medical Technology 44: 273–278

White J G 1979 Ultrastructural studies of the gray platelet syndrome. American Journal of Pathology 95: 445–462

White J G, Edson J R, Desnick S J, Witkop C J 1971 Studies of platelets in a variant of the Hermansky-Pudlak syndrome. American Journal of Pathology 63: 319–332

White J G, Burris S M, Hasegawa D, Johnson M 1984 Micropipette aspiration of human blood platelets: a defect in Bernard-Soulier's syndrome. Blood 63: 1249–1252

Wicki A N, Clemetson K J 1985 Structure and function of platelet membrane glycoproteins Ib and V. Effects of leukocyte elastase and other proteases on platelet response to von Willebrand factor and thrombin. European Journal of Biochemistry 153: 1–11

Witkop C J, Krumwiede M, Sedano H, White J G 1987 Reliability of absence of platelet dense bodies as a diagnostic criterion for Hermansky-Pudlak syndrome. American Journal of Hematology 26: 305–311

Woodcock B E, Cooper P C, Brown P R, Pickering C, Winfield D A, Preston F E 1984 The platelet defect in acute myeloid leukaemia. Journal of Clinical Pathology 37: 1339–1342

Wu K K, Le Breton G C, Tai H H, Chen Y C 1981 Abnormal platelet response to thromboxane A2. Journal of Clinical Investigation 67: 1801–1804

Yamada K, Fukumoto T, Shinkai A, Shirahata A, Meguro T 1978 The platelet functions in acute febrile mucocutaneous lymph node syndrome and a trial of prevention for thrombosis by antiplatelet agents. Acta Haematologica Japonica 41: 113–124

Yamamoto K, Yamamoto N, Kitagawa H, Tanoue K, Kosaki G, Yamazaki H 1986 Localization of a thrombin-binding site on human platelet membrane glycoprotein Ib determined by a monoclonal antibody. Thrombosis and Haemostasis 55: 162–167

Yarom R, Muhlrad A, Hodges A, Robin G C 1980 Platelet pathology in patients with idiopathic scoliosis: ultrastructural morphometry, aggregation, x-ray spectrometry and biochemical analysis. Laboratory Investigation 43: 208–216

Yoshida N, Aoki N 1978 Release of arachidonic acid from human platelets. A key role for the potentiation of platelet aggregability in normal subjects as well as in those with nephrotic syndrome. Blood 52: 969–977

Zahavi J, Marder V J 1974 Acquired 'storage pool disease' of platelets associated with circulating anti-platelet antibodies. American Journal of Medicine 56: 883–890

Zucker M B 1977 Heparin and platelet function. Federation Proceedings 36: 47–49

Zucker M B, Pert J H, Hilgartner M W 1966 Platelet function in a patient with thrombasthenia. Blood 28: 524–534

8. Disorders of red cells: I Lack of erythrocyte production

Martin J. Pippard

INTRODUCTION

Anaemia can be defined as a blood haemoglobin concentration which is more than two standard deviations below the mean for the normal population (reference ranges, and their variation with age and sex are shown in Chapter 1). This definition inevitably results in an overlap between normal and abnormal values. The significance of an individual measurement of haemoglobin concentration also has to be assessed in relation to changes from any previous values obtained in the same patient, and in relation to other determinants of oxygen delivery to the tissues (e.g. respiratory or cardiac disease). A reduced haemoglobin concentration can result from two primary pathophysiological mechanisms:

1. defective production of red cells
2. excessive loss of red cells through haemolysis or haemorrhage.

In general, the distinction between these two mechanisms is made on the basis of the reticulocyte count, the latter being appropriately increased in response to increased erythropoietin concentrations in haemolytic anaemias, but not in defects of red cell production. Correction of the percentage reticulocyte count for haematocrit or red cell number, and allowance for the increase in circulating reticulocytes caused by their early 'shift' from marrow into blood under the stimulation of high concentrations of erythropoietin, allows calculation of a reticulocyte production index (Hillman & Finch 1969). Failure to increase red cell production by more than two- to three-fold in response to anaemia suggests that defective red cell production is the main cause.

Classification of disorders of erythrocyte production

Impaired red cell production may be due to a quantitative defect (relative hypoplasia) or to a disorder of erythrocyte maturation in which there is often greatly increased but ineffective erythropoiesis with intramedullary death of the red cell precursors. Although there may be a contribution from both mechanisms in any individual case, usually one predominates; for example, early iron deficiency is associated with relative erythroid hypoplasia, but as the anaemia becomes more severe, defective haemoglobinization of the cytoplasm (a 'cytoplasmic maturation defect') leads to increasingly ineffective erythropoiesis.

The use of automated blood cell counters allows a ready measurement of red cell size, and a classification based on whether the red cells are microcytic, macrocytic or normocytic may be diagnostically useful. The approach to classification used in this chapter is shown in Table 8.1. Defects in haemoglobin production resulting in impaired cytoplasmic maturation of erythroblasts tend to give rise to microcytic red cells. Defects of DNA synthesis and thus of nuclear maturation are often associated with the production of macrocytic red cells. Marrow failure syndromes tend to give rise to normocytic red cells, though macrocytes may also be present because of elements of ineffective erythropoiesis among remaining erythroblasts. Defects in nuclear maturation are invariably associated with ineffective erythropoiesis, while defects in marrow environment or erythroid stem cells are by definition hypoplastic. The primary pathophysiological mechanism in disorders associated with defective haemoglobin synthesis varies from extreme ineffective erythropoiesis (e.g. in major thalassaemia

Table 8.1   Disorders of erythrocyte production

Defects in haemoglobin synthesis
1. Impaired haem synthesis:
   a. Iron deficiency
   b. 'Anaemia of chronic disorders'
   c. Sideroblastic anaemia*
   d. Lead poisoning
2. Impaired globin chain synthesis:
   Thalassaemia syndromes*
Defects in erythroid cell division and maturation *
1. Nuclear maturation defects:
   a. Cobalamin (vitamin B_{12}) deficiency
   b. Folate deficiency
   c. Hereditary abnormalities of cobalamin or folate
      metabolism
   d. Other metabolic defects associated with megaloblastic
      anaemia (Lesch-Nyhan syndrome, orotic aciduria,
      thiamine-responsive megaloblastic anaemia)
2. Congenital dyserythropoietic anaemias (types I, II, III)
3. Sideroblastic anaemias
Defects in marrow 'environment' or erythroid stem cells
1. Marrow failure:
   a. Aplastic anaemia } see Chs 2, 3, 4 and 12
   b. Marrow infiltration
   c. Pure red cell aplasia:
      Prolonged —Congenital
                 (Diamond-Blackfan syndrome)
               —Acquired
      Short-lived —Parvovirus infection
                  —Transient erythroblastopenia
                   of childhood
                  —Drugs
                  —Nutritional deficiencies
2. Inadequate erythropoietin production
   a. Chronic renal disease
   b. 'Anaemia of chronic disorders'
   c. Protein malnutrition
   d. Anaemia of prematurity

*Characterized by marked ineffective erythropoiesis.

syndromes) to the relative hypoplasia of early iron deficiency and the anaemia of chronic disorders.

DEFECTS IN HAEMOGLOBIN SYNTHESIS
I. IMPAIRED HAEM SYNTHESIS

Iron deficiency

Iron deficiency is the commonest cause of anaemia at all ages. It is particularly widespread in infants and young children, where rapid growth leads to large iron requirements which may outstrip the available iron in the diet. Iron deficiency can be defined as the situation in which the availability of iron limits the production of haemoglobin. However, as will be discussed below, there is much current interest in possible nonhaematological manifestations of iron deficiency which

may also be particularly important in the developing child.

Role of iron and iron-containing proteins

In order to understand the pathogenesis of iron deficiency and the tests used in its diagnosis, some understanding of the function of iron-containing proteins and the pathways of iron movement in the body is required.

The major part of body iron is in the form of haem, which is essential for oxygen delivery to the tissues by haemoglobin and myoglobin. The ability of iron to exist in both Fe(II) and Fe(III) redox states is responsible for its general role in all cells as a component of haem proteins or iron-sulphur proteins which take part in electron transfer reactions. These iron-containing enzymes include the mitochondrial cytochromes a, b and c, succinate dehydrogenase and cytochrome c oxidase, and are essential for the oxidative production of energy as adenosine triphosphate. Cytochrome P_{450} in the endoplasmic reticulum is involved in a range of drug and metabolite oxidation reactions. Other haem-containing enzymes include catalase, myeloperoxidase, and tryptophan pyrrolase: xanthine oxidase and NADH dehydrogenase contain iron-sulphur complexes. Ribonucleotide reductase, essential for DNA synthesis and cell division, is also dependent upon non-haem iron (Hoffbrand et al 1976). These widespread functions of iron mean that it would be surprising if the effects of iron deficiency were confined to the erythron (see p. 207).

The redox reactivity of iron which makes it essential for all living cells also means that in the oxygen-rich atmosphere most iron is in the form of Fe(III), which at neutral pH forms highly insoluble ferric hydroxide. Thus, despite iron being the fourth most abundant element in the earth's crust, it is relatively unavailable. As a result, living organisms have developed highly specialized iron-binding proteins, both to obtain iron from the environment and to hold ferric iron in solution while limiting its potential toxicity. Thus, in addition to the functional iron-containing compounds described above, there are a number of specialized proteins of iron storage and transport. In man, these enable iron to be transported in the plasma at neutral pH (bound to the plasma protein, transferrin), or stored within cells as ferritin or its degradation product (haemosiderin). Biochemical measurement of these proteins can provide clinically useful information about the iron status of a patient.

Iron exchange

The majority of body iron is in the form of haemoglobin, with an additional 5–30% of the total stored as ferritin or haemosiderin. Internal iron exchange is dominated by the supply of iron to the developing red cell precursors in the bone marrow, its subsequent appearance within circulating red cells, and, finally, release of the iron from the haem within macrophages at the end of the 120–day red cell lifespan (Fig. 8.1). Plasma transferrin, though it holds a tiny fraction of total body iron at any one time, plays a pivotal role in this iron exchange. Given the small size of the transferrin iron pool, and its dependence on iron supplied from donor tissues (macrophages, hepatocytes and gut mucosal cells), it is not surprising that concentrations of plasma iron may show wide fluctuations, even

within hours, in the same individual. However, in pathological states such as iron deficiency or iron overload, the plasma iron concentration tends to be consistently low or raised, respectively. Iron stores within macrophages of the reticuloendothelial system and hepatic parenchymal cells can be mobilized in response to increased demands for functional iron compounds. Where there is excessive iron input to the body, either as blood transfusions or from increased iron absorption (p. 214), the circulating transferrin becomes fully saturated with iron and there is increased parenchymal tissue uptake, initially predominantly by hepatocytes.

Biochemistry of iron

Iron taken up from the intestinal mucosal cells joins the iron recycled from haem by macrophages in being delivered to the plasma, where it is bound to transferrin. Transferrin is a single polypeptide chain which has a molecular weight of 75–80 kDa and two iron-binding sites. Transferrin is synthesized primarily by the liver, at a rate which is inversely related to iron stores (Morton & Tavill 1977). It is thus increased in iron deficiency and reduced in iron overload, but the mechanism of this iron regulation of synthesis is unknown.

Though all body cells express surface receptors for transferrin, the vast majority are normally on erythroid precursors in the bone marrow, with smaller numbers on hepatocytes. The transferrin receptor is a dimeric transmembrane protein formed from two polypeptides (MW weight 190 kDa) linked by a single disulphur bond (Trowbridge et al 1984). The mechanism by which transferrin is taken up by cells is shown in Figure 8.2. At the near neutral pH of the plasma, diferric and, to a lesser extent, monoferric transferrins have a high affinity for the transferrin receptor. The receptor–transferrin complex is internalized to an endosomal vesicle, which is then acidified to release the Fe(III) from the transferrin. At acidic pH, the apotransferrin has a high affinity for the receptor to which it thus remains bound as it is recycled back to the cell surface: there, it dissociates at neutral pH to be re-utilized for plasma iron transport. How the iron leaves the endosome is not clear. It enters a labile pool of intracellular transit

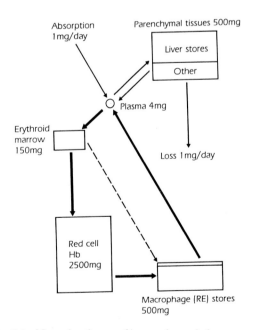

Fig. 8.1 Normal pathways of iron exchange in humans. Values for iron in each compartment are for an adult male. The dotted line represents the small amount of normal wastage erythropoiesis due to intramedullary death of erythroblasts. Reproduced from Weatherall et al 1987, by permission of Oxford University Press.

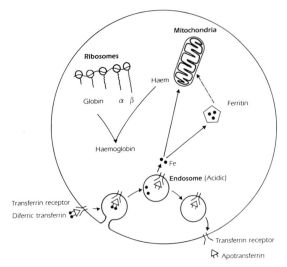

Fig. 8.2 Mechanism of cellular iron uptake. Intracellular transit iron (Fe) is available for incorporation into functional iron compounds or storage ferritin protein. It also regulates synthesis of ferritin and transferrin receptor proteins by polyribosomes (see text). Reproduced from Pippard & Hoffbrand 1989, with permission.

iron which is available for uptake by mitochondria and incorporation into haem, as well as to the main storage protein ferritin.

The greater affinity of transferrin receptors for fully saturated (diferric) rather than monoferric transferrin (Huebers et al 1983) means that the percentage saturation of the plasma transferrin (or total iron binding capacity, TIBC) has a major effect upon the availability of iron to the tissues and the rate of plasma iron turnover (Cazzola et al 1985). As a result, the measurement of plasma iron and transferrin concentrations and, particularly, the percentage saturation of the TIBC gives a measure of the iron supply to the tissues – a saturation of less than 16% is unable to support normal adult erythropoiesis (Bainton & Finch 1964). Where iron supply for mitochondrial haem synthesis is limiting, the final stage of iron incorporation into the protoporphyrin ring (Fig. 8.4, p. 212) is prevented and red cell protoporphyrin accumulates to be bound within the haem pocket of the globin chains during the life-span of the red cell. Measurement of the red cell protoporphyrin therefore provides an alternative, and relatively stable, measure of iron supply to the developing red cell.

Apoferritin is a hollow, spherical protein which can keep up to 4000 iron atoms per molecule in solution in the form of a core of iron hydroxide-phosphate. Synthesis of the 24 ferritin protein subunits on polyribosomes is increased in response to increased concentrations of intracellular transit iron. As a small amount of the newly synthesized apoferritin is glycosylated and is secreted into the plasma, immunoassay of serum ferritin can be used to give an indirect assessment of intracellular iron, and thus body iron stores (Worwood 1986). Unfortunately, ferritin protein synthesis is also increased by inflammatory disease as an 'acute phase protein', and this may increase plasma ferritin concentrations even in the absence of iron stores. In developing red cells haemoglobin synthesis predominates, but in the cells of iron storage (hepatocytes and macrophages) iron incorporation into ferritin is a major intracellular pathway for the transit iron. In these iron storage cells, continued accumulation of ferritin results in the formation of the insoluble degradation product, haemosiderin, within lysosomes. It is this insoluble material which is stained by Perls' reagent when bone marrow samples are examined histologically for the presence of iron stores.

Recent studies have provided exciting data on the regulation of intracellular iron. Both ferritin synthesis and the production of transferrin receptors is controlled by the amount of labile intracellular iron. In both cases, the regulation is at the level of control of translation of the mRNA, there being an iron regulatory element (IRE) in the 5' untranslated region of the ferritin mRNA, and in the 3' untranslated region of the transferrin mRNA (Kuhn 1991). Binding of a regulatory, probably iron-sulphur, protein to the IRE stabilizes transferrin receptor mRNA (enhancing translation), but inhibits the translation of ferritin mRNA. The regulatory IRE-binding protein can also bind labile iron, the latter inducing a conformational change which prevents attachment to the mRNA. In the presence of intracellular iron, synthesis of transferrin receptors is therefore inhibited, and ferritin synthesis enhanced. These intracellular control mechanisms enhance the understanding of intracellular iron homeostasis. They clarify the recent demonstration that circulating transferrin receptors released from the surface of proliferating cells, are increased in proportion to the amount of erythropoiesis, but also in iron deficiency

(Huebers et al 1990). Breakdown of the homeostatic mechanisms may lead to an excess of intracellular transit iron; this is responsible for much of the toxicity of iron overload, as well as being the major source of iron chelated by the drug desferrioxamine, currently used in the treatment of iron-loading anaemias (p. 221).

Food iron absorption

Regulation of body iron is exclusively dependent on iron absorption, since there is no physiological mechanism for the excretion of excess iron (McCance & Widdowson 1937). Although the uptake of iron by the intestinal mucosal cells and its transfer to the portal circulation are regulated in response to body iron stores, anaemic hypoxia, and (less well understood) the degree of erythropoietic activity (Bothwell et al 1979), the quantity and form of iron present in the diet primarily determines how much iron is available. Food iron exists either as non-haem Fe(III) complexes or, in smaller quantities, as haem proteins present in meat. Haem is absorbed intact, the iron being released within the intestinal mucosal cell, and its uptake is relatively unaffected by the rest of the gut contents. However, the availability of Fe(III) is highly dependent upon factors which maintain it in solution within the gut lumen; these include hydrochloric acid, which promotes ionisation, and dietary constituents which form soluble complexes (e.g. ascorbic acid). Many other dietary constituents (e.g. the phosphate and phytates common in vegetarian diets) form insoluble complexes with the iron, which is thus rendered unavailable. As well as containing haem iron, products of meat digestion also enhance the availability of inorganic Fe(III). Mixed, meat-containing diets therefore have a considerable advantage in terms of iron availability compared with the vegetarian diets common in much of the world.

Changes in body iron during development

During fetal development, the accumulation of haemoglobin and storage iron is relatively independent of maternal iron status, although where the mother has a severe iron deficiency anaemia during pregnancy, the newborn child can also have a slight reduction in haemoglobin concentration (Singla et al 1978). At birth, a full-term infant has a total body iron content of approximately 78 mg/kg, of which over 75% is in the form of haemoglobin (Josephs 1959). The exact amount is dependent upon the haemoglobin concentration at birth, which in turn is greatly affected by the time at which the umbilical cord is clamped: the red cell mass may increase from around 30 ml/kg to 50 ml/kg with late clamping. A low endowment of iron as haemoglobin can also result from prematurity, fetal-maternal haemorrhage at delivery, twin transfusion syndrome, or fetal blood loss during delivery.

After birth, arterial oxygen saturation increases, erythropoietin secretion declines, and there is a consequent marked fall in erythropoietic activity, with the disappearance of nucleated red blood cells and reticulocytes from the peripheral blood. Neonatal red cells have a shorter red cell survival than do adult red cells, and as they are cleared by the macrophages, haemoglobin concentration falls. The iron thus released goes to increase the iron stores within macrophages. This initial drop in haemoglobin concentration is followed after approximately 2 months by a resumption of erythropoiesis to maintain haemoglobin concentrations. The internal reutilization of iron accounts for over 95% of iron requirements in adults. However, in rapidly growing infants (tripling birth weight during the first year of life) only about 70% of the required red cell iron can be derived from senescent red cells, the remaining iron being derived from neonatal iron stores until they are exhausted, and thereafter from the diet. Iron stores are rarely depleted before 6 months in full-term infants. However, in premature infants the low birth weight means that the total iron endowment is much less, and with a more rapid rate of postnatal growth iron stores will be exhausted much more rapidly (Dallman et al 1980).

Iron deficiency is therefore most likely to occur between 6 months and 2–3 years of age (earlier in premature infants), at a time when iron stores are normally very low. However, iron deficiency is also common in preschool children where the composition of the diet may continue to limit iron availability. A further period of rapid growth during adolescence is compounded in girls by an

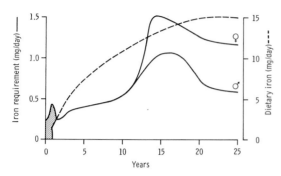

Fig. 8.3 Daily iron requirements at various ages (solid lines; upper female, lower male) in relation to the iron available in an average Western diet (dotted line). The shaded area during the first year indicates a period of negative iron balance met by utilization of neonatal iron stores. Iron balance is marginal at two critical periods of rapid growth. Reproduced from Bothwell et al 1979, with permission of Blackwell Scientific Publications Ltd.

Table 8.2   Causes of iron deficiency in childhood

Dietary insufficiency
  Early transfer from iron-fortified formula to cow's milk for
  bottle feeding
  Inadequate use of iron-fortified cereal after weaning
  Predominantly vegetarian diet
Increased physiological requirements
  Rapid growth in infancy (especially up to age 2–3 years and
  in low-birth-weight infants)
  Adolescent growth spurt (especially in girls)
Blood loss
  Perinatal: fetal-maternal, placenta, twin-to-twin
  Gastrointestinal: fresh cow's milk intolerance, parasites
  (e.g. hookworm), non-steroidal analgesics, Meckel's
  diverticulum, haemorrhagic telangiectasia, peptic ulcer,
  inflammatory bowel disease
Malabsorption
  Coeliac disease

increased requirement for the replacement of iron lost during menstruation, and leads to a further period of increased dependence upon dietary iron. Since iron in the diet is of limited, though variable, availability, these periods of rapid growth are particularly associated with the risk of developing iron deficiency (Fig. 8.3). It is not until growth stops after adolescence that iron stores begin to increase in young adult males, though in females iron stores approach adult male values only after the menopause.

Causes of iron deficiency

The factors that may give rise to iron deficiency in children are summarized in Table 8.2. The combination of rapid growth and lack of availability of dietary iron is the most common cause of iron deficiency; the possibility of a malignant cause of blood loss is less of a concern than in adults.

In mixed Western diets, there are approximately 6 mg of iron per 1000 kcal. The milk in the diet of infants contains a much lower amount of iron, around 1.5 mg per 1000 kcal in both breast milk and cow's milk. However, the iron in breast milk is much more available than that of cow's milk (Saarinen et al 1977). Though the mechanism of this enhanced availability of breast milk iron is not understood, it tends to compensate for the low concentration of iron and to give some protection against the development of iron deficiency. Iron supplementation of an infant formula based on

cow's milk (to 10–20 times the amount of iron in unfortified milk) increases the uptake of iron from this source. At weaning to solid foods, the combination of foods in the diet becomes important in determining the availability of the iron (Monson et al 1978). An iron intake of 1 mg/kg per day is recommended for full-term infants aged 0.5–3 years. This requirement could be met, and iron deficiency largely prevented, by:

1. continued breast feeding for 6 months (or the use of an iron-supplemented formula)
2. avoidance of cow's milk,
3. weaning to iron-containing foods by the age of 6 months, with the inclusion of enhancers of iron absorption (vitamin C and meat) (Burman 1982).

In low birth weight infants, recommended iron intake is greater at 2 mg/kg (maximum 15 mg) per day, starting no later than 2 months of age (American Academy of Pediatrics Committee on Nutrition 1976), and even higher amounts of iron may be required for very low birth weight infants. A summary of dietary iron recommendations for children and adults is shown in Table 8.3.

Occult gastrointestinal blood loss is commonly associated with unprocessed cow's milk feeding in early infancy (Formon et al 1981), compounding the low iron content and poor availability of the iron in cow's milk. In many parts of the world, blood loss related to hookworm is common, and proportional to the magnitude of the infestation.

Table 8.3 Recommended daily intake of iron.

	Age (years)	Recommended dietary iron (mg/day)
Infants	0.5–3	15
Children	4–10	10
Adolescents	11–18	18
Men	>19	10
Women: premenopause	19–50	18
postmenopause	>50	10

These figures (based on American Academy of Pediatrics, Committee on Nutrition, 1976, and World Health Organization Technical Report, 1972) are an approximate guide for an average 'western' diet, and will vary considerably with the composition of the diet, particularly its content of food derived from animals.

Iron deficiency itself may cause damage to the intestinal mucosa, with induction of blood loss and impaired absorption of iron (Naiman et al 1964, Kimber & Weintraub 1968), though it has sometimes been difficult to separate the effects of cow's milk intolerance from a direct effect of iron deficiency. Of the other causes of gastrointestinal blood loss in children, Meckel's diverticulum warrants special mention as a cause of painless intermittent blood loss and iron deficiency (Brayton 1964, Spencer 1964). Iron deficiency may also develop in patients with haemophilia. Malabsorption of inorganic iron rather than haem iron is common in coeliac disease (Anand et al 1977). Occasionally, iron deficiency anaemia may be the sole manifestation of coeliac disease.

In the vast majority of cases, iron deficiency in children is related to a dietary deficiency. Unless the anaemia is severe in the presence of an apparently adequate diet, or there is clinical evidence of overt blood loss or underlying disease, detailed investigation for the more unusual causes shown in Table 8.3 is not normally warranted. However, recurrent anaemia or failure to respond to iron therapy should lead to further investigation for blood loss or malabsorption.

Prevalence of iron deficiency

A recent survey in the UK showed that 26% of children aged 17–19 months were anaemic, as defined by a haemoglobin concentration of less than 11 g/dl (Aukett et al 1986). Studies in children admitted to hospital (Ehrhardt 1986) and in children attending community infant welfare clinics (Earley et al 1990) have shown a similar prevalence of 20–30% iron deficiency anaemia. The frequency was higher among children with an Asian rather than European background, a vegetarian diet being commoner among the Asian subgroup (Earley et al 1990). In US surveys, 3–24% of toddlers were found to have an iron deficiency anaemia (Oski & Stockman 1980). Socioeconomic factors are likely to contribute a major part of the risk of developing iron deficiency during the first 3 years of life. There is evidence from the US that the prevalence of anaemia among low-income children is declining, probably as a result of efforts to supplement the diet (Yip et al 1987).

Clinical features of iron deficiency

Nonspecific effects of anaemia include decreased exercise tolerance and listlessness, pallor of the mucous membranes, nailbeds and palms, and systolic cardiac flow murmurs. There may be clinical evidence of the underlying disease if iron deficiency is secondary to blood loss or malabsorption.

There has been a renewal of interest in possible nonhaematological effects of iron deficiency (Table 8.4). In addition to the well-known epithelial changes of chronic iron deficiency (including buccal mucosal atrophy and koilonychia), more subtle effects on behaviour, muscle function and immune function have been suggested. Of particular concern has been the mounting evidence that, in infants, there may be decreased responsiveness, activity and attention span in those who are iron deficient. The effect may be more profound in those with more prolonged iron deficiency (Lozoff & Brittenham 1982). Even children who have evidence of storage iron depletion but no anaemia may be at risk (Oski et al 1983). Iron therapy may improve weight gain and psychomotor development (Aukett et al 1986). The long-term consequences of iron deficiency at this early stage of brain development and growth are far from clear. However, evidence that children who were iron deficient in infancy have lower scores on tests of mental and motor functioning when they first attend school (Lozoff et al 1991) does give cause for concern, and provides an additional rationale for ensuring adequate iron nutrition during infancy.

Table 8.4 Nonhaematological effects of iron deficiency*

Target system	Effect	Possible mechanisms
Skin and gut	Koilonychia Glossitis Oesophageal web ?Achlorhydria	Poorly defined epithelial or mucosal enzyme deficiencies (e.g. of cytochrome oxidase in buccal epithelium)
	Increased absorption of lead and cadmium	Shared absorptive pathway with iron (Bothwell et al 1979)
Muscles	Diminished work performance, independent of anaemia. Rapid development of lactic acidosis on exercise (Finch et al 1979)	Mitochondrial abnormalities (Cartier et al 1986), with abnormal oxidative phosphorylation. Diminished alpha glycerophosphate dehydrogenase (Finch et al 1976)
Nervous system	Diminished attention span, and reduced cognitive performance in children (Lozoff et al 1987, Aukett et al 1986)	Deficiencies of iron-dependent brain enzymes, e.g. tyrosine hydroxylase, tryptophan pyrrolase and aldehyde oxidase (Mackler et al 1978). Reduced dopamine receptor function (Yelunda 1990)
	Pica in adults and children	
	Increased plasma and urinary catacholamines (Voorhess et al 1975)	Monoamine oxidase deficiency. Impaired conversion of tetraiodothyronine (T4) to triiodothyronine (T3) with compensatory sympathetic activity (Dillman et al 1980, Beard 1987)
Immunity	Diminished T-cell function and cell-mediated immunity (Dallman 1987)	Diminished activity of ribonucleotide reductase required for DNA synthesis during lymphocyte proliferation.
	Impaired neutrophil bactericidal activity (Chandra 1973, Walter et al 1986, Dallman 1987)	Reduced myeloperoxidase activity.

*For general reviews see Dallman et al 1978, Cook & Lynch 1986, Dobbing 1989.
Modified from Peters & Pippard 1990, with permission.

Both iron deficiency and iron excess can be associated with an increased risk of infection. Impaired lymphocyte and neutrophil function in iron deficiency may provide a basis for reports of an increased incidence of childhood respiratory tract infections and of mucocutaneous candidiasis (Higgs & Wells 1972), but this is difficult to separate from the effects of poor socioeconomic conditions, which are also associated with iron deficiency. Paradoxically, iron excess may also potentiate infection, perhaps by providing bacteria with iron that would otherwise be scavenged by the large excess of transferrin in patients with iron deficiency (Weinberg 1984). Malarial infections may be exacerbated by parenteral iron (Oppenheimer et al 1986), and it has been suggested that treatment of iron deficiency anaemia in the tropics should be accompanied by prophylactic antimalarial therapy (Fleming 1982). However, there is no evidence that iron fortification of infant formulae and foods increases the risk of infection, and the benefits of supplementation seem to outweigh any possible adverse effects (American Academy of Pediatrics Committee on Nutrition 1978).

Diagnosis of iron deficiency

During a period of progressive negative iron balance (where iron needs outstrip the dietary availability), iron stores are first utilized, and only then does the supply of iron to the tissues begin to diminish. Eventually, functional iron compounds, including circulating haemoglobin, are affected. The laboratory tests that are used for confirming the various stages of the development of iron deficiency are summarized in Table 8.5.

Where the haemoglobin is less than 10 g/dl, there is usually little difficulty in confirming the diagnosis. The red cell MCV will be reduced, and any one of the other measurements of iron status shown in Table 8.5 is also likely to be abnormal.

In mild iron deficiency, however, laboratory confirmation of the diagnosis may be more difficult. This is because not only is there an overlap between normal and abnormal haemoglobin con-

Table 8.5 Stages in the development of iron deficiency

Iron status	Test	Confirmatory results at ages (years):	
		0.5–2.0	>12
1. Loss of storage iron	Serum ferritin	<10	<10 (µg/1)
2. Impaired iron supply to tissues	Serum iron	<4*	<10 (µmol/1)
	% saturation of serum TIBC	<7*	<16 (%)
	Erythrocyte protoporphyrin	>70	>70 (µg/dl red cells)
3. Iron deficiency anaemia	Haemoglobin concentration	<11.0*	<12.0 (g/dl)
	Red cell MCV	<72*	<78 (fl)
	Blood film	Microcytic hypochromic red cells	

*Reference ranges show lower values in children compared with adults (Koerper & Dallman 1977)

centrations, but the other measures of iron status also show this overlap. Since iron stores are frequently reduced in infants over the age 6 months, the serum ferritin concentration, reflecting iron stores, may not be helpful. Serum iron concentrations are lower in infancy and childhood than in adults (Koerper & Dallman 1977), and only in anaemic patients with a low MCV does a transferrin saturation of less than 16% constitute good evidence of iron deficiency. The normally lower MCV of infants needs to be remembered (Ch. 1). In one-year-old infants with mild anaemia (Hb <11.5 g/dl), increasing the number of confirmatory tests (MCV, erythrocyte protoporphyrin, percentage saturation of TIBC and serum ferritin) increases the likelihood of being able accurately to predict a response to oral iron therapy. However, in one study, if at least two of the confirmatory tests had to be abnormal to qualify for treatment, more than half of the potential responders would have been missed, whereas if abnormality in only one confirmatory test was considered adequate, a large number of children would have been treated who did not respond (Dallman et al 1981). These findings suggest that a therapeutic trial of oral iron may be the most practical approach in mildly anaemic (haemoglobin 10.5–11.5 g/dl) children.

The possible nonhaematological effects of iron deficiency, particularly on brain development, have provoked a renewed interest in screening for iron deficiency in infants (Lancet Editorial 1987). The haemoglobin concentration has usually been

the primary screening measure, perhaps with the addition of a reduction in red cell MCV. Dallman et al (1980) point out the critical importance of defining the reference ranges for the particular population under study, and the need for great care to exclude not only patients with mild iron deficiency, but also patients carrying a thalassaemia trait or with an infection. In the UK, this is particularly relevant to recent surveys of iron deficiency in Asian compared with European children. A reduction in red cell size has been reported more often in Asian subgroups, but cannot be attributed to iron deficiency without exclusion of coincidental thalassaemia trait. While beta thalassaemia trait can be readily identified, there is no simple confirmatory laboratory test for alpha thalassaemia (see p. 218). In one study of Gujarati Asian children attending an infant welfare clinic, 21% of those showing a microcytosis (MCV less than 74 fl) were found to have a thalassaemia trait, and in half of these alpha globin gene mapping showed the presence of alpha thalassaemia (Earley et al 1990). A substantial minority of patients with thalassaemia genes may therefore be exposed to a therapeutic trial of iron therapy as a result of enthusiastic screening. This emphasizes the importance of assessing the response to a short course of oral iron and considering a thalassaemia trait in those who do not respond.

Treatment of iron deficiency

Oral iron therapy. This is to be preferred to parenteral iron therapy in virtually all cases since there is no evidence that the rate of haemoglobin response is greater with parenteral iron, and the latter has the potential for more serious adverse reactions. The object of treatment is to correct the deficit in circulating haemoglobin concentration and to replenish iron stores.

Iron is equally well absorbed from all the commonly used ferrous salts, but poorly absorbed if given as ferric iron. Children appear to tolerate iron better than do adults, and can take up to 5 mg/kg per day. Paediatric ferrous sulphate mixture BP (12 mg iron/5 ml) and ferrous fumerate mixture BP (45 mg iron/5 ml) and ferrous succinate elixir (37 mg iron/5 ml) are suitable preparations. In older children, ferrous sulphate tablets should be used.

Iron absorption is greater when the oral iron is given on an empty stomach than when administered with meals. Intolerance of such oral iron is rare in children and should be managed by reduction in dose or with the advice to take the tablets with meals. There is no point in changing to other iron preparations (e.g. slow-release forms of iron), since any adverse effects (e.g. nausea, constipation, abdominal pain) are clearly related to the dose of available iron; better-tolerated preparations are often more expensive ways to give less available iron. Iron staining of the teeth may occur with liquid preparations, but this is transient and can be prevented by using a straw or dropper to place the iron solution on the back of the tongue. Treatment should continue for 3–6 months. The peak reticulocyte response occurs at around 7–10 days in patients with severe anaemia. It is important to check the haemoglobin concentration after a month, particularly if the iron is being given to patients with mild anaemia as a therapeutic trial (see above).

Failure of response to therapy should lead to a reconsideration of the diagnosis of iron deficiency. Other causes of microcytic anaemia include chronic inflammatory disease and thalassaemia trait (see below). Less common are patients with sideroblastic anaemia, but these patients have marked ineffective erythropoiesis and are at risk of iron overload – it is therefore of vital importance to avoid inappropriate iron therapy. If iron deficiency is confirmed as the sole cause of the anaemia, the most common reason for a lack of response is that the child is not taking the iron prescribed. Alternatively, there may be continuing blood loss greater than that which can be made good by oral iron, or the iron may not be absorbed e.g. in coeliac disease.

Parenteral iron therapy. This should be considered only if there is a failure of oral iron therapy in proven iron deficiency. There are two preparations available for parenteral use, each containing 50 mg iron/ml: iron dextran injection (Imferon) and iron sorbitol injection (Jectofer). Iron dextran can be given either intramuscularly or intravenously, the latter usually as a single total dose intravenous infusion over 6–8 hours. Iron sorbitol can be given only by intramuscular injection. Both preparations give rise to skin staining

unless the intramuscular injection is deep and via a 'z'-shaped track.

A rough rule of thumb for the total dose of parenteral iron required is related to age: 100 mg iron for infants under 6 months, 200 mg for those aged 6–12 months, 300 mg for those aged 12–24 months, and 400 mg for those over 24 months. Intramuscular injections can be given as 1 ml (50 mg) at daily intervals. The total dose of iron dextran to be used as an intravenous infusion can be calculated, giving 2.5 mg iron/kg for each g/dl of haemoglobin deficit and an additional 10 mg/kg to replenish iron stores. For such intravenous infusions a small test dose must be given initially followed by a slow infusion of the total dose over approximately 6 hours. Adrenalin and hydrocortisone must be immediately available in case of anaphylactic response. Other adverse effects include transient arthralgia, fever and lymphadenopathy.

Other disorders associated with iron-deficient erythropoiesis

Anaemia of chronic disorders

Perhaps the commonest form of anaemia in hospital patients is that associated with an underlying acute or chronic inflammatory or infective disease. A normochromic normocytic anaemia in acute inflammation can progress to a more microcytic blood picture with prolonged inflammation. The anaemia is multifactorial in origin with several different effects being mediated by inflammatory mediators such as interleukin-1 (Lee 1983). Red cell survival is modestly reduced and, despite earlier conflicting results, it now appears clear that the erythropoietin response to anaemia is blunted during inflammation (Baer et al 1987). The macrophages, responsible for the shortening of red cell survival, also show trapping of iron derived from senescent red cells with diminished reutilisation of the iron. It is the subsequent fall in serum iron which is responsible for impaired haemoglobin synthesis and progressive development of microcytic red cells. Enhancement of macrophage activity appears central to these effects, and a stimulation of ferritin protein synthesis which is independent of the intracellular iron content may account for the diversion of iron to iron stores (Konijn & Hershko 1977). In the severe inflammation associated with juvenile chronic arthritis, 40% of patients were found to have a microcytic anaemia, in some cases severe (Harvey et al 1987); unlike in iron deficiency, however, the serum ferritin concentration was highest in those who were most anaemic, confirming the movement of iron from circulating red cell haemoglobin to macrophage iron stores. It may be difficult to diagnose coincidental iron deficiency in the presence of chronic inflammatory disease (Koerper et al 1978), though a serum ferritin below 50 µg/l warrants a trial of oral iron therapy. A bone marrow examination stained for macrophage iron stores may sometimes be the quickest and most certain way of determining whether these are present or absent.

Chronic renal failure

Patients with the anaemia of chronic renal failure provide a special case, in that the predominant mechanism is one of reduced erythropoietin production. However, as in other chronic disorders, the serum ferritin concentration may be within the normal range despite absent iron stores, and iron supplementation is likely to be required to compensate for the inevitable blood losses associated with regular haemodialysis. Regular monitoring of the serum ferritin is therefore required, and has become even more necessary with the advent of treatment using recombinant human erythropoietin for the anaemia. During erythropoietin treatment, the rate of mobilization of iron stores in chronic renal disease may be inadequate to prevent the development of a 'relative' iron deficiency with reduced transferrin saturation (Eschbach 1987). Although this relative iron lack can be overcome with iron supplements, slowing of the rate of haemoglobin regeneration by reducing the dose of erythropoietin may be a more appropriate therapeutic strategy. Occasionally, parenteral iron may be required (Macdougall et al 1990).

In chronic renal failure, a microcytic anaemia may also result from aluminium accumulation from dialysis fluids (Drueke et al 1986). Aluminium may inhibit erythropoiesis by an unknown mechanism involving transferrin binding of the metal (Mladenovich 1988), though inhibition of haem synthetic enzymes may be important. Reversal of this anaemia may require chelation therapy with desferrioxamine as well as removal of the aluminium from the dialysis fluid.

Unusual causes of iron-deficient erythropoiesis

Iron sequestration

In *idiopathic pulmonary haemosiderosis*, haemorrhage into the lung results in episodes of fever, cough and sometimes haemoptysis in association with evidence of iron deficiency anaemia (Apt et al 1957). The sputum contains haemosiderin-laden macrophages, and a chest X-ray during exacerbation may show diffuse opacities. Acute episodes usually last several days but may persist for several weeks. Onset is usually in childhood and the disease usually ends in a fatal acute exacerbation. A similar chest picture with localized pulmonary haemosiderosis is seen in Goodpasture's syndrome, associated with glomerulonephritis and antiglomerular basement membrane antibodies in the serum (Briggs et al 1979).

Disorders of iron transport

The extremely rare disorder of *congenital deficiency of transferrin* is associated with a hypochromic microcytic anaemia, iron loading of the liver and other tissues, and death in childhood. Increased iron absorption from the diet (Goya et al 1972) indicates that this iron uptake is not dependent upon the presence of circulating transferrin.

An acquired severe microcytic anaemia has been described in a woman with elevated serum iron and *autoantibodies to transferrin receptors* (Larrick & Hyman 1984). Although the authors postulate that the antibodies interfere with iron incorporation by erythroid precursors, this is difficult to reconcile with their finding of a greatly increased plasma iron turnover – the latter suggests a marked degree of ineffective erythropoiesis. Shahidi et al (1964) had earlier described two siblings with a hypochromic microcytic anaemia who also had an increased concentration of serum iron, with iron overload of liver parenchymal cells only and an absence of iron in either macrophages or erythroid precursors. This suggests a defective uptake of iron by erythroblasts but the mechanism is unknown.

Copper deficiency is unusual in man and gives rise to a low serum iron concentration and hypochromic anaemia in the presence of adequate iron stores (Lahey et al 1952). The mechanism is uncertain, though it has been postulated that copper's role in ceruloplasmin (ferroxidase) may be important in mobilizing iron stores. Copper deficiency tends to occur in situations of severe dietary abnormality (e.g. when omitted from parenteral feeding regimes). Leucopenia is characteristic. Treatment is with 0.2 mg/kg copper daily by mouth in the form of 0.5% copper sulphate.

Sideroblastic anaemias

The sideroblastic anaemias are a heterogenous group of disorders characterized by a major or minor population of hypochromic microcytic blood cells in the peripheral blood together with ringed sideroblasts in the bone marrow (Bottomley 1982). Ferrokinetic studies are consistent with ineffective erythropoiesis with a normal or only modestly reduced red cell survival. Ringed sideroblasts are erythroblasts with large iron (Prussian-Blue-positive) granules forming a partial or complete ring around the nucleus. These iron granules, seen on electron microscopy to be iron-laden mitochondria, need to be distinguished from the occasional granules seen in 30–60% of normal nucleated red cells (normal sideroblasts), and from the larger cytoplasmic granules seen in the thalassaemic or megaloblastic erythroblasts (Cartwright & Deiss 1975). Ringed sideroblasts occur in small numbers in several disorders of erythropoiesis, and an arbitrary definition of more than six perinuclear granules in over 10% of erythroblasts is used to define sideroblastic anaemia. The clinical features are dependent upon the severity of the anaemia, but it is important to realise that iron overload and its pathology may complicate long-standing disease.

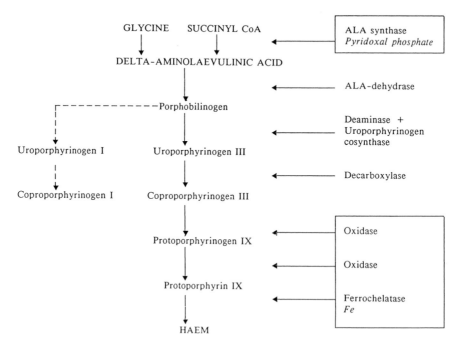

Fig. 8.4 Synthesis of haem. The enzymes shown enclosed by boxes are situated in mitochondria, whilst the others are cytosolic. The dotted lines indicate the alternative pathway followed when there is a relative lack of uroporphyrinogen cosynthase. The production of type I porphyrinogen isomers, which readily oxidize to photoactive porphyrins, is responsible for erythropoietic porphyria (accompanied by mutilating dermatitis and a haemolytic anaemia). By contrast, erythropoietic protoporphyria, presenting in childhood with skin photosensitivity, has a normal red cell survival and is due to a ferrochelatase deficiency in late normoblasts with excess production of diffusible unbound protoporphyrin.

Table 8.6 Classification of sideroblastic anaemias

Inherited
X-linked
Autosomal recessive (rare)

Acquired
Idiopathic
a. Myelodysplasia ('refractory anaemia with ringed
   sideroblasts')
b. Associated with other myeloproliferative and
   myelodysplastic disorders.

Secondary
a. Drug-induced:
      antituberculous chemotherapy
      chloramphenicol
b. Alcohol induced
c. Lead poisoning
d. Other associations (? chance):
      rheumatoid arthritis, carcinoma, myeloma, haemolytic
      anaemia, pernicious anaemia

The mitochondria are the site where haem synthesis first starts and is completed (Fig. 8.4). Failure to utilize iron for haem synthesis within the mitochondria appears to underly the iron accumulation. Impaired mitochondrial function is likely to contribute to a defect in erythroblast maturation, premature cell death, and ineffective erythropoiesis. The exact pathogenesis of the various types of sideroblastic anaemias (Table 8.6) is in many cases only partially understood.

Inherited sideroblastic anaemia

Inherited forms of sideroblastic anaemia are rare disorders usually presenting in males in childhood or adolescence. In most reported families, inheritance has followed an X-linked pattern (e.g. Rundles & Falls 1946). Female relatives may show partial expression, usually with only mild or no anaemia, though families have been described in which females are more severely affected (Lee et al 1968, Weatherall et al 1970, Peto et al 1983). This may depend on variation in the severity of the defect as well as the degree of Lyonization of the affected X-chromosome. The latter hypothesis receives some support from the presence of a true dual population of microcytic and normocytic red cells in affected females, rather than simply a widening of the red cell size distribution seen in affected males (Peto et al 1983). A few cases have been described in which the pattern of inheritance

appears to be autosomal recessive, though their clinical and haematological features were indistinguishable from the X-linked type.

In addition to the anaemia with a population of hypochromic-microcytic red cells, circulating siderocytes (with Pappenheimer bodies) are commonly seen, together with cells showing punctate basophilia. The bone marrow usually shows erythroid hyperplasia with rather ragged vacuolated cytoplasm in the erythroblasts. Storage iron is likely to be increased, and the ringed sideroblast abnormality affects large numbers of cells, particularly the late erythroblasts, though in mildly affected females only a small proportion of erythroblasts may show this change.

Clinical examination sometimes shows mild icterus in addition to pallor, and moderate splenomegaly and/or hepatomegaly may also be present. Where the disease has been longstanding, evidence of iron overload including cardiac, liver and endocrine dysfunction may be manifest. The serum iron concentration is typically increased with a reduced total iron binding capacity giving near saturation of the total iron binding capacity, indicating the risk of increased parenchymal tissue iron uptake which may eventually lead to toxic iron overload.

Acquired sideroblastic anaemia

Primary acquired sideroblastic anaemia. This is very rare before the third decade and characteristically occurs in older individuals, often in association with other evidence of myelodysplasia (Ch. 3). As in the inherited forms of sideroblastic anaemia, the severity of the anaemia is variable, but as well as a population of hypochromic-microcytic red cells, macrocytic cells usually predominate. There is a risk of transformation to acute myeloblastic leukaemia, though this is rather less than in the other myelodysplastic syndromes. As in the inherited disease, the bone marrow is usually hypercellular though there may be megaloblastic changes, and ringed sideroblasts are found in both early and late erythroblasts (Hall & Losowsky 1966). The anaemia may be stable for many years or may increase in severity so that blood transfusions become necessary. Iron overload will develop if the anaemia remains the sole manifestation of the underlying marrow disorder and the patient survives for a prolonged period.

Secondary sideroblastic anaemia. Sideroblastic anaemia may be found as a complication of antituberculous chemotherapy, particularly with the pyridoxine antagonists, isoniazid and cycloserine. It is likely that they interfere with pyridoxal phosphate function as a cofactor for ALA synthase (Fig. 8.4).

Chloramphenicol produces a dose-dependent suppression of erythropoiesis which is sometimes associated with ringed sideroblasts. The drug is a direct inhibitor of mitochondrial protein synthesis and is thought to act by causing diminished levels of ferrochelatase and thus inhibiting the insertion of iron into the protoporphyrin ring (Fig. 8.4).

Alcoholism results in a sideroblastic abnormality in up to 30% of anaemic patients, particularly when accompanied by folate deficiency and malnutrition. (Eichner & Hillman 1971). Sideroblastic change is seen only with chronic alcohol abuse and not with acute intoxication.

Lead poisoning disrupts several stages of haem synthesis, and in some cases ringed sideroblasts are visible in the marrow.

An antibody-mediated acquired sideroblastic anaemia was reported in a child who developed erythroid hypoplasia and ringed sideroblasts (Ritchey et al 1979). There are also isolated case reports in rheumatoid arthritis and juvenile chronic arthritis (Harvey et al 1987).

Pathogenesis of sideroblastic anaemia

Reduced levels of ALA synthase are described in all forms of sideroblastic anaemia (Bottomley 1982). It is easy to imagine that a defect in this mitochondrial enzyme, which is rate-limiting for haem biosynthesis, could lead to accumulation of iron in the mitochondria. ALA synthase requires pyridoxal phosphate as coenzyme and protection of a labile ALA synthase from proteolytic degradation (Aoki et al 1979), or a low affinity of the enzyme for pyridoxal phosphate (Konopka & Hoffbrand 1979) could explain the response to pharmacological doses of pyridoxine of a number of cases of inherited sideroblastic anaemia. Other haem synthetic enzymes may also be affected, and

a variable reduction of ferrochelatase activity has been found in both inherited and idiopathic acquired sideroblastic anaemias. A decreased activity of ferrochelatase could explain the elevation of free erythrocyte protoporphyrin found in most patients with the primary acquired disorder, and contrasts with the reduced free erythrocyte protoporphyrin more usual in patients with inherited forms of sideroblastic anaemia. In many cases, the defects of haem synthetic enzymes may be secondary to general disturbance of mitochondrial protein synthesis (Aoki 1980). It is possible that those patients who have a response to pharmacological doses of pyridoxine have a primary abnormality of ALA synthase itself, whereas unresponsive patients (including the majority of the idiopathic acquired disorders) may have defective mitochondrial function either secondary to a clonal abnormality of haemopoiesis or as a result of the iron accumulation itself.

Treatment of sideroblastic anaemias

In many patients, the anaemia may remain stable and asymptomatic for years. However, others may show a progressive fall in haemoglobin concentration or, being more severe from the start, require more active treatment. In all cases, a trial of oral pyridoxine (25–100 mg 3 times daily) should be given, but a clinically useful response is rare except in some kindreds with an inherited sideroblastic anaemia. In a very small number of cases, parenteral pyridoxal phosphate may be effective where oral treatment has failed. Any folic acid deficiency resulting from the erythroid hyperplasia should also be treated. Blood transfusion may be necessary and will inevitably lead to iron overload, for which iron chelation therapy using subcutaneous desferrioxamine will be required (p. 221). However, it should be noted that life-threatening iron overload may develop even without severe anaemia in patients with longstanding sideroblastic anaemia, as a result of excessive absorption of iron from the diet (Peto et al 1983). The risk of developing iron overload in the milder anaemias is directly related to the degree of erythroid hyperplasia, as has been found in a variety of other anaemias with ineffective erythropoiesis, including congenital dyserythro-

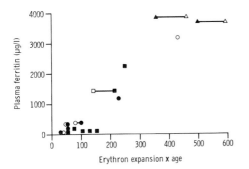

Fig. 8.5 Iron loading in untransfused dyserythropoietic anaemias is a function of erythroid expansion and age. Erythroid expansion (x normal) was assessed by ferrokinetic (black symbols), or marrow erythroid: myeloid ratios (white symbols), with paired values in some cases. ● = sideroblastic; ■ = thalassaemia intermedia; ▲ = congenital dyserythropoiesis type I.

poietic anaemias and the thalassaemia syndromes (Fig. 8.5). This emphasizes the need for careful monitoring of the saturation of the TIBC and the serum ferritin to anticipate and prevent the development of iron overload. In some cases with mild anaemia, treatment with regular phlebotomy rather than iron chelation therapy may be possible. It is of interest that improvement of the anaemia has occasionally followed phlebotomy, presumably by reversing a defect due to iron accumulation in the mitochondria (Weintraub et al 1966). Splenectomy should be avoided, since a high incidence of thrombo-embolism associated with a high postoperative platelet count may be expected.

Lead poisoning

Chronic lead ingestion is most prevalent among infants and children though it also occurs among occupationally exposed adults. Preschool children are at most risk, with their hand-to-mouth activities and ingestion of dust (e.g. from lead paint), as well as exposure to lead in the air derived from petrol engines. Lead absorption is increased by dietary deficiency of iron, common in this age group. With the additive risk from all sources it is children in poor urban environments who are at greatest risk.

In children, lead encephalopathy is the major clinical effect of lead exposure and it may give rise to an acute encephalopathy with coma and death. Anaemia is a late manifestation of lead poisoning and in children may be seen only in severe cases or in the presence of coexistent iron deficiency. Anaemia is usually normochromic or slightly hypochromic, with a shortening of red cell life-span and a mild increase in reticulocytes. Basophilic stippling is characteristic and is thought to be due to precipitation of ribosomal RNA and mitochondrial fragments, resulting from inhibition of the enzyme pyrimidine 5' nucleotidase (Paglia et al 1975). The bone marrow may show increased sideroblasts, sometimes with ringed sideroblasts. Lead is lipophilic and penetrates the red cells, so that the bulk of blood lead is within erythrocytes. Blocking of sulphydryl groups, with subsequent denaturation of structural proteins and enzymes and damage to mitochondria is likely to be the cause of the shortened red cell survival. Lead uptake by erythroblasts is followed by its concentration in the mitochondria, where delivery of iron to the protopophyrin and ferrochelatase is inhibited. This results in an accumulation of iron in the mitochondria as well as accumulation of erythrocyte protoporphyrin. The latter becomes converted to zinc protoporphyrin and remains in the red cells throughout their life-span. Fluorometric determination of zinc protoporphyrin can thus be used to screen for possible lead poisoning, with confirmation by blood lead measurement. Children with symptomatic lead poisoning require treatment which includes chelation therapy with dimercaprol (BAL) and calcium EDTA (Piomelli et al 1984).

DEFECTS IN HAEMOGLOBIN SYNTHESIS II. IMPAIRED GLOBIN CHAIN SYNTHESIS (THALASSAEMIAS)

The thalassaemias are inherited disorders of haemoglobin synthesis which result in a reduction in synthesis of one or more of the globin chains of haemoglobin. The resulting deficit in red cell haemoglobin production gives rise to microcytic and hypochromic red cells. The thalassaemias constitute one of the most frequent single-gene disorders, affecting about 4% of the world population (Thein & Weatherall, 1988). The genetic nature of the disorders means that severe thalassaemia syndromes are likely to be diagnosed in childhood, though some 'intermedia' syndromes may not be discovered until adult life and most heterozygotes are totally asymptomatic. In addition, the developmental changes in haemoglobin production during fetal and neonatal life, particularly the switch from the production of gamma globin chains and fetal haemoglobin (HbF) in utero to beta globin chains and adult haemoglobin (HbA) at around the time of birth, means that the phenotype of thalassaemia defects may change with development; for example, neonates with severe beta thalassaemia syndromes are not anaemic at birth, but become so only after the first few weeks of life, when HbA would normally have replaced the neonatal endowment of HbF.

Development changes in human haemoglobin synthesis

Human haemoglobins have a tetrameric structure consisting of two globin chains from the alpha globin gene cluster and two globin chains from the beta globin gene cluster (Table 8.7). During development, there is a single switch in production of alpha-like globin chains from zeta to alpha, while production of beta-like chains switches first from embryonic epsilon to fetal gamma and then, at around 32 weeks gestation, from gamma to adult beta chain. At the time of birth, about 60% of total haemoglobin synthesis is of HbF, though the proportion of circulating HbF remains higher at 70–90%. A slight excess of gamma over alpha chain production results in trace amounts of gamma$_4$ tetramer (Hb Bart's) even in normal babies (Weatherall 1963); in mild alpha thalassaemia syndromes, the presence of detectable amounts of Hb Bart's as a fast band on electrophoresis of cord blood haemoglobin makes confirmation of the presence of such alpha thalassaemia easier than at any time later in life (see below). After birth, the proportion of HbF in the circulating blood declines to around 5–20% at 4 months, and below 2% at one year (Huehns 1982).

Starting from the 5' end of the alpha globin gene cluster, the zeta gene is separated from two functional alpha globin genes (alpha^2 and alpha^1) by three nonfunctional pseudogenes. The normal alpha genotype can thus be written as $\alpha\alpha/\alpha\alpha$. From the 5' end of the beta gene cluster on chromosome 11, the episilon gene is followed by two gamma

Table 8.7 Haemoglobin tetramers at various stages of development. The sequential production of globin chains follows the order in which the corresponding genes are arranged (5' to 3') on chromosomes 16 and 11.

Stage of deveopment[*]	Haemoglobin	Globin chain constitution	
		From α-gene cluster (ch 16)	From β-gene cluster (ch 11)
Embryonic	Hb Gower I	$\zeta_2 \varepsilon_2$	
	Hb Portland	$\zeta_2 \gamma_2$	
	Hb Gower II	$\alpha_2 \varepsilon_2$	
Fetal	HbF	$\alpha_2 \gamma_2$ (G$_\gamma$) (A$_\gamma$)	
Adult	HbA$_2$ 2.5%	$\alpha_2 \delta_2$	
	HbA 97%	$\alpha_2 \beta_2$	

[*] The switch from embryonic to fetal haemoglobin occurs at 6–10 weeks gestation, and from fetal to adult haemoglobin at around the time of birth.

globin genes (^{G}gamma and ^{A}gamma) differing only in respect of coding for glycine or alanine at position 136 in the peptide chain. These are separated from the single beta globin gene on each chromosome by a nonfunctional pseudo-beta globin gene, and a hypofunctional delta globin gene responsible for the small output of delta chains for the minor adult haemoglobin, HbA$_2$. In both gene clusters, the genes are arranged in the same order (5' to 3') as they are expressed during development (Table 8.7). Little is known of the normal control mechanisms involved in regulating this haemoglobin switching, though hypomethylation of the promoter region 5' to each gene is likely to be involved.

Classification of the thalassaemias

The thalassaemias may be classified according to the particular globin chain which is produced at a reduced rate into alpha, beta, delta-beta, and gamma-delta-beta types. Where no alpha or beta chains are produced from the affected chromosome, the thalassaemias are described as alpha^0 or beta^0, to distinguish them from alpha$^+$ and beta$^+$ thalassaemias in which there is some synthesis but at a reduced rate. It should be noted that some structural haemoglobin variants are also synthesized at a reduced rate, the most common being HbE, and that these also may give rise to a thalassaemia phenotype. There is enormous scope for multiple interactions between different thalassaemia genes (and genes for structural haemoglobin variants).

Pathophysiology of the thalassaemias

Reduction in either alpha or beta chain synthesis, as well as giving rise to hypochromia and microcytosis of red cells, produces a relative excess of one of the globin chains. In the alpha thalassaemias, excess gamma (in fetal life) and then beta globin chains form stable tetramers called Hb Bart's (gamma$_4$) and HbH (beta$_4$) respectively. As the red cell ages and loses its antioxidant capacity these tetramers become insoluble, giving rise to inclusion bodies and subsequent trapping in the spleen, with a shortening of red cell survival. By contrast, unpaired alpha globin chains in the beta thalassaemias are highly unstable and form intracellular precipitates within developing erythroblasts in the bone marrow. These precipitates act to catalyze oxidative damage to cell membrane and contents, and result in intramedullary death and ineffective erythropoiesis. In addition, any red cells that do manage to enter the circulation are prematurely removed by the spleen. The only clinically important form of alpha thalassaemia (HbH disease) is therefore predominantly a haemolytic anaemia, whereas the major beta thalassaemia syndromes are characterized by extreme ineffective erythropoiesis, with bone marrow hyperplasia as well as shortened red cell survival.

Prevalence of thalassaemia syndromes

The thalassaemias are widely distributed through the Mediterranean, Middle East, India, South East Asia and Africa. The distribution parallels that of falciparum malaria. The cellular mechanism for a selective advantage of thalassaemia heterozygotes in protecting from malaria, particularly during early childhood, is not completely understood. Each population tends to have its own characteristic thalassaemia mutations (suggesting that these have arisen independently) and this is a factor of importance in devising strategies for the use of DNA analysis in antenatal diagnosis.

Alpha thalassaemias

The severity of the alpha thalassaemia syndromes depends upon the number of remaining functional alpha globin genes from the normal total of four (Table 8.8). The molecular defects underlying alpha thalassaemia are extremely varied, but the majority result from large deletions within the alpha gene complex. The deletion of one or other of the duplicated alpha globin genes give rise to an alpha$^+$ thalassaemia (also known as alpha thalassaemia 2). This results from misalignment and crossover during meiosis, and the expected reciprocal triplicate alpha gene arrangement has been seen in low frequency in many populations. By contrast, large deletions responsible for complete abolition of the globin output from both alpha genes, i.e. giving rise to an alpha^0 thalassaemia (also known as alpha thalassaemia 1), are more restricted in their geographical distribution, being particularly common in South East Asia

Table 8.8 The alpha thalassaemias

Functional alpha globin genes	Genotype	Syndrome	Haematological changes	Hb variants Birth	Later
4	αα/αα	Normal	None	None	None
3	−α/αα	Silent carrier or α thalassaemia minor (heterozygous α thal-2)	None or mild red cell hypochromia	Hb Bart's (1–2%)	None
2	−α/−α	α thalassaemia minor (homozygous α thal-2)	Mild anaemia with red cell hypochromia and microcytosis	Hb Bart's (2–10%)	None
	− −/αα	α thalassaemia minor (heterozygous α thal-1)			
1	−α /− −	Hb H disease	Chronic haemolytic anaemia	Hb Bart's (10–40%)	Hb H (5–40%)
	− −/αCS★				
0	− −/− −	Haemoglobin Bart's hydrops fetalis (homozygous α thal-1)	Intrauterine death or neonatal death within hours	Hb Bart's (>80%) Hb Portland Hb H	

★Gene for Hb Constant Spring (see text)

and, to a lesser extent, in the Middle East and in some Mediterranean island populations. Point mutations gives rise to the less common non-deletional forms of alpha thalassaemia; these may involve interference with gene transcription, RNA processing, or RNA translation. Hb QuongSze is a rare variant which causes the globin molecule to be unstable. A chain termination mutant which produces an alpha-globin chain with 31 additional amino acid residues (Hb Constant Spring) is common in South East Asia; the mutant chain is produced in very low quantities and thus gives rise to an alpha$^+$ thalassaemia phenotype.

The clinically important forms of alpha thalassaemia are the Hb Bart's hydrops fetalis syndrome (--/--) and HbH disease (-α/--).

Haemoglobin Bart's hydrops syndrome

Most frequent in South East Asia and in Greece and Cyprus, affected infants are usually stillborn between 28 and 40 weeks, or die within hours of birth. They are pale, with generalized oedema, massive hepatosplenomegaly and poorly expanded lungs. Nearly all their haemoglobin is Hb Bart's, which has a very high oxygen affinity and is thus nonfunctional. Survival to term is dependent upon the presence of about 20% Hb Portland, and there is a complete absence of HbF and HbA. The parents are obligatory carriers of alpha^0 thalassaemia. In the mother, there is a high incidence of toxaemia of pregnancy and other obstetric difficulties related to the large friable placenta.

A recent case report suggests that vigorous treatment with exchange transfusion very rarely may allow survival of a hydropic infant as a transfusion dependent major thalassaemia syndrome (Beaudry et al 1988). However, the report also indicates that the child had impaired mental development.

Haemoglobin H disease

With a single functioning alpha gene, there is a variable anaemia (normally in the range of 7–10 g/dl) and splenomegaly but the degree of erythroid expansion appears less than in the major beta thalassaemia syndromes (Pootrakul et al 1988). Survival into adult life is the rule, but worsening of the anaemia may result from progressive hyper-splenism and may be helped with splenectomy. Exacerbation of haemolysis commonly follows infection or exposure to oxidant drugs which increase the rate of precipitation of HbH. Patients should receive folate supplements (5 mg oral folic acid daily). Transfusion dependence is the exception rather than the rule, and severe iron overload does not usually develop.

Examination of the peripheral blood shows the thalassaemic features of hypochromia and microcytosis, as well as polychromasia and a moderate reticulocytosis. Incubation of red cells with brilliant cresyl blue demonstrates numerous inclusion bodies (HbH precipitated by the redox dye), and haemoglobin electrophoresis shows 5–40% HbH together with HbA (in neonates there are large amounts of Hb Bart's). Family studies will show that one parent is heterozygous for alpha^0 thalassaemia, and the other for alpha$^+$ thalassaemia or Hb Constant Spring.

An unusual form of acquired HbH is seen in association with myelodysplasic syndromes but this seems to be confined to the elderly. A rare association of HbH disease and mental retardation has been described in individuals who have one parent with alpha$^+$ thalassaemia with the other being normal. Here, it is thought that a new alpha^0 thalassaemia mutation has arisen on one chromosome 16 to produce HbH disease, but the mutation presumably also affects another gene important for normal mental development (Weatherall et al 1982).

Alpha thalassaemia carrier state

It can be difficult to make a positive diagnosis of an alpha thalassaemia carrier state by standard haematological studies. Loss of two alpha-globin genes usually gives rise to thalassaemic red cell indices with microcytic hypochromic red cells and an increased red cell count. Very occasional red cells containing HbH inclusions may be seen on incubation with brilliant cresyl blue. A single alpha globin gene deletion can be even more difficult to detect since the red cell indices overlap with the normal reference range. The globin chain synthesis ratios also show an overlap with normal and hence cannot be used to make a definitive diagnosis. Both forms of carrier state can be identified more easily in the newborn, where cord blood samples show a microcytosis instead of the expected macrocytosis, and the presence of Hb Bart's in small quantities. Only in the antenatal clinic, where accurate counselling of prospective parents may require differentiation from the rare normal HbA$_2$ heterozygous beta thalassaemia, is alpha globin gene mapping likely to be needed, and even this will not detect nondeletional forms of alpha thalassaemia.

Beta thalassaemias

The beta thalassaemias are a much more serious public health problem than alpha thalassaemias because individuals affected by the severe forms develop normally in utero and only become anaemic during the first few months of life. Unlike the alpha thalassaemias, the majority of beta thalassaemia genes arise from point mutations rather than gene deletion (Thein & Weatherall 1988). However, a number of gene deletions have been described, including an Indian 619-base-pair deletion from the 3' end of the beta globin gene. The nondeletional forms of beta thalassaemia include transcriptional mutations affecting promoter sequences for the beta globin gene; mutations leading to the production of nonfunctional RNA (e.g. by 'nonsense' mutations which prematurely terminate globin chain synthesis with a single base change in the RNA to form a stop codon, or by 'frame-shift' mutations which by loss or insertion of one or more bases throw the reading frame out of phase and prevent correct translation from the mRNA); and RNA processing mutants which result from faulty splicing of exons after the introns have been removed during the processing of the RNA. The latter form the majority of beta thalassaemia mutations.

The clinical expression of the beta thalassaemias ranges through thalassaemia minor (usually symptomless), thalassaemia intermedia (associated with anaemia and splenomegaly but without the need for regular blood transfusions) and thalassaemia major (a severe transfusion-dependent disorder). This variation depends upon whether the patient has inherited one or two beta thalassaemia genes as well as the severity of these particular genes. Typical findings are shown in Table 8.9.

Table 8.9 Thalassaemia involving the β globin gene cluster on chromosome 11

Type of thalassaemia	Typical findings	
	Heterozygote	Homozygote
β^0	Thalassaemia minor Raised HbA$_2$ 4–7%	Thalassaemia major* HbF 98% + HbA$_2$
β$^+$	Thalassaemia minor Raised HbA$_2$ 4–7%	Thalassaemia major HbF 30–90% + HbA + HbA$_2$
δβ	Thalassaemia minor HbF 5–15%, HbA$_2$ normal	Thalassaemia intermedia HbF only
δβ (Lepore)	Thalassaemia minor Hb Lepore 5–15%, HbA$_2$ normal	Thalassaemia major or intermedia HbF + Hb Lepore
γδβ	Neonatal haemolysis Thalassaemia minor with normal HbA$_2$ and HbF	Non-viable

* Many patients are compound heterozygotes for different molecular forms of β$^+$ and/or β^0 thalassaemia. A small proportion will have a thalassaemia intermedia syndrome by virtue of one of the reasons shown in Table 8.10.

Beta thalassaemia major

The severe homozygous or compound heterozygous forms of beta thalassaemia typically present in the first year of life with failure to thrive, poor feeding and recurrent respiratory infection. Pallor and hepatosplenomegaly are characteristic. A minority of patients present rather later in the second year of life and may have the somewhat milder clinical course of thalassaemia intermedia (see below). Haematological investigations show a severe anaemia with markedly hypochromic red cells, though the MCV is not usually as low as in heterozygous beta thalassaemias. A marked variation in red cell size and basophilic stippling is accompanied by nucleated red cells in the peripheral blood; the latter increase greatly after splenectomy. A bone marrow examination is not required for diagnosis, but there is massive erythroid hyperplasia, and many of the red cell precursors contain alpha chain inclusion bodies which can be stained with methyl violet. The serum bilirubin concentration is usually raised, reflecting the ineffective erythropoiesis and shortened red cell survival.

Although HbF production normally ceases at around the time of birth, a small proportion of erythroblasts normally retains the capacity to synthesize gamma chains. Since the pathophysiology of homozygous beta thalassaemia is related to the

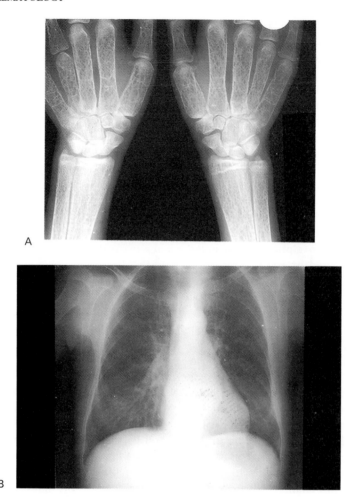

Fig. 8.6 X-ray apperances in poorly transfused β thalassaemia major. **A**. Hands showing widening of bones and lacy trabecular pattern. **B**. Chest X-ray showing 'double' heart contour – the dense shadow is a retrocardiac paraspinal extramedullary erythroid mass.

unbalanced globin chain synthesis and accumulation of excess alpha globin chains, cells with the ability to reduce this imbalance by producing gamma globin chains are more likely to survive and reach the circulation. In beta^0 thalassaemia, the only haemoglobin which can be produced is HbF, but a variable amount of HbA will be produced with beta$^+$ thalassaemia genes. It is important to carry out haemoglobin electrophoresis before blood transfusion to distinguish these two possibilities. In the absence of transfusion, death within the first two years of life is the rule. With inadequate transfusion, there is progressive splenomegaly and hypersplenism which combines with the ineffective erythropoiesis to increase the severity of the anaemia. The HbF which is produced

has a high oxygen affinity, further exacerbating the tissue hypoxia and leading to massive marrow expansion under erythropoietin drive. The bone marrow expansion leads to gross deformities of the skull, with thickening and overgrowth of the zygomata. However, these changes are widespread throughout the skeleton with a lacy trabecular pattern on X-ray (Fig. 8.6A), and spontaneous fractures may occur. Bone marrow expansion may not be confined to the skeleton, and extramedullary tumour masses, e.g. in the thorax (Fig 8.6B) and skull, can cause local complications. Intercurrent infections, leg ulcers and a hypermetabolic state with weight loss, fever and secondary gout are common. The massive bone marrow expansion is associated with an inappropriate increase in gastrointestinal iron absorption, and tissue iron loading and damage may occur in later childhood even in the absence of regular blood transfusions.

With regular blood transfusion, early growth and development is normal, but at around the time of puberty complications of iron overload (hepatic, cardiac and endocrine disturbances) begin to occur. Secondary sexual development is delayed or absent, the pubertal growth spurt does not occur, and death, usually from cardiac failure or arrhythmia, is usual by the end of the second decade in the absence of iron chelation therapy (see below).

Management. The great variety of clinical and psychological problems accompanying this chronic disorder and its management emphasize the need for joint surveillance by paediatrician and haematologist, with the support of specialist physicians to deal with, for example, endocrine, cardiac and bone problems. Regular blood transfusion, splenectomy where hypersplenism develops, and the use of iron chelation therapy form the mainstay of conventional management, while bone marrow transplantation is now being used in some cases, with the hope of a permanent cure.

Blood transfusion should maintain a haemoglobin concentration which is sufficient to permit normal growth and prevent bony deformity secondary to marrow expansion. In addition, maintenance of high haemoglobin concentrations reduces the likelihood of developing splenomegaly and hypersplenism and suppresses excess iron absorption from the gut (De Alarcon et al 1979). The expanded blood volume associated with the anaemia seems to be reduced by high transfusion regimens, and as a result the amount of blood required to maintain a haemoglobin concentration above a pretransfusion value of 10–11 g/dl may not be greater than when the haemoglobin is maintained at a lower level. A reasonable objective is to maintain the haemoglobin between 10–14 g/dl and this usually requires blood transfusion approximately every four weeks. Others have argued for maintenance of an even higher pretransfusion haemoglobin concentration (Propper et al 1980, Modell & Petrou 1983). In older children who already have evidence of cardiac damage from iron overload, more frequent,

smaller transfusions may be advisable. Plasma-reduced blood with a haematocrit of around 60% should be used, and sensitization to leucocytes, and resulting febrile reactions, can be much reduced by the use of an in-line filter to remove white cells. In some patients, transfusions lead to the development of red cell alloantibodies which may cause difficulties in crossmatching blood: it is therefore helpful to genotype the red cells of new cases before transfusion is given.

It is important to record the pre- and post-transfusion haemoglobin concentrations at each transfusion so that the mean haemoglobin maintained by transfusion can be related to the annual blood consumption and compared with a standard curve obtained in post-splenectomy patients (Modell 1977). At a mean haemoglobin concentration of 12 g/dl, the annual blood consumption in splenectomized patients is equivalent to approximately 300 ml/kg of whole prepared blood (or approximately 120 ml/kg per year of pure red cells). If the blood consumption is greater than 1.5 times the predicted amount, hypersplenism should be suspected and splenectomy considered.

Splenectomy is required less frequently since the advent of high blood transfusion regimes. Decisions about the need for splenectomy are taken on clinical grounds and on the basis of careful records of blood transfusion, since radioisotopic studies of red cell survival and sequestration are usually unhelpful. Wherever possible, splenectomy should be postponed until after the fifth year. Pneumococcal vaccine can be given before splenectomy, and prophylactic penicillin V 250 mg twice daily should be given indefinitely thereafter; the parents should be warned about the dangers of overwhelming infection.

Iron chelation therapy to prevent the complications of iron overload should be started before the third birthday; this is because iron-induced tissue damage can be detected very early in life (Iancu et al 1977). Serum ferritin concentrations should be used to monitor iron loading. They increase with blood transfusion load, though above a concentration of 4000 µg/l the simple relationship between serum ferritin and iron stores breaks down, probably because of the release of intracellular ferritin from iron-damaged cells (Worwood et al 1980).

Desferrioxamine is the only chelating agent in current clinical use, but unfortunately it is not absorbed when given by mouth. When first introduced it was given intramuscularly, and though controlled studies showed retardation of the development of hepatic fibrosis (Barry et al 1974), tissue iron concentrations remained very high. However, much greater amounts of iron are excreted in both urine and stools using continuous infusions of desferrioxamine. Overnight subcutaneous infusions of desferrioxamine, using a battery operated pump and a narrow gauge butterfly needle inserted into the subcutaneous tissues (usually of the anterior abdominal wall), are now standard treatment on at least five nights each week. For those beginning chelation in their third year, it is reasonable to start with a single vial of 0.5 g of desferrioxamine in each infusion. This represents about 40 mg/kg and is sufficient to keep pace with continuing transfusional iron loading. As the child grows and blood transfusion requirements change, the dose should be reviewed regularly aiming for a total of around 200–300 mg/kg per week. In older patients with established iron overload, the relationship between urinary iron excretion and desferrioxamine dose should be determined individually before selecting the dose to be used on a regular basis. This is because chelation continues to be efficient at higher doses than in younger children (Pippard et al 1978), and the aim is to make inroads into accumulated iron stores as well as to keep pace with the current rate of transfusion iron loading. Desferrioxamine chelates transit iron released from ferritin stores within hepatocytes (excreted in the bile) and iron from elsewhere in the body (excreted in the urine). A number of factors, including ascorbic acid depletion and the particular stage of the blood transfusion cycle, influence the total amount and route of iron excretion. Small doses of vitamin C (50–100 mg daily) increase the urinary iron excretion in response to desferrioxamine and may be given concurrently. Initial worries about possible enhancement of iron toxicity by large doses of ascorbic acid have not been borne out using these small doses. The practical issues involved in starting chelation therapy are reviewed by Pippard (1989).

With intensive iron chelation it is now clear that life expectancy is improved. Liver iron stores can be reduced to very low levels, and cardiac, endocrine and liver complications are reduced (Hoffbrand & Wonke 1989). Desferrioxamine has proved remarkably safe for a drug given in such large quantities over prolonged periods of time, but some adverse effects have been noted. These include ocular toxicity (retinal damage) and sensorineural deafness, and growth may also be retarded, all these effects being most manifest in patients with low overall body iron receiving high doses of desferrioxamine (Porter & Huehns 1989). When the serum ferritin has fallen to less than 2000 µg/l, the dose may need to be reduced (Porter et al 1989). However, potential desferrioxamine toxicity should be considered in the perspective of the undoubted fatal consequences of progressive iron overload; in patients with symptomatic cardiac damage, treatment with high-dose continuous intravenous infusions (80–100 mg/kg every 24 hours) should be considered, if necessary via an indwelling intravenous catheter.

Hormone replacement should be considered in patients with established iron overload who develop endocrine failure. Testosterone or oestrogen supplements may be needed for secondary hypogonadism, which is usually related to hypothalamic-hypopituitary dysfunction. Insulin will be required in those who develop diabetes as a result of pancreatic iron overload.

Bone marrow transplantation from an HLA-identical sibling is now a real option to be considered in the treatment of children with beta thalassaemia major. The remarkably successful programme of Lucarelli et al (1990) means that although the procedure is most successful in younger children, even those over the age of 15 now have a reasonable prospect of survival and engraftment. Conventional treatment with blood transfusions and iron chelation therapy is life-long and often traumatic for patient and family. Furthermore, noncompliance with the arduous iron chelation regimens is common, particularly in teenage children. Nevertheless, used conscientiously, conventional treatment offers the prospect of 30, and probably more, years of life. This has to be matched against the potential for cure by bone marrow transplantation but also the definite morbidity and mortality associated with the procedure and the possibility of unknown complications related to the preparative treatment with alkylating agents (Lucarelli & Weatherall 1991). Extensive counselling of parents is essential if they are to make an informed decision, which also has to take into account the possibilities of future development of alternative methods of treatment.

Future possibilities include the development of oral iron-chelating agents, a field in which there has been promising progress over the last few years (Hershko 1988), and at least one compound (a hydroxypyridone) has been found to be effective in mobilizing iron in man (Kontoghiorghes et al 1987). Attempts to increase the production of HbF by reactivating the gamma globin gene (e.g. using 5-azacytidine or hydroxyurea) have not so far been successful in thalassaemia. Ultimately, the ability to correct the thalassaemia defect with gene therapy is a real, if longer term, prospect.

Beta thalassaemia minor

Heterozygotes for beta thalassaemia genes are typically asymptomatic. They have a slightly reduced circulating haemoglobin concentration (e.g. 9–13 g/l) with a disproportionate reduction in MCH (18–22 fl) and MCV (60–70 fl). The red cell count is therefore usually markedly increased, at greater than 5.5×10^{12}/l. The most important diagnostic feature is an increase in HbA_2 (4–7%) and, in about 50% of cases, an elevation of HbF (1–3%) probably resulting from a degree of red cell selection. Rarely, the carrier state may be 'silent', with only mild microcytosis and normal levels of HbA_2. Conversely, there are uncommon beta thalassaemia genes which result in typically thalassaemic red cell indices but a normal HbA_2. Diagnosis may also be confused by co-inheritance of an alpha thalassaemia gene, giving rise to a more balanced globin chain synthesis, with better haemoglobinized red cells (Kanavakis et al 1982) and more effective erythropoiesis (Pippard & Wainscoat 1987). These less common and atypical forms of heterozygous beta thalassaemia are only important in relation to the need for accurate genetic counselling of prospective parents. In general, heterozygous beta thalassaemia is clinically relevant only as a source of confusion with iron deficiency, and thus with the potential for unnecessary iron therapy.

Gamma-delta-beta thalassaemia and hereditary persistence of fetal haemoglobin

The delta-beta thalassaemias are genetic disorders of the beta globin gene cluster, characterized by absence of both delta and beta globin chain production, and increased levels of HbF. They are much less common than the beta thalassaemia disorders. In some cases they result from gene deletion, and in others from unequal crossover between the delta and beta globin gene loci with the formation of a delta-beta fusion gene. The product of the latter when combined with alpha chains forms Hb Lepore. In both cases the heterozygotes have a thalassaemia minor blood picture (Table 8.9). There is a compensatory increase in HbF (5–15%) in heterozygotes for delta-beta thalassaemia (the HbF being heterogeneously distributed among the red cells), while in heterozygotes for Hb Lepore there is 5–15% Hb Lepore and a somewhat more consistent increase in HbF than is seen in heterozygous beta thalassaemia (Weatherall & Clegg 1981). Because of the compensatory enhancement of gamma globin production, homozygotes tend to have a more mild course than that of beta thalassaemia major, with the clinical phenotype of thalassaemia intermedia (see below).

Other, related, gene deletions involving the delta and beta globin genes give rise to hereditary persistence of fetal haemoglobin (HPFH). Most common in Negro populations, heterozygotes have a normal peripheral blood picture with 15–30% HbF evenly distributed among the red cells. However, homozygotes, who have 100% HbF, have mildly thalassaemic red cell indices, indicating some deficit in gamma chain compared with alpha chain production. Other nondeletional forms of HPFH involve mutations within the promoter region of one or other of the gamma genes and thus give rise to increased expression of either ^{G}gamma or ^{A}gamma. A nonthalassaemic HPFH results from a high HbF determinant which segregates independently from the beta globin gene cluster. Gamma-delta-beta thalassaemias have been observed only in heterozygotes,

where they are characterized by neonatal haemolysis; in later life they produce a picture of
thalassaemia minor with normal HbA_2 (Weatherall
& Clegg 1981).

Thalassaemia intermedia

The term 'thalassaemia intermedia' describes patients who are symptomatic but have a clinically
milder disorder than transfusion-dependent thalassaemia major. The molecular basis of these disorders is summarized in Table 8.10. Compound
heterozygotes of HbE (which behaves as a mild
thalassaemia gene) and beta thalassaemia have a
thalassaemia intermedia syndrome which is common in South East Asia. Co-inheritance of alpha
thalassaemia in a patient homozygous for beta+
thalassaemia (but not beta0 thalassaemia) usually
improves the balance between alpha and beta
globin production sufficiently to give rise to a clinical picture of thalassaemia intermedia (Wainscoat
et al 1983). Similarly, a gene which enhances
gamma chain production (a delta-beta thalassaemia or HPFH determinant) may also reduce the
excess of alpha chains.

Clinically, it is extremely important to identify
at presentation those patients with homozygous
beta thalassaemia who are likely to follow a milder
course and in whom regular blood transfusion and
the need for very intensive iron chelation therapy
may be avoided. Patients with a haemoglobin
below 7 g/dl are likely to prove transfusion dependent, but if the child is otherwise well a short
period of observation with folate supplements is
warranted.

The clinical variability of patients with thalassaemia intermedia is enormous (Weatherall &

Table 8.10 Thalassaemia intermedia – molecular basis

Homozygous β thalassaemia
  Coinheritance of α thalassaemia
  Coinheritance of HPFH
Inheritance of one or two mild β+ thalassaemia genes
  e.g. Portuguese β+ thalassaemia
Compound heterozygote for β thalassaemia and HbE
Severe heterozygous β thalassaemia
  Coinheritance of extra α-globin gene (αα/ααα)
δβ thalassaemia and Hb Lepore
  Homozygous δβ thalassaemia
  δβ thalassaemia + β thalassaemia
  Homozygous Hb Lepore (some cases)

Clegg 1981). Some patients are almost symptom
free, while others develop many of the problems of
erythroid expansion and skeletal deformities that
are seen in poorly transfused beta thalassaemia
major. Where a worsening anaemia develops in
later childhood or adult life (sometimes requiring
blood transfusions for the first time), folate deficiency or hypersplenism should be suspected and
dealt with appropriately. There may be an increased risk of parenchymal iron loading after
splenectomy (Pootrakul et al 1980). Intercurrent
infections, more frequent in this group of patients,
may also produce an acute exacerbation of the
anaemia and should be treated with appropriate
antimicrobial agents and careful monitoring of
haemoglobin concentration. All patients are at
risk of developing iron overload from excessive
gastrointestinal absorption (Fig. 8.4), though this
usually lags behind by a decade or so compared
with patients with beta thalassaemia major
(Pippard et al 1982). This slower rate of iron loading means that iron chelation programmes should
be tailored for each individual; in some cases, after
initial removal of accumulated iron, intermittent
desferrioxamine infusions (e.g. once a week or
even less often) may be sufficient to maintain iron
stores at a normal level.

DEFECTS IN ERYTHROID CELL DIVISION AND MATURATION I. MEGALOBLASTIC ANAEMIAS

Megaloblastic anaemia is relatively uncommon in
infancy and childhood. Worldwide, it is usually
due to dietary folate deficiency, often in combination with more general malnutrition, but a variety
of rare inherited and acquired disturbances of cobalamin (vitamin B_{12}) and folate metabolism are
most likely to present in this age group (Table
8.11), as well as other rare inborn errors of metabolism where megaloblastic anaemia is unrelated to cobalamin or folate abnormalities. The
possibility of a megaloblastic anaemia needs to be
considered wherever the red cell size is increased,
particularly where there are macro-ovalocytes and
an increase in hypersegmented neutrophils in the
peripheral blood. The bone marrow appearances
are the critical diagnostic feature – megaloblasts
are larger than normal erythroblasts, and have

Table 8.11 Disorders giving rise to megaloblastic anaemia in early life and their likely time of presentation (Chanarin 1983)

Disorder	Likely time of presentation (months)		
	2–6	7–24	>24
Folate deficiency			
Inadequate supply			
Prematurity	+		
Dietary deficiency e.g.	+		
goat's milk anaemia			
Chronic haemolysis			+
Defective absorption			
Coeliac disease/tropical sprue			+
Anticonvulsant drugs			+
Congenital folate	+		
malabsorption			
Cobalamin deficiency			
Inadequate supply			
Maternal cobalamin deficiency		+	
Nutritional cobalamin			+
deficiency			
Defective absorption			
Juvenile pernicious anaemia			+
Congenital malabsorption		+	±
(Imerslund-Grasbeck syndrome)			
Congenital absence/		+	±
nonfunctioning intrinsic			
factor			
Defective metabolism			
Transcobalamin II deficiency	+		
Inborn errors of cobalamin	+		
utilization			
Other			
Thiamine-responsive			+
megaloblastic anaemia			
Orotic aciduria	+		
Lesch-Nyhan syndrome			+

nuclei with a lacy, finely stippled, appearance even in later cells that have well-haemoglobinized cytoplasm. There is usually marked erythroid hyperplasia, and ferrokinetic studies have confirmed an ineffective erythropoiesis. Other marrow cells may also show megaloblastic changes (e.g. giant metamyelocytes), as may mucosal cells of the gastro-intestinal and genital tracts. The mechanism for megaloblastic change, presumed to be due to impaired coiling of DNA, is not understood. It does not appear to be due to hypomethylation of DNA (Perry et al 1990), though it seems likely that defective DNA synthesis in some way underlies the maturation abnormality.

Biochemistry of cobalamin and folate

Folate. Folic acid (pteroylglutamic acid) is the pharmacological form of folate which has to be reduced to tetrahydrofolate (THF) and conjugated with additional glutamic acid residues within cells to form folate polyglutamates before it is metabolically active. Folate in the diet (mainly polyglutamates) has to be converted into monoglutamates before it can be taken up by intestinal cells, mainly in the proximal small bowel. There, it is converted to methyl THF, the main circulating form of folate, before release into the portal blood. In the blood it is bound to protein, either a high-affinity, low-capacity binder, or a low-affinity binder which may be albumin. Much of the folate is cleared initially by the liver, the site of body folate stores, and undergoes an enterohepatic circulation. After uptake by cells, transfer of the methyl group to homocysteine (see below) converts it to a form (free THF or formyl THF) available for polyglutamate synthesis. Folate poly-glutamates play a vital metabolic role as cofactors in the transfer of single-carbon units in a variety of different pathways (Fig. 8.7). Serine is thought to be a major source of single-carbon units, though methionine is a source of formate (CHO). The single-carbon units are used for the synthesis of purines and thymidine, the availability of the latter being rate-limiting for DNA synthesis. The methylation of deoxyuridine to thymidine requires thymidylate synthetase and methylene THF, the latter being inactivated during the reaction by oxidation to dihydrofolate. The enzyme dihydrofolate reductase is therefore vital for maintaining cellular levels of active folate. The degree of impairment of thymidine synthesis can be assessed in the deoxyuridine suppression test for megaloblastosis: in a short term incubation of a patient's bone marrow cells, prior addition of deoxyuridine will produce less suppression of the uptake of preformed radiolabelled thymidine than normal in the presence of either folate or cobalamin deficiency. The diagnostic value of this test can be extended by assessment of correction by either folinic acid (formyl THF) or cobalamin. The suppression is restored by folinic acid alone in megaloblastic anaemias due to either cobalamin or folate deficiency, while in cobalamin deficiency cobalamin also leads to a partial correction.

Cobalamin. Cobalamin consists of a corrin nucleus containing a cobalt atom and a nucleotide

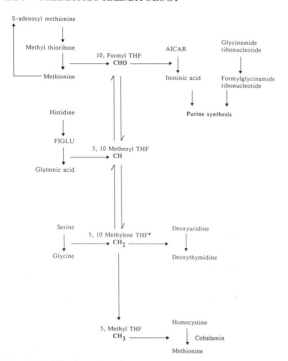

Fig. 8.7 The function of tetrahydrofolate (THF) in transfer of single-carbon units. Polyglutamates of THF accept single-carbon units from the reactions on the left, and transfer them to the reactions on the right. The state of reduction of the single-carbon units is altered by a series of interconverting enzymes: formate is required for purine synthesis, methylene for thymidine synthesis, and methyl for methionine synthesis. *THF is reduced to dihydrofolate during thymidine synthesis and regenerated by the enzyme dihydrofolate reductase. FIGLU = forminoglutamic acid. AICAR = amino imidazole carboxamide ribonucleotide.

base lying at right angles to it. Only two roles for cobalamin have been identified in mammals: the de-novo synthesis of methionine, involving methyl cobalamin, and the conversion of methylmalonic acid to succinic acid, involving adenosyl cobalamin (Fig. 8.8). The cobalt atom in the stable dietary form of hydroxocobalamin has to be reduced before it can take part in these reactions. A glycoprotein, intrinsic factor, produced by gastric parietal cells is essential for cobalamin absorption, the cobalamin-intrinsic-factor complex traversing the gut to be taken up by specific receptors in the terminal ileum. From here, cobalamin enters the portal blood bound to transcobalamin II, (TCII), for which all cells have receptors. In addition, the plasma contains a glycoprotein R-binder which binds the majority of the plasma cobalamin but as yet has no known

function. Like folate, most of the body's reserves of cobalamin are in the liver, and there is an enterohepatic circulation.

Folate/cobalamin interactions. The transfer of the methyl group from methyl THF to homocysteine (Fig. 8.8) is impaired in the absence of cobalamin. In seeking to explain the megaloblastic anaemia seen with cobalamin deficiency, it has been widely accepted that the failure of methyl transfer in this reaction creates a critical lack of the free THF needed to take part in single-carbon transfer reactions involving formate and methylene for purine and pyrimidine synthesis (Fig. 8.7): the interconversion of methylene THF and methyl THF appears essentially one-way under physiological conditions, and the methyl THF appears effectively 'trapped' (Herbert & Zalusky 1962). However, this hypothesis fails to explain the poor utilization of free THF in cobalamin-deficient cells in the deoxyuridine suppression test or by cobalamin-deficient animals. More recently, it has been suggested that the primary defect in cobalamin deficiency may be the failure of synthesis of methionine, the main supplier of formate single-carbon units (Fig. 8.7). A lack of formyl THF would have general effects on folate metabolism since this is a substrate from which the active polyglutamates are formed (Chanarin et al 1985). The lack of ability to form folate polyglutamates, which are retained within cells, probably explains the low red cell folate values which tend to occur in cobalamin deficiency. A low serum cobalamin is also seen in about one-third of patients with isolated folate deficiency. The explanation for the latter is not known, but the observation serves to emphasize that a low serum cobalamin concen-

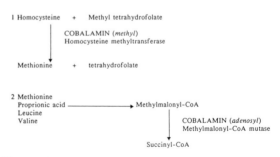

Fig. 8.8 Biochemical reactions involving cobalamin. (**1**) De novo synthesis of methionine. (**2**) Conversion of methylmalonic acid to succinate which enters Kreb's cycle.

tration alone is not enough to indicate cobalamin deficiency.

Folate deficiency

Dietary folate and folate balance

Folates are present in all foods, animal and plant, but they are labile and easily destroyed by cooking and exposure to ultraviolet light. Cow's milk contains about 50 µg folate/1, as does human breast milk. Goat's milk is a particularly poor source at 6 µg/l. Reheating pasteurized milk reduces folate content by up to 80%. In the UK, daily folate intake averages 200 µg, roughly equivalent to WHO recommendations of 3.1 µg/kg. In infancy, requirements on a weight basis are up to 10 times higher, at 20–50 µg/day.

Serum and red cell folate concentrations are high at birth (even where the mother had a marginal folate status), but decline to adult values within a few weeks. Rapid growth at this time means that folate balance is precarious and overt deficiency may result, especially in premature infants, in association with chronic infections, or with the use of heat-sterilised artificial feeds with low folate content. Adolescence does not seem to be accompanied by any increased risk of megaloblastic anaemia due to folate deficiency in developed countries.

Causes of folate deficiency

Nutritional. Dietary deficiency of folate may be the sole cause of megaloblastic anaemia, but more often than not it compounds additional factors giving rise to increased folate requirements (see below). It occurs not only in infants with general malnutrition (kwashiorkor and protein-calorie malnutrition, where over half of children may have megaloblastosis), but also in those with a particular reason for a low dietary folate, e.g. feeding with goat's milk. It may also occur in those on special diets, e.g. for the treatment of phenylketonuria (Royston & Parry 1962).

Increased requirements. Premature infants have a more marked fall in serum and red cell folate concentrations than term infants, but only a minority develop overt megaloblastic anaemia. The latter is not always related to the additional factors, such as infection, which can usually be

found in folate-deficient term infants (Hoffbrand 1970).

Haemolytic and dyserythropoietic anaemias consume folate, and a worsening of the anaemia should lead to a suspicion of folate deficiency. An aplastic crisis may be precipitated.

Infections and chronic inflammatory diseases, including tuberculosis and exfoliative dermatitis, may reduce appetite and folate intake while increasing folate demands.

In all these situations, consideration should be given to the use of prophylactic folate supplements.

Malabsorption. Coeliac disease causes malabsorption of folate (more often than of cobalamin, since the mucosal lesion is usually more pronounced in the proximal small bowel), as does tropical sprue. Loss of folate from the enterohepatic circulation may speed the development of deficiency in these conditions.

The long-term use of anticonvulsants (especially phenytoin) has been associated with megaloblastic anaemia, possibly as a result of inhibition of conversion of dietary folate polyglutamates to absorbable monoglutamates (Hoffbrand & Necheles 1968).

Inherited disorders of folate metabolism

Congenital malabsorption. This has been described as causing severe megaloblastic anaemia in eight children (for review, see Chanarin 1990). As well as failure of uptake by the enterocyte, there is impaired transport to the CNS; progressive mental impairment is usual but not invariable. Treatment requires 3 mg folinic acid by injection twice weekly.

Dihydrofolate reductase deficiency. Although one or two cases have been reported in which megaloblastic anaemia has been interpreted as due to a deficiency of this enzyme (with a therapeutic response to reduced but not unreduced THF; Walters 1967), there is considerable doubt as to whether this is a real clinical entity.

Cobalamin deficiency

Dietary cobalamin and nutritional deficiency

Cobalamin is found only in foods of animal origin, and deficiency may sometimes develop in life-long vegetarians. With a mixed diet, adults have approximately 3 mg total body cobalamin, with a daily requirement of about 1 μg – a substantial reserve of several years' supply. Neonates normally have approximately 50 μg in total. Only in unusual circumstances will uncomplicated dietary deficiency of cobalamin cause megaloblastic anaemia in childhood. One such circumstance occurs with maternal cobalamin deficiency, where the baby is born with very low cobalamin reserves (Baker et al 1962); prolonged breast feeding will provide little more in the deficient mother's milk, and megaloblastic anaemia with failure to thrive, mental regression, and involuntary movements, may occur by the end of the first year of life. A response to as little as 0.1 μg cobalamin daily by mouth (Jadhav et al 1962) suggests a daily requirement in infancy of approximately this amount.

Malabsorption of cobalamin

Juvenile pernicious anaemia. This disease is indistinguishable from the adult form and is characterized by gastric atrophy, achlorhydria, and a high incidence of antibodies to intrinsic factor. Onset is usually in the second decade of life. In some cases there may be a polyendocrinopathy syndrome with myxoedema, hypoparathyroidism or Addison's disease. Diagnosis requires demonstration of cobalamin malabsorption which can be corrected by intrinsic factor, as well as a low serum cobalamin concentration. Treatment is as for adult-onset disease, with 250–1000 μg hydroxycobalamin every 1–2 months.

Congenital vitamin B₁₂ malabsorption (Imerslund–Grasbeck syndrome). This autosomal recessive disorder is the commonest of the inherited causes of megaloblastic anaemia, and appears to be due to an abnormality of the ileal receptor for the cobalamin–intrinsic factor complex (Burman et al 1985). It is accompanied in nearly all cases by proteinuria due to an abnormality of the glomerular basement membrane. Clinical presentation is usually in the first 2 years of life, with megaloblastic anaemia, irritability, vomiting, and listlessness sometimes progressing to coma. Neuropathy may be present, with loss of tendon reflexes and vibration sense, and there may be evidence of subacute combined degenera-

tion of the spinal cord. The isolated malabsorption of cobalamin is not corrected by intrinsic factor, and lifelong cobalamin injections are required.

Congenital deficiency of intrinsic factor. Several families have been described with this autosomal recessive disorder (Heisel et al 1984). The stomach is otherwise normal and there are no antibodies to intrinsic factor. In at least one case, the disorder has been shown to be due to an abnormally functioning intrinsic factor rather than its absence (Katz et al 1972). Clinical presentation is as for congenital cobalamin malabsorption. Parenteral hydroxocobalamin is required for life.

Defects of cobalamin transport and utilisation

Transcobalamin II deficiency. Absence of the main transport protein for cobalamin, TCII, leads to a failure of transport from the enterocytes and to the tissues. Clinical presentation is usually within the first 3 months of life, with failure to thrive, diarrhoea and vomiting, glossitis and listlessness. A severely megaloblastic marrow may be associated with leucopenia and thrombocytopenia in addition to anaemia, but serum cobalamin concentration is normal (being largely dependent upon the cobalamin attached to R-binder); this suggests that uptake of cobalamin in utero must be relatively normal. Diagnosis is by demonstration of the absence of protein capable of binding radiolabelled cobalamin and migrating with TCII during chromatography or gel electrophoresis, or by the use of immunological techniques. The latter have shown the presence of nonfunctional TCII in some cases. Inheritance is as an autosomal recessive, with parents having half the normal amount of functional TCII. Treatment requires massive doses of parenteral cobalamin (1000 μg hydroxycobalamin 1–2 times weekly), allowing sufficient cobalamin to reach the cells by passive diffusion. Mental impairment is likely if treatment is inadequate or intermittent. Retrospective diagnosis after initiation of treatment requires it to be stopped for some weeks, for the treatment ensures that there will be no free binding sites on any TCII present.

Inborn errors of cobalamin metabolism. After its delivery to cells, the cobalamin must be converted into the correct form (methyl or adenosyl) at the right intracellular site for the reactions shown in Figure 8.8. Various mutants have been described (reviewed by Chanarin 1990), which give rise to: (1) methylmalonylaciduria and homocysteinuria (i.e. both coenzymes affected), most often but not invariably with megaloblastic anaemia; (2) homocysteinuria with megaloblastic anaemia (i.e. with defective methylcobalamin function), and (3) methylmalonylaciduria in the absence of megaloblastic anaemia (i.e. with defective adenosylcobalamin function).

Accumulation of methylmalonic acid leads to acidosis and ketosis, failure to thrive, lethargy and, eventually, coma. Homocysteinuria also predisposes to thrombosis. Megaloblastic anaemia presents in the first few weeks of life and may be accompanied by microcephaly, fits and delayed mental development. Diagnosis involves measurement of methylmalonic acid and homocysteine in the urine, but precise identification of the enzyme defect is dependent upon studies in skin fibroblast cultures. Treatment is with large doses of parenteral hydroxycobalamin (1000 μg 1–2 times weekly).

Other megaloblastic anaemias

A handful of patients have been described with a curious syndrome of *thiamine-responsive anaemia,* accompanied by sensorineural deafness and diabetes mellitus (Haworth et al 1982). Megaloblastic anaemia occurred in later childhood in some, but within the first 3 months of life in others. Ringed sideroblasts may also be present. The anaemia responds to treatment with large doses (up to 100 mg daily) of thiamine (Mandel et al 1984), but megaloblastic changes persist. The cause is unknown.

Orotic aciduria is a rare autosomal recessive defect of pyrimidine synthesis with failure of conversion of orotic acid to uridine and consequent excretion of large amounts of orotic acid, sometimes with crystals, in the urine. Treatment with oral uridine (1–1.5 g daily) restores normoblastic erythropoiesis.

The *Lesch–Nyhan syndrome* of mental retardation, self mutilation and choreoathetosis results from impaired synthesis of purines due to lack of hypoxanthine phosphoribosyltransferase. Some patients have a megaloblastic anaemia which responds to adenine therapy (1.5 g daily), but this has little overall clinical benefit (Van der Zee 1970).

Investigation and management

General points. In a megaloblastic anaemia, cobalamin deficiency will be suggested by a low serum cobalamin combined with a normal serum folate, but red cell folate is also commonly low. Urinary excretion of methylmalonic acid is increased, and this may be a particularly useful test in the diagnosis of inborn errors of cobalamin metabolism. Abnormal deoxyuridine suppression is partially corrected by cobalamin as well as folinic acid. A vitamin B_{12} absorption test is likely to be required in sorting out the precise cause of the cobalamin deficiency.

In folate deficiency, a low red cell folate provides unequivocal evidence of folate depletion; the serum folate is also low, but reduced levels are nonspecific, being found in most chronic illness. The serum cobalamin concentration is also sometimes reduced (see p. 226, Folate/cobalamin interactions). Urinary excretion of FIGLU after histidine loading is increased (see Fig. 8.7). In both folate and cobalamin deficiency, a clinical and haematological response to the factor involved is the final confirmatory test.

Management in the very young. The foregoing descriptions of the disorders associated with megaloblastic anaemias in the young, particularly the risk of mental impairment, emphasize the need for prompt and precise diagnosis and treatment. The age of presentation may help the physician to focus on the most likely diagnoses (Table 8.11). A history of an affected sibling should suggest an inherited disorder, and an unusual diet or other predisposing illness may also help in diagnosis. The following discussion of investigation and management in very young children is based on Chanarin (1983).

Pretreatment samples should include serum for cobalamin and folate concentrations, and whole blood for red cell folate assay. A bone marrow aspiration should be obtained to confirm megaloblastosis and, wherever possible, to carry out a deoxyuridine suppression test. A 24-hour urine collection for methylmalonic acid and homocysteine assay should be started immediately, using a metabolic cot in infants. Proteinuria will point strongly to congenital cobalamin malabsorption.

Initial treatment should begin after completion of the 24-hour urine collection. Both hydroxycobalamin (250 µg) and folinic acid (3–5 mg) should be given by intramuscular injection on alternate days pending further data. Alternatively, if the deoxyuridine suppression test has already provided evidence of cobalamin deficiency, this should be given alone. A response is indicated by rapid improvement in appetite and loss of irritability and apathy, as well as haematological improvement. In the absence of a response, urinary excretion of orotic acid should be determined.

Cobalamin deficiency will be confirmed by a low serum concentration, except in the case of TCII deficiency – measurement of TCII is therefore required in all cases to exclude deficiency. Vitamin B_{12} absorption tests, preferably using a total body counter in the very young, will allow distinction of those lacking intrinsic factor from those with congenital malabsorption of cobalamin (Imerslund-Grasbeck) or TCII deficiency where defective absorption is not corrected by exogenous intrinsic factor. Congenital folate malabsorption can be detected by the lack of any significant rise in plasma folate concentration after a test dose of 5 mg folic acid (when the concentration should rise to more than 100 ng/ml)

Treatment has been considered in the discussion of the individual disorders.

DEFECTS IN ERYTHROID CELL DIVISION AND MATURATION II. CONGENITAL DYSERYTHROPOIETIC ANAEMIAS

Two groups of congenital anaemias associated with dyserythropoiesis, the thalassaemias and congenital sideroblastic disorders, have already been considered. A further heterogeneous group of uncommon 'congenital dyserythropoietic anaemias' (CDAs) is considered here for convenience, though the biochemical nature of the disorders is not known. In-vitro culture of peripheral blood BFU-Es shows evidence of normal and abnormal erythroblast morphology within every colony, suggesting that the defects arise at the stem cell level. The CDAs are refractory to known treatments and are characterized by reticulocytopenia in the

presence of marked erythroid hyperplasia, i.e. ineffective erythropoiesis. The latter is associated with a variable unconjugated hyperbilirubinaemia leading in these often asymptomatic patients to an initial differential diagnosis of Gilbert's syndrome. Gallstones and splenomegaly are common. The major long-term complication is iron overload, usually from excessive gastrointestinal absorption (Fig. 8.5), but in a minority of patients from the need for regular blood transfusions. Iron overload can be successfully managed with iron chelation therapy, sometimes with the addition of gentle regular phlebotomy if the anaemia is mild; the principles of treatment are the same as for the iron overload in thalassaemia intermedia syndromes (p. 224). Presentation may be at any age from neonatal to late adult life. A classification of these disorders is shown in Table 8.12.

CDA type I

The peripheral blood shows a marked anisocytosis, macrocytosis and punctate basophilia, while the bone marrow is characterized by megaloblastoid hyperplasia with abnormal proliferation of polychromatophilic erythroblasts and dissociation of nuclear and cytoplasmic maturation. A small proportion (1–2%) of cells show incomplete nuclear division, others are binucleate, often with a discrepancy in the maturation of the 2 nuclei, and internuclear chromatin bridges are characteristic (Heimpel 1976). Globin chain synthesis studies on peripheral blood have shown a slight excess of alpha over beta chains in some but not all patients, with occasional alpha chain precipitates visible on electron microscopy (EM). EM studies also show a diagnostic 'Swiss cheese' ap-

Table 8.12 Classification of congenital dyserythropoietic anaemias

	Type I	Type II	Type III
Anaemia	Mild or moderate	Mild to severe	Mild
Peripheral blood	Macrocytic	Normocytic	Macrocytic
Bone marrow	Megaloblastic Internuclear-bridging and binucleate cells	Bi- and multinuclearity (10–30%)	Multinuclear 'gigantoblasts'
Inheritance	Recessive*	Recessive*	Dominant

*Known to occur in siblings of either sex

pearance to the nuclei, the affected cells showing an arrest of DNA, RNA and protein synthesis (Wickramasinghe & Pippard 1986). The anaemia is usually mild, but patients may present with symptoms and signs of haemochromatosis in adult life. Splenomegaly is common but splenectomy is not clinically unhelpful in this condition.

CDA type II (HEMPAS)

The most common of the CDAs, the anaemia is sometimes severe enough to necessitate regular blood transfusion (Verwilghen 1976); splenectomy may then reduce the need for transfusion, particularly in those with evidence of more prominent peripheral haemolysis (Barosi et al 1979). Red cells are normocytic, with nonspecific changes of poikilocytosis and punctate basophilia. The late erythroblasts in the bone marrow show binuclear and multinuclear cells with karyorrhexis. Electron microscopic studies show an excess of endoplasmic reticulum parallel to the cell membrane, giving a 'double membrane' appearance. As in CDA type I, some patients have a mild excess of alpha over beta globin chain production. The reticuloendothelial cells in the marrow contain PAS-positive needle-like inclusions, presumably a reflection of the increased catabolism resulting from the numerous erythroblasts dying within the marrow. The diagnostic finding in this disorder, which is also known as HEMPAS (hereditary erythroblastic multinuclearity associated with a positive acidified serum test), is that the red cells are lysed by around 30% of acidified sera from normal individuals, but not by their own acidified serum. This laboratory finding seems to be related to the presence in a proportion of normal sera of an IgM antibody to a 'HEMPAS antigen'. The fetal *i* antigen is also expressed more strongly than in normal individuals, or than is usual in the 'fetal' erythropoiesis that is characteristic of any 'stress' erythropoiesis. HEMPAS cells are also more readily lysed by anti-*I* sera, as they bind complement more readily than normal under these circumstances.

CDA type III

The least common of the CDAs, this disorder is characterized by a mild macrocytic anaemia with many multinucleated erythroblasts, and gigantoblasts with up to 12 nuclei, in the marrow (Goudsmit 1977). In some cases there has been hepatosplenomegaly, and bone changes related to erythroid expansion have also been reported. Any initial diagnostic worries about possible erythroleukaemia will be resolved by the stable haematological picture with normal leucocyte and platelet counts.

DEFECTS IN MARROW ENVIRONMENT OR ERYTHROID STEM CELLS

The hypoplastic anaemias to be discussed here result either from defects intrinsic to the haemopoietic stem cell, or from a marrow stromal, immune-mediated or cytokine abnormality that fails to support normal erythropoiesis. The disorders leading to generalized marrow failure (e.g. aplastic anaemia and marrow infiltrative disorders) are discussed in Chapters 2, 3, 4 and 12. The relative hypoplasia occurring in the 'anaemia of chronic disorders' and chronic renal failure has been discussed earlier in this chapter in the context of impaired iron supply, but a relative lack of erythropoietin production, possible humoral (Prouse et al 1987) or cellular inhibitors of erythropoiesis, and other effects within the cytokine network may all have a role in these secondary anaemias. The anaemia common in premature infants should also be considered under this heading (see also Ch. 10).

Anaemia of prematurity

Although the haemoglobin concentration normally falls after birth, it falls further and faster in the premature infant. The haemopoietic response is inadequate, but this does not appear to be due to a lack of erythroid progenitors or an impaired progenitor response to erythropoietin (Shannon et al 1987). Furthermore, although deficiencies of iron and folate are common in those born prematurely, their effects do not usually become manifest until after the first few weeks of life. A suboptimal production of erythropoietin is thought to be responsible, and trials of therapy using recombinant human erythropoietin are in progress in an attempt to reduce the need for neonatal blood transfusion; these trials are difficult to control and still at a pilot stage (Halperin et al 1990).

Pure red cell aplasia

Congenital red cell aplasia (Diamond–Blackfan anaemia)

This disorder usually presents in early infancy, with only a few cases being seen for the first time after the age of one year. It is characterized by a severe macrocytic or normocytic anaemia (with a haemoglobin concentration often as low as 3–4 g/dl), reticulocytopenia, and a selective deficit of marrow red cell precursors. Leucocytes are normal, and platelets normal or increased (Diamond et al 1976, Alter & Nathan 1979). The majority of cases are sporadic, but familial cases have shown either dominant or recessive patterns of transmission. There is a higher than normal frequency of 'small for dates' babies, and approximately 25% have at least one congenital abnormality (including 10% with abnormalities of the thumb). Characteristic facial features have been described, with snub nose, wide-set eyes and a thick upper lip (Cathie 1950).

The red cells contain more HbF than normal, and there is also a high level of red cell i antigen expression. Together with the tendency to macrocytosis, these features of fetal erythropoiesis are important for the differential diagnosis from other causes of childhood red cell aplasia. Increased lymphocytes may be seen in the marrow, and very occasional patients may show normal or even increased numbers of erythoblasts with evidence of a maturation arrest. Values for serum iron and transferrin saturation are increased, as in any condition of reduced erythropoiesis. Serum erythropoietin concentrations are higher than in any other form of anaemia.

The pathogenesis is unknown and, indeed, the disorder is likely to be heterogeneous in this respect. Abnormalities in purine or pyrimidine metabolism have been described, particularly increased red cell adenosine deaminase (Glader et al 1983), but their significance is not known. Cytogenetic studies are normal. Cellular and humoral inhibitors have been proposed, and the clinical response to immunosuppression has raised questions of a possible autoimmune aetiology. However, in-vitro studies of erythroid progenitors suggest that they may be normal in number but abnormally insensitive to erythropoietin (Lipton et al 1986); there was no correlation between progenitor cell numbers or sensitivity to erythropoietin, and the patient's degree of anaemia or their response to prednisolone therapy.

Treatment. About two-thirds of patients will have a useful response to prednisolone. A suitable starting dose is 2 mg/kg daily in divided doses, to be continued until the haemoglobin concentration is greater than 10 g/dl. Thereafter, a slow tapering of the dose should begin, moving from divided to single daily doses and then to alternate-day therapy. Some patients are exquisitely sensitive to small changes in dose, even when the dose is already almost 'homeopathic', and the range of maintenance doses can be from 1–40 mg on alternate days. An increase in reticulocytes is usual within a week or two of starting steroid treatment, but a rise in haemoglobin concentration may be delayed, or may not occur. A few patients have a rapid response followed by a remission independent of steroid support. However, most require continued maintenance therapy. About one-third of patients either have no response or relapse on steroids and become refractory even to increased doses of prednisolone. High doses of prednisolone (4–6 mg/kg daily) or dexamethasone should be tried before resorting to regular blood transfusions, with their attendent requirement for intensive iron chelation therapy (p. 221).

Bone marrow transplantation offers an alternative, potentially curative, option for such refractory patients, and has been carried out successfully in a small number of cases (Lenarsky et al 1988). However, there is a similar dilemma over the use of this treatment as in beta thalassaemia major (p. 222), particularly as around 20% of the steroid refractory patients may have a spontaneous remission later in life. Iron overload is the major cause of death in congenital red cell aplasia, though this may change with the use of more effective iron chelation regimens.

Acquired red cell aplasia

Pure red cell aplasia. This acquired disorder is most frequent in adults, but a small number of cases occur in adolescence. There may be an associated thymoma (5–10% of patients with thymoma develop pure red cell aplasia), and infections and a range of drugs have been implicated as aetiological agents (Alter et al 1978), though the majority of cases are idiopathic. A normochromic normocytic anaemia is the rule, with absent marrow erythroid precursors. Studies of marrow erythroid colonies suggest that some patients have serum or cellular inhibitors of erythropoiesis, and an antibody to erythropoietin has been described (Peschle et al 1975). In those with a thymoma, removal has a 25% chance of inducing remission. A number of immunosuppressive regimens have been tried, with over half of the patients responding to various combinations containing prednisolone (Clarke et al 1984). If immunosuppressive therapy fails, supportive treatment with blood transfusion and iron chelation therapy will be needed.

Parvovirus infection and haemolytic anaemias. A transient erythroid hypoplasia follows infection with parvovirus (Young & Mortimer 1984), the agent responsible for the mild childhood infection of erythema infectiosum. The virus specifically infects CFU-E and prevents their maturation. Even in normal subjects, the period of viraemia (about 1–2 weeks) is accompanied by a reticulocytopenia, but in patients with a chronic haemolytic anaemia there may be a catastrophic fall in haemoglobin concentration during this time. The aplastic crisis of sickle cell disease was the first shown to be due to parvovirus infection (Pattison et al 1981, Serjeant et al 1981), but the same pattern has now been shown in a variety of haemolytic anaemias, including hereditary spherocytosis and pyruvate kinase deficiency. Supportive blood transfusions may be needed during the short period of erythroid aplasia, but marrow recovery is then invariable. The period of viraemia is ended by the appearance of IgM antibodies to parvovirus, and these can be used diagnostically to confirm or refute recent parvovirus infection.

Transient erythroblastopenia of childhood. This disorder is characterized by the development of severe anaemia and reticulocytopenia in a previously healthy and otherwise normal child. A history of viral illness a few weeks earlier is common. The peak age of incidence is around 2 years, with a range from 1 month to 8 years (Alter 1987). Most cases occur after the first year of life, in contrast to congenital red cell aplasia.

The anaemia (haemoglobin range 3–9 g/dl) is normocytic and normochromic and the red cells do not show the 'fetal' characteristics (raised MCV, increased HbF, and high i antigen expression) seen in congenital red cell aplasia. The marrow usually shows an erythroblastopenia. However, if recovery from this transient disorder is beginning, the marrow will be hyperplastic, often with dyserythropoietic features which can lead to confusion with the congenital dyserythropoietic anaemias until the course to complete recovery is obvious. These marrow changes are nonspecific features of stress erythropoiesis, which is also responsible in the recovery phase for the transient appearance of macrocytes, F-reticulocytes and i antigen expression. Given a normal red cell survival, the red cell aplasia has presumably been present for some weeks before the child presents with the symptomatic anaemia. Steroids have no place in the management; indeed, masterly inactivity is usually the right course and blood transfusion can in most cases be avoided, despite the severe anaemia, unless there is evidence of cardiac embarrassment. The pathogenesis of transient erythroblastopenia of childhood is uncertain, though circulating immunoglobulin inhibitors of erythropoiesis have been postulated (Dessypris et al 1982).

Other causes of transient red cell aplasia. Red cell aplasia has been described in association with severe malnutrition, where a whole range of dietary deficiencies, including riboflavin, could be playing a role. A red cell maturation arrest can occur with folate deficiency, and it is of interest that severe cobalamin deficiency has been reported to give rise to severe red cell aplasia in a single child with TCII deficiency (Niebrugge et al 1982). Reversible red cell aplasia is also seen with a wide range of drugs (Alter et al 1978), and it is possible that other viruses besides the parvovirus may occasionally cause this problem (Young & Mortimer 1984).

REFERENCES

Alter B P, Potter N V, Li F P 1978 Classification and aetiology of the aplastic anaemias. Clinics in Haematology 7: 431–465

Alter B P, Nathan D G 1979 Red cell aplasia in children.

Archives of Disease in Childhood 54: 263–267

Alter B P 1987 The bone marrow failure syndromes. In: Nathan D G, Oski F A (eds) Hematology of infancy and childhood, 3rd edn. W B Saunders. Philadelphia, p 159–241

American Academy of Pediatrics, Committee on Nutrition 1976 Iron supplementation for infants. Pediatrics 58: 765–768

American Academy of Pediatrics, Committee on Nutrition 1978 Relationship between iron status and incidence of infection and infancy. Pediatrics 62: 246–250

Anand B S, Callender S T, Warner G T 1977 Absorption of inorganic and haemoglobin iron in coeliac disease. British Journal of Haematology 37: 409–414

Aoki Y, Muranaka S, Nakabayaski, Ueda Y 1979 δ-Aminolaevulinic acid synthetase in erythroblasts of patients with pyridoxine-responsive anemia. Hypercatabolism caused by the increased susceptibility to the controlling protease. Journal of Clinical Investigation 64: 1196–1203

Aoki Y 1980 Multiple enzymatic defects in mitochondria in hematological cells of patients with primary sideroblastic anemia. Journal of Clinical Investigation 66: 43–49

Apt L, Pollycove M, Ross J F, Pratt M, Sullivan J, Donovan J 1957 Idiopathic pulmonary hemosiderosis. A study of the anemia and iron distribution using radioiron and radiochromium. Journal of Clinical Investigation 36: 1150–1159

Aukett M A, Parks Y A, Scott P H, Wharton R A 1986 Treatment with iron increases weight gain and psychomotor development. Archives of Disease in Childhood 61: 849–857

Baer A N, Dessypris E N, Goldwasser E, Krantz S B 1987 Blunted erythropoietin response to anaemia in rheumatoid arthritis. British Journal of Haematology 66: 559–564

Bainton D F, Finch C A 1964 The diagnosis of iron deficiency anemia. American Journal of Medicine 37: 62–70

Baker S J, Jacob E, Rajan K T, Swaminathan S P 1962 Vitamin-B$_{12}$ deficiency in pregnancy and the puerperium. British Medical Journal 1: 1658–1661

Barosi G, Cazzola M, Stefanelli M, Ascari E 1979 Studies of ineffective erythropoiesis and peripheral haemolysis in congenital dyserythropoietic anaemia type II. British Journal of Haematology 43: 243–250

Barry M, Flynn D M, Letsky E A, Risdon R A 1974 Long-term chelation therapy in thalassaemia major: effect on liver iron concentration, liver histology, and clinical progress. British Medical Journal 2: 16–20

Beard J 1987 Feed efficiency and norepinephrine turnover in iron deficiency. Proceedings of the Society for Experimental Biology and Medicine 184: 337–344

Beaudry M A, Ferguson D J, Pearse K, Yanofsky R A, Rubin E M, Kan Y W 1986 Survival of a hydropic infant with homozygous alpha-thalassaemia-I. Journal of Pediatrics 108: 713–716

Bothwell T H, Charlton R W, Cook J D, Finch C A 1979 Iron metabolism in man. Blackwell Scientific Publications, Oxford

Bottomley S 1982 Sideroblastic anaemia. Clinics in Haematology 11: 389–409

Brayton D 1964 Gastrointestinal bleeding of 'unknown origin'. American Journal of Diseases in Children 107: 288–292

Briggs W A, Johnson J P, Teichman S et al 1979 Antiglomerular basement membrane antibody-mediated glomerulonephritis and Goodpasture's syndrome. Medicine 58: 348–361

Burman D 1982 Iron deficiency in infancy and childhood. Clinics in Haematology 11: 339–349

Burman J F, Jenkins W J, Walker-Smith J A et al 1985 Absent ideal uptake of IF-bound vitamin B$_{12}$ in vivo in the Imerslund-Grasbeck syndrome (familial vitamin B$_{12}$ malabsorption with proteinuria). Gut 26: 311–314

Cartier L J, Ohira Y, Chen M, Cuddihee R W, Holloszy J O 1986 Perturbation of mitochondrial composition in muscle by iron deficiency. Journal of Biological Chemistry 261: 13827–13832

Cartwright G E, Deiss A 1975 Sideroblasts, siderocytes and sideroblastic anemia. New England Journal of Medicine 292: 185–193

Cathie I A B 1950 Erythrogenesis imperfecta. Archives of Disease in Childhood 25: 313–24

Cazzola M, Huebers H A, Sayers M H, MacPhail A P, Eng M, Finch C A 1985 Transferrin saturation, plasma iron turnover, and transferrin uptake in normal humans. Blood 66: 935–939

Chanagrin I 1983 Management of megaloblastic anaemia in the very young. British Journal of Haematology 53: 1–3

Chanarin I, Deacon R, Lumb M, Muir M, Perry J 1985 Cobalamin-folate interrelations: a critical review. Blood 66: 479–489

Chanarin I 1990 The megaloblastic anaemias, 3rd edn. Blackwell Scientific Publications, Oxford

Chandra R K 1973 Reduced bactericidal capacity of polymorphs in iron deficiency. Archives of Disease in Childhood 48: 864–866

Clark D A, Dessypris E W, Krantz S B 1984 Studies on pure red cell aplasia XI. Results of immunosuppressive treatment of 37 patients. Blood 63: 277–286

Cook J D, Lynch S R 1986 The liabilities of iron deficiency. Blood 68: 803–809

Dallman P R, Beutler E, Finch C A 1978 Effects of iron deficiency exclusive of anaemia. British Journal of Haematology 40: 179–184

Dallman P R, Siimes M A, Stekel A 1980 Iron deficiency in infancy and childhood. The American Journal of Clinical Nutrition 33: 86–118

Dallman P R, Reeves J D, Driggers D A, Lo E Y T 1981 Diagnosis of iron deficiency: the limitations of laboratory tests in predicting response to iron treatment in 1-year-old infants. Journal of Pediatrics 98: 376–381

Dallman P R 1987 Iron deficiency and the immune response. American Journal of Clinical Nutrition 46: 329–334

De Alarcon P A, Donovan M-E, Forbes G B, Landaw S A, Stockman J A 1979 Iron absorption in the thalassemia syndromes and its inhibition by tea. New England Journal of Medicine 300: 5–8

Dessypris E N, Krantz S B, Roloff J S, Lukens J N 1982 Mode of action of the IgG inhibitor of erythropoiesis in transient erythroblastopenia of childhood. Blood 59: 114–123

Diamond L K, Wang W C, Alter B P 1976 Congenital hypoplastic anemia. Advances in Pediatrics 22: 349–378

Dillman E, Gale C, Green W, Johnson D G, Mackler B, Finch C 1980 Hypothermia in iron deficiency due to altered tri-iodothyronine metabolism. American Journal of Physiology 239: R377–R38 1

Dobbing J (ed) 1989 Brain, behaviour and iron in the infant diet. Springer–Verlag, London

Drueke T B, Lacour B, Touam M et al 1986 Effect of

aluminium on hematopoiesis. Kidney International 29: 545–548

Earley A, Valman H B, Altman D G, Pippard M J 1990 Microcytosis, iron deficiency, and thalassaemia in preschool children. Archives of Disease in Childhood 65: 610–614

Ehrhardt P 1986 Iron deficiency in young Bradford children from different ethnic groups. British Medical Journal 292: 90–93

Eichner E R, Hillman R S 1971 The evolution of anemia in alcoholic patients. Americal Journal of Medicine 50: 218–232

Eschbach J W, Egrie J C, Downing M R, Browne J K, Adamson J W 1987 Correction of the anemia of end-stage renal disease with human erythropoietin. New England Journal of Medicine 316: 73–78

Finch C A, Miller L R, Inamdar A R, Person R, Seiler K, Mackler B 1976 Iron deficiency in the rat. Physiological and biochemical studies of muscle dysfunction. Journal of Clinical Investigation 58: 447–453

Finch C A, Gollnick P D, Hlastala M P, Miller L R, Dillman E, Mackler B 1979 Lactic acidosis as a result of iron deficiency. Journal of Clinical Investigation 64:129–137

Fleming A F 1982 Iron deficiency in the tropics. Clinics in Haematology 11: 365–388

Forman S J, Ziegler E E, Nelson S E, Edwards B B 1981 Cow milk feeding in infancy: gastrointestinal blood loss ad iron nutritional status. Journal of Pediatrics 98: 540–545

Glader B E, Backer K, Diamond L K 1983 Elevated erythrocyte adenosine deaminase activity in congenital hypoplastic anemia. New England Journal of Medicine 309: 1486–1490

Goudsmit R 1977 Congenital dyserythropoietic anaemia, type III. In: Lewis S M, Verwilghen R L (eds) Dyserythropoiesis. Academic Press, London p 83–92

Goya N, Miyazaki S, Kodate S, Ushio B 1972 A family of congenital atransferrinemia. Blood 40: 239–244

Hall R, Losowsky M S 1966 The distribution of erythroblast iron in sideroblastic anaemias. British Journal of Haematology 12: 334–340

Halperin D S, Wacker P, Lacourt G et al 1990 Effects of recombinant human erythropoietin in infants with the anemia of prematurity: a pilot study. Journal of Pediatrics 116: 779–796

Harvey A R, Pippard M J, Ansell B M 1987 Microcytic anaemia in juvenile chronic arthritis. Scandinavian Journal of Rheumatology 16: 53–59

Haworth C, Evans D I K, Mitra J, Wickramasinghe S N 1982 Thiamine-responsive anaemia: a study of two further cases. British Journal of Haematology 50: 549–561

Heimpel H 1976 Congenital dyserythropoietic anaemia type I: clinical and experimental aspects. In: Congenital disorders of erythropoiesis, CIBA Foundation Symposium 37. Elsevier, Amsterdam, p 135–149

Heisel M A, Siegel S E, Falk R E et al 1984 Congenital pernicious anemia: report of seven patients, with studies of the extended family. Journal of Pediatrics 105: 564–568.

Herbert V, Zaluksy R 1962 Interrelation of vitamin B_{12} and folic acid metabolism: folic acid clearance studies. Journal of Clinical Investigation 41: l262–1276

Hershko C 1988 Oral iron chelating drugs: coming but not yet ready for clinical use. British Medical Journal 296: 1081–1082

Higgs J M, Wells R S 1972 Chronic muco-cutaneous candidiasis: associated abnormalities of iron metabolism.

British Journal of Dermatology 86 (suppl 8) 88–102

Hillman R S, Finch C A 1969 The misused reticulocyte. British Journal of Haematology 17: 313–315

Hoffbrand A V, Necheles T F 1968 Mechanisms of folate deficiency in patients receiving phenytoin. Lancet 2: 528–532

Hoffbrand A V 1970 Folate deficiency in premature infants. Archives of Disease in Childhood 4 : 441–444

Hoffbrand A V, Ganeshaguru K, Hooton J W L, Tattersall M H N 1976 Effect of iron deficiency and desferrioxamine on DNA synthesis in human cells. British Journal of Haematology 33: 517–526

Hoffbrand A V, Wonke B 1989 Results of long-term subcutaneous desferrioxamine therapy. Baillière's Clinical Haematology 2: 345–362

Huebers H A, Csiba E, Huebers E, Finch C A 1983 Competitive advantage of diferric transferrin in delivering iron to reticulocytes. Proceedings of the National Academy of Science of the United States of America 80: 300–304

Huebers H A, Beguin Y, Pootrakul P, Einspahr D, Finch C A 1990 Intact transferrin receptors in human plasma and their relation to erythropoiesis. Blood 75: 102–107

Huehns E R 1982 The structure and function of haemoglobin: clinical disorders due to abnormal haemoglobin structure. In: Hardisty R M, Weatherall D J (eds) Blood and its disorders. Blackwell Scientific Publications, Oxford, p. 323– 400

Iancu T C, Neustein H B, Landing B H 1977 The liver in thalassaemia major: ultrastructural observations. In: Iron metabolism. CIBA Foundation Symposium 51 (New series) Elsevier, Amsterdam, 293–316

Jadhav M, Webb J K G, Vaishnava S, Baker S J 1962 Vitamin-B_{12} deficiency in Indian infants. A clinical syndrome. Lancet 2: 903–907

Josephs H W 1959 The iron of the newborn baby. Acta Paediatrica 48: 403–418

Kanavakis E, Wainscoat J S, Wood W G et al 1982 The interaction of α thalassaemia with heterozygous β thalassaemia. British Journal of Haematology 52: 465–474

Katz M, Lee S K, Cooper B A 1972 Vitamin B_{12} malabsorption due to biologically inert instrinsic factor. New England Journal of Medicine 287: 425–429

Kimber C, Weintraub L R 1968 Malabsorption of iron secondary to iron deficiency. New England Journal of Medicine 279: 453–459

Koerper M A, Dallman P R, 1977 Serum iron concentration and transferrin saturation in the diagnosis of iron deficiency in children: normal developmental changes. Journal of Pediatrics 91: 870–874

Koerper M A, Stempel D A, Dallman P R 1978 Anemia in patients with juvenile rheumatoid arthritis. Journal of Pediatrics 92: 930–933

Konijn A M, Hershko C 1977 Ferritin synthesis in inflammation I. Pathogenesis of impaired iron release. British Journal of Haematology 37: 7–16

Konopka L, Hoffbrand A V 1979 Haem synthesis in sideroblastic anaemia. British Journal of Haematology 42: 73–83

Kontoghiorghes G J, Aldouri M A, Hoffbrand A V et al 1987 Effective chelation of iron in β thalassaemia with the oral chelator l ,2-dimethyl-3-hydroxypyrid-4-one. British Medical Journal 295: 1509–1512

Kuhn L C 1991 mRNA-protein interactions regulate critical pathways in cellular iron metabolism. British Journal of Haematology 79: 1–5

Lahey M E, Gubler C J, Chase M S, Cartwright G E, Wintrobe M M 1952 Studies on copper metabolism. II. Hematologic manifestations of copper deficiency in swine. Blood 7: 1053–1074

Lancet Editorial 1987 Iron deficiency – time for a community campaign? Lancet i: 141–142

Larrick J W, Hyman E S 1984 Acquired iron-deficiency anemia caused by an antibody against the transferrin receptor. New England Journal of Medicine 311: 214–218

Lee G R, MacDiarmid W D, Cartwright G E, Wintrobe M M 1968 Hereditary, X-linked, sideroachrestic anemia. The isolation of two erythrocyte populations differing in Xg^a blood type and porphyrin content. Blood 32: 59–70

Lee G R 1983 The anemia of chronic disease. Seminars in Hematology 20: 61–80

Lenarsky C, Weinberg K, Guinan E et al 1988 Bone marrow transplantation for constitutional pure red cell aplasia. Blood 71: 226–229

Lipton J M, Kudisch M, Gross R, Nathan D G 1986 Defective erythroid progenitor differentiation system in congenital hypoplastic (Diamond-Blackfan) anemia. Blood 67: 962–968

Lozoff B, Brittenham G M, Wolf A W et al 1987 Iron deficiency anemia and iron therapy effects on infant developmental test peformance. Pediatrics 79: 981–995

Lozoff B, Jimenez E, Wolf A W 1991 Long-term developmental outcome of infants with iron deficiency. New England Journal of Medicine 325 : 687–694

Lucarelli G, Galimberti M, Polchi P et al 1990 Bone marrow transplantation in patients with thalassemia. New England Journal of Medicine 322: 417–421

Lucarelli G, Weatherall D J 1991 For debate: bone marrow transplantation for severe thalassaemia. (l) The view from Pesaro (2) To be or not to be. British Journal of Haematology 78: 300–303

McCance R A, Widdowson E M 1937 Absorption and excretion of iron. Lancet ii: 680–684

Macdougall I C, Hutton R D, Cavill I, Coles G A, Williams J D 1990 Treating renal anaemia with recombinant human erythropoietin: practical guidelines and a clinical algorithm. British Medical Journal 300: 655–659

Mackler B, Person R, Miller L R, Inamdar A R, Finch C A 1978 Iron deficiency in the rat: biochemical studies of brain metabolism. Pediatric Research 12: 217–220

Mandel H, Berant M, Hazani A, Naveh Y 1984 Thiamine-dependent beriberi in the 'thiamine-responsive anemia syndrome'. New England Journal of Medicine 311: 836–838

Mladenovic J 1988 Aluminium inhibits erythropoiesis in vitro. Journal of Clinical Investigation 81: 1661–1665

Modell B 1977 Total management of thalassaemia major. Archives of Disease in Childhood 52: 489–500

Modell B, Petrou M 1983 Management of thalassaemia major. Archives of Disease in Childhood 58: l026–1030

Monsen E R, Hallberg L, Layrisse M et al 1978 Estimation of available dietary iron. American Journal of Clinical Nutrition. 31: l34–141

Morton A G, Tavill A S 1977 The role of iron in the regulation of hepatic transferrin synthesis. British Journal of Haematology 36: 383–394

Naiman J L, Oski F A, Diamond L K, Vawter G F, Schwachman H 1964 The gastrointestinal effects of iron-deficiency anemia. Pediatrics 33: 83–99

Niebrugge D J, Benjamin D R, Christie D, Scott C R 1982 Hereditary transcobalamin II deficiency presenting as red cell hypoplasia. Journal of Pediatrics 101: 732–735

Oppenheimer S J, Gibson F D, Macfarlane S B et al 1986 Iron supplementation increases prevalence and effects of malaria: report on clinical studies in Papua New Guinea. Transactions of the Royal Society of Tropical Medicine and Hygiene 80: 603–612

Oski F A, Stockman J A 1980 Anemia due to inadequate iron sources or poor iron utilization. Pediatric Clinics of North America 27: 237–252

Oski F A, Honig A S, Helu B, Howanitz P 1983 Effect of iron therapy on behaviour performance in nonanemic, iron deficient infants. Pediatrics 71: 877–880

Paglia D E, Valentine W N, Dahlgren J G et al 1975 Effects of low-level lead exposure on pyrimidine 5'-nucleotidase and other erythrocyte enzymes. Possible role of pyrimidine 5'-nucleotidase in the pathogenesis of lead-induced anemia. Journal of Clinical Investigation 56: 1164–1169

Pattison J R, Jones S E, Hodgson J et al 1981 Parvovirus infections and hypoplastic crises in sickle-cell anaemia. Lancet 1: 644–665

Perry J, Chanarin I, Deacon R, Lumb M 1990 Methylation of DNA in megaloblastic anaemia. Journal of Clinical Pathology 43: 211–212

Peschle C, Marmont A M, Marone G, Genovese A, Sasso G F, Condorelli M 1975 Pure red cell aplasia: studies on an IgG serum inhibitor neutralising erythropoietin. British Journal of Haematology 30: 411–417

Peters T J, Pippard M J 1990 Disorders of iron metabolism. In: Cohen R D, Lewis B, Alberti K G M M, Denman A M (eds) The metabolic and molecular basis of acquired disease. Bailliere Tindall, London p 1870–1884

Peto T E A, Pippard M J, Weatherall D J 1983 Iron overload in mild sideroblastic anaemias. Lancet i: 375–378

Piomelli S, Rosen J F, Chisholm J J, Graef J W 1984 Management of childhood lead poisoning. Journal of Pediatrics 105: 523–532

Pippard M J, Callender S T, Letsky E A, Weatherall D J 1978 Prevention of iron loading in transfusion-dependent thalassaemia. Lancet i: 1178–1181

Pippard M J, Rajagopalan B, Callender S T, Weatherall D J 1982 Iron loading, chronic anaemia, and erythroid hyperplasia as determinants of the clinical features of β-thalassaemia intermedia. In: Weatherall D J, Fiorelli G, Gorini S (eds) Advances in red blood cell biology. Raven Press, New York, p l03–113

Pippard M J, Wainscoat J S 1987 Erythrokinetics and iron status in heterozygous β thalassaemia, and the effect of interaction with α thalassaemia. British Journal of Haematology 66: 123–127

Pippard M J 1989 Desferrioxamine-induced iron excretion in humans. Baillière's Clinical Haematology 2: 323–343

Pippard M J, Hoffbrand A V 1989 Iron. In: Hoffbrand A V, Lewis S M (eds) Postgraduate haematology, 3rd edn. Heinemann, London

Pootrakul P, Rugkiatsakul R, Wasi P 1980 Increased transferrin iron saturation in splenectomized thalassaemic patients. British Journal of Haematology 46: 143–145

Pootrakul P, Kitcharoen K, Yansukon P et al 1988 The effect of erythroid hyperplasia on iron balance. Blood 71: 1124–1129

Porter J B, Huehns E R 1989 The toxic effects of desferrioxamine. Baillière's Clinical Haematology 2: 459–474

Porter J B, Jaswon M S, Huehns E R, East C A, Hazell J W P 1989 Desferrioxamine ototoxicity: evaluation of risk factors in thalassaemic patients and guidelines for safe dosage. British Journal of Haematology 73: 403–409

Propper R D, Button L N, Nathan D G 1980 New approaches to the transfusion management of thalassemia. New England Journal of Medicine 55: 55–60

Prouse P J, Harvey A, Bonner B, Gumpel J M, Reid C D L, Ansell B M 1987 Anaemia in juvenile chronic arthritis: serum inhibition of normal erythropoiesis in vitro. Annals of the Rheumatic Diseases 46: 127–134

Ritchey A K , Hoffman R, Dainiak N, McIntosh S, Weininger R, Pearson H A 1979 Antibody-mediated acquired sideroblastic anemia: response to cytotoxic therapy. Blood 54: 734–741

Royston N J W, Parry T E 1962 Megaloblastic anaemia complicating dietary treatment of phenylketonuria in infancy. Archives of Disease in Childhood 37: 430–435

Rundles R W, Falls H F 1946 Hereditary (? sex-linked) anemia. American Journal of Medical Sciences 211: 641–658

Saarinen U M, Simes M A, Dallman P R 1977 Iron absorption in infants: high bioavailability of breast milk iron as indicated by the extrinsic tag method of iron absorption and by the concentration of serum ferritin. Journal of Pediatrics 91: 36–39

Serjeant G R, Topley J M, Mason K et al 1981 Outbreak of aplastic crises in sickle cell anaemia associated with parvovirus-like agent. Lancet 2 : 595–597

Shahidi N T, Nathan D G, Diamond L K 1964 Iron deficiency anemia associated with an error of iron metabolism in two siblings. Journal of Clinical Investigation 43: 510–521

Shannon K M, Naylor G S, Torkildson J C et al 1987 Circulating erythroid progenitors in the anemia of prematurity. New England Journal of Medicine 317: 728–733

Singla P N, Chand S, Khanna S, Agarwal K N 1978 Effect of maternal anemia on the placenta and the newborn infant. Acta Paediatrica Scandinavia 67: 645–648

Spencer R 1964 Gastrointestinal hemorrhage in infancy and childhood: 476 cases. Surgery 55: 718–734

Thein S L, Weatherall D J 1988 The thalassaemias. In: Hoffbrand A V (ed) Recent advances in haematology 5, Churchill Livingstone, Edinburgh, p 43–71

Trowbridge I S, Newmann R A, Domingo D L et al 1984 Transferrin receptors: structure and function. Biochemical Pharmacology 33: 925–932

Verwilghen R L 1976 Congenital dyserythropoietic anaemia type II (HEMPAS). In: Congenital disorders of erythropoiesis. CIBA Foundation Symposium 37. Elsevier, Amsterdam, 151–170

Voorhess M L, Stuart M J, Stockman J A, Oksi F A 1975 Iron deficiency anemia and increased urinary norepinephrine excretion. Journal of Pediatrics 86: 542–547

Wainscoat J S, Kanavakis E, Wood W G et al 1983 Thalassaemia intermedia in Cyprus: the interaction of α and β thalassaemia. British Journal of Haematology 53: 411–416

Walter T, Arredondo S, Arevalo M, Stekel A 1986 Effect of iron therapy on phagocytosis and bactericidal activity in neutrophils of iron-deficient infants. American Journal of Clinical Nutrition 44: 877–882

Walters T 1967 Congenital megaloblastic anaemia responsive to N^5-formyl tetrahydrofolic acid administration. Journal of Pediatrics 70: 686–687

Weatherall D J 1963 Abnormal haemoglobins in the neonatal period and their relationship to thalassaemia. British Journal of Haematology 9: 265–277

Weatherall D J, Pembrey M E, Hall E G, Sanger R, Tippett P, Gavin J 1970 Familial sideroblastic anaemia: problem of Xg and X chromosome inactivation. Lancet ii: 744–748

Weatherall D J, Clegg J B 1981 The thalassaemia syndromes, 3rd edn. Blackwell Scientific Publications, Oxford

Weatherall D J, Higgs D R, Clegg J B, Wood W G 1982 The significance of haemoglobin H in patients with mental retardation of myeloproliferative disease. British Journal of Haematology 52: 351–353

Weatherall D J, Ledingham J G G, Warrell D A (eds) 1987 Oxford textbook of medicine, 2nd edn. Oxford University Press, Oxford p 19.82

Weintraub L R, Conrad M E, Crosby W H 1966 Iron loading anemia. Treatment with repeated phlebotomies and pyridoxine. New England Journal of Medicine 275: 169–176

Wickramasinghe S N, Pippard M J 1986 Studies of erythroblast function in congenital dyserythropoietic anaemia, type I: evidence of impaired DNA, RNA, and protein synthesis and unbalanced globin chain synthesis in ultrastructurally abnormal cells. Journal of Clinical Pathology 39: 881–890

Worwood M, Cragg S J, Jacobs A, McLaren C, Ricketts C, Economidou J 1980 Binding of serum ferritin to concanavalin A: patients with homozygous β thalassaemia and transfusional iron overload. British Journal of Haematology 46: 409–416

World Health Organization 1972 Nutritional anemias. WHO Technical Report Series No 503, Geneva

Worwood M 1986 Serum ferritin. Clinical Science 70: 215–220

Yelunda S 1990 Neurochemical basis of behavioural effects of brain iron deficiency in animals. In: Dobbing J (ed) Brain, behaviour, and iron in the infant diet. Springer-Verlag, London p 63–75

Yip R, Binkin N J, Flashood L, Trowbridge F L 1987 Declining prevalence of anemia among low-income children in the United States. Journal of the American Medical Association 258: 1619–1623

Young N, Mortimer P 1984 Viruses and bone marrow failure. Blood 63: 729–737

van der Zee S P M, Lommen E J P, Trijbels J M F, Schretlen E D A M 1970 The influence of adenine on the clinical feature and purine metabolism in the Lesch-Nyhan syndrome. Acta Paediatrica Scandinavia 59:259–264

9. Disorders of red cells: II Haemolysis

J. P. M. Evans

INTRODUCTION

Haemolysis is red cell breakdown resulting in a reduction in the normal red cell lifespan. Anaemia develops if the increase in marrow activity and the consequent reticulocytosis cannot compensate for this. The normal red cell lifespan in children is 120 days; however, in neonates it is 60–80 days and is even shorter in premature infants.

The diagnosis of haemolysis is usually simple and requires evidence of both increased red cell breakdown and increased marrow activity. Usually a blood film, reticulocyte count, bilirubin and urine testing for haemoglobin and haemosiderin is sufficient to confirm the diagnosis, but sometimes measurements of haptoglobins may be necessary, and occasionally assessment of red cell survival using radioisotopes.

Diagnosis

Reticulocyte count

Reticulocytes are young erythrocytes which contain the remnants of ribosomes and RNA originally present in the nucleated red cell precursors. They are detected with a supravital stain which precipitates this material in the red blood cell. It is usual to count reticulocytes manually and to report this as a percentage of the total number of erythrocytes present (normal range 0.5–1.5%); however, this method of reporting may be misleading in the presence of a reduced total number of circulating red cells and it is better to report an absolute count, the normal range being $25–75 \times 10^9/1$ after the first 3 months of life.

In the presence of anaemia, the reticulocyte count usually reflects the compensatory bone marrow response, but the count may increase to $150 \times 10^9/1$ in moderate anaemia, even without an increase in erythropoietic activity; because of prematurely released young red cells.

Total unconjugated bilirubin

Normally 1% of the red cell population breaks down each day and haemoglobin is degraded to bilirubin. An increase in unconjugated bilirubin suggests an increase in destruction of haemoglobin.

Haptoglobin

This plasma protein is produced in the liver and binds free haemoglobin to form a complex which is rapidly cleared. The level of free haptoglobin falls when production cannot match clearance of the complex and this usually occurs when the rate of red cell destruction is approximately twice normal. Whilst a low level of haptoglobins may be useful to confirm the presence of haemolysis, the result may be misleading in a number of situations, such as parenchymal liver disease, congenital ahaptoglobinemia and in neonates, where levels are low. In contrast, elevated levels arise in inflammatory disease including infection, malignancy and connective tissue disorders and in the presence of these, mild haemolysis may fail to produce the anticipated reduction in haptoglobin concentration.

Plasma and urine free haemoglobin

Free haemoglobin does not appear until all the available haptoglobin has been depleted. Haemoglobinuria is easy to detect by spot test but further tests are necessary to distinguish haemoglobinuria from haematuria. When there is more than a transient small amount of haemoglobinuria, haemoglobin is absorbed by the renal tubular epithelium and this is eventually excreted into the urine as haemosiderin when epithelial cells are shed. The presence of haemosiderin in the urine is a useful sign of intermittent chronic intravascular haemolysis, because haemosiderin will be detectable for weeks after the last haemolytic episode.

Diagnosis of haemolysis in neonates

In neonates, the diagnosis of haemolysis may be more difficult. In the newborn, anaemia, jaundice and reticulocytosis occur commonly in nonhaemolytic conditions. The red cell lifespan is shorter than in older children, and the normal haemoglobin and reticulocyte counts vary with age.

At birth, reticulocyte counts of up to $350 \times 10^9/l$ are not unusual. The level of reticulocytes decreases so that at the end of the first week of life it falls to less than $80 \times 10^9/l$. Blood taking is an important cause of anaemia in premature and sick neonates and needs to be considered in the differential diagnosis of a fall in haemoglobin. Unconjugated hyperbilirubinaemia is a feature of physiological jaundice of normal infants and is probably related to hepatic immaturity and the increase in catabolism of red cells at birth.

Haptoglobins are extremely low or even absent in the first month of life and therefore cannot be used to indicate haemolysis in this age group (Lundh et al 1970). In making a diagnosis of haemolysis in a neonate, it is crucial that all investigation results are compared to age-adjusted values and other interacting clinical factors.

Differential diagnosis

Once a diagnosis of haemolysis has been made, the determination of its cause is usually simple. The clinical history may provide many important clues as to whether it is a congenital or acquired problem, and whether it is recurrent or chronic. A family history of anaemia, jaundice, gall stones or splenectomy are suggestive of a congenital cause. It is also important to determine whether there have been previous miscarriages, anaemia or jaundice in other children. It is always useful to know whether the child has had a previous normal blood count and whether there were any neonatal problems with jaundice or blood transfusion.

Clinical examination may show splenomegaly or signs of haemopoietic hypertrophy such as frontal bossing; neurological abnormalities may be associated with kernicterus and also some of the inherited enzyme anomalies.

Anaemia is a common finding in haemolysis, but if mild may be compensated by an increase in erythropoiesis. The MCV is often slightly raised in the presence of a brisk reticulocytosis. Examination of the blood film may show simple polychromasia or abnormalities associated with specific disorders, such as spherocytes, red cell fragments or the 'bite' cells associated with unstable haemoglobins or glucose-6-phosphate dehydrogenase (G6PD) deficiency.

More specific investigations to determine the cause of haemolysis may be undertaken in the light of these findings and are discussed later in the context of each individual disorder.

General features of haemolysis

In haemolytic anaemias, the maintenance of a stable haemoglobin concentration is dependent upon an increase in bone marrow erythropoiesis. Suppression of the bone marrow, often due to viral infections, may cause a sudden fall in haemoglobin.

Parvovirus B19 has now been shown to be a common cause of temporary reticulocytopenia. It is a common viral infection in normal children, causing a mild illness which may be asymptomatic or may cause a characteristic facial rash ('slapped face') associated with arthralgia (so-called 'fifth disease'). In children with chronic compensated haemolysis, the reticulocytopenia which results from this infection may produce a sudden and dramatic anaemia. Because of the greater requirement caused by increased erythropoiesis, it is common practice to give folic acid supplements to all patients with chronic haemolytic anaemias.

A simple classification of childhood haemolytic anaemias is given in Table 9.1. Some examples are considered in more detail below.

MEMBRANE ABNORMALITIES

The red cell membrane is vital to the oxygen transport function of the red cell. In order to pass through

Table 9.1   Classification of childhood haemolytic anaemias

A. *Inherited*
  I Defects in the structure and function of the red cell
    membrane
        Hereditary spherocytosis
        Hereditary elliptocytosis
  II Defects of erythrocyte metabolism
        Glucose 6-phosphate dehydrogenase deficiency
        Pyruvate kinase deficiency
        Other enzyme disorders
  III Qualitative haemoglobin disorders
        Stable variants – sickle cell disease
        Unstable variants
  IV Quantitative haemoglobin disorders
        Impaired globin chain synthesis
        The thalassaemias (Ch. 8)
B. *Acquired*
  I Immune
        Autoimmune
        Alloimmune (neonatal)
  II Non-immune
        Infection
        Mechanical – microangiopathic haemolytic anaemia
        Drug-induced
        Paroxysmal nocturnal haemoglobinuria

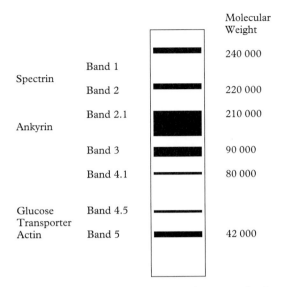

Fig. 9.1   SPS PAGE gel electrophoresis pattern of major red blood cell membrane proteins

the microcirculation, the red cell needs to have enormous deformability. In addition, the membrane needs to allow oxygen to diffuse yet maintain the concentrations of intracellular glucose and ions. Abnormalities of the red cell membrane are an important cause of both congenital and acquired haemolysis. In order to understand these, an appreciation of the basic structure and function of the normal red cell membrane is important.

The normal red cell membrane

The red cell membrane is composed of a lipid bilayer and membrane proteins.

The membrane skeleton is a protein lattice attached to the cytoplasmic side of the red cell membrane. It contains four major proteins: spectrin, actin, protein 4.1 and ankyrin. Spectrin is the most abundant of these proteins and is composed of two chains, alpha and beta, which are twisted into a heterodimer and joined head-to-head to form an elongated tetramer. The distal end of these tetramers is linked to actin and the junction is strengthened by protein 4.1. This protein skeleton is attached to the membrane by ankyrin, which connects the spectrin beta chain to the major transmembrane protein band 3. Figure 9.1 shows the polyacrilamide gel electrophoretic (PAGE)

pattern of the normal red blood cell skeleton. Figure 9.2 is a diagram of a cross section of the red cell membrane.

The genes of some of the main membrane proteins have now been mapped: the spectrin alpha chain to chromosome 1, the spectrin beta chain to chromosome 14, ankyrin to chromosome 8, band 3 to chromosome 17, band 4.1 to chromosome 1, and glycophorin B to chromosome 2 (Pekrun & Gratzer 1990). An increasing number of the known genetic abnormalities of the red cell membranes are now being defined as being caused by abnormalities or deficiencies of the proteins of the membrane skeleton.

Of equal importance in terms of membrane function is the lipid component of the membrane, which is organized into a lipid bilayer. The predominant lipids are phospholipids and cholesterol. The major classes of phospholipids are choline-containing (phosphatidyl choline and sphingomyelin) and the amino phospholipids (phosphatidyl ethanolamine and phosphatidyl serine). They are distributed asymmetrically between the bilayer leaflets; the outer leaflet is enriched with the choline phospholipids and the inner leaflet is enriched with the amino phospholipids. Membrane ATP has an absolute requirement for phospholipids in order to function. The precise role of the specific phospholipids in membrane struc-

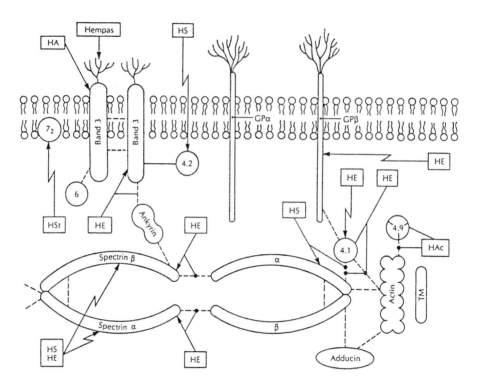

Fig. 9.2 Schematic representation of the organization of the red cell membrane and its membrane skeleton. Only the major structural proteins are shown. The membrane skeletal network is composed of spectrin, mainly in the form of tetramers, each containing two αβ dimer units. They are attached at their extremities to junctions, containing short actin filaments (protofilaments). Six spectrin molecules, on average, are attached to each junction, each interaction being stabilized by a 4.1 molecule. Two molecules of tropomyosin and one trimeric 4.9 are bound to the photofilaments, and some junctions also have an attached adducin dimer. The known interactions between different protein components are denoted (*broken lines*). The transmembrane proteins are shown as passing through the lipid bilayer. Glycophorin-α and glycophorin-β are the major sialoglycoproteins (also called glycophorins A and C). Band 6 is glyceraldehyde-3-phosphate dehydrogenase, and Tm is tropomyosin. Arrows denote a protein in which a genetic anomaly is expressed, and closed circles indicate the protein-protein interaction affected by the mutation. The straight line between HAc and 4.9 denotes a reported phosphorylation anomaly; bent arrows denote a protein with reduced abundance in certain genetic states. The clinical manifestations of the indicated anomalies are shown. HA—hemolytic anaemia, associated with premature appearance of the senescence antigen; HAc—hereditary acanthocytosis; HSt—hereditary stomatocytosis; HEMPAS—dyserythropoietic anaemia (congenital dyserythropoietic anaemia II).
From: Pekrun & Gratzer 1990, with permission.

ture and function is still being elucidated, but their interaction with both skeletal and integral proteins suggests that they are intimately involved in maintaining the structural integrity and permeability properties of the erythrocyte membrane.

The intracellular concentration of sodium and potassium is a critical determinant of the red blood cell water content, volume and hence deformability. A number of cation transport systems maintain sodium and potassium concentrations, including membrane ATPase. Calcium regulation, also via a membrane ATPase, is also of critical importance in the regulation of cell volume and membrane structure.

Disorders of the membrane skeleton

Hereditary spherocytosis (HS)

Probably the most common haemolytic anaemia

in people of North European extraction, hereditary spherocytosis (HS) has a frequency of 1 in 5000 in this population, but it appears to be less common in other races and ethnic groups. The majority of cases are inherited in an autosomal dominant fashion and this can be shown in approximately 75% of cases. In 25% of cases the mode of inheritance is less clear, possibly that of an autosomal dominant characteristic of reduced penetrance, an autosomal recessive one or possibly due to a new mutation (Smedley & Bellingham 1991).

Clinical features. The severity of haemolysis varies from very mild to very severe, although the majority are moderate (Krueger & Burgert 1966). Anaemia, jaundice and splenomegaly are characteristic. The disease can present at any time but usually presents in childhood. Anaemia is the most common presentation but children may be asymptomatic. Most children suffer intermittent jaundice which is often associated with a mild viral infection. The jaundice is associated with a raised unconjugated bilirubin. The spleen is palpable in the majority of children and most adults. Most older children and adults have compensated haemolysis with little or no anaemia. The reticulocyte count is almost always raised. The anaemia is usually mild but, as with any other chronic haemolytic anaemias, a sudden exacerbation may occur, usually due to an increased rate of haemolysis or transient marrow aplasia. Pigment gall stones occur in up to 85% of adults and have been described in children as young as 5 years of age (Mackinney 1965).

Neonatal hereditary spherocytosis. Jaundice is very common during the neonatal period, and 30–50% of children with hereditary spherocytosis have a history of significant neonatal jaundice (Trucco & Brown 1967). This usually becomes evident in the first 48 hours but may manifest later. Exchange transfusion is occasionally thought necessary. There is no evidence that those who are symptomatic as neonates have more severe hereditary spherocytosis.

Pathophysiology. As red cells circulate, they become more spheroidal as a result of loss of membrane and there is a progressive decrease in surface area. Spherocytosis probably results from more than one mechanism. There is loss of both lipid and protein. Increased permeability to cations

is also probably a consequence of the lesion within the membrane, but whether this plays a significant role in the loss of surface remains uncertain.

The major site of destruction of red cells appears to be the spleen. Spherocytes are poorly deformable and are probably physically trapped in the splenic cords and sinuses because of their inability to squeeze through them. The relative hypoxia and acidity in the splenic structure may lead to further lipid loss, and the failure of the cation pumps allow sodium and water to accumulate. The way in which haemolysis is increased by viral or bacterial infections is not clear, but hyperplasia of the spleen may be an important factor.

The molecular basis of hereditary spherocytosis. Spectrin deficiency has been described in the majority of patients. Reduction to a level of approximately 50% was first noted in severe haemolytic spherocytosis inherited in an apparently recessive fashion, and the level of spectrin deficiency appears roughly to correlate with the severity of haemolysis and, possibly, the response to splenectomy.

A milder degree of spectrin deficiency has been shown in the majority of patients with typical autosomal dominant hereditary spherocytosis. The molecular basis of this spectrin deficiency is unknown, but is possibly due to a decrease in synthesis, an unstable mutant or defective binding of the beta spectrin to its major binding proteins 4.1.

Ankyrin deficiency has also been described in severe spherocytosis (Coetzer et al 1988). The role of the membrane skeletal defect in the surface area loss is unclear, but one possible explanation is that the membrane skeleton is organized as a monomolecular gel with the individual skeletal elements in close contact with each other. Consequently, a decrease in spectrin content leads to a decrease in surface area occupied by the skeleton.

In addition to a loss of surface area, several other abnormalities have been described in HS cells these include altered cation permeability, and also a beta spectrin defect resulting in defective spectrin:protein 4.1 interaction and subsequent increase in ATP utilization (Palek 1987). This may be secondary to the underlying skeletal defect leading to a decrease in the activity of the sodium/potassium pump.

Diagnosis of spherocytosis. The diagnosis is

essentially one of exclusion, but is usually straight-forward, and spherocytes are easy to find in the majority of cases on a blood film. The increase in osmotic fragility in a formal osmotic fragility test correlates with the degree of spherocytosis. The test is more sensitive after incubation of the sample for 24 hours, because the metabolically depleted cells suffer a further loss in surface area. Diagnosis in the neonatal period may be difficult. Fetal cells are more osmotically resistant than adult cells, but in neonatal HS the incubated osmotic fragility is usually abnormal.

The major diagnostic problem in the newborn is to distinguish HS from ABO incompatibility; occasionally in neonates, bacterial sepsis can also cause spherocytosis. The differentiation from these acquired conditions is helped by family studies and also by the course of the disease. It should be noted that increased osmotic fragility per se is not diagnostic of HS and will be seen in other haemolytic anaemias where spherocytes are present.

Treatment. The majority of patients benefit from splenectomy, which prolongs the red blood cell survival. Following splenectomy, the red cell abnormalities persist, but haemolytic and aplastic crises cease and the risk of traumatic rupture of an enlarged spleen is abolished. The main benefit of splenectomy is that, as a result of the greatly reduced haemolytic rate, the risk of development of gall stones becomes much less, but the most serious side-effect is the risk of postsplenectomy sepsis. The risk of pneumococcal infection can probably be reduced by the administration of prophylactic penicillin and pneumococcal vaccine. Splenectomy is indicated in all but very mild spherocytosis, but should be postponed until late childhood unless the disease interferes with normal growth and development. Occasional severe forms where repeated transfusions are required justify splenectomy in infancy.

Hereditary elliptocytosis (HE)

This disorder rarely results in measurable haemolysis despite the dramatically abnormal blood film. Anaemia is not usually a feature, and the degree of reticulocytosis, if any, is very mild. The majority of cells are elliptocytic. The disease only presents a clinical problem in the unusual haemolytic variants, and also in the very rare homozygous form of hereditary elliptocytosis where haemolysis is severe and may require blood transfusion therapy (Evans et al 1983)

Mild HE with transient poikylocytosis. Patients with mild HE sometimes show a more severe haemolytic anaemia in the neonatal period and this may be sufficiently severe to require transfusion (Austin & Desforges 1969). The appearance of the blood film is not characteristic of mild HE, and numerous poikylocytes and pyknocytes are seen. The appearance of the blood film gradually improves, eventually becoming identical to that seen in mild HE. This disorder can be difficult to distinguish (in the neonatal period) from more severe haemolytic anaemias. A study of family members may be very useful, revealing typical mild HE in one or other parent.

Hereditary pyropoikylocytosis. This unusual condition presents in the neonatal period. The blood film is very abnormal, showing the presence of elliptocytes, spherocytes, fragments and some red cells with bud-like projections. The disease is defined on the basis of the red blood cell response to heating in vitro, and the pyropoikylocytes undergo budding or fragmentation at a temperature several degrees below that at which normal blood cells fragment (Palek 1987). The condition was initially described in Negro patients, but its occurrence in Caucasians has now been reported. It may be difficult to distinguish from homozygous HE or more severe cases of HE with transient poikylocytosis and pyropoikylocytes. The inheritance of hereditary pyropoikylocytosis is unclear, and family studies may not be helpful, in that parents and siblings of patients may have mild HE.

Pathophysiology of HE. Despite the rarity of clinical problems in common HE, the disorder has proved very useful in providing insight into the structure and abnormalities of the red cell cytoskeleton, and a variety of skeletal defects have been described.

Up to 30% of HE patients and all HPP patients have defects in the association of spectrin dimers into tetramers and oligimers. This may be due to spectrin alpha chain or beta chain problems, whilst deficiency of protein 4.1 may also contribute to the disorder (Pekrun & Gratzer 1990).

Treatment. The vast majority of cases of common HE require no treatment or follow-up. Hereditary pyropoikylocytosis and homozygous hereditary elliptocytosis may respond to splenectomy, and the management is as for hereditary spherocytosis.

Acquired disorders of the red cell membrane

Liver disease results in changes of plasma lipid composition and lipid composition of the red cell membrane. Haemolysis is not usually a clinical problem, except in the presence of severe liver disease.

Hereditary acanthocytosis (abetalipoproteinaemia)

In this rare condition, there is a deficiency of low density lipoproteins, red cells show bizarre spiny deformities, but haemolysis is typically mild.

DISORDER OF RED CELL METABOLISM

The mature red cell is dependent on the anaerobic metabolism of glucose to meet its energy requirements. Mitochondria and the capacity for oxidative phosphorylation are lost at the reticulocyte stage of erythroid development. Adenosine triphosphate [ATP] is necessary for the red blood cell to maintain its shape (see Red cell membrane

section). Cation transport is also involved in the synthesis of glutathione (GSH) and the supply of NADH which participates in the reduction of methaemoglobin to functional haemoglobin. Glycolysis also generates the high levels of 2,3 diphosphoglycerate (2,3DPG) that modulate haemoglobin oxygen affinity.

Other important metabolic pathways in the red blood cell include the aerobic hexose monophosphate shunt that is *not* involved in the generation of ATP but in the formation of both reduced nicotinamide adenine nucleotide (NADPH) and pentose sugars. NADPH has an important role in glutathione metabolism. Reduced glutathione is present in relatively high concentrations in normal red blood cells, and is an important intracellular reducing agent. Oxidants such as superoxide and hydrogen peroxide are generated within the red cell, and glutathione has an important antioxidant function, preventing oxidation of the red cell membrane or haemoglobin. The Rapoport-Leubering shunt is responsible for maintaining high concentrations of 2,3DPG. The major pathways of red cell metabolism are summarized in Figure 9.3. It must be noted that the profile of enzyme activities of the red cell in the first few weeks of life differs significantly from that of the adult and older child (Stockman & Osti 1978, Konrad et al 1972).

Table 9.2 Clinical features of some enzymopathies

Embden-Meyerhof pathway enzyme deficiency	Mode of inheritance	Neonates	Clinical features	Red cell appearances
Pyruvate kinase (PK)	Autosomal recessive	Anaemia and jaundice common. May require exchange transfusion	Moderate to severe haemolytic anaemia. Splenectomy often helps	Basophilia in occasional cells
Glucose phosphate isomerase (GPI)	Autosomal recessive	Jaundice common	Acute haemolytic crises may be associated with infection	No characteristic features
Triose phosphate isomerase (TPI)	Autosomal recessive	Severe jaundice reported	Progressive neurological disorder develops after 6 months of age. Death in early childhood. Increased susceptibility to infection	"
Hexokinase (HK)	Autosomal recessive	Jaundice	Moderate haemolysis	"
Phosphoglycerate kinase (PGK)	X-linked	Neonatal jaundice usual	Moderate to severe neuropsychiatric disability. May have rhabdomyolysis and muscle weakness	"
Phosphofructokinase (PFK)	Autosomal recessive (Jewish ancestry)	Usually mild	Exertional myopathy, muscle cramps, myoglobinuria	"

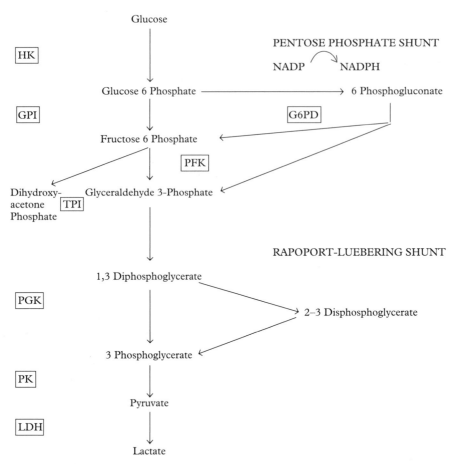

Fig. 9.3 Schematic diagram of the major pathways of red cell metabolism. Key enzymes are indicated by boxed initials and include: HK = Hexokinase; G6PD = Glucose-6-phosphate dehydrogenase; GPI = Glucose phosphate isomerase; TPI = Triose phosphate isomerase; PK = Pyruvate kinase; LDH = Lactic dehydrogenase; PFK = Phosphofructokinase; PGK = Phosphoglycerokinase.

The most common enzyme deficiency is G6PD deficiency but, except in very unusual cases, this is not a cause of a chronic haemolytic anaemia, presenting rather as acute haemolytic episodes. Enzyme abnormalities are a rare cause of chronic haemolytic anaemia, pyruvate kinase [PK] deficiency being the most common.

Haematological features. In general, there are no specific abnormalities of red cell morphology associated with the majority of enzymopathies. Patients with G6PD deficiency during episodes of haemolytic crisis may show the presence of 'bite cells', and also Heinz bodies may be demonstrated after oxidant stress. Basophilic stippling is a feature of pyrimidine 5' nucleotidase deficiency. Echi-

nocytes or sputnik cells are seen in PK deficiency and in other glycolytic enzymopathies. Red cell morphology becomes much more strikingly abnormal after splenectomy.

Inheritance. The majority of enzymopathies are inherited as an autosomal recessive trait, although G6PD and phosphoglycerokinase (PGK) (Fig. 9.3) are X-linked. This distinguishes them from membrane disorders and unstable haemoglobins, which are usually inherited in a dominant fashion.

Clinical features. Apart from general features of haemolytic anaemia, some of the enzymopathies have specific features (Table 9.2). Favism (haemolysis after ingestion of fava beans) or the precipitation of haemolysis by oxidant drugs is suggestive of G6PD deficiency.

Nervous or muscle disease is associated with some of the rarer abnormalities of the Embden-Meyerhof pathway. Cyanosis may be due to methaemoglobinaemia, in turn due to methaemoglobin reductase deficiency or to one of the M type haemoglobinopathies. Exertional myoglobinuria is characteristic of phosphofructokinase (PFK) deficiency.

Glucose-6-phosphate dehydrogenase (G6PD) deficiency

Biochemistry. The enzyme G6PD catalyses the conversion of glucose-6 phosphate to 6-phosphogluconate. This is the first enzyme reaction of the hexose monophosphate shunt. NADP is a cofactor which is reduced to NADPH and is vital in maintaining glutathione in its reduced state.

More than 300 types of G6PD have been described. Most of these variants are enzymatically normal and are not a cause of clinical problems. G6PD B is the normal enzyme found in Caucasians and many Negroes. G6PD A is the most common variant associated with haemolysis, and is found in 10–15% of American Negroes (Dacie 1985). It is unstable and its activity is decreased in older red cells. G6PD Mediterranean is the most common abnormal variant in Caucasians of Mediterranean origin, and has a markedly reduced catalytic activity. G6PD Canton has enzymatic properties similar to those of G6PD Mediterranean, and is the most common cause of G6PD-deficiency in Asians. In the case of G6PD variants associated with chronic haemolysis, there is no single biochemical abnormality which has been identified.

When G6PD-deficient red cells are exposed to oxidants, the major intracellular antioxidant GSH is depleted. Oxidation of haemoglobin leads to denaturation and Heinz bodies, and oxidation of the membrane leads to the accumulation of membrane polypeptide aggregates due to disulphide bond formation between spectrin molecules and between spectrin and other membrane proteins. This results in rigid red cells that are susceptible to entrapment and destruction by splenic macrophages.

Cells that are less severely damaged may have part of the red cell membrane removed in the spleen, and this is thought to be the cause of the characteristic 'bite cells' seen in G6PD deficiency.

Clinical features. G6PD deficiency is the most common red blood cell enzyme abnormality which is associated with haemolysis and affects millions of people in the Mediterranean, Africa and China. The worldwide distribution is similar to that of malaria, and it appears that G6PD deficiency may protect against this infection to some extent. As G6PD is X-linked, haemolysis is a problem mainly in male subjects, although it can occur in females, due either to homozygous inheritance of an abnormal G6PD gene or, more commonly, to extreme lyonization.

G6PD does not normally cause chronic anaemia, and in the steady state the blood picture looks normal. Acute haemolytic episodes may be caused by oxidant drugs (Table 9.3). Although many drugs have been implicated in causing haemolysis in G6PD-deficient subjects, the evidence in many cases is unclear. Infections such as hepatitis, salmonellosis and pneumonia may also provoke haemolysis.

Haemolysis following exposure to fava beans occurs in G6PD-deficient Caucasians and Asians but is not seen in Negroes. It does not occur in all susceptible G6PD-deficient individuals, and the exact factor causing haemolysis is unclear.

Haemolysis in the neonatal period is relatively common. In one study from Greece, approximately 30% of all exchange transfusions for hyperbilirubinaemia were carried out in G6PD-deficient infants.

Diagnosis. The diagnosis of G6PD deficiency is aided by a typical clinical history of episodic haemolysis associated with drugs, infections or fava beans. 'Bite cells' are often seen during acute episodes and brilliant cresyl blue supra vital stains of blood may show Heinz bodies on such occasions. Specific enzyme assay measures the rate at which NAPDH is generated when glucose-6-phosphate and NADP are added to a haemolysate (Beutler 1984). The level may appear to be falsely high during a haemolytic crisis, due to the relatively higher enzyme concentration present in reticulocytes. A repeat assay when the haemolytic episode is over is often necessary to determine the severity of deficiency and to make the diagnosis.

Management. Supportive care is the approach

Table 9.3 Drugs and chemicals associated with significant haemolysis in subjects with G6PD deficiency

Drugs	Definite association	Possible association*	Doubtful association
Antimalarials	Primaquine		Quinacrine
	Pamaquine	Chloroquine	
	Pentaquine		Quinine
Sulfonamides	Septrin (Sulfamethoxazole)		Sulfisoxazole
	Sulfanilamide	Sulfamethoxazole Pyridazine	Sulfoxone
	Sulfacetamide	Sulfadimidine	Sulfadiazine
	Sulfapyridine		Sulfamerizine
Sulfones	Dapsone (Thiazolesulfone Diaminodiaphenylsulphone, DDS)		
Nitrofurans	Nitrofurantoin		
Antipyretic/ analgesics	Acetanilide		Amiopyrine
			Acetominophen
			Phenacetin
			Aspirin
Others	Nalidixic acid	Chloramphenicol	PAS
	Naphthalone	Vitamin K Analogues	L-Dopa
	Niridazole		Vitamin C
	Phenylhydrazine		Dimercaprol
	Toluidine blue		Doxorubicin
	Trinitrotoluene (TNT)		Probenecid
	Methylene blue		
	Phenazopyridine		

*These agents will cause clinically significant haemolysis but only when given in larger than therapeutic doses, or to subjects with severe variants or to neonates.

to acute haemolytic episodes; blood transfusion may be necessary when anaemia is severe. When the diagnosis has been made, further episodes of haemolysis may be prevented by education and the avoidance of provoking factors, particularly drugs.

Pyruvate kinase deficiency

Approximately 300 cases of pyruvate kinase deficiency have been described, making it the second most common enzymopathy; it is particularly common in Northern Europeans. The disease has a variable clinical course.

About one-third of cases present during the newborn period, and one-third of these require transfusion. In some patients, the anaemia improves as the child gets older. Children with milder forms of the disease may not be picked up until late childhood or even adult life.

Biochemistry. The conversion of phosphoenol pyruvate to pyruvate is catalyzed by pyruvate kinase and this reaction generates ATP. When depleted of ATP, pyruvate-kinase-deficient red cells leak potassium and water, becoming dehydrated.

The red cell membrane appears to become more rigid and this may explain the consequent susceptibility to entrapment within the spleen.

Diagnosis. The clinical features of pyruvate kinase deficiency are not very specific. Red cell morphology is often normal, although it is usually possible to find an occasional echinocyte. Definitive diagnosis requires the assay of red cell pyruvate kinase activity.

In anaemic homozygotes or compound heterozygotes, enzyme activity ranges from 0–50% of normal, and in heterozygotes is usually between 40 and 60%. There is a poor correlation between the degree of pyruvate kinase activity and the severity of haemolysis.

Treatment. Severely affected patients sometimes benefit from splenectomy, particularly by the elimination of the need for transfusion support.

Diagnosis of enzymopathies

The concentrations of major red cell metabolites can be measured to assist in the diagnosis of enzymopathy. Increased 2,3DPG levels occur in

Table 9.4 Disorders of purine and pyrimidine metabolism

Enzyme defect	Mode of inheritance	Neonates	Clinical features	Red cell appearances
Pyrimidine 5' nucleotidase deficiency	Autosomal recessive	Neonatal jaundice may occur	Splenomegaly, hepatosplenomegaly Moderate haemolysis	Basophilic stippling conspicuous
Adenosine deaminase overproduction	Autosomal dominant	Mild haemolysis	Mild to moderate haemolysis	No characteristic features
Adenylate kinase deficiency	Unknown	Mild haemolysis*	Mild*	No characteristic features

* Role in haemolytic anaemia controversial

most anaemias but are also present in hypoxia, alkalosis and hyperphosphataemia. The greatest increase is noted in pyruvate kinase deficiency, and in this condition the DPG:ATP ratio may be very useful. Paradoxically, low concentrations of 2,3DPG are a useful indicator of a disorder affecting the beginning of the glycolytic pathway, and suggest deficiency of hexokinase, phosphofructokinase (PFK) or glucose phosphate isomerase (GPI; Lestas & Bellingham 1990).

Glycolytic intermediates

Glycolytic intermediates may be affected by metabolic blocks, and perturbations in their concentrations can give useful diagnostic information. In pyruvate kinase deficiency, in addition to the elevated levels of 2,3DPG, phosphoenol pyruvate (PEP), 2-phosphoglycerate (2PG) and 3-phosphoglycerate (3PG) are also all elevated. Low levels of all intermediates, especially glucose-6-phosphate and fructose 1,6 diphosphate (F1,6PD), suggest hexokinase deficiency. It is important to confirm the diagnosis with specific enzyme assays, which are usually done in specialized laboratories. When assaying glycolytic intermediates, it is vital to run appropriate controls. Ideally, these should include control samples with an equivalent reticulocytosis, as well as samples from carefully age-matched normal controls. The normal neonatal ranges of practically all enzymes and intermediates are different from adults, and changes occur continuously during the first year of life.

Prenatal diagnosis of triose phosphate isomerase (TPI) pyruvate kinase (PK) and glucose phosphate isomerase (GPI) deficiency are all possible.

Enzyme disorders of purine and pyrimidine metabolism

Maturation of the reticulocyte requires disposal of ribosomal RNA which is no longer needed for protein synthesis. Pyrimidine 5' nucleotidase is essential for this process, otherwise pyrimidine nucleotides accumulate in the cell; why such cells are destroyed prematurely is not known. The clinical features of the disorder, together with those of two other extremely rare disorders of protein synthesis, are indicated in Table 9.4.

HAEMOGLOBIN VARIANTS

Haemolysis due to unstable haemoglobin variants

Unstable haemoglobins are variants which denature either spontaneously or in response to oxidant stress. They are usually inherited in an autosomal dominant fashion.

Clinical features. The clinical picture is variable and ranges from a complete lack of symptoms to a severe transfusion-dependent haemolytic anaemia. The most severe cases present during infancy, but less severe cases can be diagnosed in late childhood or adult life, sometimes presenting with gallstones.

The unstable haemoglobins may have other functional abnormalities, such as high or low oxygen affinity. Patients with a low-affinity variant show a lower haemoglobin than expected for the degree of haemolysis. The higher-affinity variants may be associated with a higher haemoglobin level, and variants which produce methaemoglobin may produce clinical cyanosis.

Unstable haemoglobins may be due to abnormalities of either the alpha chain or the beta chain. Beta-chain variants present only after the switch from fetal to adult haemoglobin, at about 6 months of age.

Alpha-chain variants may present at any time

after birth. Only one unstable haemoglobin has been shown to be due to an abnormality of the gamma chain of haemoglobin (Lee-Potter et al 1975), and this is a clinical problem only during the first few months of life. The majority of variants involve the beta chain.

Laboratory features. The blood film is often not specific, although anisocytosis and basophilic stippling may be present. Occasionally, 'bite cells' are seen. Heinz bodies are found only after splenectomy or during an acute exacerbation of haemolysis. The abnormal haemoglobin may not be detectable by routine electrophoresis. A heat denaturation test and the isopropanol precipitation test are good screening tests for unstable haemoglobins, but precise identification of the variant requires amino acid analysis.

Management. Treatment is essentially supportive. Splenectomy has been found to be useful occasionally in some cases, although often not in those with the most severe disease. It should perhaps be avoided in childhood.

Haemolysis due to stable haemoglobin variants

Sickle cell disease

Sickle cell disease primarily affects people of African, Afro-Caribbean, Middle Eastern, Indian and Mediterranean descent. The important sickling syndromes are homozygous sickle cell disease [HbSS] and the double heterozygous states haemoglobin SC disease [HbSC] and sickle beta thalassaemia [Sβthal]. Eight per cent of American Negroes have sickle cell trait, and in parts of Africa one-third of all births are AS heterozygotes.

Pathophysiology. Sickle cell disease is caused by a single-base mutation of adenine to thiamine which results in a substitution of valine for glutamic acid at the sixth codon of the β-globin chain. Concentrated solutions of sickle haemoglobin form a gel when deoxygenated, and this is thought to be the basis of sickling and the subsequent red cell membrane damage. The rigid sickle cell may then cause blockage to blood flow in the microcirculation.

The propensity of sickle haemoglobin to form a gel is inversely correlated with its concentration. This may explain the observed reduction in disease severity associated with high levels of haemoglobin F.

Diagnosis. The diagnosis of homozygous HbSS sickle cell disease is usually straightforward, and sickle cells, target cells and polychromasia are seen on the blood film. Haemoglobin electrophoresis demonstrates more than 80% haemoglobin S. Investigation of double heterozygous states producing sickle cell disease may be more difficult, and family studies may be necessary, but it is essential, both for treating the patient and counselling the parents, that the precise diagnosis is obtained.

Antenatal diagnosis is possible by chorionic villous biopsy in the first trimester of pregnancy, and it is important that good, nondirective counselling is available for affected couples, taking account of the variable clinical course.

Clinical features. The typical features are chronic haemolytic anaemia complicated by infection and sickle cell crises.

Some patients have repeated hospital admissions with frequent vaso-occlusive crises. Others remain asymptomatic and are only affected late in life. The major problems for infants and young children with sickle cell disease are overwhelming infection, particularly with *Pneumococcus* and *Haemophilus influenzae*, and acute splenic sequestration, where a precipitous fall in haemoglobin is associated with a rapidly enlarging spleen (see below). Patients do not usually present clinically until the switch from fetal to adult-type haemopoiesis is advanced. However, the risk of overwhelming sepsis appears to start early on. The highest mortality is in the first 5 years of life. In a Jamaican study, 10% of cases died in the first year, 5% in the second and 3% in the third (Serjeant 1985).

Infection. The increased risk of infection in sickle cell disease appears to be due to hypersplenism, defective opsonization mechanisms and probably other, ill-defined factors. Affected patients are particularly prone to infections with *Pneumococcus*, *Haemophilus influenzae* and *Salmonella*. The risk of infection by *Pneumococcus* has been shown to be at least 600 times that in a normal population, with the greatest risk in the first 3 years of life. It has been clearly shown that prophylactic penicillin results in an 80% reduction in the infection rate in infants aged between 3 and 36 months (Gaston et al 1986), and so penicillin prophylaxis should be started in all sickle children by the age of 4 months.

The role of antipneumococcal vaccine in the prevention of infection has not yet been so clearly defined, but there is some evidence of both serological response and efficacy in children with sickle cell disease over the age of 2 years (Ammann 1982).

Acute painful crises. This results from vaso-occlusive episodes and may be provoked by infection, dehydration or cold. Pain may occur anywhere, and is most frequently seen in bones, muscles and abdomen. Young children suffer the 'hand-foot' syndrome, dactylitis due to infarction of the metacarpals and metatarsals with resultant painful swelling of the hands and feet.

There is no specific treatment for painful crises, and the child should be supported by fluid replacement, pain relief and antibiotics. It is always important to look for a focus of infection and then treat this appropriately. Joint effusions and swelling of tissues over infarcted bones are not infrequently seen. There is an increased risk of osteomyelitis often caused by *Salmonella*. This may be multifocal and difficult to distinguish from infarction.

Splenic sequestration. This is the other major cause of mortality in the early years. It is characterized by the sudden onset of pallor, breathlessness, abdominal pain and splenic enlargement. Rapid sequestration of red cells in the spleen leads to sudden anaemia. Urgent transfusion is sometimes indicated and it may even be necessary to use un-cross-matched blood on rare occasions.

Splenic sequestration crises often recur, and it is common practice to carry out elective splenectomy after a child has recovered from an episode. In children under the age of 2 years, recurrence can be prevented by regular blood transfusions; this allows a delay in splenectomy until the patient is older. It is probably of benefit to teach parents of young children with sickle cell disease to examine regularly for splenomegaly.

Acute chest syndrome. This is more common in older children and adults and is characterized by lung consolidation on the chest X-ray which may be bilateral. The cause is complex and ill understood but includes infection and infarction. Chest pain and breathlessness may occur but the physical signs may be unimpressive. Patients may deteriorate rapidly. Transfusion should be given if the haemoglobin concentration is falling, and exchange transfusion may be necessary in severe cases. It is one of the commoner causes of death in sickle cell disease.

Stroke. Cerebrovascular occlusions are one of the most feared complications of sickle cell disease and one of the few indications for immediate exchange transfusion. The risk of recurrence is very high, and a programme of regular transfusion should be embarked upon to prevent it. The exact period of transfusion therapy is unknown but should probably last at least 3 years. Apart from major lesions, there is also some evidence of more subtle neurological damage in sickle cell disease (Pavelkis et al 1989).

Anaemia. The haemoglobin concentration is reduced in patients with sickle cell disease but tends to remain stable in any individual case. Children with haemoglobin SC disease have higher haemoglobin concentrations, which may be near the normal range. A fall in haemoglobin results from a variety of causes, including splenic sequestration or reduced marrow activity resulting from virus infections, particularly parvovirus.

Blood transfusions. There is little evidence that blood transfusion during a simple painful crisis either reduces its severity or curtails its length. Repeated transfusions to suppress erythropoiesis and keep the haemoglobin S concentration less than 30% may be used to prevent complications. However, children receiving regular blood transfusions will require iron chelation treatment, as otherwise iron overload develops. Exchange transfusion may be indicated to prevent sickling in acute conditions, such as chest syndrome or stroke, and occasionally it is helpful in the preparation of a patient for elective surgery. The risks of blood transfusions, including reaction, sensitization and infection and iron overload, need to be balanced against any potential benefits.

Development. Many children with sickle cell disease are thin, and puberty and its growth spurt may be delayed, although the final height is usually normal.

Enuresis is a common problem, probably as a result of high fluid intakes and urinary volumes.

Sickle cell variants

Sickle/thalassaemia syndrome. Sickle beta thalassaemia (HbS-β_0 thalassaemia), in which no HbA is present, is more severe than HbS β_+ thalassaemia, in which a small amount of HbA is present. Both tend to be milder than HbSS. Microcytosis is a characteristic finding.

Haemoglobin SC disease. This also tends to be a milder disease than the homozygous form, but any individual can suffer any of the complications described for HbSS. Proliferative retinopathy in older patients with SC disease is a greater problem than in HbSS.

Sickle cell trait. Sickle cell trait is not usually associated with morbidity, and life expectancy of affected individuals is normal. Some renal abnormalities have been described, including a concentration defect and microscopic haematuria.

When people with sickle cell trait are exposed to extreme hypoxic conditions, sickling infarcts can occur, in particular in the spleen, and the trait may also carry a slightly increased risk of some thrombotic complications.

Other stable abnormal haemoglobins producing haemolysis

Outside the context of double heterozygosity with HbS, other qualitative haemoglobin disorders are rarely associated with clinically important haemolysis.

Haemoglobin C. Homozygotes have a mild anaemia, with a haemoglobin concentration usually in the range of 9–12 g/dl. Anaemia can be exacerbated, for example by infection. Splenomegaly develops during childhood, and one in four or five patients will develop clinical hypersplenism. The blood film typically shows 30–90% target cells and microspherocytes. Heterozygotes are clinically normal but have target cells on their blood films.

Haemoglobin D. Several forms of HbD exist, the commonest being D Punjab. Relatively few homozygotes have been described. Some show target cells, reduced osmotic fragility and compensated mild haemolysis.

Haemoglobin E. HbE is probably the commonest structural haemoglobin variant in the world, with an estimated 28 million carriers

in South East Asia alone (Wong & Kham 1984). The heterozygous state is asymptomatic, with haematological features similar to those of thalassaemic trait. Homozygotes have a mild haemolytic anaemia, microcytosis and a relative erythrocytosis.

The most important clinical syndrome associated with HbE is the double heterozygous state of HbE/β thalassaemia, which produces a severe transfusion-dependent anaemia similar to β thalassaemia major. The syndrome is most often seen in children from India or Bangladesh.

ACQUIRED DISORDERS LEADING TO HAEMOLYSIS

Paroxysmal nocturnal haemoglobinuria (PNH)

This is extremely uncommon in childhood (Miller et al 1967, Forman et al 1984) and is mainly a disease of adults. It does occasionally arise in children, with manifestations similar to those in adults. Acquired chronic intravascular haemolysis with haemosiderinuria, pancytopenia and thrombosis are the main clinical features. The diagnosis is made by the acidified serum lysis test, as the red cells are peculiarly sensitive to complement. It is a stem-cell disorder, and is associated with marrow hypoplasia in some patients. There is also an ill-understood but well-recognized predisposition to venous thrombosis, particularly in the hepatic portal system.

Haemolysis secondary to infection

Infections may cause haemolysis by a variety of mechanisms. Bacterial sepsis may provoke micro-angiopathy as a result of subacute intravascular coagulation. Viral infections can precipitate autoimmune haemolytic anaemia, and in the congenitally infected neonate hyperplasia of the reticuloendothelial system is probably the major mechanism.

Malaria

On a worldwide basis, malaria is a very important cause of haemolysis. It is predominantly due to infection with *Plasmodium falciparum* but the de-

Table 9.5 Autoimmune haemolytic anaemia in children

Type	Features	Associated conditions	Antibody specificity	Treatment
Warm	Acute or chronic Mild or severe Pallor, jaundice (Renal failure)	Idiopathic Systematic lupus erythematosus Rheumatoid arthritis Hodgkin's disease ITP – Evans' syndrome Methyldopa therapy	Usually auto-pan agglutinin, occasionally some incomplete anti-Rhesus or other specificity (anti-e)	Steroids (Dialysis)
Cold: DL type	Haemoglobinuria after exposure of extremities to cold Acute, self limiting	Non-specific viruses Measles vaccine Varicella	Usually anti-P, biphasic D L type	None, other than supportive
Cold: other	Mild anaemia Jaundice (Raynaud's) Acute, self-limiting	Mycoplasma Infectious mononucleosis	Anti-I Anti-I	None, other than supportive.

*Any autoimmune haemolytic anaemia may require transfusion in the face of a rapid fall in haemoglobin and symptoms. If no compatible blood can be found, the least incompatible should be given.
ITP = Immune thrombocytopenic purpura; DL = Donath Landsteiner; (Brackets) indicate 'occasionally'.
From: Lilleyman J S 1991. Current Paediatrics.

gree of anaemia in malaria is frequently disproportionate to the degree of parasitaemia. A multiplicity of factors have been implicated. These include haemolysis (due to parasites, hyperactivity of the reticuloendothelial system and autoimmunity), depression of erythropoiesis and ineffective erythropoiesis (Abdalla et al 1980, Perrin et al 1981).

A positive direct antiglobulin test has been found in up to 50% of children with *Plasmodium falciparum* malaria although this is not universally correlated with significant haemolysis. In endemic areas, up to 10% of all newborns have malarial infection which may be accompanied by severe anaemia.

Congenital infections

Cytomegalovirus, herpes simplex, rubella, toxoplasmosis, and syphilis may all be associated with haemolysis. There may be an associated thrombocytopenia, and in the case of syphilis the presence of a Donath-Landsteiner antibody (see below) may contribute to the haemolytic process.

Autoimmune haemolytic anaemia (AIHA)

AIHA is uncommon in childhood and tends to be acute and self-limiting. It may occur at any age, and often there is evidence of preceding or concurrent viral infection, particularly of the upper respiratory tract. It usually resolves within 3 months.

In older children, autoimmune haemolysis may be a manifestation of multisystem autoimmune disease, and systemic lupus erythematosus should be considered. The clinical features of the main types of AIHA are shown in Table 9.5. There are few large studies of childhood AIHA, but the presence of cold antibodies appears to be rare. In contrast, the Donath-Landsteiner antibody has been documented in approximately 40% of children (Nordhagen et al 1984, Sokol et al 1981). This is a biphasic antibody usually demonstrating anti-P specificity. Fixing to red cells in the cold, it generates complement-mediated lysis when the temperature rises to 37°C, causing paroxysmal cold haemoglobinuria (PCH). Classically associated with congenital syphilis, it is much more commonly encountered in children after some non-specific virus infection. PCH is an essentially benign and self-limiting condition requiring only supportive therapy. Warm-type AIHA is less common but can occasionally be severe and life-threatening. The clinical features of the main types of AIHA are shown in Table 9.5. Very occasionally, autoimmune haemolysis may be associated with the administration of drugs, and this possibility should be considered when anaemia develops in a child being treated with high doses of penicillin.

Management

For patients who require treatment, high-dose

oral steroid therapy (2–4 mg/kg) should be the first line of treatment. Once a response has been obtained this should be gradually reduced until the lowest alternate day maintenance dosage has been established. Patients who do not respond to steroids, or whose disease progresses to chronicity and who cannot be maintained on acceptable doses, present a therapeutic problem. In older children with chronic AIHA, splenectomy may be of benefit and should be considered. There is some equivocal evidence that high-dose intravenous immunoglobulin may reduce the rate of haemolysis (Berkman et al 1988), and anecdotal reports of efficacy of other immunosuppressive drugs, such as azathioprine, cyclophosphamide and vincristine, have been published. Severely anaemic children may require careful transfusion, though compatibility testing will be difficult and often the least incompatible blood has to be given.

Microangiopathic haemolytic anaemia

This condition refers to red cell fragmentation and damage in the microcirculation and appears to be the result of small-vessel disease in part due to endothelial damage and the presence of fibrin strands. In children, the most common cause is the haemolytic uraemic syndrome, although it is also occasionally seen in children with burns, and similar abnormalities may be found following the insertion of some types of heart valve prostheses.

The haemolytic uraemic syndrome (see also Ch. 6)

The haemolytic uraemic syndrome is characterized by renal failure, thrombocytopenia and microangiopathic haemolytic anaemia. It commonly follows an episode of diarrhoea, which may be bloody. Recently, verotoxin-producing E. coli (E. coli 0157) has been shown to be associated with the epidemic form of this disorder. The sporadic variety may be more serious and has no known cause. Treatment for both is supportive, and may include renal dialysis.

Haemolytic disease in the newborn (HDNB)

Alloimmune haemolytic anaemia due to placental transfer of maternal antibody is an important cause of haemolysis in the neonatal period, but as a result of prophylactic passive immunization programmes for at-risk mothers it is becoming much less common. Haemolysis is maximum at the time of birth, and diminishes as the concentration of maternal antibody in the infant circulation declines. The presence of a positive direct antiglobulin test (where there is feto-maternal incompatibility) does not make the diagnosis, since some patients with positive tests do not haemolyse. Ninety nine percent of haemolytic disease in the newborn is due to anti-Rhesus-D. Fifty percent of cases need some sort of treatment, and death occurs in 10–20% of cases. There is a wide spectrum of disease severity ranging from mild jaundice on day 2 onwards to death in utero. Severely affected fetuses develop hepatosplenomegaly and hydrops fetalis due to ascites and oedema.

Severe HDNB may be complicated by disseminated intravascular coagulation. The strength of positivity of the Coombs tests gives no indication of the expected severity of haemolysis. It is rare for severe HDNB to complicate the first incompatible pregnancy.

Haemolytic disease of the newborn due to other blood group antibodies

The reduction in the incidence of anti-D following the introduction of passive immunization programmes has resulted in other antibodies becoming relatively more important, although they rarely cause disease as severe as that due to anti-D. Anti-c is the next most important (Hardy & Napier 1981), and approximately 30% of affected babies require exchange transfusion in the postnatal period. Others tend to be mild. Anti-MNS may cause disease of a similar severity to ABO incompatibility (see below). Anti-Le[a] and anti-PI are almost invariably IgM antibodies which do not cross the placenta and have not been shown to cause HDNB.

ABO haemolytic disease

ABO disease is due to IgG anti-A or anti-B crossing the placenta and causing haemolysis in an ABO incompatible fetus. It is usually only a problem in mothers with blood group O, and occurs in up to 20% of pregnancies where it is possible (3% of all births). It is rare for babies to have clinical problems, and the necessity for exchange transfusion is unusual (perhaps 1%). Phototherapy is usually sufficient. Stillbirth is unreported; first babies may be affected and there is no evidence of an increase in severity in subsequent pregnancies.

The A and B antigens are not well developed in infants and this probably explains some of the mildness of the clinical course.

The diagnosis is usually straightforward. Mother's blood group is O, and IgG anti-A or anti-B titres are usually in excess of one in 1000. The baby is usually group A and has anaemia, spherocytes and jaundice. The direct antiglobulin test is often paradoxically negative or only weakly positive.

Haemolytic disease in the newborn resulting from maternal autoimmune haemolytic anaemia

Any pregnant woman suffering with chronic autoimmune haemolytic anaemia due to an IgG antibody can potentially transmit that antibody transplacentally and produce alloimmune haemolysis in the fetus (Chaplin et al 1973, Sokol et al 1982). The same is true if acute acquired maternal AIHA arises during pregnancy. Such patients should be carefully monitored.

REFERENCES

Abdalla S, Weatherall D J, Wickramasinghe S N ,Hughes M 1980 The anaemia of falciparum malaria. British Journal of Haematology 46: 171–183

Ammann A J 1982 Current status of pneumococcal polysaccharide immunization in patients with sickle cell disease or impaired splenic function. American Journal of Pediatric Hematology and Oncology 4: 301–306

Austin R F, Desforges J F 1969 Hereditary elliptocytosis: an unusual presentation of haemolysis in the newborn associated with transient morphological abnormalities. Pediatrics 44: 196–200

Berkman S A, Lee M L, Gale R P 1988 Clinical use of intravenous immunoglobulins. Seminars in Hematology 25: 140–158

Beutler E 1984 Red cell metabolism, 3rd edn. Grune and Stratton, New York

Chaplin H Jr., Cohen R, Bloomberg G, Kaplan H J, 1973 Pregnancy and idiopathic haemolytic anaemia: a prospective study during 6 months gestation and 3 months post partum. British Journal of Haematology 24: 219–229

Coetzer T L, Lawler J, Lui S C, Prchal J 1988 Partial ankyrin and spectrin deficiency in severe atypical hereditary spherocytosis. New England Journal of Medicine 318: 230–234

Dacie J V 1985 The hereditary haemolytic anaemias, part 1. In: The haemolytic anaemias, vol. 1. Churchill Livingstone, Edinburgh

Evans J P M, Baines A J, Hann I M, Al-Hakim I 1983 Defective spectrin dimer-dimer association in a family with transfusion-dependent homozygous hereditary elliptocytosis. British Journal of Haematology 54: 163–172

Forman K, Sokol R J, Hewitt S, Stamps B K 1984 Paroxysmal nocturnal haemoglobinuria: a clincopathological study of 26 cases. Acta Haematologica 71: 217–226

Gaston H, Verter J, Woods G 1986 Prophylaxis with oral penicillin in children with sickle cell anaemia: a randomised trial. New England Journal of Medicine 314: 1593–1599

Hardy J Napier J A F 1981 Red cell antibodies detected in antenatal tests on Rhesus positive women in south and mid-Wales, 1948–1978. British Journal of Obstetrics and Gynaecology 88: 91–100

Konrad P M, Valentine W M, Paglia D E 1972 Enzymatic activities and glutathione content of erythrocytes in the newborn: comparison with red cells of older normal subjects and those with comparable reticulocytosis. Acta Haematologica 48: 193–201

Krueger H C, Burgert E O Jr 1966 Hereditary spherocytosis in 100 children. Mayo Clinic Proceedings 41: 821–830

Lee-Potter J P, Deacon Smith R A, Simpkiss M J, Kamuzora H 1975 A new cause of haemolytic anaemia in the newborn. A description of an unstable foetal haeoglobin: F Poole, $\alpha_2\gamma_2$ 130 tryptophan-glycine Journal of Clinical Pathology 28: 317–320

Lestas A N, Bellingham A J 1990 A logical approach to the investigation of red cell enzymopathies. Blood Reviews 4: 148–157

Lundh B, Oski F, Gardner F H 1970 Plasma haemopexin and haptoglobin in haemolytic disorders of the newborn. Acta Paediatrica Scandanavica 59: 121–126

Luzzatto L, Mehta A 1989 Glucose 6-phosphate dehydrogenase deficiency. In: Scriver C R, Beaudet A L, Sly W S, Valle D(eds) Metabolic basis of inherited disease, 6th edn. McGraw Hill, New York, 2237–2265

Mackinney A A 1965 Hereditary spherocytosis. Archives of Internal Medicine 116: 257–265

Miller D R, Baehner R L, Diamond L K 1967 Paroxysmal nocturnal haemoglobinuria in childhood and adolesence. Pediatrics 39: 675–688

Nordhagen R, Stensvold K, Winsnes A, Skyberg D 1984 Paroxysmal cold haemoglobinuria – the most frequent acute autoimmune haemolytic anemia in children? Acta Paediatrica Scandanavica 73: 258–262

Palek J 1987 Hereditary elliptocytosis, spherocytosis and related disorders: consequences of a deficiency or a mutation of membrane skeletal proteins. Blood Reviews 1: 146–168

Pavelkis S G, Protivnik I, Promdi S, De Viro D C 1989 Neurological complications of sickle cell disease. Advanced Pediatrics 36: 247–276

Pekrun A, Gratzer W 1990 Disorders of the red cell membrane. Current Opinions in Pediatrics 2: 116–120

Perrin L M, Machay L J, Miescher P J 1981 The hematology

of malaria. Seminars in Hematology 19: 70–82

Serjeant G R 1985 Sickle cell disease. Oxford University Press, Oxford

Smedley J C, Bellingham A J 1991 Current problems in haematology 2: hereditary spherocytosis. Journal of Clinical Pathology 44: 441–444

Sokol R J, Hewitt S, Stamps B K 1981 Autoimmune haemolysis: an 18 year study of 865 cases referred to a regional transfusion centre. British Medical Journal 282: 2023–2027

Sokol R J, Hewitt S, Stamps B K 1982 Autoantibodies, autoimmune haemolysis and pregnancy. Vox Sanguinis 43: 169–176

Stockman J A III, Oski F A 1978 Erythrocytes of the human neonate. Current Topics in Hematology 1: 193–232

Trucco J I, Brown A K 1967 Neonatal manifestations of hereditary spherocytosis. American Journal of Diseases in Children 113: 263–270

Wong H B, Kham S K Y 1984 Screening for haemoglobinopathies/thalassaemia utilizing haematologic indices. Journal of the Singapore Paediatric Society 26: 170–175

10. Disorders of red cells: III Red cells and oxygen transport

J. G. Jones   B. M. Holland   C. A. J. Wardrop

Four important parameters of blood determine adequacy of tissue oxygenation:-

1. Concentration of haemoglobin
   a. erythropoiesis
   b. blood losses and haemolysis
2. Haemoglobin-oxygen affinity
   a. oxygen affinity of abnormal haemoglobins
   b. oxygen affinity of normal haemoglobins
3. Red cell volume and blood volume
   a. measurement of RCV in preterm neonates
4. Blood viscosity
   a. plasma viscosity
   b. haematocrit
   c. red cell deformability and filterability
   d. red cell aggregation
   e. leukocyte rheology

CONCENTRATION OF HAEMOGLOBIN

Erythropoiesis

Once the cell mass of the embryo grows too large to be oxygenated by simple diffusion, an oxygen transporting system becomes essential. This transporting system is the protein haemoglobin contained within a highly specialized and flexible mature red blood cell – the erythrocyte. The erythrocytes develop from progenitor cells that are also the primary source of leukocytes and platelets and are hence termed pluripotent haematopoietic stem cells. The pluripotent stem cells are capable of both self renewal and of progressive differentiation in more than one direction. The differentiation procedure leads ultimately to a wide spectrum of mature blood cells that have lost the ability to replicate. The earliest recognizable erythrocyte precursor is the normoblast, that matures, without replication, to a reticulocyte and finally to the mature erythrocyte. The normoblast is itself preceded by at least three distinct and committed cell lines that are still capable of replication: the early and late erythroid burst forming units [BFU-e] and the erythrocyte colony-forming units [CFU-e]. The proposed sequence of events is depicted diagrammatically in Figure. 10.1

The earliest BFU-e respond to high concentrations of erythropoietin in vitro but many not do so in vivo. As these colonies mature, they become less proliferative and more responsive to erythropoietin. The resulting CFU-e are again significantly less able to replicate and are totally dependent on erythropoietin for further maturation, and the production of this hormone, mediated through hypoxia, is the major controlling influence on erythropoiesis by the fetus, neonate and adult.

Earlier stages in the linear maturation process are sensitive to other regulators (Fig. 10.1). The yolk sac is the initial site of erythropoiesis which begins at about 3 weeks' gestation. This pattern of erythropoiesis is termed 'primitive' as the products are megaloblastic and nucleated cells that do not develop further. This short-lived form of erythropoiesis is replaced at about 6 weeks by a hepatic 'definitive' erythropoiesis that produces macrocytic but enucleated cells that develop further to more mature erythrocytes with advancing gestation. In the human fetus, the 'definitive' erythropoiesis shifts from the liver to the bone marrow from 20 weeks' gestation, and this process is completed soon after birth. It is probable that this maturation progression of haematopoiesis from extramedullary organs to the bone marrow requires communication between the different organs, and this is provided by the circulating blood.

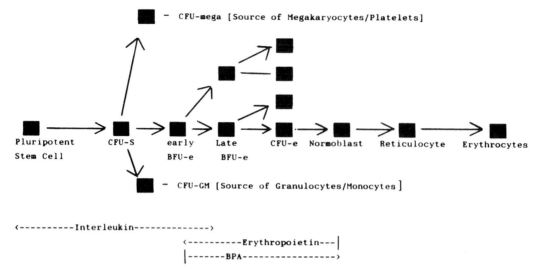

Fig. 10.1 Diagrammatic representation of the erythroid cell line. The possible hormonal regulation pattern is depicted at the bottom of the diagram. BPA = burst promoting activity. (Adapted from Brown 1988.)

Hence, normal fetal and neonatal (but not adult) blood contains immature erythrocyte precursors and their progenitors in measurable numbers.

Our rapidly expanding knowledge of haematopoiesis has arisen from modern techniques of molecular biology and culture techniques for assessing colony stimulating factors (CSF) and this approach has elevated the science from a descriptive to a mechanistic discipline (Christensen 1989). These recent advances offer tremendous potential for development in clinical management of conditions such as neonatal neutropenias, hyporegenerative anaemias, haemoglobinopathies and thalassaemias.

Erythropoietin has been a prime target for this exploitation of modern techniques of molecular biology, combined with those of biotechnology. Erythropoietin is a glycoprotein produced by adult kidneys and fetal livers in response to declining venous Po_2 in those organs. Although maternal erythropoietin, at normal concentration, does not cross the placental barrier, the developing fetus is able to respond to a maternal hypoxaemia through its own production of the hormone. When the fetus is born to the extrauterine oxygen-rich atmosphere, the levels of erythropoietin decline rapidly, with a half-life of approximately 4 hours. This is accompanied by a more gradual decline in the concentration of circulating erythrocytes. Erythropoietin from adult kidneys is a protein of

molecular mass of 30,400 daltons. It is heavily glycosylated, with carbohydrate accounting for over 30% of its mass. This carbohydrate is not essential for the stimulation of erythrocyte synthesis, but prolongs the half-life of the hormone in vivo. The amino acid sequence of the protein is known and, through a corresponding cDNA, the erythropoietin gene has been identified, isolated and cloned, and expressed in a biologically active form in Chinese hamster ovary cells. This recombinant human erythropoietin is virtually identical with that isolated from human urine and is now available for clinical use.

In general, paediatric anaemia that is marked by low serum erythropoietin concentrations affects the preterm infant or the child with chronic renal failure. The first reflects developmental immaturity of the preterm infant's erythropoietic response through postnatal life, while the second represents impairment in the production of the hormone due to renal tissue damage. Recombinant human erythropoietin has been used successfully to correct anaemia in patients with renal disease that requires chronic haemodialysis, and with adequate iron stores, the response is dose dependent. A similar successful outcome may be possible with the anaemia of preterm infants, given sufficient nutritional support to meet the production of about 90 ml of erythrocytes as the baby grows from 1 kg to 3 kg. This volume of red cells is normally produced during growth in utero over the same period.

Red blood cell production thus begins early in the embryo, and the haemoglobin concentration is typically around 9 g/dl by 10 weeks' gestation. This concentration rises to about 15 g/dl at 24 weeks, and reaches term levels of about 16–17 g/dl by the middle of the third trimester. Alterations in oxygen delivery to the fetus have a profound effect on this normal pattern of development. Hence, elevated levels of haemoglobin are found at birth in growth-retarded infants, infants of smoking or diabetic mothers and infants gestating at high altitudes.

Immediately after birth, there is usually an increase in haemoglobin concentration; this is due to a contraction in plasma volume and depends on the amount of placental transfusion (see below). An initial increase of about 10% in the concentration of haemoglobin stabilizes by about 10 hours after birth. In term babies, erythropoiesis stops in the first week, and there follows a sharp decline in circulating haemoglobin which reaches a nadir of about 11 g/dl at 8–10 weeks. By 6 months it increases to 12 g/dl and gradually climbs during childhood to reach adult values by puberty.

The erythrocytes produced by the human fetus differ from adult cells in the type of haemoglobin, enzyme content, membrane characteristics and blood group antigens. They also show curtailed survival in the circulation postnatally, as compared with adult cells.

Blood losses and haemolysis

Perinatal spontaneous haemorrhages and, inevitably, later blood sampling losses make major impacts on the amount of blood in the preterm infant's circulation (Blanchette & Zipursky 1984, Obladen et al 1988). Most such infants therefore become multitransfused, with many 'donor-exposures', imposing infective and, perhaps, immunological risks. It is very common for intensively-managed infants to receive, in aggregate, the equivalent of more than one exchange transfusion. Examination of the balance between losses and replacement transfusions suggests that losses tend to exceed replacements (Fig. 10.2). Thus, in present practice, infants may often be managed with oligovolaemia and recurring anaemia. Advice on 'how much' and 'when' to transfuse such babies varies greatly (Holland et al 1987).

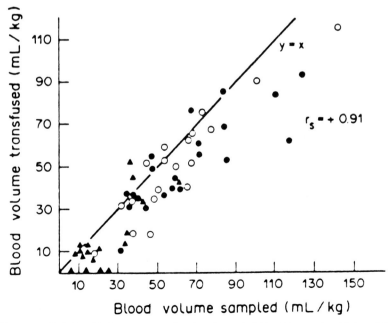

Fig. 10.2 Relationship between transfused and sampled blood in very low birth-weight infants. (Adapted from Obladen et al 1988.)

HAEMOGLOBIN–OXYGEN AFFINITY

In addition to changes in the concentration of haemoglobin seen before and after birth, there are also changes in the type of circulating haemoglobin. The synthesis of haemoglobin is the subject of other chapters in this book, but a brief summary is included here as it is relevant to understanding changes in oxygen transport during development from the embryo to the fetus, through childhood and puberty to adulthood. Six genetic variants of haemoglobin are produced during normal human development. All these haemoglobins are tetrameric proteins and composed of two identical dimers, each of which is synthesized from one α-like globin chain (alpha (α), zeta (ζ)) and one β-like globin chain (beta (β), gamma (γ), epsilon (ϵ)). In normal circumstances, no homopolymers are formed and no tetramers are formed from just α-like globins or just β-like globins. Each globin is coded for by a specific gene, with α-like genes clustered on chromosome 16, and β-like genes clustered on chromosome 11. The expression of each gene is carefully controlled and is switched on or off at appropriate times to give a specific sequence of tetramers with properties that are designed for each stage of development. The arrangement of the genes and the sequence of appearance of the various haemoglobins are depicted diagrammatically in Figure 10.3. The symbols ψ and θ refer to pseudogenes which may be remnants of once active genes that are no longer expressed in protein synthesis.

Synthesis of fetal haemoglobin [HbF; $\alpha_2\gamma_2$] begins at about 5 weeks postconception, and rep-

resents about 90% of the haemoglobin produced by the fetus. The remaining 10% is an adult haemoglobin [HbA; $\alpha_2\beta_2$]. HbF is itself heterogeneous, being composed of two different variants of the γ-chain. The predominant variant [Gγ] represent 75% of the total and contains a glycyl amino acid residue in position 136 of the protein chain; the remaining 25% of the γ-chain [Aγ] contains an alanyl residue in this position. The synthesis of the major form of adult haemoglobin [HbA] begins at about 34 weeks' gestation when the expression of the γ-gene is gradually replaced by expression of the β-gene. This phenomenon, termed 'switching', proceeds with a half-life of approximately 6 weeks until, at 1 year, a constant (1% or less) of the haemoglobin synthesized is HbF. Synthesis of a minor (5–10%) variant of adult haemoglobin [HbA$_2$; $\alpha_2\delta_2$] begins at birth and is maximal at about 1 year.

Oxygen affinity of abnormal haemoglobins

Failure to express any of the globin genes leads to a deficiency of the corresponding globin chain (subunit) of haemoglobin and to different forms of thalassaemia. However, single-base substitutions in a gene may lead to nothing more drastic than a single amino acid substitution in the corresponding globin chain. Most of the recorded substitutions affect surface residues of the protein, which retain normal physiological properties. However, a considerable number of abnormal haemoglobins with a single amino acid substitution exhibit clinical manifestations. In order to understand the possible consequences of such a substitution on the physiological function of the haemoglobin

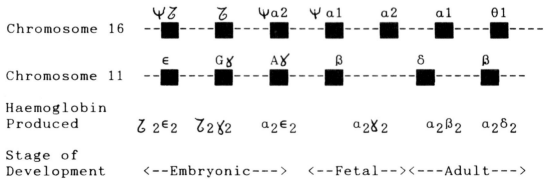

Fig. 10.3 Genetic variants of human haemoglobin. (Adapted from Thein & Weatherall 1988.)

requires some knowledge of the allosteric structure and properties of the final tetramer.

Each subunit of haemoglobin carries an iron-containing haem group which binds one molecule of oxygen. The intrinsic affinity of each subunit for oxygen depends critically on the orientation of each haem group with respect to the protein. In addition, the binding of oxygen to each haem is influenced by the 3-dimensional (quaternary) structure of the entire tetramer, and each successive oxygen is bound more tightly to the protein. This cooperative binding is manifested as a sigmoidal haemoglobin-oxygen binding curve (see below), and a molecular model for it was proposed by Monod, Wyman & Changeaux in 1965. These authors also introduced the term 'allosteric' to describe the properties of proteins such as haemoglobin. All these proteins contained binding sites for competitive inhibitors that were not 'isosteric' with the primary ligand – oxygen in the case of haemoglobin. As this phenomenon was new to protein-ligand equilibria at that time, the term 'allosteric' was introduced to distinguish these inhibitors from conventional competitive inhibitors that 'competed' with a primary ligand for the same binding site on the protein. Haemoglobin, like all other allosteric proteins, exists in two different conformational states – the T (tense)-state with a low affinity for oxygen, and R (relaxed)-state with a high affinity for oxygen. Both forms exist in an equilibrium that favours the T-state in the absence of oxygen, the R-state in the presence of excess oxygen. Inhibitors of oxygen binding have a higher affinity for the T-state. The key to understanding the allosteric properties of haemoglobin lies in the molecular changes during the T to R transition, and the extra chemical bonds that stabilize the T-state but are broken in the transition when oxygen binds to one of the subunits. There are two areas on the protein that are crucial for these stabilizing forces for the T-states, another area that is important during the reversible transition between the two states and a further area that is responsible for the proper alignment of each haem group:

1. The $\alpha_1\beta_2$ site. This is the area of contact between the two dimeric halves of the protein, and involves some 19 hydrophobic amino acid residues. It is the major area of contact in the protein that 'slides' during the T to R transition. Abnormalities in this site will affect this transition and hence the affinity of the protein for oxygen.

2. The C-terminal site. The C-terminal amino acids of both the α and β subunits are basic amino acids and contribute one +ve and one –ve group to electrostatic bonds that stabilize the T-state but are absent from the R-state. Abnormalities of the C-terminal region will destabilise the T-state and increase the affinity of the protein for oxygen.

3. The BPG-binding site. This important regulatory site consists of three positively charged amino acids on each of the two β chains. These six +ve groups interact strongly with the four –ve charges that exist on 2,3-bisphosphoglycerate (2,3BPG) at physiological pH. The 2,3BPG-binding site exists in a crevice down the centre of the molecule that is accessible only to dissolved molecules when the protein is in the T-state. BPG is therefore an inhibitor of oxygen binding to haemoglobin, and any modification to this important site will alter the degree of inhibition. It is difficult to imagine an improvement of the 2,3BPG-binding, and proteins modified in this site are likely to have a high affinity for oxygen. The amino acid sequence of the γ-chain of HbF differs from the β-chain, and this difference includes the replacement of one of the +ve groups of the 2,3BPG- binding site with a hydrophilic serine residue. This reduces the affinity of fetal haemoglobin for 2,3BPG and hence increases its affinity for oxygen.

4. The haem-binding pocket. Each haem group is tightly wedged in a hydrophobic pocket formed from different parts of the polypeptide chain. The iron is bonded to the proximal histidine of each subunit, and the sixth coordination position is free or bound to oxygen. The orientation of the haem group is carefully engineered to allow free entry and egress of oxygen to and from its binding site – the iron. Any changes in the hydrophobic amino acids that bind the periphery of the haem will change this access route and alter the affinity of that subunit for oxygen.

Table 10.1 shows examples of haemoglobins with abnormal binding affinities for oxygen, resulting from a single amino acid substitution in one of the four important contact sites described above.

The physiological response to a high-affinity

Table 10.1 Some abnormal haemoglobins with altered oxygen affinity due to a single amino acid substitution

Abnormal haemoglobin	Affected region of molecule	Amino acid substitution
A. Increased affinity		
Chesapeake	$\alpha_1\beta_2$	α Arg → Leu
Yakima	$\alpha_1\beta_2$	β Asp → His
Kempsey	$\alpha_1\beta_2$	β Asp → Asn
Radcliffe	$\alpha_1\beta_2$	β Asp → Ala
Brigham	$\alpha_1\beta_2$	β Pro → Leu
Ranier	C-terminal	β Tyr → Cys
Andrew (Minneapolis)	C-terminal	β Lys → Asn
Syracuse	BPG-site	β His → Pro
Rahere	BPG-site	β Lys → Thr
Providence	BPG-site	β Lys → Asp
B. Decreased affinity		
Kansas	$\alpha_1\beta_2$	β Asp → Thr
Denmark Hill	$\alpha_1\beta_2$	α Pro → Ala
Heathrow	Haem-pocket	β Phe → Leu

*Adapted from Smith et al 1983

haemoglobin is stimulation of erythropoiesis and polycythaemia. Conversely, low-affinity haemoglobins are usually, but not invariably, associated with mild anaemia. Some of the abnormalities listed in Table 10.1 involve the α-globin but most are found in the β-globin; both will be apparent at birth. However, to our knowledge, there are no recorded clinical problems during infancy and childhood that can be attributed to the altered oxygen affinity of the haemoglobins. Nevertheless, it is one parameter in the multifactorial process of oxygen delivery to tissue.

Other amino acid substitutions can affect the stability of the protein, enhance oxidation to methaemoglobin or alter the solubility of the protein. The most prevalent of all abnormal haemoglobins – HbS, the haemoglobin of sickle cell disease – falls in this last category. In HbS, a negatively charged glutamate residue (β6) is replaced by a hydrophobic valine, and this creates a 'sticky patch' on the T-state of the protein that leads to polymerization of deoxyhaemoglobin and precipitation within the cell. Although the affinity for oxygen is decreased, the major clinical problems arise from the extreme rigidity of the sickled cells, which leads to acute and extreme ischaemia in affected tissues.

Oxygen affinity of normal haemoglobins

The switching from HbF to HbA synthesis is under careful genetic control; this is unaffected by preterm delivery, but can be delayed by environmental factors such as maternal hypoxia or diabetes, and in infants that are small for gestational age. In all these cases, the pattern of synthesis is restored to normal at birth. The cause for this delay is unknown, but seems to be related to stress erythropoiesis, which is known to increase the production of HbF-containing cells in infants and adults. There are also genetic defects that affect the switching and give rise to a hereditary persistence of fetal haemoglobin (HPFH). This is a form of $\delta\beta$ thalassaemia, where a failure to synthesize both of these adult globins leads to a variable persistence of γ-chain synthesis. The underlying genetic defects range from a single point mutation on chromosome 11 (nondeletion forms), to large scale deletions in the $\delta\beta$ cluster of genes (deletion forms). The reasons for the failure to switch off expression of the γ-gene in these conditions remains a matter of conjecture, but is of more than academic interest. A controlled clinical switch from β-chain to γ-chain synthesis would be advantageous in sickle-cell disease, where clinical problems associated with ischaemia coincide with the polymerization of the deoxygenated form of an abnormal haemoglobin (HbS). The underlying abnormality in HbS is a single amino acid substitution in the β-globin. This abnormality does not, of course, affect the γ-globin. A total switch to HbF synthesis would not be necessary for a significant clinical improvement, as a relatively small amount of this tetramer ($\alpha_2\gamma_2$) will prevent polymerization of the abnormal HbS. A knowledge of 'switching' is also relevant to the understanding of oxygen delivery during the first few weeks of life, and how this is altered in preterm infants who may live for 4–6 weeks ex utero before operation of the 'switch' and therefore with a sustained high level of circulating HbF.

In normal term infants, the inevitable decline in the concentration of haemoglobin is offset, in part, by an increase in the ratio of HbA:HbF due to the 'switch' described above. HbF differs from HbA in its lower affinity for 2,3BPG, which is an important inhibitor of oxygen-binding by both forms of haemoglobin (see above). In the presence of 2,3BPG, HbA has a lower affinity for oxygen than does HbF; this has a marginal effect on oxygen loading in the lungs, but a significant effect on the unloading of oxygen to respiring tissues. As 98% of arterial oxygen is bound to haemoglobin, it may seem at first glance that the concentration of haemoglobin should be an adequate guide to the oxygen-delivering capacity of blood, and that the affinity, provided it is high enough for saturation in the lungs, should be of secondary importance. However, the apparently insignificant amount of oxygen dissolved in plasma provides the concentration gradient that drives oxygen from blood into tissues. Hence a high blood oxygen content is of little value if the corresponding concentration in plasma is too low to sustain an adequate rate of tissue perfusion with the gas.

To complicate matters further, the relationship between the amount of oxygen in plasma and that bound to haemoglobin is not linear. The true relationship is sigmoidal and conventionally expressed as the haemoglobin-oxygen dissociation curve, which relates the oxygen saturation in blood, and oxygen tension in free solution in plasma (Fig. 10.4). The partial pressure of oxygen (PO_2) corresponding to a 50% saturation of haemoglobin

with oxygen is the P_{50} value and is about 3.6 kPa (27 torr) in adult blood at pH 7.4 and a Pco_2 of 5.3 kPa (40 torr). The P_{50} value in vivo is controlled by pH, Pco_2 and 2,3BPG, as all three are inhibitors of oxygen-binding to haemoglobin. The inhibition of oxygen-binding to haemoglobin by a decrease in pH or an increase in Pco_2 or 2,3BPG is expressed as an increase in P_{50} which is a right shift of the dissociation curve shown in Figure 10.3. The P_{50} value for blood from a preterm infant born at 30 weeks' gestation is about 2.7 kPa (20 torr).

A realistic expression of the likely physiological consequences of these complex changes in the circulating haemoglobin of the neonate requires a calculation based on the amount and properties of that haemoglobin. 'Available oxygen' (AO; Jones et al 1979) has proved to be a useful measure of the ability of blood to deliver oxygen to tissues. Available oxygen is the calculated oxygen content of blood between the measured, or assumed, arterial Po_2 and a chosen central venous Po_2 of 2.67 kPa (20 torr). The AO represents the amount of oxygen that can be released to the tissues before the need arises for an increase in cardiac output to cope with extra oxygen demands. An example calculation of the effect of a change in P_{50} on the calculated AO is given in Figure 10.4. Data are now available that allow estimation of the likely AO for infants of different gestational age:

$$AO \text{ (ml/g Hb)} = 0.54 + 0.005 \times \text{total age [weeks]} \quad (1)$$

The 'total age' is the sum of the gestational age at birth and the postnatal age. This increase in AO with age helps to offset the effect of a declining haemoglobin concentration during the first 2–3 months of life.

The AO should not be, but often is, confused with a similar parameter 'oxygen release capacity', which is calculated in the same way but using 5.33 kPa (40 torr) as the central venous Po_2. The essential difference between the two calculations is that the former incorporates the physiologically important steep portion of the haemoglobin-oxygen dissociation curve, while the second does not. The oxygen release capacity is chosen to represent the oxygen delivery status of an infant under normal conditions of oxygen consumption and at rest. Table 10.2 shows changes in the AO

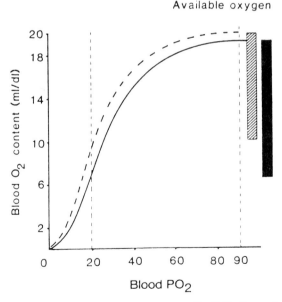

Available oxygen

Blood O_2 content (ml/dl)

Blood PO_2

Fig. 10.4 Effect of fetal haemoglobin on 'Available Oxygen' in preterm infants. Oxygen availability is represented diagrammatically by the vertical columns (– – ■ = adult blood, P_{50} 27 mmHg) and (– – ▨ = preterm infant, P_{50} 23 mmHg). Haemoglobin concentration is assumed to be 15 g/dl and PaO_2 100 mmHg. Note, however, that haemoglobin may be as low as 7–10.5 g/dl in the infant. (Adapted from Holland et al 1987.)

Table 10.2 Changes in the concentration of haemoglobin and calculated values for available oxygen and oxygen release capacity in a preterm infant

Age (Weeks)	[Hb] (g/dl)	p50 (kPa)*	Oxygen release capacity (ml/dl)*	Available oxygen (ml/dl)†
0	16.6	2.61	2.3	10.2
4	11.3	3.17	2.7	8.9
10	8.8	3.23	2.3	7.0

* Data from Brown 1988
† Calculated according to Wardrop et al 1978

and oxygen release capacity in a preterm infant during the initial postnatal decline in the concentration of haemoglobin and while HbF is gradually replaced by HbA. The oxygen release capacity shows that the infant can compensate for the decline in the oxygen content of blood and maintain oxygen delivery at rest. However, the infant is still disadvantaged during periods of raised oxygen demands and this is reflected in the calculated AO.

With the advent of noninvasive means of measuring oxygen consumption and cardiac output in infants at rest, a functional 'Oxygen Reserve' can be defined as:

$$
\begin{aligned}
\text{Oxygen reserve} = {} & \text{available oxygen (ml/dl)} \\
& \times \text{cardiac output (dl/min)} \\
& - \text{oxygen consumption (ml/min)}
\end{aligned}
\tag{2}
$$

This oxygen reserve will represent the oxygen available to cope with demands in excess of normal resting consumption and before the need arises for an increase in cardiac output.

The worst possible scenario, in terms of an anaemic hypoxia, is apparent in infants born before 30 weeks' gestation when the nadir of their haemoglobin level occurs before 'switching' from fetal to adult haemoglobin synthesis. The combination of low haemoglobin level and a low P_{50} can tip the balance to clinical signs of anaemic hypoxia. A similar problem may arise in neonates with a high-affinity haemoglobin (see above) but no specific case has been recorded. In a group of preterm infants born between 28 and 30 weeks' gestation, there were clinical signs of hypoxia when the nadir of haemoglobin occurred at 5–6 weeks with a mean AO of only 6.0 ml/dl of blood. In a matched group of infants, with no recognized clinical signs of hypoxia, the mean AO was 7.1

ml/dl (Wardrop et al 1978). This difference was statistically significant and was not matched by a similar difference in the concentration of haemoglobin. However there was a considerable overlap in the values for AO found in the symptomatic and asymptomatic babies. This, at the time disappointing, overlap points to another important variable in the ability of blood to oxygenate all tissues in neonates – the variable relationship between the concentration of haemoglobin (or haematocrit) and the total volume of circulating red cells and hence the blood volume.

RED CELL VOLUME AND BLOOD VOLUME

Red cell volume (RCV) during the first day of life in preterm infants predicts their outcome in terms of duration and intensity of respiratory support necessary, and of clinical complications of preterm delivery (Hudson et al 1990). The postnatal RCV depends critically on the amount of placental blood received by the infant at birth, i.e. by the handling of the umbilical vessels. Typically, a RCV of about 33 ml/kg results from immediate cord-clamping compared with 50 ml/kg after a delay of 0.5–1 minute (Linderkamp 1982). In most obstetric/neonatal units, immediate cord-clamping is performed to prevent risks of circulatory overload from excessive volume-transfer of placental blood, and to expedite the resuscitation and transfer of the newborn to the neonatal intensive care unit. Clinical practice varies, however, and there is no general agreement on the practice to secure optimal red cell endowment by the placenta. This vital clinical-physiological option seems generally to have been overlooked, but evidence is emerging that allowing a controlled placental transfusion lessens intrapulmonary shunting and thereby reduces dependence on respiratory support in preterm infants. This benefit was achieved, in a controlled study, by delaying cord-clamping for approximately 30 seconds, with the infant held 20 cm below the placenta in vaginal delivery cases (Kinmond et al 1990). In these cases, there were no adverse effects of placental transfusion, and the infants suffered fewer complications of preterm delivery. Further work in this area should allow the tactic to be developed so as to allow optimisation of blood volume parameters ab initio for the circulation in general and oxygen transport in particular.

Red cell volume is, of course, a major part of total blood volume (BV) which is also a vital variable influencing the efficacy of the circulation and hence the transport of oxygen. In routine clinical practice, both in infants and in older children, blood volume is assumed to be optimal, normal or otherwise appropriate in patients with adequate or acceptable values for haematocrit and/or concentration of circulating haemoglobin. Again, in critical care situations, blood volume is accepted as adequate in patients who lack clinical signs of shock and exhibit acceptable values for blood and/ or central venous pressure. Estimation of plasma and red cell volume in sick neonates suggests a wide variation of blood volume which is not predictable from the haematocrit in individual patients. Although the information is limited, there

is a tendency to oligovolaemia in sick newborns, and in older infants with the refractory early anaemia of prematurity. It is therefore pertinent to examine this variable relationship between the various components that comprise total blood volume.

In general, the relationship between measured haematocrit (Hct) and total circulating red cell volume (RCV) in adults (Bentley & Lewis 1976) and neonates (Jones et al 1990) is hyperbolic and described by the equation:

$$Hct = \frac{RVC}{(RVC + PV)} \qquad (3)$$

where PV is total plasma volume, within which red cells are distributed.

Individual data points show a wide scatter around this general relationship (Fig. 10.5) and, with a small number of patients, the hyperbolic relationship can seem extremely tenuous. The main

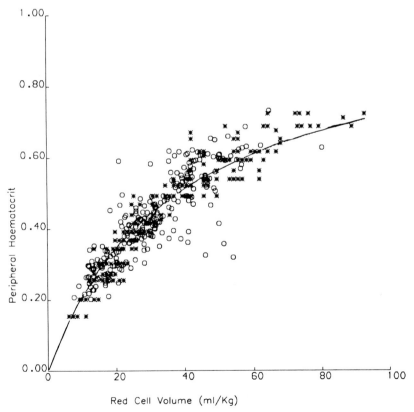

Fig. 10.5   Relationship between RCV and Hct in adults (*) and neonates (o). The points are measured and the line is the least-squares fit to equation (3) with a mean PV of 38 ml/kg. (From Jones et al 1990.)

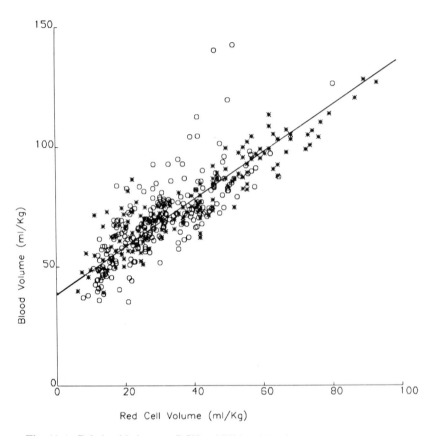

Fig. 10.6 Relationship between RCV and BV in adults (*) and neonates (o). The points are measured and the line is the least-squares fit to the equation BV = RCV + PV (38 ml/kg). (Data from Jones et al 1990.)

reason for this scatter seems to be individual variation in the ability to maintain a normal plasma volume, and there is little evidence of general or significant compensatory rises in PV in response to a low RCV. Individual fluctuations in plasma volume will produce changes in the measured Hct that do not reflect changes in RCV, which tend to be less erratic and usually gradual and/or predictable. It is therefore a tenable argument that RCV, as the relatively more stable element of the Hct, may be a better guide to a 'time-averaged' Hct, and therefore become the primary target during blood transfusion of neonates showing signs of anaemic hypoxia.

A second consequence of the relationship described in (3) is a linear correlation between RCV and BV and, allowing for individual scatter, a low RCV is generally associated with hypovolaemia (Fig. 10.6). A reduction in blood volume is accompanied by a decrease in venous compliance, and hence capacity, that is not uniform. This uneven response through vasoconstriction leads to redistribution of blood away from areas such as the splanchnic circulation, and towards tissues such as heart and brain. This protection of 'preferred' tissues avoids major responses, such as an increase in cardiac output, until the anaemia becomes severe. The resulting chronic hypoxia of other tissues is therefore often overlooked, and may be critical in preterm neonates requiring intensive clinical management. In these circumstances, there is a need for a rapid and reliable measurement of blood volume parameters, and the therapy for the anaemia may be directed to restoring red cell volume to an appropriate level. It is important that the patient has sufficient red cells to maintain a minimal cardiac output at rest and provide sufficient reserve to meet increased oxygen demands.

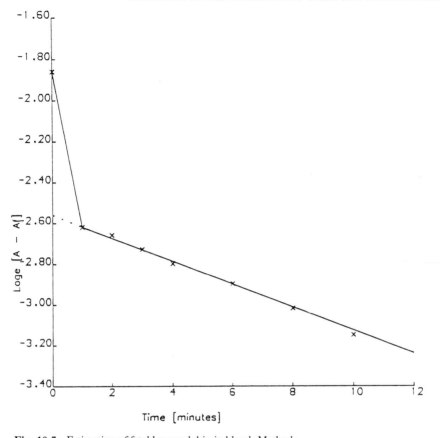

Fig. 10.7   Estimation of fetal haemoglobin in blood. Method:
1. Add 10 μl of blood to 3.0 ml of ammonia (25 mM)
2. Read absorbance at 540 nm (A) (Ao = A × 3.0/3.1)
3. Add 0.1 ml NaOH (4 M) and read absorbance at 540 nm for 12 min (At). The final absorbance can be read after 30 min *or* calculated from Ao/2.5 (Af)
4. Plot log (At – Af) versus time
5. Extrapolate linear portion of graph (2–12 min) to zero time (A' – Af)
6. %F = 100 × (A' – Af)/(Ao – Af) = 53%.

These demands are commonplace in critical care neonates, due to infections, heart and lung disease and even the act of venepuncture, which has been shown to increase oxygen demand. In this context, the neonatologist is in a uniquely advantageous position when compared with other clinicians, as the measurement of RCV (Phillips et al, 1986) is relatively easy in infants requiring transfusion.

Measurement of RCV in preterm neonates

Adult haemoglobin denatures very rapidly in dilute alkali, while fetal haemoglobin denatures at a significantly slower rate. Both denaturation reactions can be followed spectrophotometrically, and the proportion of each haemoglobin in the parent sample of blood can be calculated by simple graphical means. The test can be performed with 10 μl of anticoagulated blood, and an example calculation is described in Figure 10.7. When adult blood is transfused into an infant, the proportion of adult/fetal haemoglobin will alter and, from the magnitude of the change and the volume of adult cells administered (V), the total circulating volume of red cells can be calculated from:

$$\text{RCV} = \frac{\text{V} \times \% \text{ HbF (Post-Tx)}}{[\% \text{ HbF (Pre-Tx)} - \% \text{ HbF (Post-Tx)}]}$$

This simplified calculation, which ignores the difference in MCHC between adult and neonatal red cells, can be applied at the first required transfusion of blood and is therefore an attainable objective (Phillips et al 1986). Calculations show that a reasonable RCV to aim for during the first week of life is about 45 ml/kg, which is close to that reported in healthy term infants. This amount of red cells corresponds to a 'whole body available oxygen' of 24 ml/min/kg. With a resting oxygen consumption of 7 ml/min/kg this allows a 'whole body oxygen reserve' of 17 ml/min/kg.

The intensive care neonatologist is therefore in a position to examine some important clinical anomalies. Why are signs and symptoms of anaemic hypoxia not related to Hct alone and only loosely correlated with a calculated AO, which allows for variation in haemoglobin-oxygen affinity? Again, an elevated pulse rate and/or cardiac output, at rest, is not related to Hct (Alverson et al 1988, Keyes et al 1989), but is correlated with RCV at values below about 20 ml/kg in preterm neonates (Hudson et al 1990). These data imply that a low red cell volume is not accompanied by an equal expansion in plasma volume and, in addition to a reduction in blood oxygen content, the perfusion of tissues such as gut and liver will be impaired due to the oligovolaemia (Dallman 1981). The onset of clinical signs is then likely to coincide with the simultaneous decline in both Hct and BV due to a diminished RCV.

This conclusion can be inferred from findings in patients who have suffered acute blood loss and also in those suffering from a more insidious anaemia, such as early refractory anaemia of prematurity, where the circulating RCV is reduced. It is now possible to measure RCV, Hct and, from (3), BV. The discrepancy claimed between peripheral and whole-body Hct, due largely to inappropriate measures of PV based on the volume of distribution of molecules such as albumin, that are considerably smaller than red cells, is relatively trivial. Provided care is taken in drawing blood from a well warmed heel (or directly from an artery or a vein), the peripheral Hct can safely be used for this purpose. The method described above, for measuring RCV in neonates can be made sufficiently 'user-friendly' to become part of routine clinical investigation. Future work could well be directed towards seeking a multiple correlation between measures of hypoxia and both AO

and BV. For most practical purposes, a measured Hct can be allowed to replace the estimated AO. A combination of Hct and RCV could now become the centrepieces for investigation in sick preterm infants, and RCV may become the logical target in any transfusion regimen of acutely ill individuals. The contrast, mentioned earlier, between the failure to correlate increases in cardiac output with Hct and the positive correlation found between cardiac output and RCV is now easily understood. The stimulus to cardiac output is probably the hypoxia resulting from a combination of anaemia and hypovolaemia, and RCV is the one quantity that influences both variables.

Similar considerations are relevant in the clinical management of polycythaemia in young children, which is defined, in general, as an elevated haematocrit or haemoglobin concentration. The distinction between a true erythrocytosis and contracted plasma volume, essential in adult haematological diagnosis, is not realized in neonatal practice. In these older patients, the dilution of endogenous fetal haemoglobin by transfused adult haemoglobin cannot be used to assess RCV, and other dilution techniques must be sought. The dilution of biotin-labelled cells is a possibility and has proven to be effective both in adults and in preterm infants (Hudson et al 1990b). The method is, however, laborious and time consuming, but should nevertheless be seriously considered as an investigative tool by research workers with the skilled staff and appropriate technology – a fluorescence activated cell sorter (FACS).

BLOOD VISCOSITY

Blood circulation in the fetus and the neonate is characterized by high flow with low vascular pressure and resistance. Any disturbance of the normal rheology of blood in these conditions is therefore likely to have important clinical consequences. Indeed, hyperviscosity is reported in about 1–5% of all infants and clinical manifestations must be expected in about 2% of them. Blood viscosity is determined by plasma viscosity, haematocrit, red cell deformability and aggregation. Blood flow through the microcirculation is further affected by leukocyte rheology.

Table 10.3   Rheological data on plasma from neonates and adults*

Gestational age (weeks)	24–30	31–36	38–41	Adults
Protein (g/l)	45 ± 4	51 ± 5	58 ± 6	74 ± 8
Fibrinogen (g/l)	17.1 ± 5.2	23.3 ± 5.4	25.2 ± 6.0	34.6 ± 5.5
Plasma viscosity (mPa.s)	1.04 ± 0.06	1.16 ± 0.08	1.25 ± 0.09	1.46 ± 0.11

*Data from Linderkamp 1987

Plasma viscosity

Plasma viscosity is directly proportional to the concentration of proteins and is particularly sensitive to high-molecular-weight proteins such as fibrinogen. Table 10.3 shows data on the concentration of plasma proteins and measured plasma viscosity in adults and in neonates at different gestations. There are no pathological disturbances of plasma viscosity in neonates.

Haematocrit

The increase in haemoglobin concentration during fetal development was mentioned earlier and has a profound effect on blood viscosity. Approximately 34% of infants with hyperviscous blood are in fact polycythaemic. At a high shear rate of 230/s, blood viscosity depends on the haematocrit but is typically 10 times that of plasma. The relationship between haematocrit and blood viscosity is similar in neonates and adults and can be expressed by:

$$Ln\ Viscosity = k.[Hb]/Ln\ (MCH) + Ln\ (plasma\ viscosity)$$

Ln = logarithm, where [Hb] is the concentration of haemoglobin, MCH = mean corpuscular haemoglobin, and k is a shear-dependent constant.

At a given Hct, blood viscosity is lower in neonates due to the lower plasma viscosity and larger cells (expressed here as MCH). The Hct of blood is not constant during circulation but changes in vessels of different diameter. Plasma can flow into narrow capillaries faster than cells and hence the Hct drops as the vessel diameter decreases below 500 μm. More surprisingly, the viscosity of blood, at a given Hct, is lower in the narrower tubes, and this has been termed the Farrhaeus-Linqvist effect. The decrease in viscosity in narrow tubes is greater with neonatal red cells and this is attributed to their larger volume.

In terms of oxygen delivery, there is a delicate balance between blood oxygen content and blood flow – an increase in Hb concentration will increase the first but decrease the latter through an increase in viscosity. Calculations and experimental measurements show that the concentration of haemoglobin for optimum 'oxygen flow' is at a Hct of 0.5 in neonates, compared with 0.4 in adults (Fig. 10.8).

There are recognized disturbances of blood rheology associated with an elevated haematocrit. These are evident in infants with inappropriately late cord clamping, asphyxia, intrauterine growth retardation and diabetic mothers. The treatment in pathological cases is haemodilution.

Red cell deformability and filterability

The average deformation of red cells from fetuses,

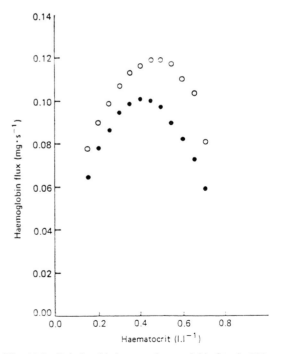

Fig. 10.8   Relationship between haemoglobin flow in 100 um tubes and haematocrit in neonates (o) and adults (•). (From Linderkamp 1987.)

Table 10.4 Rheological data for red blood cells from neonates and adults*

	Preterm infants (gestational age = 24–30 weeks)	Term infants	Adults
Deformability (rheoscope)	0.41 ± 0.04	0.42 ± 0.04	0.43 ± 0.03
Filtration rates (μl/s/per cm$^{2)}$)	32.3 ± 5.3	44.7 ± 6.8	55.3 ± 7.9
MCV (fl)	122.7 ± 11.6	108.1 ± 5.3	89.6 ± 4.1

Deformability measured at a shear stress of 54 dyn/cm^2
Filtration measured at 10 cm H_2O pressure
*Data from Linderkamp 1987

neonates and adults are the same when measured under defined shear conditions with instruments such as the rheoscope, ektacytometer or rotational viscometer. However, the distribution of values is marginally higher in fetuses and neonates. The filterability of red cells through membranes with pore diameters of 3–6 μm is lower in neonates than in adults, and is inversely related to gestational age in the neonates. Aspiration of individual cells into micropipettes of similar diameter is also more difficult with neonatal than with adult cells. Regression analysis of the filterability of red cells versus the mean corpuscular volume (MCV) is a continuum from the large cells of the youngest neonates to the small cells of adult blood. The recorded differences in the flow of red cells from neonates and adults into and through narrow capillaries has therefore been attributed entirely to the size of the cells. Table 10.4 compares the rheological properties of red blood cells from neonates and adults.

There are small differences between the mechanical properties of the membranes from neonatal and adult red cells. Neonatal cell membranes extend and bend more easily, but take longer to deform and to recover from deformation.

Decreased red cell deformability is seen in septicaemia, necrotizing enterocolitis, exposure to oxidizing agents during vitamin E deficiency, acidosis, growth retardation and maternal diabetes.

Red cell aggregation

The aggregation of near-stagnant red blood cells is of paramount importance in haemorrheology, as it is a major determinant of blood viscosity at low shear rates. Red cell aggregation increases with gestational age, and is less in neonates than in adults. It is sensitive to macromolecules such as fibrinogen or artificial dextrans, and the decreased aggregation seen in neonates has been attributed to the different properties of fetal fibrinogen. In fact neonatal and adult cells show similar aggregation properties with adult fibrinogen and this has led to the view that the intrinsic properties of the cells are not important factors in cell aggregation, which is envisaged as a non-specific adsorption of macromolecules to cells in a cross-linking configuration. However, both the extent and strength of aggregation is less for neonatal than for adult cells at high concentrations of artificial aggregating agents, and this difference is confined to the older cells of each population. This and other similar data have led in recent years to more emphasis on the intrinsic properties of the red cells as important determinants of aggregation, and osmotic forces, rather than molecular interactions, are seen as stabilizers of the aggregates.

Leukocyte rheology

The transit time of adult leukocytes through 5-μm pores is greater than that for adult erythrocytes by almost three orders of magnitude. Hence, leukocytes in adult blood slow down filtration rates through 5-μm membranes by about 50%. The flow properties of adult granulocytes and lymphocytes are approximately the same, while the larger monocytes are significantly slower. The rheology of neonatal leukocytes, relative to that of their red cells, is similar, but with two important differences: neonatal blood contains more leukocytes than does adult blood, and there is a higher preponderance of immature granulocytes that have rheological properties similar to the monocytes. Hence, leukocytes in neonatal blood are likely to exert a greater effect on blood flow through microcapillaries than those in adult blood.

SUMMARY

New and rational approaches are being developed worldwide to describe anaemia and polycythaemia in quantitative, dynamic and pathophysiological terms as disorders of oxygen transport by the blood. A better understanding of these disorders will allow more rational and effective prophylaxis and treatment. These new approaches are particularly relevant in preterm infants under intensive care. From the beginning of life ex utero, the preterm infant faces many problems that may be exacerbated by an inadequate oxygen-transporting capability. Correction of this one defect serves to minimize complications that are so prevalent in this group of infants. Means of achieving this end include proper placento-fetal transfusion and, when necessary, donor red cell transfusion. A new and exciting prophylactic possibility is the use of recombinant human erythropoietin to stimulate the production of endogenous red blood cells (Phibbs et al 1989). This approach, made possible by modern advances in molecular biology and biotechnology, is of proven efficacy in older children with the anaemia of renal disease. Clinical trials are currently underway to estimate its value in the immature infants that are known to be low in serum erythropoietin. A successful outcome of these studies would allow maintenance of blood parameters which are optimal for oxygen transport and for tissue perfusion. This kind of therapy could avert the hazards of donor cell transfusion in a group of intensively-managed and high-risk populations, both in the early days following delivery and later in the refractory early anaemia of prematurity.

In all three of these possible approaches it is important to define a clear target that will benefit the patient with minimum risk. At present, this target is the measured peripheral haematocrit and/or concentration of circulating haemoglobin. This latter point is now under scrutiny in patients requiring intensive management of their clinical problems, and a new target may well be on the horizon. The detailed knowledge gained about the synthesis of different forms of haemoglobin, modulation of their affinity for oxygen, the relationship between total circulating red cell volume and blood volume and the viscosity of blood drives us to two very simple and equivalent conclusions:

1. To meet normal oxygen demands and allow an adequate oxygen reserve, a neonate at birth requires a total circulating red cell volume of about 45 ml/kg in a total blood volume of 85 ml/kg. These numbers represent a required Hct of 0.53. The corresponding values for adults are an RCV of 30 ml/kg and Hct of 0.43.

2. The flow of blood, at a given arterial pressure and resistance, depends on its viscosity, and this in turn depends on the Hct and the size of the cells. In terms of 'haemoglobin flow', there is an optimum Hct of 0.5 in neonates and 0.4 in adults.

The similarity of these conclusions from two disparate lines of argument may be more than mere coincidence. Evolution has probably perfected the roles of haemoglobin and red cells in fulfilling the different needs of the fetus and of the child developing into adulthood. An imbalance in the functional properties of the haemoglobin and the flow of blood through the vasculature will demand compensatory responses from the individual. Changes in the viscosity of blood, in the amount and/or properties of the haemoglobin or in the oxygen demands of an infant should all therefore command clinical attention – intervention is then a matter of judgement. In this context, laboratory measurements are useful guides, provided they are used for the correct purpose. Present practice seems to weigh heavily on a measured Hct which, as a major determinant of viscosity and AO, and as a derivative of RCV, is a sensible choice. However, there is a tendency to consider the optimum Hct as a maximum, and the target aimed for is usually considerably lower than the optimum. In neonates requiring transfusion, it is now an easy matter to measure RCV and thus deduce the total blood volume from the peripheral Hct. Transfusion and erythropoietic stimulation regimens should be directed towards achieving an adequate RCV within the limitations of a maximum Hct which is appropriate to the age of the infant and a necessity to avoid risks of hyperviscosity syndromes.

REFERENCES

Alverson D C, Isken V H, Cohen R S 1988 Effect of booster blood transfusions on oxygen utilisation in infants with broncho-pulmonary dysplasia. Journal of Pediatrics 113: 722–726

Bentley S A, Lewis S M 1976 The relationship between total red cell volume, plasma volume and venous haemoatocrit. British Journal of Haematology 33: 301–307

Blanchette V, Zipursky A 1984 Assessment of anaemia in newborn infants. Clinics in Perinatology 11: 489–510

Brown M S 1988 Fetal and neonatal erythropoiesis. In: Stockman J A, Pochedly A (eds) Developmental and neonatal haematology. Raven, New York, p 39–56

Christensen R D 1989 Haematopoiesis in the fetus and neonate. Pediatric Research 26: 531–535

Dallman P R 1981 The anaemia of prematurity. Annual Reviews of Medicine 32: 143–160

Holland B M, Jones J G, Wardrop C A 1987 Lessons from the anaemia of prematurity. In: Oski F A (ed) Hematology/ Oncology Clinics of North America 1: 355-366

Hudson I, Cooke A, Holland B et al 1990a Red cell volume and cardiac output in anaemic preterm infants. Archives of Disease in Childhood 65: 672–675

Hudson I R B, Cavill I A J, Cooke A, Holland B M, Turner T L, Wardrop C A J 1990b Biotin labelling of red cells in the measurement of red cell mass in preterm infants. Pediatric Research 28: 199–202

Jones J G, Holland B M, Veale K E A, Wardrop C A J 1979 'Available Oxygen', a realistic expression of the ability of the blood to supply oxygen to tissues. Scandinavian Journal of Haematology 22: 77–82

Jones J G, Holland B M, Hudson I R B, Wardrop C A J 1990 Total circulating red cells versus haematocrit as the primary descriptor of oxygen transport by the blood. British Journal of Haematology 76: 288–294

Keyes W G, Donohue P K, Spivak J L Jones M D, Oski F A 1989 Assessing the need for transfusion of premature infants and role of haematocrit, clinical signs and erythropoietin level. Pediatrics 84: 412–417

Kinmond S, Hudson I R B, Aitchison T et al 1990 Placento-

fetal transfusion in preterm infants. Early Human Development 22: 175

Linderkamp O L 1982 Placental transfusion: determinants and effects. Clinics in Perinatology 9: 559–592

Linderkamp O L 1987 Blood rheology in the newborn. In: Lowe G D O (ed) Baillière's Clinical Haematology 1: 801–826

Monod J, Wyman J, Changeaux J P 1965 On the nature of allosteric transitions: a plausible model. Journal of Molecular Biology 12: 88–118

Obladen M, Sachsenweger M, Stahnke M 1988 Blood sampling in low birth weight infants receiving different levels of intensive care. European Journal of Pediatrics 147: 399–404

Phibbs R H, Shannon K, Mentser W C 1989 Rationale for using and recombinant human erythropoietin to treat the anaemia of prematurity. In: Baldamus C A, Scigall P, Wieczorek L, Koch K M (eds) Erythropoietin: from molecular structure to clinical application. Karger, Basel, p 324–329.

Phillips H M, Holland B M, Abdel-Mois A et al 1986 Determination of red cell mass in assessment and management of anaemia in babies needing blood transfusion. Lancet 1: 882–884

Smith E L, Hill R L, Lehman I R, Lefkowitz R J, Handler P, White A 1983 Principles of biochemistry: mammalian biochemistry, 7th edn. McGraw Hill, Auckland

Thein S L, Weatherall D J 1988 The thalassaemias. In: Hoffbrand A V (ed) Recent Advances in Haematology 5: 43–74

Wardrop C A J, Holland B M, Veale K E A, Jones J G, Gray O P 1978 Non-physiological anaemia of prematurity. Archives of Diseases in Childhood 53: 855–860

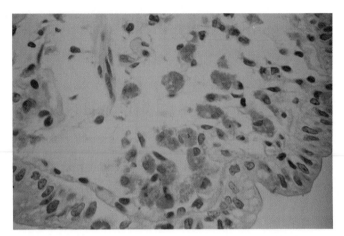

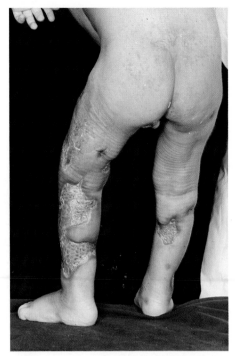

Plate 1 Small intestinal mucosa in a girl with severe combined immunodeficiency disease. This jejunal biopsy of a 6-months-old girl with SCID shows the typical morphology with a reduced cellularity (lack of plasma cells) of the lamina propria with patchy infiltration of the villus tip with macrophages. Morphometry can be normal. (× 400, H&E stain.)

Plate 2 Deep leg ulcerations after recurrent pseudomonas skin infections in a boy aged 18 months with X-linked hypogammaglobulin-aemia.

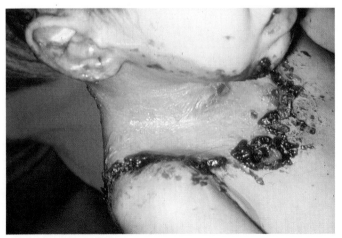

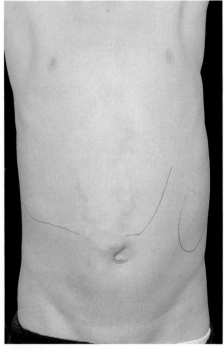

Plate 3 Severe skin ulceration after radiation therapy for enlarged lymph-nodes in a child with ataxia telangiectasia, demonstrating the exquisite sensitivity to ionizing radiation.

Plate 4 Massive hepatosplenomegaly, convoluted superficial veins and ascites in a 9-year-old boy with hyper IgM syndrome and primary sclerosing cholangitis.

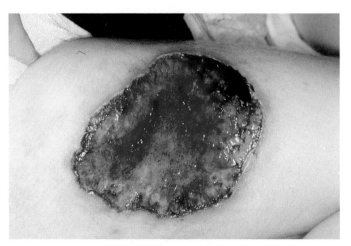

Plate 5 Necrotizing fasciitis in a 13-year-old child with moderately severe lymphocyte adhesion molecule deficiency (CD 18 expression approx. 3–5%.)

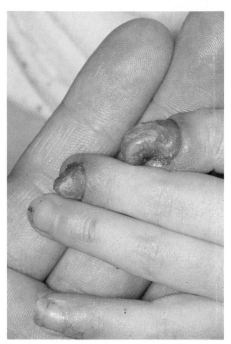

Plate 6 Severe fungal nail infection in a girl with chronic mucocutaneous candidiasis. Fungal hyphae were identified from nail scrapings.

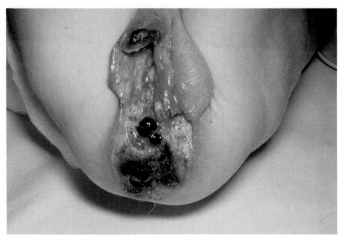

Plate 7 Severe recto-vaginal ulceration in a 4-month-old girl with hyper-IgE syndrome. (The patient made a complete recovery without persistent scar formation. Follow-up 10 years.)

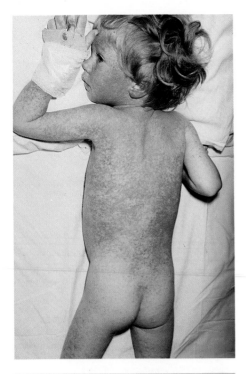

Plate 8 Acute graft-versus-host disease grade III-IV. Widespread maculo-papular rash covering over 75% of the body in a child with PNP deficiency and transfusion-associated graft-versus-host disease.

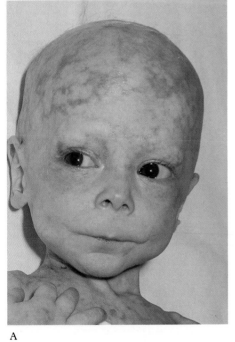

A

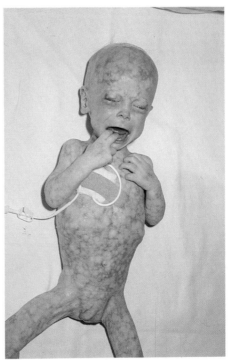

B

Plate 9 Chronic graft-versus-host disease. Reticular-vasculitic distribution of chronic, intermittently ulcerating skin lesions and alopecia in a 9-month-old boy after haploidential transplantation for reticular dysgenesis.

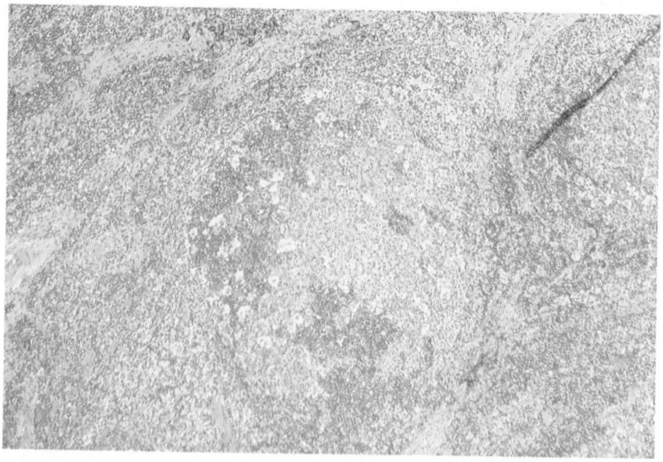

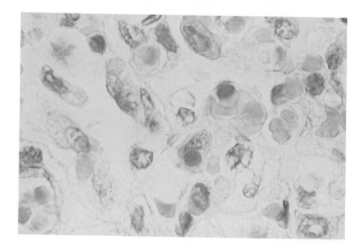

Plate 10 Lymph-node histology of 5-year-old child with AIDS. The section shows a follicular hyperplasia with disruption of germinal centres by small lymphocytes. (× 300, H&E stain.)

Plate 11 Cytomegalovirus pneumonitis. Typical viral inclusion bodies and multinucleated cells in a lung biopsy specimen obtained for diagnostic purposes in a child with HIV infection and pneumonitis. (× 250, H&E stain.)

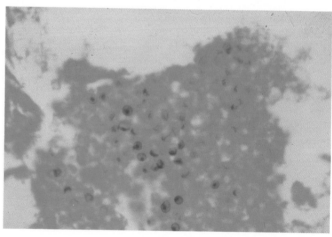

Plate 12 *Pneumocystis carinii* 'cysts' in the lung tissue of a child with pneumonitis and HIV infection (Grocott-Gomori methamine silver nitrate stain).

11. Nonmalignant disorders of lymphocytes: primary and acquired immunodeficiency diseases

Stephan Strobel

A BRIEF ONTOGENY OF T- AND B-LYMPHOCYTE DEVELOPMENT

The pivotal role of the thymus for the development of a functioning immune system has been recognized since 1961 (Miller 1991). The exact mechanisms and pathways of T lymphocyte differentiation are, however, still a matter of continuing research and controversy (Boyd & Hugo 1991). The immune system employs two broad lineages of lymphocytes, B- and T-cells. They are derived from a small number of pluripotent hematopoietic stem cells. B (bursa equivalent) and T (thymus derived) cells react specifically with antigen and mediate specific immunity. In response to inductive signals, the stem cell generates an enormous number of lymphocytes (and other hemopoietic cells) through a process which involves multiplication, growth and differentiation (Fig. 11.1). These steps are controlled by a continuously expanding number of recently discovered cytokines (interleukins), which act during the developmental process often in conjunction with others. This developmental process is controlled by a huge number of regulatory and structural genes which leave a great potential for a functional abnormality of the immune system.

T-lymphocytes

The development of the lymphoid system occurs along two pathways, the T- and B-cell pathways. The thymus, derived from the entodermal cells of the 3rd, 4th pharyngeal pouch, is the development and education site for the T-lymphoctye, the effector for cell-mediated immune responses.

The thymic epithelium is considered to be the organ in which major parts of the crucial self/nonself discrimination process takes place. Within the thymic environment, autoreactive T-cell clones are eliminated, and nonreactive clones are released into the periphery. The majority of these cells use the αβ chain of the mature T-cell receptor (TCR2).

As T-cells mature in and outside the thymus, they express a variety of unique membrane-bound glycoproteins (cell surface receptors) which can be distinguished and identified with monoclonal antibodies and visualized with immunofluorescent staining techniques.

Differentiation within the thymus

It seems that direct contact of lymphocytes with the thymic epithelium during ontogeny is required for the generation of functional T-cells. T-lymphocytes populate the thymus at approximately 7–8 weeks of gestation. The medullary, cortical and subcapsular epithelium all express HLA class I and II antigens, whereas the elements of mesenchymal origin, the pathognomonic Hassall's corpuscles, do not. The role of peptides produced by the thymus (thymic hormones – thymosin, thymulin, thymostimulin, etc.) in the development of lymphocytes and their biologic activity *in vivo* is uncertain. Long-term benefits of thymic hormone administration in humans for correction of an underlying immunodeficiency *in vivo* have not been reported.

T-cell receptor diversity

The nature of the T-cell receptor (TCR) has been defined by genetic analysis in humans and mice. The T-cell antigen receptor is a polymorphic disulphide-linked heterodimer of a 50 000 dalton

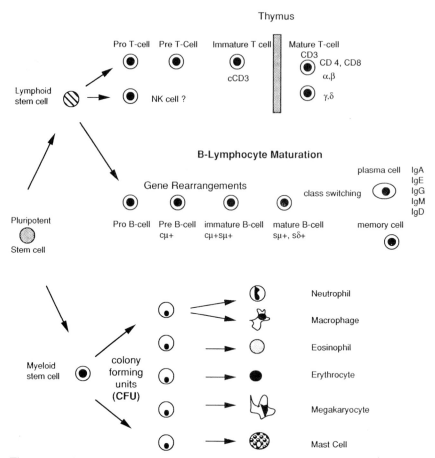

Fig. 11.1 Schematic diagram of lymphocyte development. Highly simplified diagram of T- and B- cell development from a multipotent haematopoietic stem cell (including differentiation and maturation pathways of the myeloid lineage). All growth, differentiation and proliferation steps are under the control of multifunctional cytokines. The thymus is the major site of T-lymphocyte development, whereas B-cell maturation takes place in the bone marrow. Self/nonself discrimination in the thymus leads to elimination of self-reactive cell clones. The majority of nonengaged cells die a programmed cell death (apoptosis). (c = cytoplasmic, s = surface, $\mu+$ = IgM, $\delta+$ = IgD expression.)

α and a 40 000 dalton β subunit (Fig. 11.2). Four T-cell gene families (alpha, beta, gamma, delta) that rearrange during somatic T-cell development have been identified and found to have variable joining and constant elements which express a 20–50% homology to those of the immunoglobulins.

The α, β chains of the receptor encoded by genes located on chromosomes 7 and 14 are closely related to the immunoglobulin chains, and form part of the immunoglobulin superfamily (Acuto & Reinherz 1985). An alternative heterodimer the γ,δ T-cell receptor (TCR1) has recently been described and is predominantly expressed on cells with the CD3, but not CD4 or CD8 cell surface receptors. Its function is still hypothetical. Early reports describe antigen specificity for an acute phase protein (heat shock protein), tuberculin (PPD), and a role in the mucosal immune system (Spencer et al 1989) as well as in infectious diseases and inflammatory processes (Haas et al 1990). The heterodimeric TCR proteins appear to function as recognition molecules in close collaboration with the major histocompatibility complex (MHC), whereas the noncovalently linked CD3 complex seems to be responsible for signal transduction to the nucleus. Antigen receptor

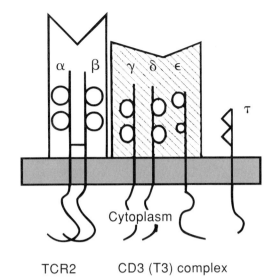

TCR2   CD3 (T3) complex

Fig. 11.2   T-cell antigen receptor complex (TCR/CD3). The TCR2 receptor consists of α, β heterodimer and a disulphide linkage. The TCR1/CD3 subunit (γ,δ,ε) comprises three noncovalently linked heterodimers. The function of the τ-chain and the conformation of the whole complex is not known.

interaction leads to an increase in cytosolic free calcium and activation of the protein kinase C system. This stage is followed by expression of previously untranscribed genes encoding for the cytokine IL2 and the IL2 receptor.

Chromosomal location of T-cell receptor chains

The T-cell receptor chains have been located as follows:

T-alpha chain: 14q11 (long arm)
T beta chain: 7q32 (long arm)
T delta chain: 7p15 (short arm)
T gamma chain: 14q11 (long arm)

These gene families are generally rearranged in a certain order (e.g. α before β), and use specific genes for specific immunological functions.

B-lymphocytes

Human B-lymphocytes develop initially in the fetal liver but in adult life they are produced in the bone marrow from B precursor cells. The B-cell development occurs generally in three phases. Committed pre B-cells (B-cell precursors) re-

arrange their heavy and light chain genes in a series of events involving DNA re-arrangement, transcription, splicing, translation and assembly of heavy and light chains. This leads to the expression of membrane bound IgM, the initial antigen receptor. At this stage cells can differentiate into different B-cell subsets. In a second phase which is generally antigen dependent, B-cells populate secondary lymphoid tissues and undergo immunoglobulin class switching to IgG, IgA or IgE. These events are regulated by a multitude of B-cell growth and differentiation factors.

Once the B-cells are differentiated into antibody producing cells (plasma cells) they have lost the majority of their surface antigen receptors. Memory B-cells are most likely derived from B-cells which have once been driven into proliferation and have subsequently reverted to the quiescent phase. A characteristic of these memory cells is that they respond to a small antigenic stimulus and can generally not be tolerised.

EVALUATION OF CHILDREN WITH SUSPECTED IMMUNODEFICIENCY

Clinical features

Recurrent and/or severe infections, failure to thrive, diarrhoea and concomitant skin changes are the main, at times rather nonspecific, clinical signs of an underlying immunodeficiency in the young infant. Infections in patients with a *humoral immunodeficiency* are often manifest between 3 and 6 months of age, at the nadir of the maternally transmitted immunity (IgG). These patients have an increased incidence of infections with encapsulated bacterial pathogens (*Pneumococcus*, *Haemophilus influenzae*, *Streptococcus*, *Meningococcus*) which ultimately leads to chronic sinopulmonary infections, septicaemias, meningitis, osteomyelitis and/or severe necrotizing skin infections.

Abnormalities of *cell-mediated immunity* predispose to a variety of fungal, viral and parasitic infections in addition to those mentioned for humoral deficiencies. Disseminated viral infections (e.g. adenovirus, influenza, cytomegalovirus, poliovirus) are fatal in most infants with severe combined immunodeficiency diseases (SCID; see below).

Restoration of the immune system, preferably with a matched bone marrow transplant, can save infants with SCID and disseminated diseases (e.g. disseminated BCG after vaccination).

A careful family history exploring unexplained early (male) deaths, consanguinity, etc. can raise the awareness of a possible underlying immuno-deficiency and vaccination may need to be postponed until after the exclusion of an immuno-deficiency disease.

Central nervous system (CNS) involvement is frequently seen as a primary complication in Di George syndrome (hypocalcaemic fits), ataxia telangiectasia (ataxia, choreoathetosis, drooling), purine nucleoside phosphorylase deficiency (PNP; cerebral palsy), or as a secondary complication in antibody deficiencies (e.g. meniningoencephalitis due to echovirus) and in Wiskott–Aldrich syndrome (intracranial haemorrhage, lymphoma).

In some previously healthy older children with a short history of recurrent infections the possibility of an underlying systemic autoimmune disease (systemic lupus erythematosus (SLE), panarteritis nodosa, systemic vasculitis) has to be excluded. Vertical transmission of HIV infection, now the major route of HIV infection in childhood, can cause early clinical symptoms similar to those of a congenital SCID within the first 6 months of life, and has to be considered in the differential diagnosis. Infants with a severe combined im-munodeficiency generally do not reach their second birthday untreated except in the rare case of a slowly evolving severe combined immuno-deficiency due to absence of enzymes of the purine salvage pathway (adenosine-deaminase (ADA), purine nucleoside phosporylase (PNP)).

Humoral (antibody) deficiencies usually mani-fest before the fourth year of life. Later first manifestations in previously healthy, agamma-globulinaemic, children have been described.

Autoimmune phenomena, anaemia, thrombo-cytopenia, neutropenia, allergic manifestations, arthritis, short stature and lymphoreticular malig-nancies in association with an undue susceptibility to infection should alert one to the possibility of an underlying immunodeficiency.

Initial laboratory investigations

A provisional diagnosis of an underlying immuno-deficiency disease can often be made on the basis of the medical history and a thorough physical examination, taking into account the laboratory and microbiological investigations listed below:

1. Culture for viruses, bacteria, fungi and parasites: nasopharyngeal aspirate, saliva, stool, urine
2. Total and differential blood count: platelets, neutrophils, lymphocytes, eosinophils, monocytes
3. Erythrocyte sedimentation rate
4. Direct Coombs test
5. Immunoglobulins (G, A, M, E): serum levels and function
6. IgG subclass analysis (in infants > 6 months)
7. Isohaemagglutinins (IgM)
8. Vaccination antibody titres
9. Other specific antibody titres against respiratory viruses or recently encountered pathogens
10. Complement analysis (C_3, C_4, CH_{50})
11. Bone marrow aspiration (indicated in cytopenic infants without autoimmune features.

If there is no clear clinical picture emerging and/or confirmation of the suspected diagnosis is in-dicated, further investigations of T- and B-cell numbers, subsets and function should be per-formed in specialized (paediatric) immunologic reference laboratories.

SPECIFIC IMMUNODEFICIENCY DISEASES

In view of the rather heterogeneous clinical and immunological expression of immunodeficiency diseases, a classification into disorders affecting mainly the T-cell, or B-cell (and/or T-cell) line-ages is inaccurate and an oversimplification. For didactic reasons the description of specific immunodeficiencies is separated into disorders mainly affecting the function of T-lymphocytes, B-lymphocytes or both cell types. The WHO classification of primary immunodeficiency dis-eases is given in Table 11.1

Combined immunodeficiencies

Combined immunodeficiency diseases (CID) are

Table 11.1 WHO classification of primary immunodeficiency diseases

A **Combined immunodeficiencies**

Designation	Serum Ig	Circulating B-cells	T-cells	Presumed pathogenesis	Inheritance	Associated features
1. Severe combined immunodeficiency (SCID):						
a) X-linked	Decreased	Normal or increased	Markedly decreased	Primarily maturation defect of T cells	XL	–
b) Autosomal recessive	Decreased	Markedly decreased	Markedly decreased	Maturation defect of both T and B cells	AR	–
2. Adenosine deaminase (ADA) deficiency	Decreased	Progressive decrease	Progressive decrease	T cell and B cell defects from toxic metabolites	AR	Cartilage abnormalities
3. Purine nucleoside phosphorylase (PNP) deficiency	Normal or decreased	Normal	Progressive decrease	T cell defect from toxic metabolites (e.g. dGTP) due to enzyme deficiency	AR	Anemia
4. HLA class II deficiency	Normal or decreased	Normal	Normal	Defect of regulatory gene for transcription of MHC class II molecules	AR	–
5. Reticular dysgenesis	Decreased (maternal)	Markedly decreased	Markedly decreased	Defective maturation of T and B cells and myeloid cells (stem cell defect)	AR	Pancytopenia

B **Predominantly antibody deficiencies**

Designation	Serum Ig	Circulating B cells	Presumed pathogenesis	Inheritance	Associated features
1. X-linked agammaglobulinemia	All isotypes decreased	Markedly decrease Absent	Intrinsic defect pre-B to B cell differentiation	XL	–
2. X-linked hypogammaglobulinemia with growth hormone deficiency	All isotypes decreased	Decreased	Unknown	XL	Short stature
3. Ig deficiency with increased IgM ('hyper IgM syndrome')	IgM increased and IgD increased or normal, other isotypes decreased	IgM and IgD-bearing cells normal, others absent	Isotypes switch defect	Various: XL, AR, unknown	Autoimmune neutropenia; thrombocytopenia; hemolytic anemia
4. Ig heavy chain gene deletions	IgG1 or IgG2, IgG4 absent and in some cases IgE and IgA2 absent	Normal	Chromosomal deletion at 14q32	AR	–
5. κ chain deficiency	Ig(κ) decreased: antibody response normal or decreased	Normal or decreased κ-bearing B cells	Point mutations at chromosome 2p11 in some patients	AR	–
6. IgA deficiency	IgA1 and IgA2 decreased	Normal	Failure of terminal differentiation of IgA + B cells	Various: AR, unknown	Autoimmune and allergic disorders;
7. Selective deficiency of IgG subclasses (with or without IgA deficiency)	Decrease in one or more IgG isotypes	Normal	Defects of isotypes defferentiation	Unknown	–
8. Common variable immunodeficiency (CVID)	Variable reduction of Ig isotypes	Normal or decreased	Faulty B cell maturation associated with: intrinsic B cell defects; low B cell numbers; defective T helper function; antibodies to B cells; augmented suppressor function	Various: AR, AD or unknown	See text

Table 11.1   (*contd*)

Designation	Serum Ig	Circulating B cells	Presumed pathogenesis	Inheritance	Associated features
9. Transient hypogammaglobulinemia of infancy	IgG and IgA decreased	Normal	Differentiation defect: delayed maturation of helper function in some patients	Unknown	Frequent in families with other IDs

C Other well-defined immunodeficiency syndromes

Designation	Serum Ig and antibodies	Circulating B-cells	T-cells	Presumed pathogenesis	Inheritance	Associated features
1. Wiskott-Aldrich syndrome	Decreased IgM: antibody to polysaccharides particularly decreased	Normal	Progressive decrease	Cell membrane defect affecting hematopoietic stem cell development	XL	Thrombocytopenia; small defective platelets; eczema; lymphoreticular malignancies
2. Ataxia telangiectasia	Often decreased IgA, IgE and IgG subclasses; increased IgM monomers; antibodies variably decreased	Normal	Decreased	Unknown: presumed defect in DNA repair	AR	Ataxia; telangiectasia; defective chromosomal repair; increased alpha fetoprotein; lymphoreticular malignancies
3. 3rd and 4th pouch/arch syndrome (Di George)	Normal or decreased	Normal	Decreased	Embryopathy: thymic hypoplasia or aplasia	Unknown	Hypoparathyroidism: cardiac outflow tract malformation; abnormal facies

D Syndromes associated with immunodeficiency

Chromosome abnormalities
    Bloom syndrome
    Fanconi anemia
    Down syndrome
Multiple organ system abnormalities
    Partial albinism
    Short-limbed dwarfism
    Cartilage hair hypoplasia
    Agenesis of the corpus callosum
Hereditary metabolic defects
    Acrodermatitis enteropathica
    Type 1 orotic aciduria
    Biotin dependent carboxylase deficiency
Hypercatabolism of Ig
    Familial hypercatabolism of Ig
    Myotonic dystrophy
    Intestinal lymphagiectasia

a heterogenous group of (mostly) genetic diseases which are characterized by gross anatomical and functional impairment of cell-mediated and humoral immunity. Less severe forms with residual functional immunity can be distinguished from the severe combined immunodeficiency diseases (SCID) which have a poor prognosis. However, the latter disorders can be corrected by marrow transplantation (BMT).

SEVERE COMBINED IMMUNODEFICIENCY DISEASE (SCID)

Severe combined immunodeficiency diseases

(SCID) are caused by a functional failure of cellular and humoral (antibody mediated) immunity. This group of disorders can be divided into:

1. SCID with haemopoietic hypoplasia (e.g. reticular dysgenesis)
2. SCID without T- and B-cells (T⁻,B⁻)
3. SCID without T but with B cells (T⁻,B⁺) (most common form)
4. SCID due to adenosine deaminase deficiency (ADA)
5. SCID due to purine nucleoside phosphorylase deficiency (PNP)
6. SCID due to defective HLA class II (and/or class I) expression
7. SCID due to other functional T-lymphocyte defects.

SCID with haemopoietic hypoplasia and bone marrow failure (syn. Reticular dysgenesis)

This most severe form of SCID is due to a developmental defect of the (haemopoietic) stem cell which leads to a global deficiency of the immune system which can also affect nonspecific immunity because of agenesis of granulocytic precursors in the bone marrow (De Vaal & Synhaeve 1959, Ownby et al 1976).

The gene location is not known; the inheritance is autosomal recessive and/or sporadic. Prenatal diagnosis is possible via second-trimester fetal blood sampling and analysis of immunity in a fetus at risk (i.e. where there is a previously affected sibling).

Pathogenesis. The disease is thought to be caused by an interruption of normal marrow differentiation at about the 10th week of gestation. A metabolic defect interfering with lymphocyte maturation has been postulated (Ownby et al 1976). Autopsy findings are similar to those found in SCID. The marrow usually contains erythroid precursors, macrophages and megakaryocytes.

Clinical features. Infants usually present in the first few days or weeks of life with severe infections, vomiting, diarrhoea and early failure to thrive. Clinical presentations up to 3 months of age have been reported.

Laboratory findings. A marked neutropenia or total absence of neutrophils are the most consistent findings. Haemoglobin and platelets are initially normal but are severely reduced in the later stage of this rapidly progressing disease. Lymphocytes can be seen in normal numbers and can display normal cell surface markers as assessed with monoclonal antibody analysis in vitro. These T-cells are, however, unresponsive to mitogens. Normal IgG levels in these infants reflect maternal transfer; serum IgA and IgM levels are reduced.

Treatment. The only therapeutic options are vigorous supportive therapy dealing with the acute clinical symptoms (infections, failure to thrive) until restoration of immune function can be successfully achieved with a BMT. All blood transfusions containing immunocompetent cells (i.e. red cells, platelets, fresh plasma) need to be irradiated to prevent fatal graft-versus-host disease.

SCID with varying degrees of T- and B-cell involvement

This is a severe combined immunodeficiency syndrome due to a hereditary deficiency of both the T- and B- cell system, associated with lymphoid aplasia and/or thymic hypoplasia.

Autosomal-recessive, X-linked and sporadic forms have been described. The chromosome location for X-linked SCID is Xq 13 (Conley et al 1990). Chorionic villus sampling and subsequent prenatal diagnosis can only be performed in informative X-linked families using specific cDNA probes. The carrier status of the mother can be investigated by analysis of maternal lymphocytes, which are screened for non-random X-inactivation (Puck et al 1987). If the mother is a carrier, only male pregnancies have a 50% risk of being affected. Second trimester fetal blood sampling remains an additional method of carrying out prenatal-diagnosis if the phenotype of the previously affected sibling is well documented.

Pathogenesis. T⁻B⁻ SCID (Swiss-type hypogammaglobulinaemia; reviewed by Hitzig et al 1971) is thought to be due to a failure of lymphoid stem cell development. The lack of response to thymic hormone therapy or thymic transplantation argue against a primary thymus defect in these patients.

T⁻, B⁺ SCID, in which there are very low T-cell numbers and normal or increased numbers of B-cells, is more common (Conley et al 1990). In-vitro co-culture experiments have demonstrated that the B-cells of these patients can synthesize normal amounts of immunoglobulins when cultured with normal T-cells (Seeger et al 1976, Griscelli et al 1978). One might be justified in assuming that the basic defect is at the level of the T-cell (T-helper cell) which does not provide the necessary help signal to respond to antigenic contact with immunoglobulin production.

Whether a syndrome described by Nezelof (1964) is a separate disease entity is questionable. It may be a variant of a T⁻B⁺ SCID with normal serum levels of nonfunctional (or minimally functional) immunoglobulins and has phenotypic similarities with the purine nucleoside phosphorylase (PNP) deficiency syndrome (Hitzig 1971).

Histology. The lymphoid system shows a general hypoplasia. Thymic hypoplasia/aplasia with rudimentary Hassall's corpuscle formation is a constant feature. Lymph nodes lack germinal centres, and the T-cell areas are depleted. The gut-associated lymphoid tissues are also depleted, and the intestinal mucosa lacks plasma cells and often shows a patchy macrophage infiltrate (Plate 1).

Frequent clinical manifestations of SCID

A positive family history with a previous early death of a sibling (? male) in healthy, possibly consanguinous parents, should alert one to the possibility of an underlying inherited severe immune problem in an infected infant. The early onset of refractory oral thrush and diarrhoea are associated with complex T-cell deficiencies. Severe recurrent episodes of bacterial pneumonia and severe ear, nose and throat infections are often signs of a B-cell (antibody) deficiency, and usually commence during the nadir of maternally transmitted IgG at around 3–6 months of age.

Pulmonary symptoms are common and severe pneumonias with *Pneumocystis carinii*, respiratory or enteroviruses (measles, influenza, parainfluenza, echo, adeno) are often fatal. Systemic dissemination after BCG vaccination can present in a similar way to the above infections, and needs to be considered in the infant at risk (Heyderman et al 1991).

Neurological complications (chronic encephalopathy and progressive multifocal leukencephalopathy) are less frequent but can be the first sign of CNS infection due to the immunodeficiency and need to be ruled out before a bone marrow transplant with cytoreductive preparative therapy is considered.

Gastrointestinal manifestations and complications can be life-threatening and frequently necessitate total parenteral nutrition. Chronic, often multiple virus infections (cytomegalovirus, rotavirus, adenovirus, astrovirus) or infections with helicobacter, cryptosporidium, clostridium and *Giardia lamblia* need to be specifically ruled out.

Skin disorders are common, and severe (seborrhoeic) dermatitis can cause differential diagnostic problems with graft-versus-host disease. An early or slowly developing desquamating erythroderma is compatible with intrauterine acquired graft versus host disease, Omenn's syndrome (see below), or with Langerhans cell histiocytosis. Therapy-resistant, often ulcerating and superinfected napkin dermatitis (e.g. *Pseudomonas, Candida* and herpes simplex) can also be an early non-specific manifestation of a combined immunodeficiency.

The lymphoid system is generally hypoplastic, and tonsils are absent. Lymphadenopathy is seen in infants with Omenn's syndrome or graft versus host disease induced by engraftment of maternal cells.

Short limbed skeletal dysplasias and cartilage hair hypoplasias can also be associated with SCID (Cederbaum et al 1976).

Frequent laboratory findings

Reduced levels of immunoglobulins IgG, A, M are the most consistent findings in infants with SCID. At an early clinical presentation (2–3 months), normal IgG levels reflect maternal transfer, while IgA and IgM are reduced. A blood lymphopenia (N.B.: normal values are age dependent) may be present; however, a normal count in the young infant does not rule out a combined immunodeficiency. Monoclonal antibody analysis of mononuclear cells demonstrates generally reduced mature T-lymphocyte levels (CD3, 4,8). Circulating B-cell numbers (CD19,CD20) can be increased in the T⁻B⁺ (mostly X-linked) variant, and are decreased or absent in the T⁻B⁻ (often autosomal-recessive) variant. Specific antibody

Table 11.2 Summary of CD molecules expressed on leucocytes

Antigen	Distribution	Description
CD1a	Langerhans' cells, thymocytes	
CD2	T-cells, NK cells	Sheep erythrocyte receptor
CD3	T-cells	T-cell receptor complex
CD4	T-cell subset (helper)	MHC class II restricted recognition
CD5	T-cells, B-cell subset	
CD7	T-cells	?IgM Fc receptor
CD8	T-cell subset (cytotoxic/suppressor)	MHC class I restricted recognition
CD11a	Leucocytes	α chain of LFA-1 adhesion molecule
CD11b	Monocytes, granulocytes	α chain of LFA-1 (CR3) molecule
CD11c	Monocytes, granulocytes	α chain of adhesion molecule 150.95
CD14	Monocytes (granulocytes)	
CD16	Granulocytes, NK cells	FcR γIII (low affinity) receptor
CD18	Leucocytes	β chain of LFA-1 molecule
CD19	B-cells	
CD25	Activated T-cells, B-cells	Il-2-receptor (low affinity chain)
CD45RO	T subset, B-cells, granulocytes	UCHL-1, memory T-cell subset (?)
CD45RA	T subset, B-cells, granulocytes	Naïve T-cell subset (?)
CDw52	Leucocytes	Campath-1

titres against viral or bacterial pathogens are absent in the older infant – or, if present, reflect maternal transfer.

The ability of the lymphocytes to respond to PHA, anti-CD3 or other mitogens in vitro is absent or markedly reduced.

Allogeneic stimulation in a mixed lymphocyte culture with parental or third-party lymphocytes is usually absent. Residual immunocompetence of T-lymphocytes can exist in the mixed lymphocyte reaction (MLR). This is an important finding and has to be taken into account when considering a bone marrow transplant and the most appropriate preparative regimen.

SCID due to Adenosine deaminase deficiency

A distinct variant in approximately 25–50% of the autosomal recessive forms of SCID is due to deficiency of adenosine deaminase, an enzyme required in the purine salvage pathway (Fig. 11.3).

The ADA gene has been cloned, the approximate gene localization being at chromosome 20q13qter. First-trimester diagnosis is now possible by chorionic villus sampling, and measurement of the enzyme activity in specialized laboratories. Second-trimester fetal blood analysis is an alternative.

Pathogenesis. The enzyme ADA catalyzes the conversion of adenosine to inosine, and of deoxyadenosine to deoxyguanosine. It is thought that

the accumulation of the deoxyguanosine-triphosphate (DGTP) which accumulates in ADA-deficient lymphocytes finally results in cessation of DNA synthesis and cell death. ADA deficiency is an example of a disorder in which there is a progressive decline of immune competence. Some patients initially retain some lymphoid

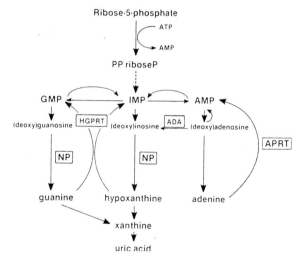

Fig. 11.3 Diagram of the purine salvage pathways. ADA = adenosine deaminase; NP = nucleoside phosphorylase; ATP = adenosine triphosphate; AMP = adenosine monophosphate; IMP = inosine monophosphate; GMP = guanosine monophosphate; HGPRT = hypoxanthine-guanine phosphoribosyl transferase; APRT = adenine phosphoribosyl transferase; PP ribose P = phosphoribosyl pyrophosphate. (From Amman & Hong 1989, with permission of W.B. Saunders, Philadelphia)

development and mitogen responsiveness (Amman et al 1983). Patients also exhibit a defect in cartilage formation, which is demonstrated by concavity and flaring of the anterior ribs, and pelvic abnormalities.

Histology. The thymus shows lymphoid depletion and rudimentary or absent Hassall's corpuscles.

Clinical features. The clinical manifestations are those seen in other forms of SCID, but may have a later onset due to the progressive nature of the immunodeficiency.

Laboratory findings. With time, these patients develop a severe lymphopenia and the features of a T⁻B⁻ or T⁻B⁺ SCID. Enzyme analysis of blood cells, and the lack of uric acid in the urine, confirm the diagnosis. Previous blood transfusions as an exogenous source of ADA, a high-purine-containing diet, and chemotherapeutic agents (e.g. cotrimoxazole) can interfere with the enzyme analysis. For these reasons, it is advisable to verify the parent's heterozygote carrier state by the concomitant measurement of red cell enzyme activity and/or uric acid metabolites.

Treatment. During severe infectious episodes and before performing a BMT, ADA activity can be supplied by irradiated blood transfusions. This partially restores immunocompetence in patients who still have sufficient numbers of circulating lymphocytes. BMT is the only long-term life saving therapeutic intervention with an approximately 50% success rate (haploidentical, mismatched BMT; Report of the European Bone Marrow Transplant Group, Fischer et al 1990). A major risk factor for BMT failure in these patients is graft rejection. Another recent therapeutic approach is the administration of bovine ADA conjugated to polyethylene glycol (PEG ADA) to increase the enzyme half-life in vivo. Long-term results of its efficiency are outstanding. Near complete restoration of immunity in some of these patients for up to 3 years has been reported. Skin test (delayed type hypersensitivity) is poorly restored with this form of therapy (Levy et al 1988).

SCID due to purine nucleoside phosphorylase (PNP) deficiency

A rare variant of SCID is due to a deficiency of the enzyme purine nucleoside phosphorylase (PNP) which leads to a progressive T-cell immunodeficiency state although B-cell function is intact.

The inheritance is autosomal recessive and the gene is localized close to chromosome 14q13. Enzyme analysis is possible in the first trimester by chorionic villus sampling. This method of prenatal diagnosis is superior and less invasive than second trimester fetal blood sampling and analysis of enzyme and T-lymphocyte levels. Estimation of T-lymphocyte numbers in the fetal blood at this stage in development can lead to falsely negative results, since cell numbers can be normal in affected children.

Pathogenesis. In the purine salvage pathway, PNP catalyzes the degradation step after ADA (Giblett et al 1972, Fig. 11.3). A deficiency of PNP leads to increased amounts of lymphocytotoxic breakdown products, e.g. deoxyguanosine, which accumulates as deoxyguanosine-triphosphate (DGTP), inhibits DNA synthesis and leads to subsequent cell death.

Clinical features. The clinical presentation of children with this disease is variable and is possibly dependent on the extent of residual enzymic activity. Some infants present in a similar way to those with SCID having early failure to thrive, severe cytomegalovirus and varicella infections, recurrent pneumonia and ENT infections. More often, however, these patients can be relatively infection free for 1–2 years, and the first sign of the disease is a cerebral palsy (Hirschhorn 1977), which can be nonprogressive and mild (author's observation in two patients with PNP deficiency) and is associated with recurrent upper respiratory tract infections. The cause for the cerebral palsy is unknown. Patients may recover normally from measles and chickenpox if infected before the development of the full blown immunodeficiency. Although this is a rare disease, children with a progressive lymphopenia, and haematological, autoimmune and neurological abnormalities up to 4–6 years of age require specialist immunological investigation in order to rule out PNP deficiency. Skin test reactivity to previously encountered pathogens (delayed hypersensitivity) is reduced or absent.

Laboratory findings. Infants with PNP defi-

Table 11.3   T-cell subset and PHA responsiveness in children with severe combined immunodeficiency disease at the time of diagnosis

Diagnosis		T-, B-	T-, B- (maternal graft)	T-, B+ (X-linked)	ADA-Deficiency (T-, B-)	T-, B+	PNP Def.	X-linked SCID (T-/B+ (mat. graft)	Omenn's syndrome
T cell subsets (%*):									
CD2	(> 60)	49	nd	0	0	1	51	24	94
CD3	(? 55)	0	23	4	0	0	34	42	94
CD4	(35 ± 10)	0	13	3	0	0	22	7	79
CD8	(20 ± 10)	20	33	3	0	0	22	36	20
CD14	(12 ± 8)	0	16	44	51	1	21	3	9
CD16	(10 ± 5)	7	71	14	nd	nd	19	nd	9
CD19	(11 ± 9)	0	0	39	0	17	40	65	0
CD25	(¶ 5)								87
HLA DR	(20 ± 7)								57
PHA S. I.	(> 20)	1.6	18	0.5	0	0	14	0	16
Age (months)		6	6	0.8	0.2	4	78	3	4

* Normal values (mean ±1 Standard Deviation). (Mean values differ slightly for the age ranges covered in this Table and % should only be taken as a guidance.) (Age related normal ranges have to be established for all age groups in each laboratory.) Highlighted T-cell counts are suggestive of maternal engraftment in these patients. (nd = not done.)

ciency may have normal or decreased quantitative and/or qualitative levels of IgG, A and M. Autoantibodies to erythrocytes and platelets are common. Analysis of circulating lymphocytes with monoclonal antibodies using fluorescence activated cell sorter analysis, reveals reduced mature T-lymphocyte numbers (CD3) with normal B-cell (CD19, 20) distribution. In-vitro mitogen responsiveness is absent or markedly reduced (Table 11.3).

Treatment. Supportive therapy consists of antibiotic therapy, *Pneumocystis carinii* prophylaxis with cotrimoxazole, and short-term substitution of PNP activity and correction of anaemia and thrombocytopenia with irradiated blood products. Children who present later than the common age range for SCID may have transfusion-acquired GVHD which is universally fatal (Strobel et al 1989). Matched BMT is the therapy of choice.

SCID due to defective HLA class II (and/or class I) expression (bare lymphocyte syndrome, MHC class II deficiency)

A combined immunodeficiency of varying severity due to defective expression of HLA class II (DP, DR, DQ) and/or, rarely, of class I (HLA-A, B, C) has been described (Touraine et al 1978, Schuurman et al 1979).

HLA genes are situated on chromosome 6. The inheritance is autosomal recessive, and most cases have been described in North Africa (Touraine 1981) although there are also patients known in Central Europe. Prenatal diagnosis has been performed in the second trimester by fetal blood samples and analysis of HLA molecules on lymphocytes.

Pathogenesis. The HLA antigens are of major importance as recognition molecules on the surface of lymphocytes, antigen-presenting cells and epithelia. Thus, their defective expression leads to a combined immunodeficiency, which is characterized by absence of delayed hypersensitivity, in vivo or in vitro, to previously encountered antigens. Despite this deficiency, some patients may respond in an allogeneic mixed lymphocyte reaction (MLR). It is unclear whether this reactivity is correlated with residual HLA class II expression or is due to HLA class I antigens. HLA class II deficiency is the first immunodeficiency to have been linked to a defect of an immunoregulatory protein. The defect has been shown to be the consequence of an abnormal DNA-binding protein (RF-X) which binds to the X-Box located at the 5' end of all HLA class II genes (Reith et al 1988, Griscelli et al 1989).

Clinical features. All patients described so far have suffered from severe repeated infections and diarrhoea within the first year of life. The presentation is similar to that of a child with a severe combined immunodeficiency or hypogammaglobulinaemia with protracted diarrhoeal disease.

Viral pneumonitis (also *Pneumocystis carinii*), bronchitis and bacterial septicaemia are common. Persistent thrush and/or intestinal infections (cryptoporidiosis) are often responsible for the marasmic state. Intestinal biopsy shows a partial to subtotal villus atrophy with an inflammatory cell infiltration and/or plasma cells. Common viruses affecting the respiratory tract are adenovirus, herpes simplex, respiratory syncytial virus and cytomegalovirus (CMV). Polio and coxsackie have been responsible for meningoencephalitis (Hadam et al 1984, Griscelli et al 1989). There is a risk of disseminated polio virus infection after oral vaccination, as in all severe immunodeficiencies.

Laboratory findings. Most patients are hypogammaglobulinaemic and show normal numbers of lymphocytes in the differential blood count. (Occasionally, normal immunoglobulin levels have been noted); (Griscelli et al 1985). Specific vaccination antibodies are absent. Low serum antibody levels have been observed after prolonged clinical infections. Delayed hypersensitivity responses (intradermal skin test) are absent.

In-vitro analysis of mononuclear cells shows that HLA class II antigens are absent (< 1%) on all cells which normally express them (B-lymphocytes, monocytes, PHA-stimulated lymphoblasts). CD3-positive T-cells and B-cells (CD19) are normal in numbers, CD4-positive lymphocytes are often decreased, whereas CD8-positive lymphocytes are increased, possible independent of the clinical status. Mitogen responsiveness in vitro is normal.

Treatment and prognosis. Adequate antimicrobial therapy accompanied by nutritional support, including total parenteral nutrition in severe intestinal disease, are first line treatment options. A BMT is the only long-term curative measure and has been successfully attempted (Fischer et al 1990). Recombinant gamma-interferon therapy aimed at induction of HLA class II expression is theoretically appealing but has not been successful clinically.

Reported death rates within the first 5 years are over 60%. The long-term prognosis is very poor in the nontransplanted patient.

SCID due to other functional T-lymphocyte defects

A number of children with features of combined immunodeficiency remain undiagnosed with currently available routine immunologic diagnostic tests, and may require more sophisticated molecular immunological analysis. Recently, T-lymphocyte deficiencies affecting the CD3 τ (theta) chain, the expression of interleukin-2 receptors, CD4 expression and intracellular signalling molecules have been described (Alarcon et al 1988, Chatila et al 1989).

PREDOMINANTLY ANTIBODY DEFICIENCIES

Clinical syndromes due to disorders of the B-cell system are primarily associated with deficiences of antibody production. It must be emphasized that a clear distinction between humoral or cellular deficiencies is artificial, in view of the close collaboration of T- and B-cells seen in a variety of immune responses, notably in antigen presentation and antibody production. Many humoral deficiency syndromes exhibit variable degrees of associated T-cell abnormalities.

X-linked agammaglobulinaemia

X-linked agammaglobulinaemia (XLA), also known as Bruton's agammaglobulinaemia (Bruton 1952), is an inherited humoral immunodeficiency affecting males and characterized by absent or low levels of immunoglobulins A,M,G,D and of circulating B cells.

The gene is localized on the long arm of the X-chromosome, close to Xq22.

Prenatal diagnosis of an affected male fetus is possible in most families with an affected index child, using a combination of currently available gene probes and gene tracking methods. Carrier detection is possible because B-lymphocytes from a carrier mother show a nonrandom X-inactivation pattern of B-cells. This finding is restricted to affected B cells only; T-cells show normal random inactivation patterns.

Pathogenesis. The primary defect appears to be a block in the differentiation of the pre-B-cell to those B-cells which express IgM on their cell surface.

Associated findings. The thymus morphology and T-cell dependent areas of the lymphoid system are normal. Lymphoid tissues lack plasma cells, and lymph nodes – usually small – fail to develop germinal centres after antigen stimulation. This leads to a general reduction of lymphoid tissues, specifically affecting tonsils and the Peyer's patches of the gut.

Clinical features. Patients with XLA are generally protected during the first 3–6 months of life through placentally transferred maternal immunoglobulins. Although most infants present nowadays between 6 months and 2 years of age with repeated infections, early (< 6 months) and late presentations (> 4 years) are not uncommon. The diagnosis can be delayed for several years due to the frequent use of antibiotics in a child with recurrent or chronic sinopulmonary or ear infections. Total immunoglobulins should be measured in any child who suffers from recurrent (bacterial) upper respiratory tract infections. Physical findings in children with XLA are often unremarkable, apart from the site of infection and possible associated growth failure. Hepatosplenomegaly and lymphadenopathy are absent in the uncomplicated patient.

Most children present with acute or chronic bacterial ENT and lung infections, pyodermas, septicaemias and also osteomyelitis. Infections are commonly due to encapsulated bacteria including *Pneumococcus, Streptococcus, Meningococcus, Haemophilus influenzae, Staphylococcus aureus*, and *Pseudomonas aeruginosa* (Plate 2). Mycoplasma infections are also a cause of significant morbidity. Immunity to viruses is generally intact. Severe disseminated disease with echovirus, polio and other enterovirus infections are rare, but life-threatening complications. Echovirus infection can be associated with tissue dissemination, myositis, hepatitis, myocarditis and arthritis. Further spread can lead to infection of the brain ultimately leading to cortical atrophy and death. High dose intravenous immunoglobulin (i.v.Ig) and also intrathecal application of i.v.Ig have been reported to affect the outcome favourably in some cases (Mease et al 1981). *Pneumocystis carinii* pneumonitis is not generally associated with XLA (see Hyper-IgM syndrome), but should be considered

in infants presenting with severe lung infection at an early age.

As a consequence of repeated lung infections, secondary bronchiectasis is a serious complication which influences the long-term prognosis. Irreversible lung damage is seen in about 10–15% of children under 10 years of age. Higher i.v.Ig replacement therapy (Sorensen & Polmar 1984, Roifman et al 1987) may be capable of reducing this rather disappointing rate of pulmonary complications.

Gastrointestinal symptoms are usually not as severe as in patients with common variable hypogammaglobulinaemia. Chronic rotavirus and *Giardia lamblia* infestations can lead to protein losing enteropathy and a malabsorptive state. 'Intractable' diarrhoea can complicate the management of these patients; the exact cause is unknown, and viral, bacterial and fungal cultures are commonly negative.

About 50% of all patients complain of joint pains, which have been linked in earlier reports to inflammatory changes which responded to immunoglobulin therapy. Occasionally painful sterile serous effusions of large joints (mostly knee) can persist for months and do not easily respond to i.v.Ig. These effusions do not usually cause functional deficiencies. Patients with XLA have a slightly increased risk of developing a malignancy (Spector et al 1978) in a similar way to other patients with immunodeficiencies.

Laboratory findings. Characteristic findings are low (< 2 g/l) or absent serum IgG levels associated with absent levels of IgA, M and D. Serum IgE levels are variable. The global failure of antibody production after antigenic stimulation can be assessed by measuring antibody responses to vaccinations or to commonly encountered infectious pathogens, e.g. respiratory viruses. Blood group antibodies (isohaemagglutinins, IgM) are generally absent. Delayed-type hypersensitivity responses are normal. Analysis of blood lymphocytes demonstrates the lack of mature B-cells (CD20) or early B cells (CD19). Pre-B-cells can be identified in the bone marrow. Analysis of T-cell function is normal.

Antibiotic treatment. Few patients would survive their initial bacterial infections without antibiotic therapy. Despite a considerable reduction of antibiotic use due to the administration of intravenous immunoglobulin preparations (i.v.Ig), antibiotics are frequently needed as an adjunct or as prophylactic therapy in the severe forms of the disorder. As a general rule, the antibiotic dose has to be higher and given over longer periods than comparable infections in the non-immuno-deficient patient. Whenever possible, the pathogen should be cultured and identified, and antibiotic therapy adjusted accordingly. In culture-negative infections of the respiratory tract, sinuses and ears, cotrimoxazole and amoxicillin for 10–14 days are usually adequate. The response to therapy has to be closely monitored in order to decide whether there is a need for i.v. antibiotic therapy. Severe lung infections must be treated with intravenous broad-spectrum antibiotics which cover *Haemophilus*, *Staph. aureus*, *Strep. pneumoniae* and mycoplasma. When cultures are negative, a third-generation cephalosporin is a possible choice. The addition of erythromycin, high-dose cotrimoxazole (to cover pneumocystis pneumonitis) and/or an aminoglycoside is dependent on clinical presentation, X-ray changes and the extent of previous antibiotic therapy.

Prophylaxis. Some patients need continuous cotrimoxazole prophylaxis during the winter months (e.g. November–April) at half of the normal treatment dose (e.g. 20–24 mg cotrimoxazole (TMP/SMX)/kg/day) in addition to i.v. immunoglobulin administration.

Immunoglobulin treatment. Regular intravenous replacement therapy with human IgG preparations is the therapy of choice and markedly reduces the frequency of bacterial infections. It is also likely to prevent early bronchiectasis and chronic damage to other target organs. Polyspecific IgG preparations which leave the functional activity of the molecule intact have a half-life of about 3 weeks. Initial 3-weekly replacement doses of 0.2–0.4 g/kg body weight are generally required, but doses should be adjusted to the age-specific normal IgG levels *and* to clinical response. Serum level adjustments can be achieved by a variation of the infusion interval (2–4 weeks) or by a dose increase (0.3 g–0.6 g/kg). Chronic sinusitis, bronchitis and possibly a deterioration of pulmonary function may be prevented by aiming for upper normal age-related serum levels in patients with pre-existing damage (Roifman et al 1987). Serum IgG levels of inpatients, e.g. at diagnosis and/or during acute life-threatening infections, can be normalized by two infusions of 1 g/kg body weight over 24 hours.

Side-effects. The start of i.v.Ig therapy in the infected child needs to be carefully monitored in hospital, since the initial infusions of IgG can lead to antigen–antibody complex formation, and complement and neutrophil activation. Clinical signs are fevers, chills, flush, pallor, rigor and occasional bronchoconstriction. Prevention of these at times severe reactions can be achieved by: (1) reduction of infusion flow rate (4–6 hours); (2) premedication with steroids and/or administration of an antihistame. Fever and headaches can occur several hours after an infusion, and often respond to symptomatic therapy with paracetamol.

Patients with low or absent serum IgA levels can occasionally develop IgE anti-IgA antibodies after infusion with IgA-containing IgG preparations, and may develop anaphylactic-type reactions during therapy. Most IgG preparations contain trace amounts of IgA. If side-effects are proven to be due to anti-IgA antibodies, specific non-IgA-containing preparations can be obtained from some manufacturers.

Intramuscular Ig preparations (i.m.Ig). Intramuscular Ig represents a possible alternative for some patients living in conditions where i.v.Ig administration is not feasible for logistic reasons or because it is too expensive. Intramuscular Ig doses are: 0.3 ml/kg every 2 weeks (16.5% solution) or 0.6 ml/kg every 4 weeks. Because of the difficulties in achieving adequate serum levels by i.m. injections, and injection associated pains, more frequent weekly administration is advisable.

Safety of i.v.Ig and supervision of XLA-patients. The manufacturing process for i.v.Ig is certainly virucidal for HIV. Rare transmissions of non-A, non-B hepatitis have been reported. For this reason, liver function has to be assessed regularly. In the case of a significant rise in liver enzymes, e.g. twice normal levels of AST, the administration of i.v.Ig has to be terminated and the manufacturer informed to avoid possible further spread *if* an infusion-associated hepatitis is the most likely cause of deranged liver function. Rare cases of fulminant liver failure have been described in infusion-associated non-A, non-B hepatitis. Trough Ig levels have to be measured regularly before each infusion until the individual requirements of the patients are stable and known. I.v.Ig requirements can vary during infectious episodes.

Lung function. Lung function has to be carefully monitored by X-ray and functional tests, since a major cause for chronic morbidity in XLA is due to irreversible lung damage.

Vaccination. Children with XLA should not receive oral, live attenuated, polio vaccines because of the low risk of disseminated central nervous system infection. MMR vaccine in patients on i.v.Ig therapy is not indicated, since these children are likely to have acquired protective antibody levels through the replacement therapy.

Parent support group. Helpful information for XLA-sufferers and infants with other forms of immunodeficiencies can be obtained from national support groups (UK HGG Society for Immunodeficiency Diseases).

Immunoglobulin deficiency with normal or increased IgM (hyper-IgM syndrome)

This is a rare immunodeficiency syndrome characterized by normal or increased serum IgM (+IgD) with a concomitant reduction of IgG, IgA and an increased incidence of autoimmune diseases (Rosen et al 1961).

The disease is mainly X-linked, but autosomal recessive) and sporadic cases have been noted. The gene for the X-linked form has been mapped to Xq 24–27 (Mensink et al 1987). Prenatal diagnosis is impossible due to insufficient linkage data.

Pathogenesis. A developmental defect in immunoglobulin isotype switching from IgM-bearing B-lymphocytes to IgG and IgA or IgE seems to be the underlying abnormality. A deficiency of immunoglobulin isotype 'switch T-cells' has also been proposed and demonstrated in vitro (Mayer 1986), and would suggest that this syndrome is not an inherent B-lymphocyte abnormality. There are thought to be no gene defects in the switch region sites of B-cells for IgG or IgA-production. Congenital rubella infection during the complex isotype switching process may interfere with fetal development and has been implicated in the development of a hyper IgM syndrome.

Clinical features. Recurrent bacterial sinopulmonary infections as well as mouth ulcers, gingivitis and stomatitis are leading clinical symptoms, especially when neutropenia is present. Pneumonitis due to *Pneumocystis carinii* has been the presenting infection in three of our patients. In contrast to children with XLA with acute or chronic infections, infants with the hyper IgM syndrome often show a marked lymphoid enlargement, with liver and spleen involvement.

Complications. Recurrent interstitial *Pneumocystis carinii* infections and autoimmune features such as haemolytic anaemia, thrombocytopenic purpura, neutropenia, arthritis and primary sclerosing cholangitis (Plate 4) are known complications which can severely affect the prognosis of this disease.

Laboratory findings. Low or absent serum IgG, A and E levels, and an increased (to over 3–10 g/l) or normal IgM (and IgD) with normal levels of isohaemagglutinin titres are key findings. T-lymphocyte analysis and response to mitogens are usually normal; the rare finding of a reduced in vitro PHA response indicates an associated T-cell abnormality. Surface IgG or IgA-bearing B-lymphocytes are absent or, sometimes, low. Associated autoimmune features can manifest as Coombs-positive haemolytic anaemia, neutropenia and thrombocytopenia.

Treatment and prognosis. Immunoglobulin replacement therapy as in XLA is the appropriate treatment and reduces increased IgM levels in some patients by preventing recurrent infections. The associated neutropenia responds, in some cases to increased i.v.Ig substitution. Attention to good antiseptic mouth care (e.g. chlorhexidine) reduces the risk of prolonged episodes of gingivitis and mouth ulcers in neutropenic patients. Patients should receive pneumocystis prophylaxis with cotrimoxazole (48 mg/kg on 3 days a week in two doses).

The overall good prognosis is dependent on the control of autoimmune complications and on the extent of the neutropenia. Late and severe complications are intestinal B-cell lymphoma and primary sclerosing cholangitis.

SELECTIVE IMMUNOGLOBULIN CLASS DEFICIENCIES

Selective IgA deficiency

Selective IgA deficiency is generally defined by serum concentrations of < 0.05 g/l with normal total IgG and IgM levels. Secretory IgA is also absent (Rockey et al 1964). It is the most common immunodeficiency, with an incidence of 1:320 to 1:700 in blood donors of Caucasian background.

There is no clear genetic pattern. The disease is mostly sporadic: autosomal dominant or recessive inheritance has been described.

Pathogenesis. The pathogenesis of the patient's failure to produce IgA is unknown. Patients with IgA-deficiency seem to have a defect of the B-cell/plasma cell system without a recognizable T-cell abnormality. A firm genetic linkage has not been established, although some studies suggest that an HLA-associated gene (possibly class III) is responsible for the disease (Schaffer et al 1989). Gene deletions as a cause of IgA deficiency are rare (1/20 000–30 000 blood donors).

Function of IgA. IgA (together with IgM) is the secretory immunoglobulin of all mucosal surfaces, and is especially important for the gastrointestinal tract and the respiratory system. Secretory IgA is produced in subepithelial plasma cells as a monomer, this joins together to become a dimer (J-chain) and is then taken up by the secretory piece, which acts as a poly Ig receptor at the basolateral side of the epithelial cell; from there, it is transported onto the mucosal epithelium. Serum and secretory IgA consist of two subclasses – IgA1 and IgA2 – which have different resistances against proteases, with IgA2 being the more resistant subtype. The immunological function of the IgA is directed towards prevention of adhesion, and neutralization of invading organisms. IgA antibody–antigen complexes do not generally activate the complement cascade, and provide a means of mucosal or reticuloendothelial clearance without activation of inflammatory pathways (Brandtzaeg 1987).

Clinical features. Despite the great number of healthy IgA-deficient individuals, there is a clear association with:

1. autoimmune diseases

2. recurrent pulmonary infections and allergy
3. gastrointestinal disorders, e.g. coeliac disease
4. possible malignancies (Amman & Hong 1971).

Autoimmune diseases. The aetiology remains speculative (Amman & Hong 1970). Increased antigen access into the circulation and the subsequent production of antibodies that crossreact with human tissue or trigger other immunological events has been suggested. An increased rate of infection may also lead to an increased rate of tissue damage, leading to an altered self with a subsequent increase in autoantibody production. The autoimmune diseases most commonly associated with IgA deficiency are listed: Table 11.4.

Gastrointestinal disorders. Gastrointestinal symptoms are frequent in patients with IgA deficiency. Symptoms range from nonspecific colitis to coeliac disease, intestinal nodular hypertrophy (see CVID) and inflammatory bowel disease (ulcerative colitis, Crohn's disease). Coeliac patients with IgA deficiency have a compensatory increase of serum IgM and IgM-producing plasma cells in the gut. A gluten-free diet normalizes the abnormal IgM findings. A possible association with humoral and cellular immunodeficiencies needs to be considered (Brandtzaeg et al 1985).

Recurrent pulmonary infection and allergy. The incidence of IgA deficiency is higher in patients with recurrent infections and allergic symptoms of the respiratory tract. The pulmonary disease may present as recurrent pneumonia, bronchitis and/or obstructive lung disease. If family history, clinical symptoms (asthma, allergic rhinitis) and radiographic changes suggest an atopic disease, treatment follows anti-allergic therapeutic principles. Persistence of recurrent infections involving

Table 11.4 IgA deficiency and associated autoimmune diseases

Rheumatoid arthritis	Chronic active hepatitis
Juvenile rheumatoid arthritis	Autoimmune haemolytic
Systemic lupus erythematosus	anaemia
Thyroiditis	Idiopathic thrombocytopenic
Transfusion reactions due to	purpura
anti-IgA antibodies	Addison's disease
Pernicious anaemia	Positive serum
Dermatomyositis	autoantibodies:
Sjögren syndrome	anti-endocrine glands
	anti-nuclear (ANA)
	anti-DNA (DNA)
	Inflammatory bowel disease

ear, nose and throat suggests an additional immunodeficiency, e.g. IgG subclass deficiency (Oxelius et al 1974).

Laboratory findings. The serum IgA-level is below 0.05 g/l. Patients with higher levels but which are below 2 standard deviations of the age-related normal levels are also often referred to as IgA-'deficient' patients. Measurements in this grey area should be repeated because of the great variability of immunoglobulin estimations in different laboratories. Patients above the 0.05 g/l level do not usually follow the same clinical course as those with lower levels. An association with an IgG subclass deficiency needs to be ruled out in all patients with low IgA levels. There is an increased incidence of the HLA B8, DR3 tissue type in IgA deficiency and in coeliac disease.

Autoantibodies. Autoantibodies are directed against rheumatoid factor (30%), smooth muscle, mitochondria, thyroglobulin, basement membrane, parietal cells, single- and double-stranded DNA. Anti-cow, -sheep and -goat (20%) antibodies might cause false positive hepatitis B surface antigen (HBsAg) and high IgA serum levels if bovidae antisera are used. The source of sensitization in patients is usually unknown, but it may be related to abnormal gastrointestinal permeability and antigen handling. T-cell immunity can be abnormal. If such an abnormality is present, other primary immunodeficiencies with IgA deficiency need to be considered, e.g. ataxia teleangiectasia and cellular immunodeficiencies with abnormal immunoglobulin synthesis.

Treatment and prognosis. There is no IgA

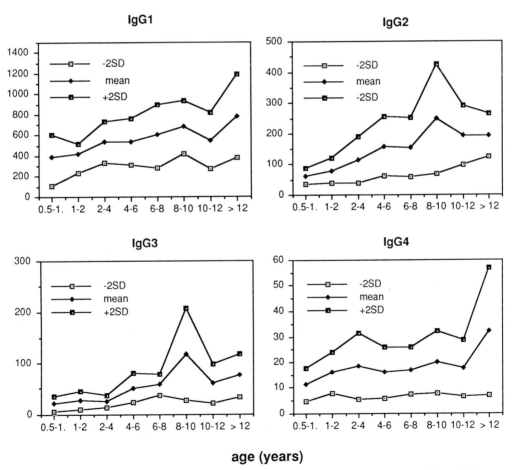

age (years)

Fig. 11.4 Age related normal IgG subclass serum levels in children. Normal values obtained from 24–40 children; each age group (radial immunodiffusion). Data from Institute of Child Health, Department of Immunology, London.

replacement option and symptomatic therapy for the underlying disease is the first step, e.g. gluten-free diet in coeliac disease, hormone replacement and/or immunosuppressive therapy. Children with very low levels of IgA have the risk of developing anti-IgA antibodies, which can be responsible for anaphylactic reactions (IgE, immune-complex-mediated) after plasma or i.v.Ig infusions. Once anti-IgA antibodies have been demonstrated, great care should be taken to avoid accidental infusion of IgA-containing blood products. Blood should be given as washed and packed red cells. If i.v.Ig is clinically indicated (see IgA and associated IgG deficiencies) and the patient reacts to the infusion, a preparation made from an IgA-deficient donor pool should be used and can be provided by some manufacturers.

Selective IgA deficiency is the mildest form of a primary immunodeficiency disease and the good prognosis is only slightly affected by the development of an autoimmune disease. The finding of an IgA deficiency in a healthy child should prompt the search for associated diseases during long-term follow-up.

Selective deficiencies of IgG subclasses

IgG subclass deficiency is characterized by an absence or low level of any subclass alone or a combination with any other subclass (Schur et al 1970, Oxelius 1974). The age-related normal IgG subclass levels in children are shown in Fig. 11.4, and the biological properties of the IgG subclasses, in Table 11.5.

Inheritance has been described as sporadic, X-linked or autosomal recessive.

Pathogenesis. A selective deficiency or low level of immunoglobulin G subclasses can derive from a wide range of disturbances. The most common defect is an intrinsic secretory B-cell abnormality which cannot be corrected in vitro by co-culture experiments with normal T-cells. Subclass deficiencies due to gene deletions and lack of IgG-subclass-committed precursor B-cells have very rarely been reported.

Clinical features. Most clinical symptomatic patients (sex ratio 3:1 in childhood) with subclass deficiencies present with recurrent sinopulmonary infections, otitis media and/or allergic symptoms, such as asthma, hayfever and food allergic disease (Fig. 11.5). In a study of a highly selected group of children seen in a paediatric immunology unit, 24–40% of subclass-deficient children presented with recurrent infections with or without allergic symptoms, or with allergy alone (Goldblatt et al 1989).

Some children present in a manner similar to hypogammaglobulinaemic patients, with recurrent severe lung infections, bronchiectasis and a persistent productive cough.

Laboratory findings. Total serum IgG levels can be low or at the lower limit of normal, normal or increased in subclass-deficient patients. IgA deficiency is a leading finding and is associated with IgG2/4 deficiency in 40–50% of patients. IgA deficiency can co-exist with any subclass deficiency, and always necessitates subclass analysis in the symptomatic child. Subclass estimations can vary in children for several reasons:

1. there is a maturational delay of IgG2 and IgG4 production in infancy
2. intercurrent infections can lead to higher than normal levels
3. variability of the analytical method.

It is important to establish and use age-related

Table 11.5 Biological properties of IgG subclasses

Property	IgG1	IgG2	IgG3	IgG4
Production in the first 2 years of life	+++	+	+++	±
Serum concentrations (%)	65–75	15–20	5–10	1–5
Antibody specificity exposure	Not restricted	Capsulated bacteria	Viruses	Persistent
Fc receptor binding	High	Medium	High	Low
Complement activation	+++	+	+++	–
Biological half-life	21	21	7–10	21
Placental transfer	+++	+(+)	+++	+++

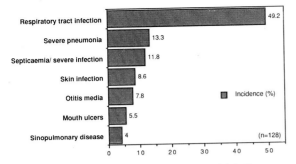

Fig. 11.5 Clinical presentation of children with IgG subclass deficiencies.

normal values. Reduced subclass levels in children need to be confirmed before they can form the basis for long-term clinical management. IgG subclass estimations are not helpful before 6 months of age, due to maternally transmitted immunoglobulins.

Patterns of subclass deficiencies

IgG1. IgG1 represents two-thirds of serum IgG, and a lack of this subclass – often in association with another subclass – can present clinically as hypogammaglobulinaemia. However, compensatory increased production of nonaffected subclasses may lead to the picture of an antibody deficiency with hypergammaglobulinaemia. Severe IgG1 deficiency leads to an increased incidence of severe pyogenic infections and progressive lung disease.

IgG2. IgG2 deficiency is frequently associated with IgG4 and IgA deficiency. This is thought to be due to a close linkage of the heavy chain genes for both IgA and IgG on chromosome 14. Clinical symptoms include chronic lung disease, and recurrent meningitis due to meningococci and pneumococci. Total serum IgG levels are often normal. Children do not respond to polysaccharide vaccines unless linked to a protein conjugate, which induces IgG1 antibody production. The protective efficacy in IgG2-deficient patients is unknown.

IgG3. Recurrent bacterial sinopulmonary infections and viral-like syndromes have been reported in a pedigree with isolated IgG3 deficiency due to a gene deletion on chromosome 14. It is unclear what distinguishes patients with IgG3 deficiency with clinical symptoms from those which are entirely healthy.

IgG4. The significance of an isolated IgG4 deficiency – that is with a serum level of < 0.05 mg/l – is unclear. Some 10–20% of a normal population have IgG4 serum levels undetectable by radial immunodiffusion.

Treatment. Once the diagnosis of a subclass deficiency has been established, severe clinical symptoms similar to X-linked agammaglobulinaemia (XLA) need to be treated with antibiotic prophylaxis and/or i.v.Ig replacement therapy, according to the principles outlined for XLA. Recurrent, less severe infections can often be managed by early antibiotic therapy during upper respiratory tract infections. Children with IgG2 deficiency and meningitis or septicaemia with encapsulated bacteria (i.e. *pneumococcus, meningococcus*) should receive long-term penicillin prophylaxis. A regular (every 6-12 months) analysis of IgG subclass levels in deficient children is advisable until a clear pattern emerges, and to identify patients with a spontaneous recovery or a maturational delay of immunoglobulin production.

Common variable immunodeficiency

Common variable immunodeficiency syndrome (CVID) describes a highly heterogeneous group of patients with late-onset hypogammaglobulinaemia and decreased ability to produce antibodies after antigenic stimulation; there are variable degrees of T-cell impairment (Wedgwood et al 1975).

Originally considered as an acquired or sporadic immunodeficiency, family studies now seem to indicate a genetic basis for this disease (Friedman et al 1977). According to in vitro findings, CVID can broadly be divided into groups with:

1. primarily B-cell abnormality
2. primarily T-cell immunoregulatory abnormality
3. autoantibodies against T- or B-cells.

B-cells can be absent (as in XLA), or fail to proliferate or differentiate into plasma cells, or fail to secrete immunoglobulins. Normal T-cell function can be affected by abnormal T-suppressor activity, lack of T-helper cells and/or autoantibody production against T- (and B-) cells.

Histopathology. Lymph node histology reveals a hypoplasia of the B-cell-dependent germinal centre and a lack of plasma cells. A coeliac disease-like intestinal mucosal villus atrophy in the absence of plasma cells must alert one to the possible diagnosis of CVID. Severe combined immunodeficiency and X-linked agammaglobulinaemia also have to be considered when intestinal biopsies are shown to lack plasma cells and have reduced or absent numbers of T-lymphocytes on immunohistochemical analysis.

Clinical features. Patients with CVID can present in infancy and childhood or during the second and third decades of life. The leading clinical manifestations are recurrent sinopulmonary infections, pneumonia and/or bronchiectasis.

Relatively sparse lymphoid and tonsilar tissues contrast clinically with the recurrent sinopulmonary and ENT infections. Hepatosplenomegaly and lymphadenopathy can signal a severe infectious mononucleosislike picture caused by EBV or cytomegalovirus infection. Digital clubbing and altered thorax dimension indicate chronic lung changes.

Microbiological findings. Common pathogens responsible for recurrent infections include *Pneumococcus, Staphylococcus, haemophilus influenzae* and *Mycoplasma pneumoniae*. There is increased evidence of interstitial pneumonitis due to *Pneumocystis carinii*. Lung changes due to *M. tuberculosis* and fungal pathogens need to be considered. Gastrointestinal pathogens include *Giardia lamblia, helicobacter jejuni, Clostridium* and *Cryptosporidium*.

Laboratory findings. Hypogammaglobulinaemia with serum IgG levels of 2–3 g/l and usually low or absent IgA and IgM are the leading findings. Serum IgE is normal or elevated in about 10% of patients. Isohaemagglutinin titres are reduced or absent. T-cell analysis in some patients with T-lymphocyte dysfunction demonstrates decreased numbers of CD3 and CD8 cytotoxic/suppressor T-cells leading to an *increased* CD4: CD8 ratio (Cunningham-Rundles 1989). B-cell numbers can be normal, increased or absent. Delayed-type hypersensitivity responses and in vitro mitogen responsiveness are reduced in 30% of these patients.

Complications. *Gastrointestinal complications* are seen in about 10% of patients and are more frequent than in XLA. A coeliac-like syndrome with diarrhoea or steatorrhoea, mucosal enzyme

deficiencies, protein-losing enteropathy and villus atrophy is often due to giardiasis, helicobacter or clostridium infections (Ament et al 1973). A gluten-free diet is unhelpful, and therapy must be directed against the cultured pathogen. In culture-negative patients, jejunal juice or mucosal tissue culture and histology may be needed to identify the infectious organism. Mucosal abnormality returns to normal after eradication of the pathogen.

Intestinal lymphoid hyperplasia of the small bowel is a diagnosis often suggested by typical X-ray changes and is thought to be an abortive attempt by the lymphoid tissue to produce antibodies in the lamina propria. These features are seen in other diseases and are not of specific diagnostic significance.

Autoimmune phenomena. Despite the inability of CVID patients to produce antibodies against infecting pathogens, they are capable in some instances of producing autoantibodies. Coombs-positive autoimmune haemolytic anaemia, idiopathic thrombocytopenic purpura, and autoimmune neutropenia are the major manifestations of autoimmune disease in the CVID patient (Conley et al 1986).

Joint pains. Joint pains can be the leading symptom in CVID and can present with a monoarthritis of a large joint similar to a seronegative juvenile rheumathoid arthritis; likewise, hand, foot, and knee joints can be affected.

A tenosynovitis can also be present. These symptoms often subside on i.v.Ig therapy. Septic arthritis, e.g. due to *haemophilus influenzae*, mycoplasma and ureaplasma, need to be ruled out in some cases by needle aspiration and microbiological investigation. Patients usually respond to i.v.Ig and appropriate antibiotic therapy.

CNS. Viral meningoencephalitis due to enteroviruses needs to be considered in patients with neurological symptoms (Fig. 11.6).

Nonspecific granulomata. Lung changes similar to those of sarcoidosis can be seen, and are caused by noncaseating granulomata. Liver, spleen and skin can also be affected. The aetiology is unknown; biopsy cultures are negative. The changes usually respond to steroid therapy.

Treatment. The main therapeutic option is i.v.Ig therapy, as in X-linked hypogammaglobulinaemia. Adjuvant antibiotic therapy in chronic disease is frequently needed, since i.v.Ig is not

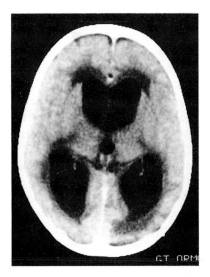

Fig. 11.6   Meningoencephalitis in common variable immunodeficiency disease. CT Scan shows extensive hydrocephalus after a meningoencephalitis due to echo- and adenovirus. The boy is well after ventriculo-peritoneal shunting and high dose i.v. Ig substitution.

always sufficient to reduce recurrent infections (e.g. bronchiectasis). The *antibiotics* of choice are cotrimoxazole, amoxycillin, cephalosporins, and tetracycline in the patient over 12 years of age. Whenever possible, antibiotic therapy during acute infections or exacerbation of the lung disease should be adjusted to pathogen sensitivity.

Gastrointestinal complications. Extensive diagnostic efforts, including jejunal biopsy and/or colonoscopy must be directed at identifying the possible infectious cause of the malabsorptive state, so that adequate treatment can be initiated *Giardia lamblia, helicobacter fetus* and also *Cryptosporidium* are known pathogens in these patients. Treatment of cryptosporidial disease is often unsatisfactory. A trial of spiramycin therapy (or with newer macrolid compounds) is indicated in addition to high-dose i.v.Ig substitution. The effects of oral immunoglobulin therapy e.g. 50 mg/kg per day in 4–6 doses, is unproven in prospective randomized clinical trials. Anecdotal reports indicate some usefulness in the severely affected infant.

Noninfectious causes of malabsorptive states and steatorrhoea have been described on the basis of an underlying autoimmune disease and/or fibrosis of the small bowel mucosa.

Autoimmune phenomena. Autoimmune phenomena can often be managed by an increase in i.v.Ig substitution in order to achieve serum IgG levels in the upper two-thirds of the normal range, by an increase of the administered dose or by reduction of the dosage interval. Demonstration of autoantibodies without clinical symptoms should not be taken as an indication to initiate high dose i.v.Ig therapy. Control of idiopathic thrombocytopenic purpura (ITP)-like features and also associated neutropenias have been achieved by an increase in substitution therapy. For ITP, a 5-day loading regimen 0.4 g/kg per day (i.e., a total of 2 g/kg) is often needed in addition to the continuing replacement therapy. If the patient does not respond to i.v.Ig therapy, corticosteroid administration (2 mg/kg prednisolone) should be tried. In the frequently relapsing steroid-dependent patient, an increase of maintenance i.v.Ig may reduce the steroid requirements and associated side-effects.

Transient hypogammaglobulinaemia of infancy

Transient hypogammaglobulinaemia of infancy (THI) is a rare disorder which is diagnosed retrospectively. There is a transient hypogammaglobulinaemia which persists beyond the physiological nadir of serum IgG levels at 4–6 months of age (Tiller & Buckley 1978).

Pathogenesis. The pathogenesis is unclear but thought to be due to delayed maturation of T-helper function for B-cell differentiation and immunoglobulin production.

Clinical features. There are two broad categories of patients. In the first group, the children are asymptomatic and the diagnosis is made by chance or because of a family history of recurrent infection and/or a minor immunodeficiency. The second group clearly has an increased rate of recurrent pyogenic infections of ears, bronchopulmonary system and skin.

Laboratory findings. Serum IgG levels can be as low as 1–4 g/l, with associated slightly low levels of IgA and IgM. Patients with this disease can produce isohaemagglutinins and generally do respond to diphtheria and tetanus vaccination. Transient hypogammaglobulinaemia is a rare disease, and low total serum IgG levels found in children between 4 and 12 months of life are more often the first signs of a permanent hypogammaglobulinaemia. Lower levels may also be found in prematurely born (<32 weeks of gestation) infants, whose physiological nadir is lower than normal because of lower serum IgG levels at birth and in whom it may take longer to achieve 'normal' levels.

Vaccination. The diagnosis of transient hypo-gammaglobulinaemia is a retrospective one, and these infants have to be treated as being hypo-gammaglobulinaemic until normal immunoglo-bulin production is demonstrated. During this period they should receive killed vaccines; this avoids the rare complication of paralytic or cerebral poliomyelitis which can be seen as a severe complication in XLA and common variable immunodeficiency states.

Treatments and prognosis. Most infections do respond to antibiotic therapy. Intravenous or i.m.IG is only very rarely required.

The prognosis is excellent. Children usually recover in the second year of life.

OTHER WELL DEFINED IMMUNODEFICIENCY SYNDROMES

Wiskott–Aldrich syndrome (WAS)

Wiskott–Aldrich syndrome (WAS) is an X-linked disease characterized by eczema, thrombocytopenia, reduced platelet size, recurrent infections a variable degree of immunodeficiency and an increased incidence of lymphoid malignancy. (Wiskott 1937).

The gene has been localized to the short arm of the X chromosome (Xp11) (de-Saint Basile et al 1987). Prenatal diagnosis and carrier detection are possible in about 98% of fully informative families, with the use of hypervariable probes in specialized genetic departments. Analysis of non-random X-inactivation of mononuclear cells can be used for carrier detection.

Pathogenesis. Until recently, there was no underlying hypothesis which could explain the existence of immunological and haematological abnormalities in WAS. A deficiency of a cell membrane glycoprotein (sialophorin) as a result of a defect in the glycosylation of membrane proteins has been described on T-lymphocytes (Gp115, CD43) and platelets (GpIB⁻). However, the gene for this glycosylation defect has been localized to

chromosome 14 and clearly indicates that this abnormality cannot be the sole primary defect (Remold-O'Donnell & Rosen 1990).

Clinical features. Petechiae, gastrointestinal bleeding episodes, occasionally intracranial haemorrhages, and extensive eczema are often the first clinical manifestations in the neonatal period. Some 20% of patients die during acute bleeding episodes. Signs of immunodeficiency, indicated by recurrent infections, often become obvious at about 6 months of age. Common pathogens isolated from lung, blood, cerebrospinal fluid and ears include *Haemophilus influenzae*, *Pneumococcus*, *Meningococcus* and *Pneumocystis carinii*. Severe viral and fungal infections are an indicator of progressive decline of immune function, seen with increasing age.

Eczema-like skin changes can involve the whole body (erythroderma) and are not always responsive to topical treatment. Some patients with debilitating eczema require systemic steroid therapy, which makes patients even more prone to overwhelming viral (e.g. Varicella zoster, Herpes simplex) and fungal (*Candida*, *Aspergillus*) infections. Autoimmune disorders may have the appearance of cutaneous or generalized vasculitides (including cerebral and coronary arteries), rheumatoid arthritis and haemolytic anaemia. The occurrence in about 20% of patients of leukaemia and Hodgkin's disease are manifestations of an increased risk of lymphoreticular malignancies in these patients (Spector et al 1978, Penn et al 1988).

Laboratory findings. A reduction in platelet numbers to 5–10 × 10⁹/l, and in platelet size to about 50% of normal, are consistently found. Functional platelet aggregability is reduced. Serum immunoglobulins in the second half of the first year show normal, or often elevated, levels of IgA and IgE, and reduced IgM. The inability to produce antibodies after exposure to polysaccharide antigens, and the absence of isohaemagglutinins in infants (over 6 months of age) provide an important diagnostic clue. Monoclonal IgG proteins are an additional feature. T-cell immunity, including T- and B-cell numbers and subpopulations, as well as PHA responsiveness, are initially normal. Lymphopenia and reduced T-cell function are signs of a progressive immunodeficiency which is often manifest after six years. Mixed lymphocyte responsiveness of WAS patients *in vitro* is a more sensitive marker of immunocompetence than the response to mitogens. Reduced cytotoxic activity of lymphocytes and a reduction of FcRI receptor expression on monocytes are *in-vitro* signs of the increased susceptibility to severe virus infections in later life. A reduced expression of the CD43 marker (see above) on T-lymphocytes is helpful as a diagnostic tool in the very young patient who presents with thrombocytopenia and eczema, and where WAS has to be considered in the differential diagnosis.

Differential diagnosis. Idiopathic thrombocytopenic purpura or autoimmune thrombocytopenia through transfer of maternal antibody during pregnancy can be distinguished from WAS by normal platelet size, normal or hyperactive bone marrow and the absence of serum immunoglobulin abnormalities. Thrombocytopenia with absent radius (TAR syndrome) is occasionally part of the differential diagnosis (see Ch. 6).

Treatment. Platelet survival in WAS is variable, but acute bleeding episodes usually respond to platelet transfusions which should be irradiated (> 30 Gy) to prevent graft-versus-host disease until the cellular immunity of the patient has been assessed. Thrombocytopenia is at times responsive to low-dose steroids. Long-term steroid therapy enhances the underlying immunodeficiency, increasing the risk of overwhelming infections, and splenectomy should be considered in highly steroid-dependent patients' and/or those with frequent severe bleeding episodes. Splenectomized patients need lifelong penicillin prophylaxis. Prophylactic antibiotic therapy with cotrimoxazole needs to be considered in patients with severe recurrent infections. Antibiotic therapy should be started early and in adequate doses, to prevent overwhelming septicaemias, lung infections and their sequelae. Therapy with topical fluorinated steroid preparations is often required to control the at times debilitating skin changes.

Bone marrow transplantation. There is a low risk of malignancies developing in recipients of matched BMT. More recently, a matched unrelated donor (MUD) transplant in these patients has become a possible therapeutic option in the absence of a matched sibling. The clinical experience with haploidentical mismatched BMT

is disappointing due to the increased incidence of EBV associated lymphomas. The variability of the disease makes it difficult to decide which treatment option (and at what time during the disease) to pursue. Whether the risk of malignancies decreases after BMT is currently not known.

Prognosis. The overall life expectancy in WAS has increased due to 'aggressive' antibiotic therapy and BMT. Early deaths are usually due to bleeding episodes. Overwhelming infections with increasing age are the cause of death in 60%. Lymphoreticular malignancies and leukaemias are responsible for 5–10% of deaths. Survival into the second and third decade is not uncommon. It is not clear whether long-term survivors represent incomplete forms of this heterogeneous syndrome.

Ataxia telangiectasia

Ataxia telangiectasia (AT) (Louis Bar syndrome) is a clinical syndrome characterized by telangiectasia, recurrent sinopulmonary infections, progressive ataxia, combined immunodeficiency (IgA- and T-lymphocyte deficiency) endocrine abnormalities and increased susceptibility to ionizing radiation (Plate 4).

Extensive genetic heterogeneity is supported by the existence of five different complementation groups. One affected gene is localized to chromosome 11q22–23 by linkage analysis. Stable translocations involving chromosomes 7,14 and the X-chromosome have been described (Gatti et al 1988). Recently, first trimester diagnosis has been accomplished by investigation of increased radiation-induced chromosomal breaks of cultured fibroblasts obtained at chorionic villus sampling. Mid-trimester diagnosis is also feasible, by analysis of chromosomal breakages in lymphoblastoid cells after low-dose ionizing irradiation.

Pathogenesis. There seems to be no unifying hypothesis which can explain the clinical symptoms and the extreme sensitivity of AT cells to radiation. A DNA-repair defect associated with abnormal gene control seems likely. This may also account for the high serum levels of alpha-fetoprotein and carcino-embryogenic antigen (CEA). Progressive atrophy of the brain Purkinje cells, testes and ovaries, thymus and lymphoid tissue is common.

Clinical features. Onset of the disease is variable, occurring usually within the first 2 years of life with the features of ataxia, unsteady gait and posture, drooling, recurrent infection, and a mask-like facies. Cerebellar, extrapyramidal and posterior column signs develop during the disease. Recurrent infections of the sinopulmonary system and development of bronchiectasis due to bacterial and viral organisms are a common problem. Puberty is delayed, males are often infertile, and growth failure becomes apparent with disease progression. A markedly increased rate of acute lymphocytic leukaemias and lymphomas in children, and of epithelial malignancies in young adults has been reported in patients and, to a lesser extent, in family members (Boder 1985).

Laboratory findings. Raised alpha-fetoprotein (AFP) serum levels together with an unsteady gait is highly suggestive of the disease. Below the age of one year, the AFP levels may initially be normal. Signs of immunodeficiency progress with time. Lymphopenia, IgA deficiency (associated with IgG2 deficiency) low IgE levels and varying degrees of impaired T-cell functions (reduced mitogen responsiveness and low or absent delayed hypersensitivity responses) are found in 50–70% of affected infants.

Chromosomal studies reveal translocations involving common breakpoint sites 14q32, 14q11, 7q5, 7q12, close to the gene sites for immunoglobulin heavy chains and the T-cell receptor chains. An increased expression of the 'immature' TCR1 γ, δ receptor has been demonstrated on T-lymphocytes. Endocrine dysfunction, autoantibody production and chronic active hepatitis are associated findings.

Treatment and prognosis. There is no curative therapy, and attempts to restore the underlying immunodeficiency by transplantation have not halted the progressive neurological disease. Early antibiotic therapy and i.v.Ig replacement in hypogammaglobulinaemic patients are indicated. Patients with AT are extremely radiosensitive, and dose reduction of radiomimetic drugs or radiation is advisable (see Fanconi syndrome). Blood transfusions in the immunocompromized child should be irradiated to 30 Gy and bCMV-negative.

The prognosis is very variable with early deaths but also patients surviving until the third or fourth decade. Supportive therapy does not alter the CNS progression to severe mental and physical disability.

DI GEORGE SYNDROME (also known as thymic hypoplasia, and immunodeficiency with hypoparathyroidism and congenital heart disease)

The Di George syndrome is a congenital immunodeficiency with variable expression, characterized by hypocalcaemic seizures (hypoparathyroidism) congenital heart disease (mostly involving the right-sided aortic arch, and the tetralogy of Fallot) with unusual facies and increased susceptibility to infections. It was first described in three infants by Di George in 1965.

Most cases are sporadic, but familial occurrences are known; the gene is localized on chromosome 22. In view of the sporadic nature of the syndrome and its variable expression, prenatal diagnosis is not possible.

Pathogenesis

In the 6th to 10th week of intrauterine life, the thymus, thyroid, parathyroid glands and certain vascular and facial structures develop from the 1st–6th branchial pouch area. The Di George syndrome most likely results from an intrauterine disturbance before the 12th week of gestation, mainly affecting the above structures. The cause of the failure of orderly embryogenesis is unknown. It has been associated with chronic alcoholism of the mother during pregnancy (Amman et al 1982) and/or with a microdeletion on chromosome 22 (Kelley et al 1982).

Clinical features

Complete forms of this syndrome are most often recognized by the characteristic facial abnormalities, including hypertelorism, cleft lip or palate, low-set ears, a blunted nose, short philtrum of the lips and antimongoloid slant of the eyes. Additional abnormalities, such as oesophageal atresia or imperforate anus, are rare. Urinary tract abnormalities have been described (Conley et al 1979). The following cardiovascular abnormalities are common in the complete form, although patients without them have been described:

1. right sided aortic arch
2. tetralogy of Fallot
3. atrial septal defect
4. ventricular septal defect
5. hypoplastic pulmonary artery
6. pulmonary artery atresia.

Hypocalcaemic seizures are often the first clinical features, presenting within the first 24–48 hours of life. Additional hyperphosphataemia, absent parathormone levels and evidence of thymic deficiency in association with facial and cardiac abnormalities are diagnostic. Rarely, a Zellweger syndrome has to be considered in the differential diagnosis of parathyroid and thymic deficiencies (Amman & Hong 1989).

Laboratory findings

Children with congenital heart disease and/or with congestive heart failure can have a transient hypocalcaemia. The presence of low calcium and elevated phosphorus levels which are *unresponsive* to therapy in a patient with congenital heart disease are suggestive of the disease.

The total lymphocyte count can be decreased, normal or increased. The percentage of circulating mature lymphocytes is usually decreased, as is their response to phytohaemagglutinin (PHA). Analysis of other factors of immune function have been performed; their results have been very variable and inconsistent, and are probably dependent on the degree of thymic involvement (Muller et al 1988, 1989).

Rare complete forms fail to express the α,β heterodimer of the CD3/TCR2 receptor complex, but express the (thymus-independent) receptor TCR1 instead (γ,δ).

Treatment

Initial management is directed towards control of the hypoparathyroidism and prevention of graft versus host disease (GVHD) during cardiopulmonary bypass surgery.

Hypoparathyroidism (and hypocalcaemic seizures): intravenous calcium gluconate infusions followed by oral calcium supplements and 1,25 dihydrocholecalciferol supplementation. (1–2 mg/kg per day). Parathormone therapy is not generally needed.

Prevention of graft-versus-host disease (during cardiopulmonary bypass surgery or cellular blood product support): Once a Di George syndrome is suspected, and when full assessment of immune competence cannot be accomplished before surgery, all cellular blood products have to be irradiated > 3000 rad (30 Gy) to avoid the occurrence of GVHD in an immunocompromized child.

Immune reconstitution. In complete Di George syndromes, fetal thymic tissue transplantation (10th gestational week) has been advocated as the therapy of choice for primary thymic deficiency. Long-term immunological reconstitution has been reported via intraperitoneal and intramuscular thymic transplants (Cleveland et al 1968). A (matched) bone marrow transplantation is, however, the current therapy of choice, and carries a better long-term out look with regard to the persistence of normal immune function (Borzy et al 1989). Clinical variability and partial deficiency states are major difficulties in assessing earlier reported effects of thymic transplantation and hormone therapy. Partially affected neonates usually regain their full immunity within 1–2 years, and can be kept infection-free by appropriate supportive and anti-infectious therapy.

Prognosis

Spontaneous improvements in T-cell immunity and correction of hypoparathyroidism have been reported. The prognosis is good for the far more common infants with a partial Di George syndrome, and is mainly dependent on the underlying cardiac abnormality. The *in-vitro* features of a cellular immunodeficiency are transient and are only rarely responsible for an increased rate of infection during the first year of life. Mental retardation is common as the result of neonatal seizures. Major prognostic factors are the severity of the underlying heart disease and the extent of hypoparathyroidism.

Follow up

Follow-up management after discharge from hospital must be dependent on first line treatment and the extent of the immunodeficiency, and close collaboration between cardiologists, immunologists and endocrinologists (hormone replacement therapy) will be required. Live vaccines should be withheld in infants with initial signs of a cellular immunodeficiency until the immune function is normal.

LFA-1 deficiency (Leukocyte adhesion deficiency (LAD), delayed cord separation syndrome.)

Leukocyte adhesion deficiency (LAD) disease is characterized by recurrent necrotic soft tissue infections, impaired pus formation despite marked granulocytosis, peridontitis and gingivitis, and delayed cord separation associated with a severe reduction or absence of the adhesive glycoproteins of the LFA-1 integrin family on neutrophils and lymphocytes.

The disease is autosomal recessive and occurs most often in children of North African origin. It has also been reported in infants of Central European origin. The gene location of the β-chain of the LFA-1 heterodimer is on chromosome 22 q 22.3. Prenatal diagnosis can be achieved by second trimester fetal blood sampling and analysis of leukocyte adhesion molecules with monoclonal antibodies.

Pathogenesis. LAD disease results from defective expression of three leukocyte adhesion molecules – LFA-1 (Gp 80 kDa) Mac-1 (Gp165 kDa) and p150.95 (Gp150 kDa) – which belong to the integrin family (Springer 1990). The absence or abnormal expression of the β-chain leads to abnormal expression of the functionally necessary α/β heterodimers. A mature β-chain appears to be required for normal subunit maturation, intracellular transport and cell surface assembly of the transmembrane heterodimer. The consequences of defective leukocyte adhesion molecule expression are now well understood for granulocytes and lymphocytes. Clinical symptoms are mostly due to defective neutrophil function. Neutrophils of affected individuals show defective migration and impaired adhesion-dependent chemotaxis and aggregation. Neutrophils are unable to phagocytose iC3b-opsonized particles, and thus fail to generate the respiratory burst. Adherence-independent functions and release of neutrophil granule content triggered by soluble stimuli are preserved, including the killing of microorganisms. The consequences for lymphocyte function are less well understood. Altered migration to lymphoid organs and reduced cell-mediated cytotoxicity are part of the disease spectrum.

Clinical features. Infants with a severe adhesion molecule deficiency (leukocyte adhesion molecule expression < 1%) frequently present with delayed cord separation (> 3 weeks), omphalitis, septicaemia or soft tissue infections in the neonatal period. The infections are very similar to those seen in granulocytopenic patients. LAD patients are functionally neutropenic despite a marked granulocytosis up to $4–8 \times 10^9/l$. *Staphyloccus aureus*, Gram-negative enteric bacteria and fungi (*Candida* and *Aspergillus*) are frequently encountered pathogens. Death in the severe form of the disease is often due to overwhelming infections at between 2 and 4 years of age. Patients with a moderate phenotype (see below) are also at risk of recurrent necrotizing soft tissue infections (Plate 5). Their leukocytes retain some functional activity. Patients with this phenotype have an unpredictable clinical course and may well reach the second or third decade, but usually need constant clinical attention for treatment of infections and/or skin grafting because of impaired wound healing. Patients are generally not prone to severe viral infections (Anderson et al 1985).

Laboratory findings. In the absence of immunofluorescence techniques, a provisional diagnosis can be made by clinical observations, the demonstration of a marked leucocytosis, deficient granulocyte chemotaxis, adherence and spreading behaviour on glass slides. A differential NBT test using particulate (abnormal response) or soluble stimuli (normal) can be diagnostic. Confirmation of the suspected diagnosis by FACS analysis demonstrates a lack of CD18 (β chain) and CD11a (LFA-1 α chain) on neutrophils and lymphocytes (Fig. 11.7). Reduced levels above 1% up to 15% indicate a moderate deficiency.

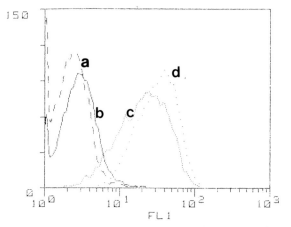

Fig. 11.7 Analysis of CD18 expression in leucocyte adhesion deficiency (LAD). LFA-1 β chain expression (CD18) on lymphoblastoid cell lines from: (a) patient with a severe LAD phenotype (CD18 < 0.5%, background); (b) patient with moderately severe LAD phenotype (CD18 3–5%); (c) obligate heterozygote mother of (b) with CD 18 expression within the normal range (~80%) but slightly lower than (d); (d) normal control. (FACS analysis, arbitrary fluorescent units (FL) log scale).

Obligate heterozygote levels (parents) can vary between 20 and 80% of normal.

Treatment. Supportive antibiotic therapy, with occasional surgical intervention in the case of deep seated or necrotic lesions with or without skin grafting, is needed but not curative. Children on prolonged antibiotic therapy may benefit from prophylactic antifungal therapy. The only curative therapy is a BMT. Engraftment has been achieved with identical and HLA-mismatched donors (LeDeist et al 1989).

X-linked lymphoproliferative syndrome

X-linked lymphoproliferative syndrome, also known as Duncan's disease (first reported kindred) and Purtilo syndrome (Purtilo et al 1975), is a mostly fatal X-linked disease caused by an abnormal immune response to an infection with Epstein-Barr virus (EBV) with subsequent features of immunodeficiency.

The gene has been mapped to Xq24–27 in several linkage studies. Prenatal diagnosis of potentially affected children in families at risk is not possible since the underlying immunodeficiency is unknown and only becomes manifest after EBV infection.

Pathogenesis. The pathogenesis is still unclear; patients at risk of developing this syndrome,

exhibit normal immune function before infection (Sullivan et al 1983). Rare survivors develop varying degrees of immunodeficiency with hypogammaglobulinaemia and a tendency to secondary malignancies (Sullivan & Woda 1989).

Clinical features. The disease can present clinically as:

1. infectious mononucleosis (75%)
2. aplastic anaemia (20%, in association with infectious mononucleosis), usually fatal
3. hypogammaglobulinaemia
4. malignant B-cell lymphoma (30%)
5. a combination thereof (Purtilo et al 1982).

About 65% of patients with the infectious mononucleosis type of onset die of liver failure and the associated bleeding disorder.

Laboratory findings. Patients initially show a normal response to EBV, with production of anti-VCA (virus capsid antigen) and EBNA (Epstein-Barr nuclear antigen) antibodies despite diminished overall antibody responses and hypogamma-globulinaemia. The CD4:CD8 ratio is reversed (below 1.0), as in other (severe) virus infections. The presence of the virus can be demonstrated by DNA-hybridization techniques in CNS, liver, spleen and lymph nodes. Autopsy findings show inflammatory and histiocytic cell infiltration and severe lymphocytic depletion of the above organs. Unaffected female carriers often display high anti-EBV antibody titres. This feature can be helpful in the differential diagnosis of a child with a severe EBV infection who is otherwise unaffected.

Treatment and prognosis. The treatment is unsatisfactory in this disorder and can only be symptomatic, that is, by replacement of deficient serum proteins, e.g. i.v.Ig in the hypogamma-globulinaemic child and administration of plasma products in liver failure. A malignant lymphoma may develop and show initial response to conventional chemotherapy. Intravenous acyclovir therapy has been tried in some patients but is of no proven benefit.

About 80% die of the primary infection; the development of a lymphoma carries a bad prognosis.

Prophylaxis. i.v.Ig may be used as prophylaxis in unaffected male siblings of a previously diagnosed patient (Sullivan & Woda 1989).

OTHER SYNDROMES ASSOCIATED WITH IMMUNODEFICIENCY

Nezelof syndrome (syn. cellular immunodeficiency with normal serum immunoglobulin levels)

This heterogeneous syndrome is characterized by lymphopenia, a cell-mediated immunodeficiency, and lymphoid and thymic hypoplasia associated with a variable degree of (specific) antibody deficiency (Nezelof et al 1964). Its relationship to PNP deficiency (see above) is unclear but several clinical features are similar.

Both X-linked and autosomal recessive inheritance patterns have been reported. The disease is generally not amenable to second-trimester prenatal diagnosis because of variable T-cell involvement.

Pathogenesis. The aetiology of the thymic dysplasia is unknown. The thymus maintains an embryonal architecture with few lymphocytes, poorly developed medullary/cortex differentiation and absence of Hassall's corpuscles. The humoral immunodeficiency seems to be secondary to abnormal T-cell regulation. The lymph node architecture shows an absence of follicle and germinal centre formation.

Clinical features. The clinical presentation, with recurrent viral, bacterial and fungal infections, is similar to that of infants with (S)CID. Moderate lymphadenopathy and hepatomegaly can be present.

Laboratory findings. Patients are often lymphopenic, with a reduction of mature (CD3) T-cells. In-vitro functional T-cell analysis is abnormal, and the patients are skin-test anergic. B-cell studies show normal numbers, but frequently an inability to respond to neoantigens (e.g. tetanus toxoid).

Serum immunoglobulin levels are normal, but IgE is frequently increased.

Treatment and prognosis. Supportive therapy consists of intensive antibiotic therapy and immunoglobulin substitution because of the lack of specific antibody production. Unirradiated blood transfusions and live vaccines must be avoided.

The variable nature of this immunodeficiency allows some infants to survive slightly longer than SCID patients (up to 4 years). There is no long-term survivor without a BMT (see SCID).

Familial reticuloendotheliosis (Omenn's syndrome)

Familial reticuloendotheliosis is a rare, often fatal, poorly defined combined immunodeficiency syndrome characterized by a widespread skin rash and marked generalized lymphadenopathy with histiocytic infiltration and blood eosinophilia (Omenn 1965).

Sporadic and autosomal recessive cases have been reported. Prenatal diagnosis is not available.

Pathogenesis. The pathogenesis is unknown. Lymph nodes show a marked histiocytic infiltration and absence of germinal centres. The dysplastic thymus lacks Hassall's corpuscles. The presentation is similar to GVHD (Jouan et al 1987). However, recent DNA studies of activated lymphocytes of one patient have failed to confirm this hypothesis (cited in Heyderman et al 1991).

Clinical features. Skin changes with alopecia, generalized lymphadenopathy and hepato(spleno)-megaly are the most constant clinical signs.

Laboratory findings. A high total white cell count (20–60 × 10^9/l) is mainly due to a marked eosinophilia and is at times associated with a normal or high lymphocyte count. Lymphopenia is rare. Immunoglobulin levels are normal or decreased. T-cell subset analysis shows an almost normal T-lymphocyte distribution (Table 11.3), except for a high incidence of T-cell activation. Phytohaemagglutinin responsiveness of T-cells is suboptimal but usually not completely absent.

Treatment and prognosis. Short-term clinical improvement can be achieved with cyclosporin A, which reduces the state of T-cell activation (and T-cell numbers) and can also improve the skin symptoms. The only curative therapy is bone marrow transplantation, which is very difficult but has been successfully performed in one patient (Heyderman et al 1991).

Immunodeficiency with thymoma

A combined immunodeficiency associated with a benign or malignant thymic tumour, mostly seen in adults between 40–70 years of age, has been described (Good 1954).

Pathogenesis. Numerous studies over the last 10 years show patients with an increased number of CD8+ cells. These cells possess an increased in-vitro suppressor activity on normal B-cell differentiation and proliferation, though these findings are not present in all patients. Auto-immune mechanisms in the pathophysiology of this evolving immunodeficiency have also been proposed. Thymic epithelial tumours may be encapsulated (two-thirds) or invasive (one-third). There is no correlation of any one type of tumour with the extent of immunodeficiency. Some 50% of tumours are of the round cell epitheloid type, 25% of spindle cell, and 25% of mixed type (Gray & Gutowsky 1979).

Clinical and laboratory findings. Recurrent sinopulmonary infections, chronic diarrhoea, septicaemia, urinary tract infections and aplastic anaemia are presenting signs. A thymoma can be present before the onset of a severe hypogamma-globulinaemia. A common finding is a lack of pre-B-cells in the marrow, and of B-cells in the periphery. The CD4:CD8 ratio is reversed in some patients. Associated findings include anaemia, myasthenia gravis, thrombocytopenia and arthritis (Hayward et al 1982).

Treatment and prognosis. The prognosis of a thymoma *with* associated immunodeficiency or other complications is poor. Thymectomy, which is often curative in benign thymomas without complications, seems not to improve the immunodeficiency, but may ameliorate the red cell aplasia or symptoms of myasthenia gravis. Intravenous immunoglobulin therapy and antibiotic therapy are indicated in hypogammaglobulinaemic patients (Batata et al 1974; see CVID).

Chronic mucocutaneous candidiasis (CMC)

Chronic mucocutaneous candidiasis (CMC) is a heterogeneous cell-mediated immunodeficiency syndrome mainly affecting the immune defences against *Candida albicans*. CMC is characterized by persistent *Candida* infection of the skin, nails, scalp and mucous membranes, with or without an associated autoimmune endocrinopathy (Herrod 1990).

Autosomal dominant, autosomal recessive and sporadic forms have been reported. Prenatal diagnosis is not available.

Pathogenesis. The exact pathogenesis is unknown but a primary cellular defect in the response to *Candida* seems to be likely. Reduced T-cell responses to mitogens and *Candida*, deficient cytokine production and serum inhibitory factors, and defective T-cell regulatory mechanism have all been described. Some of these abnormalities may return to normal with efficient antifungal therapy, which suggests that some of the observed changes are epiphenomena. Endocrinopathies are autoimmune in origin and not a consequence of *Candida* infection of the endocrine glands. A current hypothesis assumes an autoimmune disorder directed against the lymphoid system causing a cell-mediated deficiency which, through its functional abnormality, leads to *Candida* infection and endocrinopathies.

Clinical features. The disorder can present as typical mucocutaneous candidiasis or mainly as an endocrinopathy. The most severe form of CMC presents within the first year of life and develops an endocrinopathy in about 50%. *Candida* infections of skin, mucous membranes and nails (Plate 6), often resistant to topical antifungal therapy, are common. Despite high serum antibody titres against *Candida*, patients are anergic to this antigen and do not respond to intradermal *Candida* stimulation. Chronic persistent infection can lead to granulomatous skin changes. Failure to thrive can occur through oesophageal reflux and recurrent vomiting on the basis of *Candida* colonization of the oesophagus and oropharynx.

Less severe forms of late onset may only affect the nails and the oral mucosa. The commonest endocrinopathy is hypoparathyroidism, and can manifest as hypocalcaemic seizures. Addison's disease, hypothyroidism and diabetes mellitus are less common but need to be considered with increasing age. Viral infections may precede the discovery of an endocrinopathy.

Laboratory findings. Cutaneus anergy to *Candida* and failure of T-lymphocytes to respond in vitro to *Candida* represent the most common immunological abnormalities. Total lymphocyte numbers, mitogen responsiveness and alloreactivity in mixed lymphocyte culture are generally unaffected. Serum immunoglobulin levels are normal or increased, and autoantibodies to endocrine organs are frequently present. The detection of antibodies may precede the clinical manifestation of an endocrine deficiency. CMC patients with hepatitis B, cirrhosis, chronic pulmonary fibrosis and renal disease have been reported. The differential diagnosis of chronic mucosal candidiasis encompasses a multitude of T-cell-mediated immunodeficiencies and, to a lesser extent, malignancies.

Treatment and prognosis. The treatment is supportive and has to be tailored to the severity of the disease and to the possible side-effects of systemic antifungal therapy. Mild forms may respond to topical treatment (nystatin, amphotericin, clotrimazole). More severe forms with clinical evidence of systemic (e.g. lung) spread may respond to oral and/or i.v. systemic ketoconazole. New antifungal agents such as fluconazole can also be administered i.v. or orally, and lend themselves to continuous prophylaxis because of reduced liver toxicity. The patient's individual response to antifungal therapy is not predictable, and some may fail to respond to one agent but show complete clearance with another. In patients refractory to imidazole derivatives, amphotericin B is the treatment of choice. Resistant nail (bed) infection has responded to topical ticonazole treatment. Interestingly, patients with CMC do not have an increased risk of *Candida* septicaemias. Anecdotal reports describe improvement of mucosal colonization after zinc, vitamin A or biotin supplementation. Immunostimulants have been ineffective in achieving long-term improvements. Because of the clinical variability of the disease, and the often good prognosis BMT is generally not indicated. A successful BMT in one patient with CMC complicated by severe aplastic anaemia has been reported (Deeg et al 1986).

Patients with early onset and severe forms rarely reach the third decade of life, and acute Addisonian crisis remains a high risk in the older patient. Mild forms do not affect life expectancy.

Hyper-IgE syndrome with recurrent infections (HIE); Job's syndrome, Buckley's syndrome) (see also Ch. 5)

This rare, primary immunodeficiency syndrome is characterized by extremely high serum IgE levels, chronic eczematoid dermatitis, and recurrent serious infection of the skin and respiratory system

associated with a coarse facies (Davis al 1966, Buckley et al 1972).

There are rare reports of familial occurrences; the inheritance is possibly autosomal dominant. Prenatal diagnosis is neither feasible nor indicated.

Pathogenesis. The pathogenesis is unclear. A defect in T-cell regulation of IgE production, a decrease of CD8+-T-cells, a defect in polymorphonuclear chemotaxis, a decreased IgG response to encapsulated bacteria and a reduced cellular response to *Candida* and tetanus toxoid have been described in some patients, but not in others.

Clinical features. In most patients, clinical symptoms start early in life, although a specific diagnosis may often be delayed. Skin infections (cellulitis, furunculosis) and repeated lung infections due to *Staphylococcus aureus* and secondary pneumatoceles are common manifestations. Anogenital ulcerations (Plate 7), scalp, neck and face abscesses, septicaemias, joint empyema, osteomyelitis, ear and eye infections have all been described. Pruritic dermatitis is common, and the important differential diagnosis between severe atopic dermatitis or HIE is not always easy (Table 11.6). Additional infectious pathogens are *Haemophilus influenzae*, pneumococci, Gram-negative bacteria, and fungal infection with Candida. The formation of 'cold abscesses' is seen in about 30%. The abscess contents consist mainly of eosinophils and necrotic material; neutrophils are sparse due to reduced chemotaxis (review by Geha & Leung 1989).

Laboratory findings. The most consistent finding is an enormously increased IgE level

Table 11.6 Differential diagnosis of hyper IgE syndrome and atopic disease

Feature	Hyper-IgE syndrome	Atopic dermatitis
Family history of atopy	Normal (~15%)	Very common
Probability of disease	Rare	High
Age of onset	Early, < 2 months	Later, > 2 months
Dermatitis	Atypical eczema; often clear skin	Typical atopic dermatitis
Serum IgE	High	High
Specific anti-staph IgE	Present	Usually absent
Eosinophilia	Often	Often
Staph. aureus infection	Deep seated	Superficial
Positive skin tests	Low incidence	High incidence
Respiratory allergy	Rare	Common
Coarse facies	Often present	Rare

(up to 20 000–100 000 IU/l), eosinophilia and specific IgE anti-staphylococcal antibodies. IgE levels in the young infant are around 2000 IU/l, but HIE infants with a level of 250 IU/l have been described. When measuring specific anti-staphylococcal IgE, care has to be taken to avoid nonspecific protein A binding, by choosing a protein-A-negative variant staphylococcal strain as capture antigen. Serum immunoglobulin levels are normal or increased following frequent infectious episodes. IgG subclass estimations may reveal an IgG2 deficiency and this should be excluded, especially in patients with recurrent serious or deep-seated infections. Anamnestic antibody responses to bacterial antigens may be reduced. Phagocyte chemotaxis may be reduced, but phagocytosis and killing functions are usually normal. Cell-mediated immunity in vivo and in vitro to ubiquitous antigens is reduced in up to 50% of patients (reviewed by Geha & Leung 1989).

Treatment and prognosis. The cornerstone of clinical management during acute infections in the younger child is the i.v. administration of an anti-staphylococcal penicillin (e.g. flucloxacillin). The risk of infections with flucloxacillin-resistant organisms, especially in children who have had antibiotic prophylaxis, is increased in severely ill patients. These children must receive additional i.v. broad-spectrum antibiotic therapy until microbiological culture results are available. Imaging techniques (bone scan, CT scan) are helpful to diagnose an eventual haematogenous spread to bones and abdominal organs. Lobectomy and/or surgical excision of bronchiectases and pneumatoceles are required in some patients.

A high clinical suspicion for the possibility of an underlying *Candida* (or *Aspergillus*) infection is warranted in patients with long-term antibiotic prophylaxis and/or irreversible lung damage. In patients with frequent breakthrough infections on prophylactic flucloxacillin, a change to cotrimoxazole is indicated and usually effective. Antibiotic prophylaxis often leads to reduction of the enormously increased IgE levels. Similar effects have been achieved with H2-receptor antagonists (i.e. cimetidine, ranitidine). Controlled prospective randomized clinical trials of their overall effectiveness are awaited. In clinical practice, antibiotic prophylaxis with or without addi-

tion of an H2 antagonist reduces high IgE levels and results in good control of the disease.

Patients with early diagnosis and appropriate treatment carry a good prognosis. In patients with chronic lung disease, the prognosis is dependent on the control of infections and prevention of further deterioration of lung function.

Immunodeficiency with transcobalamin II (TCII) deficiency

Immunodeficiency due to the absence of transcobalamin II is rare. Children present usually before 6 months of age with megaloblastic anaemia, chronic diarrhoea, failure to thrive and low serum immunoglobulins. The pathology mainly affects rapidly dividing cell populations such as gastrointestinal mucosa, lymphoid tissue and the hematopoietic system. Children respond rapidly to intravenous and/or oral vitamin B_{12} substitution (Seeger et al 1980, author's observation 1989).

BONE MARROW TRANSPLANTATION FOR PRIMARY IMMUNODEFICIENCY DISORDERS

Prior to the discovery of the human major histocompatibility complex 25 years ago, bone marrow transplantation (BMT) had been generally unsuccessful except in identical twins. The introduction of HLA typing and assessment of mixed lymphocyte responses between donor and recipients has considerably increased the numbers of successful matched BMT in children with a variety of immunodeficiency diseases (reviewed by O'Reilly et al 1989, Fischer et al 1990). Major problems associated with BMT, either matched (non-T-cell depleted) or mismatched (T-cell depleted,) are (1) rejection (2) graft-versus-host disease (GVHD) and (3) infections. Immunocompetent cells of the recipient (T-lymphocytes, NK-cells) may reject the donor cells and prevent engraftment (rejection). On the other hand, mature immunocompetent cells in the donor marrow may recognize the recipient as non-self, and cause GVHD which may also lead to graft failure. Severe infections are still a major cause of death even in the engrafted patient and are likely to contribute to the GVHD.

Prevention of rejection

Engraftment on the one hand, and rejection on the other are influenced by the immunocompetence of the recipient, MHC disparity, the size of marrow inoculum, the extent of preparative immunosuppressive therapy given (recipient) and whether an unfractionated or a T-cell depleted marrow has been infused (Fig. 11.8). Even unfractionated MHC-compatible marrow will be rejected if the recipient is not sufficiently immunosuppressed or is severely immunodeficient (SCID).

Preparative therapy

All transplant recipients, except for identical twins and, under certain circumstances, infants with SCID, undergo cytoreductive and marrow ablative preparative therapy to avoid donor cell injury in the broadest sense. Preparative regimens vary according to the disease and the preference and experience of the centre. In Europe standardized protocols for immunodeficiency diseases (and leukaemias) are currently used by members of the European Bone Marrow Transplantation Group (EBMT). The agents most widely used are total body irradiation (TBI) in children over 2 years of age, busulfan, cyclophosphamide, procarbazine, antithymocyte globulin (ATG) and etoposide (VP16). TBI is generally used in BMT for malignant disease and leukaemia, but is not needed in nonmalignant conditions such as SCID. The

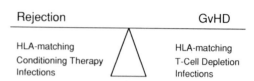

Fig. 11. 8 Factors contributing to engraftment and rejection after bone marrow transplantation.

doses of cytotoxic drugs and ionizing irradiation in Fanconi's anaemia and ataxia telangiectasia need to be reduced due to the patient's exquisite sensitivity to these forms of therapy.

Bone marrow transplantation for SCID

Matched bone marrow transplantation

Matched non T-cell depleted bone marrow transplants from sibling donors are associated with over 90% full immunological reconstitution and cure.

Haploidentical (mismatched) BMT

A matched donor is not available in about 75% of cases, and in this situation a T-cell-depleted haploidentical, parental BMT is the therapy of choice in patients with SCID. Depletion of mature T-cells from the donor's marrow has been in use since 1980 (Reisner et al 1981, 1983), and more than 100 BMT with this technique have

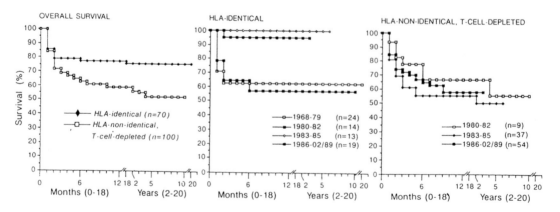

Cumulative probability of survival in SCID patients treated by BMT.

Fig. 11. 9 Survival after matched and haploidentical, T-cell-depleted marrow transplantation for severe combined immunodeficiency. (From: Fischer et al 1990, with permission of the Lancet and the author.)

been reported. Resistance to engraftment, graft loss due to unstable chimaerism and abnormalities of B-cell development and function are major factors which prevent the total success of bone marrow transplantation. Despite these problems, long-term survival and engraftment can now be achieved in over 60% of haplo-identical BMT for severe immunodeficiencies (Fig. 11.9).

Methods of T-cell depletion

The following methods of T-cell depletion are available:

1. Sheep red blood cell (SRBC) — rosetting and soybean-lectin agglutination
2. Mouse monoclonal antibody and rabbit complement (CD2, CD3) lysis.
3. CAMPATH I (CDw52) rat monoclonal antibodies and human complement lysis.
4. Immunomagnetic separation with monoclonal antibodies coupled to magnetic beads.

All the above methods remove T-cells, and some also remove B-lymphocytes, monocytes and neutrophils. The range of T-cell depletion of the marrow inoculum is 100–1000 fold.

In order to achieve complete early T and B engraftment of the donor tissue-type and improved T- and B-cell cooperation after BMT (e.g. immunoglobulin production), most European transplant centres use immunosuppressive and ablative therapy prior to BMT. This regimen also reduces the possibility of rejection in a T-cell-depleted marrow. As a general rule, the chances of rejection of donor marrow can be said to be directly related to the degree of T-cell depletion, i.e. the lower the numbers of residual T-cells in the marrow, the higher the risk of rejection and the greater the need for immunosuppression.

Transplant procedure

At the end of the preparative protocol which typically lasts around 10 days, the donor is admitted to hospital for bone marrow (BM) harvest under general anaesthesia. BM is taken in small volumes (× 2 ml) with heparinized syringes from both of the iliac crests and placed into blood collecting bags via a filter, e.g. a blood giving set. A harvest of 1×10^{10} nucleated cells/kg of recipient is generally sufficient to achieve a cell dose of 2–5×10^8 kg of mononuclear cells after T-cell depletion. Engraftment with unfractionated marrow in matched transplants can be achieved with lower cell doses, in the range of 10^7/kg. Extent of engraftment of T-cells and other leukocytes can be followed by DNA analysis. This method can also be used for detection of maternal engraftment in patients with severe combined immunodeficiencies (Fig. 11.10).

The use of monoclonal antibodies in BMT

Monoclonal antibodies were first used as a more effective and time-saving means of T-cell depletion in vitro. Their use has recently been extended to

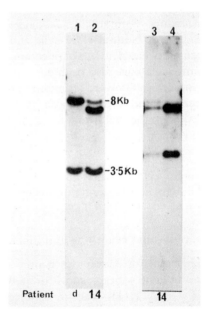

Fig. 11.10 DNA analysis of an infant with severe combined immunodeficiency disease and perinatal engraftment of maternal T-lymphocytes. Whole blood from the patient (14, track 2) and her mother (track 1) has been digested and probed. The two maternal alleles plus the paternal allele are clearly visible in the patient's DNA. Lymphocytes and granulocytes were analysed separately (tracks 3 and 4). The lymphocyte fraction shows both the maternal and paternal allele (track 3), whereas the granulocyte fraction shows one maternal and one paternal allele (track 4). This method can also be used to check engraftment after transplantation or presence of chimaerism. (Modified after Katz et al 1990)

clinical, in-vivo applications. Anti-CD3, CD4, CD7, and CD8-antibodies have been used as additional immunosuppression prior to transplantation, or as debulking agents (CD7) in leukaemias and leukaemic BMT (reviewed by Waldman 1989). An additional indication for the in-vivo use of monoclonal antibodies in the recipient is to enhance engraftment by preventing rejection. Candidate antibodies which are currently in use are anti-LFA-1 and anti-CD2. The rationale behind their use is to block the responses which depend on LFA-1-mediated adhesion and recognition. A broad range of immune responses, such as T-cell-mediated killing, natural killer activity, and antibody-dependent cytotoxicity mediated by monocytes and granulocytes, are dependent on receptor/ligand (LFA-1/ICAM) interactions (Springer 1990). They can be inhibited by daily administration of anti-LFA-1 monoclonal antibodies. Infusion of anti-CD2 antibodies interferes with adhesion of activated T-cells (CD2/LFA3) and can reduce natural killer activity of cells expressing CD2. Natural killer cells and activity have been implicated in graft rejection. Monoclonal antibodies have also been administered in vivo during severe GVHD. Therapeutic regimens have been tailored around those pathogenetic principles, and the following monoclonal antibodies have been used:

1. T-cells — CD2, CD3, CD4, CD 8
2. activated T-cells — CD7, CD25
3. cell adhesion and prevention of recognition of neoantigens — CD18, CD25.

Graft-versus-host reactions and disease

GVHD is the major barrier which prevents engraftment and more widespread use of haploidentical BMT (Fig. 11.11). The immunological response triggered during GVHD involves T-cell activation, release of cytokines and cell-mediated cytotoxicity. The severity depends on HLA disparity, age of recipient, pre-existing infections and also sex differences of the donor/recipient pair.

Acute GVHD. Symptoms of acute GVHD can begin as early as 4 days, though more typically 2–3 weeks after transplantation or transfusion of nonirradiated blood products. Symptoms are low-grade fever, maculo-papular erythematous rash

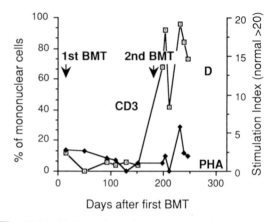

Fig. 11. 11 Failure of engraftment after first bone marrow transplantation, and signs of acute graft-versus-host disease after second (haploidentical) transplantation. (D = death.)

(Plate 8) mainly affecting the face, palms and soles of the feet, and often profuse diarrhoea. Eosinophilia, sudden lymphocytosis with mature (CD3) lymphocytes, and liver function abnormalities can be demonstrated in the blood. If the GVHD is not self-limited or is unresponsive to therapy, it can progress to marrow aplasia, hepatosplenomegaly, exfoliative dermatitis, protein-losing enteropathy and to an increased risk of infection. Differential diagnosis of GVHD in the severely immunosuppressed patient includes severe organ infections, septicaemias and drug reactions. A skin biopsy is often helpful in the differential diagnosis (Fig. 11.12).

Although the histological changes are not totally specific, the findings of Langerhans cell depletion, singe-cell necrosis, basal vascular degeneration, spongiosis and dermal perivascular round cell infiltration strongly suggest acute GVHD.

Chronic GVHD. The transition from acute to chronic GVHD is not inevitable, but is dependent on the underlying disease, preparative therapy, HLA disparity and on the extent of T-cell depletion. If features of GVHD persist for more than 100 days, the term 'chronic GVHD' is used. Depending on the series, chronic GVHD can be seen in up to 40% of patients receiving unfractionated matched bone marrow, but in only 15–20% of infants with SCID receiving T-cell-depleted marrow; female-to-male transplants carry the highest risk – up to 35% (Fischer et al 1990). Chronic GVHD can also manifest without an episode of acute GVHD.

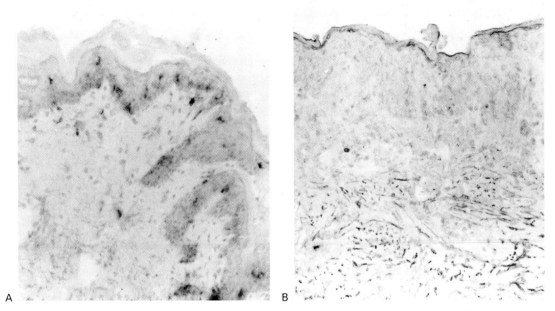

Fig 11. 12   Skin biopsy histology in graft-versus-host disease. **A**. Normal CD1a staining pattern of Langerhans' cells in the epidermis. **B**. Absence of CD1a-positive cells in a child with grade II-III skin graft-versus-host disease. (× 300, immunohistochemistry on a frozen section.)

Many clinical features of chronic GVHD are related to skin, gut, liver, and also to lung involvement.

Skin changes resemble scleroderma, with hair loss, hyperkeratosis, reticular hyperpigmentation, atrophy, ulceration and, occasionally, a vasculitic pattern (Plate 9). Impaired joint movements due to skin disease can lead to contractures.

Liver involvement is common, with increased levels of AST, gamma GT and, occasionally, increased alkaline phosphatase levels due to destruction of the bile ducts.

Intestinal involvement is characterized by diarrhoea, severe failure to thrive, and a partial or subtotal villus atrophy morphologically comparable with the histology of coeliac disease. Immunohistochemistry of the gut biopsy shows increased and aberrant (crypt region) HLA-DR expression, activated T-lymphocytes and macrophages. Coexisting virus infections need to be considered before the diagnosis of gut GVHD is made (Fig. 11.13).

Lung involvement can lead to fibrosis and chronic obliterative bronchiolitis with increasing interstitial changes and oxygen dependency. Once established, chronic obliterative bronchiolitis is often therapy-resistant and carries a fatal prognosis. In exceptional circumstances, heart-lung transplantation can be attempted and may be the only therapeutic option left in these patients.

Other clinical complications during engraftment. Immune dysregulatory processes akin to autoimmune diseases are frequent in recipients of HLA-disparate fractionated marrow grafts.

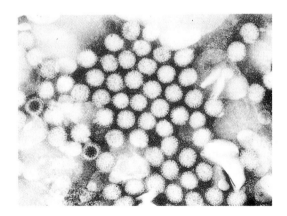

Fig. 11.13   Electronmicroscopic analysis of a stool sample of a child with diarrhoea after a bone marrow transplant for severe combined immunodeficiency, demonstrating rotavirus under negative-staining conditions. (× 3000. Kindly provided by Dr A. Phillips, electronmicroscopist, Hospitals for Sick Children (Queen Elizabeth Hospital), London, UK.)

Autoantibody production with or without organ specificity, autoimmune cytopenias and EBV-associated lymphoproliferative syndromes are clinical indicators of these complications. Some 50% of SCID patients develop autoantibodies, mainly against nuclear antigens (ANA), without clinical significance. Autoimmune cytopenias develop in up to 20% of marrow recipients, necessitating immunosuppressive therapy for 1–2 years. Long-term maintenance therapy is usually not required, and the disease does not recur in later life. EBV-associated lymphoproliferative disorders (B-cell lymphomas) carry a high mortality rate and are resistent to chemotherapy and radiation. A recent study has shown clinical benefits after infusion of a B-cell-specific monoclonal antibody. Prophylaxis with acyclovir, an agent which blocks the EBV DNA polymerase in vitro has been used successfully in patients receiving a bone marrow graft.

Differential diagnosis. The diagnosis of acute GVHD is made on the basis of acute skin and associated symptoms (see above) once possible drug reactions and viral infections have been ruled out. The diagnosis of chronic GVHD is mainly clinical and is based on the history of immunodeficiency disease, BMT and typical organ involvement, and exclusion of an underlying infection.

Laboratory findings. Increased T-lymphocyte activation markers, CD25, DR and CD23 are frequently demonstrated. A rapid and unexpected increase in mature CD3+, CD25+ T-lymphocytes shortly after a haploidentical BMT is a laboratory indicator for acute GVHD. Urinary neopterin levels are elevated during GVHD, but also during coexisting viral infections.

Treatment of GVHD. Prevention is best treatment for GVHD. A commonly used Seattle protocol uses 15 mg/m^2 methotrexate on day one, and 10 mg/m^2 on the 3rd, 6th and 11th days, in combination with daily cyclosporin A administration for approximately 6 months. SCID patients do not generally require GVHD prophylaxis in addition to T-cell depletion.

Established GVHD poses a therapeutic dilemma, since the treatment adds to the existing immunosuppression of the recipient. The armamentarium available is as follows:

1. Steroids. Methylprednisolone 5–10 mg/kg every 12 h for 48–72 h as a pulse, followed by 2 mg/kg prednisolone with slow reduction over weeks or months depending on response.

2. Cyclosporin A. According to therapeutic levels. 10–12.5 mg/kg/day orally, 3 mg/kg/day i.v. (approximate starting doses).

3. Antithymocyte globulin (ATG). Repeated courses, dose according to clinical response (2 mg/kg/day) (N.B. Serum sickness can occur during immune reconstitution!)

4. Monoclonal antibodies. Monoclonal antibody infusions are an experimental form of treatment but have already been used successfully in steroid-resistant cases. Rodent anti-CD7, –CD3, -CDw52, -CD25 and -CD18 are under clinical evaluation. The beneficial effects are often short lasting, and infusions need to be maintained for approximately 10 days and must be followed by conventional immunosuppressive therapy to prevent relapse. The possibility of an antiglobulin response limits their usefulness. Transferring the rodent antigen binding site on to a human IgG molecule might overcome these disadvantages.

Infections in the BMT recipient

Due to poorly developed host responses, neutropenia, and the presence of indwelling catheters, BMT recipients are susceptible to viral, fungal, bacterial, opportunistic and facultative intracellular organisms. Bacterial and fungal infections usually respond to appropriate treatment if diagnosed early (Table 11.7). A major threat still derives from formerly untreatable, sometimes pre-existing, virus infections, such as enteroviruses, adenovirus, Epstein-Barr virus, cytomegalovirus and parainfluenza. New antiviral drugs, such as gancyclovir, with activity against cytomegalovirus, and ribavirin with in vitro activity against adenovirus and parainfluenza III are currently being evaluated. Prophylactic use of acyclovir to prevent systemic herpes simplex infections may also have a significant effect on the reduction of systemic cytomegalovirus infections (Meyers et al 1988), but more studies are needed. Intravenous immunoglobulin substitution, which is effective practice in patients with SCID, may

Table 11.7   Treatment of infections common in bone marrow transplant recipients

Organism	Treatment
Bacteria Gram +ve and Gram −ve	According to sensitivities or a combination of piperacillin/aminoglycoside or ceftazidime/aminoglycoside

Fungi
    Candida
    Aspergillus
    Pneumocystis carinii
	Amphotericin, fluconazole
	Amphotericin, itraconazole, amphotericin + 5-flucytosine in combination
	cotrimoxazole, pentamidine

Viruses
    Cytomegalovirus
    Herpes simplex
    Varicella
    Parainfluenza, RSV
    Measles, adenovirus
 	
    EBV
 	
    Symptomatic rotavirus (or other viral infections of the gastrointestinal tract)
	Gancyclovir
	Acyclovir
	Acyclovir (higher dose for varicella)
	Ribavirin is active in vitro
	Anecdotal reports of successful therapy in some immunodeficient humans
	Prophylactic effects of acyclovir reported in BMT recipients
	Consider oral immunoglobulin therapy

Protozoa *Cryptosporidium*	Spiramycin

also afford protection against infections and acute GVHD in patients transplanted for haematological malignancies (Sullivan et al 1990). The incidence of bacterial and fungal infections is increased during the neutropenic period which can last up to 8 weeks after transplantation. Pre-existing viral infections may recur during preparative therapy or early after transplantation at the time of maximum immunosuppression. Cytomegalovirus pneumonitis is a rare but often fatal complication occurring 3–4 months after BMT in children who need continuin immuno-suppression as part of the GVHD prophylaxis protocol or for treatment of ongoing GVHD. Successful control of viral infections can be expected only after full immune reconstitution.

Immune reconstitution

The time to immune reconstitution varies according to HLA disparity, concomitant infections and evidence of GVHD.

HLA-identical (matched) BMT

Immune reconstitution with an unfractionated

stem cell graft in uncomplicated SCID patients is rapid. Normal in-vitro T- and B-cell functions develop between 10–21 days and up to 8 weeks after BMT (Fig. 11.14). Deviations from this rule are not uncommon and wide fluctuations are seen. Immunological reconstitution in leukaemic or aplastic patients or infants requiring preparative therapy or GVHD prophylaxis can be delayed for over 3–4 months. Recovery can present with normal T-cell subset patterns, or with a CD4 deficiency combined with an increased CD8

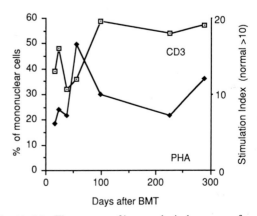

Fig. 11. 14   Time course of immunological recovery after matched bone marrow transplantation.

lymphocyte population. NK cell numbers and activity are usually increased during early engraftment.

Haploidentical (mismatched) BMT

The natural course of immune reconstitution after a T-cell-depleted BMT differs from that of an unfractionated marrow. Mature T-lymphocytes in normal numbers are not seen until about 3–4 months after transplantation. Early engraftment with demonstration of low numbers of donor-type-specific T-cells can often be detected after 3–6 weeks with sensitive DNA techniques. Cytoreductive therapy in SCID leads to haematopoietic recovery of donor origin. T-lymphocyte development is comparable to that in patients without cytoreductive therapy.

B-cell immunity

The development of normal humoral immunity is dependent on effective T- and B-cell cooperation. Whereas full T-cell immunity is seen in the majority of patients, only 59% of patients develop normal humoral immunity. This antibody deficiency is most likely the result of a failure of donor B-cell precursors to engraft. Myeloablative therapy increases the chances of full B-cell engraftment. Although, in most cases, B-cells and antigen-presenting cells remain of host origin, most haploidentical T-lymphocytes developing in SCID infants are capable of effective cooperation with B-cells of host origin for antigen presentation and antibody production at a later stage. A failure of antibody production after BMT can be due to a subclinical form of GVHD and/or a less well defined suppressor mechanism. Normalization of B-cell function can take as long as 2–4 years, during which some infants need i.v.Ig substitution (reviewed by Buckley et al 1986, O'Reilly 1989). Children with minor IgG subclass deficiencies may do well on oral cotrimoxazole prophylaxis. Recovery of immunoglobulin production in the transplant recipient on i.v.IG can be judged by the recovery of IgA and IgM production, since these immunoglobulin isotypes are not present in standard i.v.Ig preparations.

HUMAN IMMUNODEFICIENCY VIRUS (HIV) INFECTION IN CHILDREN

Shortly after description of the acquired immune deficiency syndrome (AIDS) in young homosexual men in 1982 (Center for Disease Control, Atlanta 1982), paediatric AIDS was described (1982, 1983) in infants of intravenous drug-using, HIV-infected mothers (Rubinstein et al 1983). Since then, the understanding of the disease – and unfortunately also the numbers of those individuals infected with HIV – has increased exponentially, with a doubling of reported AIDS cases between every 1–3 years, depending on country and population. In the UK 16 828 cases of HIV infection had been reported to the end of 1991. Of 370 HIV-infected children, 76 had developed AIDS and 44 had died. Of 345 children born to HIV-infected mothers, 107 are known to be infected, 93 are not infected and the status of the remainder is not known (CDR, AIDS and HIV-1 infection in the United Kingdom, 1992).

The nature of the major transmission route in infancy – i.e. from infected mother to child – makes it essential that there should be close collaboration between *all* health professionals involved in the care of the whole family. Paediatric AIDS, which is the end point of paediatric HIV infection, differs in major aspects from AIDS in adults. The following section will summarize current knowledge and approaches to paediatric HIV infection and AIDS, and will provide references for more in-depth information on selected topics. It does not attempt to cover all aspects of this world-wide epidemic with approximately 200 000 reported AIDS cases from 152 countries and 5–10 million harbouring the virus (WHO 1990 estimate).

Definition and classification

Infection with the HIV virus is confirmed by anti-HIV antibody production, HIV-core antigenaemia (P24 antigen), Western-blot analysis, virus isolation and/or HIV genomic amplification with the polymerase chain reaction. A working classification of HIV infection in children under 13 years of age is given in Table 11.8.

The varied prevalence of HIV infection in certain populations (high in Hispanics and

Negroes; lower in Caucasians) has been linked to social disadvantages, sexual preferences, and drug use. It is, however, conceivable that HLA patterns might also influence the rate of transmission (Jeannet et al 1989).

Aetiology

Infection with the human immunodeficiency virus (HIV) is a sine qua non for the development of the acquired immunodeficiency syndrome. Paediatric AIDS is a distinct entity and accounts for 1–2% of all cases.

The virus

HIV – previously known as human T-cell lymphotropic virus type III (HTLVIII) or as lymphadenopathy associated virus (LAV) – is a retrovirus (Fig. 11.15). So far, the HIV retrovirus family, which belongs to the group of lentiviruses, contains two members – HIV 1 and HIV 2. They do not share significant homology with HTLVI,

which is associated with a neurodegenerative disease called tropical spastic paresis (TSP) in which a myopathy can also occur. HTLVII has been isolated from patients with hairy cell leukaemia. HIV 2 has been identified in residents of western Africa and is also associated with an AIDS-like picture with evidence of vertical transmission. HIV 2 is closely related to a simian T-lymphotropic virus which has been reported to cause an AIDS-like disease in nonhuman primates.

HIV is an enveloped virus which contains genomic RNA, core proteins and the reverse transcriptase that can assemble DNA from the RNA template for viral replication (Fig. 11.16). The HIV genome incorporates genes coding for the core protein (gag), for the reverse transcriptase protein (pol) and the envelope glycoproteins (env). Several other, less well understood genes regulate HIV synthesis and determine latency and infectivity (reviewed by Wong-Staal & Gallo 1985, Varmis 1988).

Table 11.8 CDC classification system for HIV in children

Class P-0. Indeterminate infection
Infants < 15 months born to infected mothers but without definitive evidence of HIV infection or AIDS

Class P-1. Asymptomatic infection

Subclass A:	Normal immune function
Subclass B:	Abnormal immune function: hypergammaglobulinemia, T4 lymphopenia, decreased T4: T8 ratio, or absolute lymphopenia
Subclass C:	Immune function not tested

Class P-2. Symptomatic infection

Subclass A:	Nonspecific findings (> 2 for > 2 months): fever, failure to thrive, generalized lymphadenopathy, hepatomegaly, splenomegaly, enlarged parotid glands, persistent or recurrent diarrhea
Subclass B:	Progressive neurologic disease: loss of developmental milestones or intellectual ability, impaired brain growth, or progressive symmetrical motor deficits
Subclass C:	Lymphoid interstitial pneumonitis
Subclass D:	Secondary infectious diseases
Category D-1:	Opportunistic infections in the CDC case definition
Bacterial:	Mycobacterial infection (noncutaneous, extrapulmonary, or disseminated); nocardiosis
Fungal:	Candidiasis (esophageal, bronchial, or pulmonary), coccidioidomycosis, disseminated histoplasmosis, extrapulmonary cryptococcosis, *Pneumocystis carinii* pneumonia
Parasitic:	Disseminated toxoplasmosis with onset ˜ 1 month of age, chronic cryptosporidiosis or isosporiasis, extraintestinal strongyloidiasis
Viral:	Cytomegalovirus disease (onset ˜ 1 month of age), chronic mucocutaneous/disseminated herpes (onset ˜ 1 month of age), progressive multifocal leukoencephalopathy
Category D-2:	Unexplained, recurrent, serious bacterial infections (2 or more in a 2-year period): sepsis, meningitis, pneumonia, abscess of an internal organ, bone/joint infections
Category D-3:	Other infectious diseases: including persistent oral candidiasis, recurrent herpes stomatitis (˜ 2 episodes in 1 year) multidermatomal or disseminated herpes zoster
Subclass E:	Secondary cancers
Category E-1:	Cancers in the AIDS case definition: Kaposi's sarcoma, B-cell non-Hodgkin's lymphoma, or primary lymphoma of brain
Category E-2:	Other malignancies possibly associated with HIV
Subclass F:	Other conditions possibly due to HIV infection: including hepatitis, cardiopathy, nephropathy, hematologic disorders, dermatologic diseases

Risk factors

Intravenous-drug-using mothers, prostitution, bisexual fathers, multiple sexual partners, unprotected intercourse, blood transfusion from HIV-infected donors (before October, 1985) and multiple transfusions of blood products, as in haemophiliacs, prematurity and during cardiopulmonary bypass surgery, have all been identified as risk factors.

Routes of transmission in children

The major route of paediatric infection is vertical transmission from mother to child. The other important route of transmission, via contaminated blood products, has become almost negligible since the introduction of routine HIV antibody screening of blood donors and heat treatment of some blood products in 1985. Hospital outbreaks with devastating effects due to contaminated needles have been reported from Eastern Europe with some 800 infected children in one setting. There is a small and probably negligible risk of transmission of HIV via screened blood products if the blood has been donated during the "window" period between infection and HIV-antibody production. Rare transmissions via breast milk have been reported. In countries where there is a suitable, hygienic and affordable alternative to breast feeding, infant formulae should be given. Prospective studies in children from HIV-infected mothers in Europe show a transmission rate of about 13–16% after 3 years of follow-up (European Collaborative Study Group 1991). Higher vertical transmission rates, of 30–50%, have been reported from Africa.

Precautions. All children in hospital should be treated as if they could be carrying blood-borne infections, and 'universal precautions' (washing of hands and handling of blood-containing materials with gloves) are sufficient for infants or children with HIV infection. Infants with severe diarrhoea, bleeding episodes, vomiting and oozing skin diseases should be isolated in separate rooms under infectious (hepatitis B) precautions. Transmission of the virus into all body fluids has been reported. The risks of infection with HIV through secretions is lower than in hepatitis B. Contrary to hepatitis B transmission, nosocomial infections in institutions accommodating children with HIV infection have not been reported except where syringes have been shared.

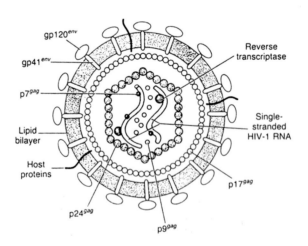

Fig. 11.15 Schematic diagram of the HIV-1 virion. Each of the virion proteins making up the envelope (gp 120^{env} and gp41^{env}) and nucleocapsid (p24^{gag}, p17^{gag}, p9^{gag}, and p7^{gag}) is identified. In addition, the diploid RNA genome is shown associated with reverse transcriptase, and RNA-dependent DNA polymerase. From: Greene 1991, reprinted with permission of The New England Journal of Medicine.

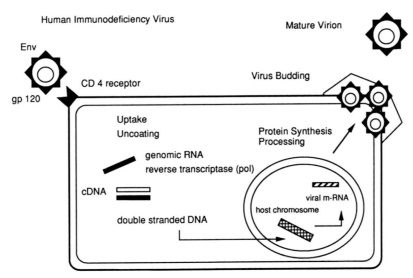

Fig. 11. 16 Life cycle of the human immunodeficiency virus. HIV attaches mainly to cells via the external envelop glycoprotein gp 120 to cells expressing the CD4 molecule. Once the virus is internalized and uncoated, the reverse transcriptase converts the single-stranded viral RNA into double-stranded linear DNA, which is then translocated into the nucleus and incorporated into the host chromosome. Viral transcripts are translated into protein synthesis of env, gag and pol, which form part of the mature infectious virion.

Rare HIV infections after needle stick injuries and injection of small amounts of contaminated blood have been described with an approximate rate of 0.4% of all injuries. Recent United States guide-lines advocate the immediate (within 1 hour) administration of oral AZT (1.2 g/day in 6 divided doses) for 2–3 days until the HIV status in an at-risk patient is known. If the blood is infected, AZT should be continued for 6 weeks, with close monitoring of serology and drug-related side-effects. The efficacy of this procedure has not been established (CDC 1990).

Immunological effects of paediatric HIV infections

The major route of entry of the HIV into cells is via the CD4 receptor, which is expressed by T-helper lymphocytes and, in lower density, by a number of other cells. A selective loss of CD4+ helper cells in the late stages of the infection in adults, i.e. in the AIDS related complex (ARC) or AIDS, is well documented and is used as a marker for diagnosis and progression of the disease. Immunologic abnormalities seen in children below 1 year after vertical transmission often differ from those seen in adults or older children. A normal absolute CD4 lymphocyte count (Fig. 11.17) is frequently seen in young infected infants. The differences are not always clear cut, but typical adult presentation with reduced CD4:CD8 ratios and lymphopenia are seen in children above 1 year of age (Fauci 1988, Nadal et al 1989).

HIV effects on immunocompetent cells

CD4-bearing T-lymphocytes, macrophages, monocytes and those of the microglia in the CNS are the main target of the virus. In infants, B-lymphocyte dysfunction usually precedes T-cell abnormalities. B-cells can be activated to produce immunoglobulins by specific antigen, by polyclonal activators and by stimulated T helper lymphocytes. Humoral immunity is incomplete at birth (low IgA levels, delayed maturation and production of IgG2, 4), and it is thought that maturation of antigen-specific IgG responses are triggered by cytokines released by intact CD4+ helpers cells (Lane et al 1983, Bernstein et al 1985). Maternal immunodeficiency and *in utero* infection may interfere with normal fetal B-cell maturation.

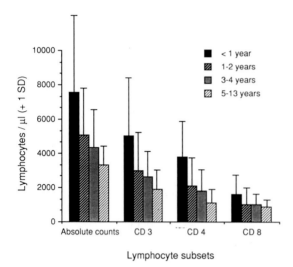

Fig. 11.17 Age-dependent differences in lymphocyte subset counts. Modified from Yanase Y 1986 Journal of Pediatric Research 20: 1147–1151.

Disturbed fetal B-cell activation and differentiation can result in hypo- (3–5%) or hypergammaglobulinaemia (>90%) as a presenting sign in children (Pahwa et al 1987). Most frequently, hypergammaglobulinaemia is associated with defective production of antigen-specific immunoglobulins. Elevated concentrations of IgG and IgA (also IgM, IgD) are seen in infants prior to any other manifestations of immunodeficiency, even without reversal of the CD4:CD8 ratio. Other B-cell abnormalities include: IgG subclass deficiencies (IgG2 and IgG4), autoimmune phenomena (e.g. autoimmune thrombocytopenic purpura ITP), Coombs red cell autoantibodies, and elevated circulating immune complexes (Ellauri et al 1988).

T-lymphocyte abnormalities

Apart from severe CD4+ lymphopenia in the later stages, several functional defects of T-cells have been demonstrated in asymptomatic HIV infection. Major deficiencies include reduction of T-cell proliferative responses to viral and soluble antigens, decrease of interferon production, and a loss of proliferation after stimulation with anti-CD3 antibodies.

Lymphoid tissues

The lymph node architecture in children with

AIDS is similar to that of adults, and shows germinal centre hyperplasia, destruction of follicular architecture and depletion of CD4+ cells (Plate 10).

Infants infected in utero often exhibit a small thymus gland with depletion of lymphoid elements involving, in severe cases, the thymic cortex and medulla, the epithelial cells and the Hassal corpuscles. The dysplastic thymus resembles other congenital immune deficiencies which are part of the differential diagnosis, e.g. severe combined immunodeficiency or Nezelof syndrome (see p. 299 above). Some of the above features are non-specific and can also be seen in children with intrauterine infections, such as rubella and hepatitis, and GVHD (Joshi et al 1990).

Laboratory findings

The laboratory diagnosis of HIV infection in infants under 18 months of age is made difficult by the following features:

1. persistence of maternally transferred anti-HIV IgG for up to 18–20 months
2. absent or very short period of anti-HIV-IgM response in the infant
3. defective humoral responses with delayed or absent specific HIV antibody production
4. unreliability of HIV p24 capture assays, culture assays and polymerase chain reaction in the presence of maternal antibody and/or cells.

Despite problems in diagnosing an asymptomatic infection earlier, antibody persistence beyond 18 months of age must be taken as a strong indicator of HIV infection. A further pointer to an infection is the persistence of hypergammaglobulinaemia (>125% of normal) in young infants, affecting IgG and IgA responses. These features, together with a positive HIV antibody test, make an infection highly likely (European Collaborative Study Group 1991).

Evaluation of immune function

Apart from specific serological, virological and also confirmatory tests (Western blot) tests, a likely laboratory diagnosis of HIV infection can be assisted by specific assays.

pneumococcal polysaccharides are helpful in investigating B-cell responses *in vivo*.

Lymphopenia

Infants with clinical symptoms of AIDS may have normal levels of circulating lymphocytes. However, application of age-related lymphocyte levels in infants may reveal a higher incidence of lymphopenia than previously reported. HIV-infected neonates may have a lymphocyte count of $2 \times 10^9/$l, which is normal in older children or adults but represents lymphopenia in the neonatal age group (lymphocytes $> 3.5 \times 10^9/l$; see Figure 11.17).

B-cell dysfunction

B-cell dysfunction is indicated by depressed *in-vitro* lymphoproliferative responses to B-cell mitogens, e.g. pokeweed mitogen (PWM). Primary and secondary antibody responses to vaccination antigens (diphtheria, tetanus toxoid) or

T-lymphocytes

Proliferative responses *in vitro* are frequently normal in early HIV infection or AIDS, even in the presence of a marked CD4:CD8 inversion. A CD4:CD8 inversion in infants is indicative of a viral infection, but is not necessarily diagnostic for an HIV infection. If the clinical presentation make HIV disease a distinct possibility, HIV antibody measurements, virus isolation and/or p24 measurements must be performed in mother and/or child after appropriate counselling and consent.

Differential diagnosis

HIV infection in early life must be distinguished from other known congenital or acquired immunodeficiencies e.g. due to rubella, hepatitis, cytomegalovirus, herpes simplex, varicella zoster,

Table 11.9 Differential diagnosis of HIV infection in childhood

Illness	Distinguishing features
Combined immunodeficiencies	
Severe combined immunodeficiencies (and variants)	
Graft-versus-host disease	
DiGeorge syndrome	See text
Wiskott–Aldrich syndrome	
Chronic mucocutaneous candidiasis	
X-linked lymphoproliferative disease	
Secondary immunodeficiencies	
Protein-losing enteropathy	Intestinal biopsy, lymphopenia, hypogammaglobulinaemia (CD4/CD8 ratio generally normal)
Severe diarrhoea	Positive culture, microscopy
Malnutrition	Low transferrin, albumin
Congenital infections	
Cytomegalovirus	CMV (in urine and blood), antibody
Rubella	IgM anti rubella antibody, clinical features
Syphilis	VDRL serology
Hepatitis B	HBsAg
Herpes simplex, varicella zoster	Isolation of virus from skin, CSF
Toxoplasmosis	IgM anti-toxoplasma antibody
Haematological disorders	
Idiopathic thrombocytopenic purpura	Anti-platelet antibodies, no other immunological abnormalities
Malignancies (e.g. lymphoma)	Diagnostic biopsies

measles, syphilis and EBV. Children at risk – i.e. children from HIV-positive or drug-using parents, haemophiliacs, thalassaemic patients and others frequently exposed to blood products, especially during 1978–1985, or patients sexually exposed to HIV – need to be further investigated. In general, immunodeficiency or other disease caused by HIV infection can be distinguished from other congenital infections, primary immunodeficiencies, haematologic disorders and/or secondary immunodeficiencies (Table 11.9).

Clinical features

Most children are congenitally infected, and in 50% of patients the diagnosis of AIDS or AIDS-related diseases is made during the first year of life. About 80–90% of cases are diagnosed by 3–4 years of age. The commonly reported AIDS indicator diseases are shown in Figure 11.18. Some infected infants present with fulminant disease between 4 and 8 months, whereas others have a more indolent course and present after 1 year. The mean survival of HIV infected infants after presentation is shown in Figure 11.19. The interval from infection to the onset of symptoms seems to be shorter in children than in adults, and shorter in congenitally infected infants than in those infected by transfusions. The mean incubation period, in perinatally acquired infections according to mathematical modelling, is thought to be 3–5 years. The progression to AIDS has been estimated at 8–10% year (based on a retrospective analysis of New York paediatric patients). This would indicate that all neonatally infected

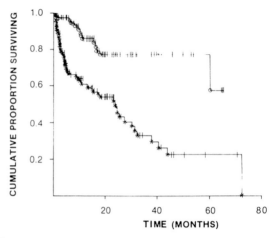

Fig. 11.19 Comparison of survival in children with HIV-1 infection diagnosed at less than 1 year of age (lower curve) with those greater than 1 year of age at diagnosis (upper curve). Age of the patient of the time of analysis is indicated by placement of the circles and lines. Circle = death; Line = survival. From Scott et al 1989, with permission of The New England Journal of Medicine.

children have developed AIDS at the age of 12–13 years (Auger et al 1988).

The mean survival of vertically HIV-infected children who present with severe opportunistic infections is considerably shorter (18–24 months) than in children who present with lymphoid interstitial pneumonitis (60 months; Fig. 11.20).

The clinical spectrum of HIV disease in childhood is vast, and discussion of all reported clinical symptoms in HIV disease would be far beyond the scope of this chapter. Emphasis is therefore laid on the more common manifestations and infections, and the principles of therapy. Lymphadenopathy, resistant oral candidiasis, hepatosplenomegaly, fever, failure to thrive, diarrhoea, weight loss and eczema are frequent findings in HIV disease (Falloon et al 1989, Pizzo 1990).

Encephalopathy

A high proportion of congenitally infected children develop a characteristic encephalopathy with developmental delay, loss of milestones, diplegia, ataxia, pseudobulbar palsy, occasional seizures, peripheral neuropathy, microcephaly and behavioural abnormalities. CSF examination shows normal cell numbers or a mild pleocytosis. CT scans show mild atrophy, basal ganglia enhancement

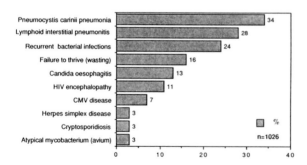

Fig. 11. 18 Commonly reported AIDS indicator diseases for perinatally acquired AIDS (reported AIDS cases, USA 1988–89)

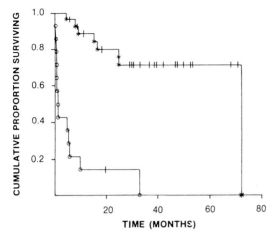

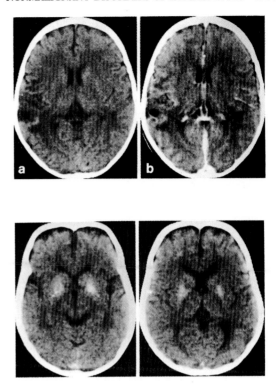

Fig. 11. 20 Comparison of survival in children with lymphoid intestinal pneumonitis (upper curve) or *Pneumocystis carinii* pneumonia (lower curve) as initial presentation. Age of patient of the time of analysis is indicated by placement of the circles, stars and lines. Circle or star = death; line = survival from diagnosis. From: Parks et al 1990 Pediatric AIDS: prospects for prevention. In: Pappas T (ed) Gene regulation and AIDS. The Woodlands, TX, Portfolio Publishing, p 247–253. Reprinted with permission of the publishers.

Fig. 11. 21 CT scan of a 22-month-old child with multiple leukencephalopathy due to vertically transmitted HIV infection. A. Scan showing multiple areas of low attenuation in the cortical white matter of both cerebral hemispheres without calcification. B. CT scan enhanced. The lower panel demonstrates symmetrical calcification in the lentiform nucleus and evidence of cortical atrophy in another child. From: Habibi et al 1989 European Journal of Pediatrics 148: 315–318 with permission of the publishers.

and white matter attenuation, or pictures resembling multifocal leukencephalopathy (Fig. 11.21).

The encephalopathy is thought to be a direct result of HIV infection of the brain. The mechanism by which HIV causes neuropathology remain uncertain, but candidates include (Belman et al 1989):

1. infection of cerebral endothelial cells with disruption of blood brain barrier
2. infection of glial cell and neurons
3. direct damage by the HIV envelope protein gp120.

Bacterial infections

Serious and recurrent bacterial infections represent a significant cause of morbidity. Septicaemia, meningitis, pneumonia, recurrent otitis media, skin abscesses, and cellulitis are often (75%) seen before other manifestations of HIV disease. The frequency of infections with common pathogens is high. *Strep. pneumoniae, Haemophilus influenzae, Salmonella, Staph. aureus*, and meningococci are major causes of serious infections (Fig. 11.22). Gram-negative bacteraemias with *Pseudomonas, Klebsiella* and *E. coli* are more frequent in children

on long-term antibiotic prophylaxis, and these organisms have to be covered in HIV-infected septicaemic patients until culture results are available. Concomitant infections with more than

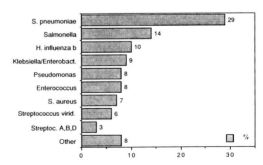

Fig. 11.22 Frequently encountered causes of bacteraemias in children with AIDS. N = 65. Modified after: Krasinski K et al 1988 Journal of Pediatric Infectious Diseases 7: 323–328, and Bernstein et al 1985.

one organism are not uncommon, and micro-biological culture results have to be interpreted accordingly.

Viral infections

Persistent EBV infections are frequent in children with HIV. EBV can be detected by in-situ hybridization in a variety of tissues (lung, lymph node) and is associated with two clinical conditions:

1. lymphoid interstitial pneumonitis/pulmonary lymphoid hyperplasia
2. generalized lymphadenopathy.

Other viral infections are also important causes of morbidity and mortality: primary varicella, herpes simplex, rubella and measles can be unusually severe and/or atypical in their presentation (without a skin rash). A sizeable proportion of HIV-infected children will excrete cytomegalovirus in their urine, e.g. during episodes of pneumonitis. However, this cannot be taken as sole clinical evidence that it is also the organism responsible for the lung changes. A lung biopsy with in-situ hybridization or detection of cytomegalovirus early proliferation antigens with immunohisto-chemical methods (DEAF test) in lung tissue is necessary to distinguish pathogen from com-mensal (Plate 11). Endoscopic broncho-alveolar lavage with positive immunohistochemical identi-fication of cytomegalovirus-infected cells (alveolar macrophages) is an alternative diagnostic ap-proach in the older child (over 3 years of age).

Opportunistic infections

Pneumocystis carinii pneumonia is the most common opportunistic infection in children (50–65%). Physical examination reveals wheezing, intercostal recession, rales and tachypnoea, and arterial blood gases show hypoxia. Chest X-ray changes can be minimal but often show an interstitial pattern, signs of air trapping and ground glass appear-ances. The diagnosis can be established with bronchoalveolar lavage, biopsy with appropriate histological stains (Plate 12) and/or immunofluo-rescence detection with monoclonal antibodies.

The prognosis after presentation with pneumo-cystis pneumonitis is not good. Clinical symptoms of other opportunistic infection include gastro-enteritis, malabsorption, pneumonia, hepatitis, chronic anaemia, fevers, night sweats and ab-dominal pain. Opportunistic infections have to be considered and excluded in all children with unexplained clinical symptoms. Other important organisms include *Cryptosporidium*, *Candida*, *Cryptococcus*, *Toxoplasma*, atypical *Mycobacterium avium intracellulare* (rare in children), and chronic infections with viruses of the herpes group (cytomegalovirus, varicella zoster, herpes simplex).

Lymphoid interstitial pneumonitis (LIP)

This is a characteristic feature of HIV in children and needs to be distinguished from opportunistic infection and tuberculosis. In general, a history of longstanding severe radiographic lung changes unresponsive to conventional therapy, and only a gradual decline in the child's activity with early signs of digital clubbing and generalized lymphaden-opathy, make lymphoid interstitial pneumonitis likely. The chest X-ray shows a widespread nodular pattern reminiscent of miliary tuberculosis, with nodular infiltrates mostly over 1 mm in diameter (Fig. 11.23). X-ray changes are often diagnostic. A lung biopsy should be considered in the case of an unusual presentation or for exclusion of tuber-culosis or additional viral and bacterial superinfec-tions. The biopsy shows a diffuse infiltrate of the alveolar septal and peribronchial areas by T-lymphocytes (mainly CD8) and plasma cells. Nodular lymphoid aggregates with occasional ger-minal centres are seen in the peribronchiolar lym-phoid tissue (Rubinstein et al 1986, Bernstein et al 1989). The clinical features of LIP and *Pneumo-cystis carinii* pneumonia are compared in Figure 11.24.

Neoplasias

These are rare in children, but Kaposi's sarcoma has been described. More common malignancies include B- and T-cell lymphomas of liver, spleen, kidneys, bone marrow and CNS. Temporary response of B-cell lymphomas to radiotherapy has been reported.

Blood abnormalities

Thrombocytopenia is a frequent haematologic

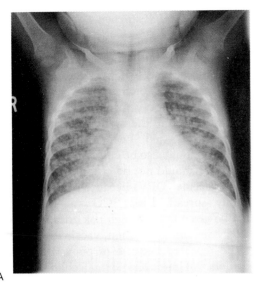 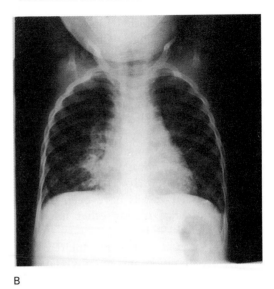

A   B

Fig. 11.23   X-ray appearances of LIP and response to zidovudine therapy. A. Widespread nodular X-ray changes reminiscent of miliary tuberculosis in an infant with LIP and vertically transmitted HIV infection. B. Marked prolonged improvement after zidovudine (AZT) therapy. (The child also responded initially to corticosteroid therapy.)

complication of HIV infection in childhood. It occurs in about 10% of children with clinical symptoms and can be the first sign of HIV disease. Other autoimmune features, such as Coombs positive anaemia and immune neutropenia, have been reported. A persistent neutropenia can limit the therapy with various antiviral agents such as azidothymidine (AZT) and gancyclovir. Where the neutropenia is directly related to the effects of HIV infection, therapy with azidothymidine can improve the neutrophil count (Rubinstein 1986).

Manifestations of HIV disease in other organ systems

Abnormalities due to HIV infections can be seen

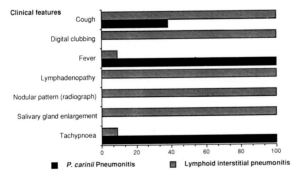

Fig. 11.24   Comparison of presenting clinical signs in lymphoid intestinal pneumonitis or *Pneumocystis carinii* pneumonia. (Modified after Rubinstein et al 1986).

in virtually all organ systems; the more common ones are summarized briefly below.

Acute HIV infection, with acute neurologic symptoms, aseptic meningitis, encephalitis or focal neurological signs, together with myalgia, arthralgia, fever, pharyngitis, skin rash, lymphadenopathy and malaise, is rare in childhood (Cooper et al 1986).

Liver. Hepatic changes suggestive of a chronic active hepatitis with elevated serum transaminase levels but without a clearly identifiable (additional) viral or opportunistic infection have been reported (Duffy et al 1986).

Pancreas. Elevated serum amylase levels are more often seen in adults but have been reported in children. Raised serum amylase levels are also seen as a side-effect of AZT therapy. Iso-enzyme estimations in patients with amylasaemia can be helpful in identifying whether the source is pancreatic or salivary (Torre et al 1987).

Kidney disease. A nephrotic syndrome, with proteinuria and raised serum creatinine levels, which can progress to renal failure is not uncommon. Biopsy pathology shows focal and segmental glomerular sclerosis. This progressive nephropathy does not generally respond to AZT or steroid therapy. Anecdotal reports mention some improvement of the azotaemia after AZT therapy without improvement in the extent of proteinuria (Rao et al 1987).

Heart. A congestive cardiomyopathy can lead to death from heart failure. Clinical manifestations are cardiomegaly, tachyarrhythmia and tachypnoea. Right ventricular hypertrophy (cor pulmonale) is seen in children with lymphoid interstitial pneumonitis or in patients who suffer, from chronic pulmonary disease, e.g. *Pneumocystis carinii* pneumonia (Steinherz et al 1986).

Eye disease. Although common in adults, cytomegalovirus retinitis is not a common feature in childhood HIV disease. However, perivascular lesions of the retinal vessels have been demonstrated in the absence of any other infectious cause (Kestelyn et al 1985).

Skin disease. Skin disorders in children with HIV disease are common and mainly related to bacterial, fungal and viral infections and scabies. Common skin affections seen in healthy children are often more extensive and treatment-resistant in HIV-infected infants. A specific HIV exanthema (infectious mononucleosis-like) described in recently infected adults has not been reported in children (Prose 1990).

HIV-associated myopathy. A rare, HIV-associated myopathy can precede the diagnosis of AIDS but arises more often during the progression of the disease. Its onset is generally subacute, with proximal muscle weakness and elevated creatine kinase (CPK) levels similar to those seen in polymyositis (inflammatory myopathy). Electromyographic pictures and biopsy histology are typical of the above. AZT-induced myopathy needs to be considered especially in children treated longterm (more than 2 years) (Dalakas & Pezeshkpour 1988) and CPK levels monitored regularly.

Treatment

Immunization

The decisions for or against immunizations in children with congenital HIV infection are complex, and general recommendations will remain controversial and are bound to change with increasing clinical experience. Important factors to be considered in HIV infection are the risk of acquiring a common childhood disease, the potentially inappropriate antibody response, and the risk of live (viral) vaccines for the HIV-infected child. Present recommendations:

Asymptomatic HIV infection

Children receive all routine vaccinations – diphtheria, tetanus, pertussis and haemophilus conjugate vaccine, when available – except oral polio vaccine, which should be replaced by the inactivated vaccine. The use of MMR is recommended in the asymptomatic or minimally symptomatic child. Pneumococcal and influenza vaccines should also be considered. Healthy family members should not be given live attenuated oral polio vaccine (OPV) because of the risk of intra-family spread. Live BCG vaccination should not be given even in high risk groups. In order to offer adequate protection, vaccinations may need to be repeated because of poor B-cell function. Evidence of immunization in a child should not be seen as evidence for the presence of protective antibody levels (Advisory Committee on Immunisation Practices, USA 1990).

Passive immune prophylaxis

Due to increasing B-cell dysfunction with progressive HIV disease, children immunized against measles should receive immunoglobulin (exposure) prophylaxis (iv.) after acute measles contact. Varicella zoster immunoglobulin should be administered after each acute exposure to this virus. (See also Management of viral infections).

Intravenous immunoglobulin therapy

The protective role and safety of i.v.IG therapy in a dose of 0.4 mg/kg every 28 days in children with symptomatic HIV disease and recurrent bacterial infection has recently been confirmed in a double blind trial in 372 children with a mean age of 40 months (The National Institute of Child Health and Human Development Intravenous Immunoglobulin Study Group 1991). Earlier single centre, non-randomized studies have also demonstrated a decreased incidence of septicaemias and an additional improvement in T-cell function on i.v.Ig replacement therapy (Ochs 1987). It seems appropriate to consider early i.v.Ig administration (0.3–0.5 g/kg/3–4 weeks) in children with a demonstrated B-cell deficiency (e.g. lack of vaccination antibody titres) and/or recurrent bacterial infections despite adequate antibiotic prophylaxis.

Bacterial infections

Antibiotic therapy in the febrile HIV-infected child with suspected community acquired infection or septicaemia needs to cover the most common (encapsulated) pathogens and must be broad spectrum until culture results are obtained. Frequent pathogens are: *Strep. pneumoniae*, *Haemophilus influenzae*, staphylococci, and Gram-negative enteric rods. Infections with *E. coli*, *Klebsiella* and *Pseudomonas* need to be considered in children who have been on long-term antibiotic therapy. *Salmonella* septicaemias (5–10%) are problematic in children with chronic *Salmonella* gastroenteritis. Resistance to therapy develops fast, and chronic carrier states are frequent. Chloramphenicol, ampicillin and ciprofloxacin have been used, although successful eradication of the organism in HIV disease is difficult. Anecdotal reports describe termination of a *Salmonella* carrier state after ciprofloxacin administration (Jacobson 1989).

Viral infections (other than HIV)

There are few effective antiviral drugs, and treatment for severe viral infections is often unsatisfactory. The clinical course of varicella zoster infections and varicella pneumonitis is unpredictable (fatal in 10%), even in HIV-infected children who show normal laboratory parameters of immunocompetence. Immediate i.v. treatment with acyclovir (1.5 g/m^2 per day) for 10 days is appropriate. Oral acyclovir administration fails to reach virucidal serum levels in varicella zoster infections. It is our policy to treat patients with AIDS and fresh herpes zoster lesions with intravenous acyclovir until no new lesions have appeared for 3–4 days followed by oral therapy. Recurrent oral or skin herpes simplex infections do respond to oral therapy (up to 2.4 g/m^2 per day). Frequently relapsing patients benefit from prophylactic treatment.

Cytomegalovirus is often excreted in urine and saliva without clinical symptoms of disease. It is less often isolated from the buffy coat of HIV-infected children. Cytomegalovirus can be the underlying cause for retinitis, pneumonitis, gastrointestinal disease and hepatitis. Gancyclovir i.v. 7–15 mg/kg per day is the treatment of choice.

Since the drug has only a suppressive effect on cytomegalovirus, treatment in proven infections must be continued long-term and/or in course form (e.g. in 5 out of 7 days) in relapsing patients. Toxic effects of gancyclovir include bone marrow suppression and neutropenia. An alternative drug is foscarnet (60 mg/kg per day i.v.), which has similar side-effects.

Fungal infections

Oral thrush and mucosal candidiasis are frequent symptoms in congenitally infected infants. These infections respond initially to oral treatment with nystatin, clotrimazole and other antifungal agents unless it spreads to other areas. Intermittent or oral fluconazole or itraconazole therapy is being investigated in ramdomized trials to see whether it will prevent disseminated fungal infection. Intravenous therapy with amphotericin B and fluconazole have been successful in treating disseminated disease and/or meningitis. *Cryptococcus neoformans* infections can cause meningeal (mild CNS pleocytosis), pulmonary or disseminated mycosis. The therapy of choice is intravenous amphotericin B, but recent reports indicate a potential role for fluconazole in cryptoccocal disease (review by Walsh & Butler 1990).

Pneumocystis carinii pneumonitis is the most common opportunistic infection in HIV-infected children. The differential diagnosis in a child with diffuse pulmonary infiltrates is wide and ranges from chronic lymphoid interstitial pneumonitis to acute bacterial, viral, fungal or pneumocystis pneumonia. Sputum specimens obtained by inhalation of nebulized hypertonic saline can also be used as a diagnostic procedure once the method has been evaluated in comparison to standard techniques, such as bronchoalveolar lavage and/or lung biopsy.

The therapy of choice is cotrimoxazole (trimethoprim/sulfamethoxazole (TMP/SMX) 20/100 mg/kg per day) i.v. or orally for at least 14–21 days. Adverse side-effects, such as skin rash, neutropenia, thrombocytopenia, fever and hepatitis, are less frequent in children than in adults. Children not responding to therapy within 5–7 days or patients with adverse reactions can be treated with pentamidine (4 mg/kg per day i.m. or i.v.). Side-effects of pentamidine therapy include thrombocytopenia, neutropenia, uraemia, hypotension, diabetes mellitus or other disturbances of glucose metabolism, and hepatitis. Alternative, mainly prophylactic, drugs currently under evaluation include trimethoprim-dapsone, trimetrexate, daily aerosolized pentamidine and pyrimethamine-sulfadiazine, which have been shown in adults to be active. *Pneumocystis* persists in the lung after treatment and recurrence is frequent without prophylactic treatment. The best mode of prevention in children is not established. Alternate-day (48 mg/kg) or once-daily (24 mg/kg) cotrimoxazole treatment are accepted regimens in children who tolerate this drug.

Positive effects of short term adjunctive corticosteroid administration (2 mg/kg prednisolone per day for one week, to be reduced to 1 mg/kg per day thereafter) for the duration of chemotherapy in *adult* AIDS patients with *Pneumocystis* pneumonitis have recently been described and shown to decrease the oxygen requirements and ventilation time (Gagnon et al 1990). This form of therapy has not yet been established in children. However, a short course of steroids in the severely ill child with ventilatory problems is certainly justified. Infections with acid-fast atypical mycobacteria (*M. avium intracellulare, M. fortuitum, M. kansasii*) and, more often, with the typical *Mycobacterium tuberculosis* need to be considered early in pulmonary infections. 'Atypical' lung infections are rare in children. Amikacin, clofazamine, ansamycin, cotrimoxazole and rifampicin have activity against atypical mycobacteria, but the clinical success rate has been limited. The sensitivities of the fast growing atypical mycobacteria should be assessed by appropriate reference laboratories. Antituberculous therapy follows established guidelines with a triple-agent therapeutic regimen at the beginning for approximately 2 months (pulmonary tuberculosis).

Antiretroviral therapy

The clinical efficacy of zidovudine (AZT) as an antiretroviral agent has been established in adults in multicentre trials (Young et al 1987) and by i.v. infusion in children (Pizzo et al 1988). Zido-vudine is a nucleoside analogue which is activated by cellular enzymes and inhibits the reverse transcriptase and/or leads to chain termination after it has been incorporated into the viral DNA. The optimal dose in children is not yet established, but doses of 120–180 mg/kg every 6 hours have been used in controlled studies. Its penetration into the CNS is good. Therapy has been reported to decrease lymphadenopathy and to increase appetite and CD4-(helper) cells. Toxic side-effects are anaemia, macrocytosis and neutropenia. Clinical trials to prevent or ameliorate these side-effects by injection of haematopoietic growth factors – erythropoietin (EPO) and granulocyte colony-stimulating factor (G-CSF) – are underway. Other anti-retroviral drugs, such as 2,3 dideoxycytidine (ddC) and 2,3, dideoxyinosine (ddI), are currently under evaluation and it is hoped that they might have lesser side-effects because of their in-vitro activity at lower doses. Zidovudine (AZT)-resistant HIV strains have been reported, and multiple anti-retroviral drug regimens may have to be devised in the future. Treatment of children with HIV infections should be coordinated in collaboration with regional or national referral centres to encourage optimal clinical management. This is needed not only to facilitate the early clinical introduction of newly developed drugs but also to increase the study size, which will allow earlier statistical evaluation of the effects of the drugs under evaluation.

Prevention of congenital infection (vertical transmission)

The efficacy of prophylactic use of zidovudine in order to prevent infection in infants born to HIV positive mothers is not established, and the results of current studies are awaited. Transmission of HIV can occur in the first trimester of pregnancy, and early antiretroviral therapy could carry embryopathic risks.

HIV vaccine

The development of an AIDS vaccine is of intense interest. Problems associated with the development of a successful vaccine are:

1. genomic variability of the virus
2. lack of knowledge of the protective role of neutralizing antibodies and the role of cell-mediated immunity
3. lack of a suitable animal model
4. inability to clearly identify (?gp 120) the protective immunodominant epitope of HIV
5. difficulties in studying the preventive effects of the vaccine.

Despite these difficulties, phase I trials with a genetically engineered gp120 loop sequence are currently under way. Protective immunity has been achieved in one study with subhuman primates. (Zagury et al 1988, reviewed by Sonigo et al 1989).

Psychosocial issues

The psychosocial implications of this disease impose a heavy burden on the child, parents, social workers, health professionals and a multitude of other agencies involved in the care of the HIV family. Major problems are associated with coping with the diagnosis of a potential fatal disease, and with the emotional and financial aspects of a chronically ill child, as well as facing social ostracism from family members and the community. Children and families with HIV infection have special needs which require interactions with a complex team. The multidisciplinary team involves counsellors, social workers, psychologists, dietitians, teachers, occupational therapists and other health care professionals. This team has to provide not only a structured approach to therapy and information about the various disease aspects, but also help and information for appropriate agencies which are needed for optimal care. School admission and decisions on possible isolation of children with an inability to control body fluids, biting behaviour and bleeding or oozing skin lesions and infectious diseases (chickenpox) have to considered in the best interest of the affected family and child and of the community. HIV infection alone should not prevent attendance at school or day care facilities. The introduction of mother and child clinics should be encouraged to improve medical care and communication between all the individuals involved in adult and paediatric care of HIV-infected individuals and their families.

REFERENCES

Acuto O, Reinherz E L 1985 The human T-cell receptor: structure and function. New England Journal of Medicine 312: 1110–1111

Alarcon B, Regueiro J R, Arnaiz-Villena A, Terhorst C 1988 Familial defect in the surface expression of the T-cell receptor CD3 complex. New England Journal of Medicine 319: 1203–1209

Ament M E, Ochs H D, Davis S D 1973 Structure and function of the gastrointestinal tract in primary immunodeficiency syndromes. A study of 39 patients. Medicine 52: 227–248

Ammann A J, Hong R 1971 Selective IgA deficiency: presentation of 30 cases and a review of the literature. Medicine 50: 223–236

Ammann A J, Cowan M J, Martin D W, Wara D W 1983 Dipyridamole and intravenous deoxycytidine therapy in a patient with adenosine deaminase deficiency. Birth Defects 19: 117–120

Ammann A J, Hong R 1970 Selective IgA deficiency and autoimmunity. Clinical and Experimental Immunology 7: 833–838

Ammann A J, Hong R 1989 Disorders of the T cell system. In: Stiehm E R (ed) Immunologic disorders in infants and children. W B Saunders Company, Philadelphia, p 257–315

Ammann A J, Wara D W, Cowan M J, Barrett D J, Stiehm E R 1982 The Di George syndrome and the fetal alcohol syndrome. American Journal of Diseases of Children 136: 906–908

Anderson DC, Schmalstieg F C, Finegold M J et al 1985 The severe and moderate phenotypes of heritable MAC-1 and LFA-1 deficiency: their quantitative definition and relation to leucocyte dysfunction and clinical features. Journal of Infectious Diseases 152: 668–689

Auger I, Thomas P, Gruttola V 1988 The incubation period for paediatric AIDS patients. Nature 330: 575–577

Batata M A, Martini N, Huvos A G, Aguilar R I, Beattie E J 1974 Thymomas: clinicopathologic features, therapy and prognosis. Cancer 34: 389–396

Belman A L, Diamond G, Dickson D, Horoupian D, Llena J, Rubinstein A 1989 Pediatric AIDS: neurologic syndromes. American Journal of Diseases of Children, 142: 29–35

Bernstein L J, Bye M R, Rubinstein A 1989 Prognostic factors and life expectancy in children with acquired immunodeficiency syndrome and pneumocytis carinii pneumonia. American Journal of Diseases of Children 143: 775–778

Bernstein L J, Ochs H D, Wedgwood R J, Rubinstein A 1985 Defective humoral immunity in pediatric acquired immunodeficiency syndrome. Journal of Pediatrics 107: 352–357

Boder A T 1985 Ataxia telangiectasia: an overview. Kroc Foundation Series 19: 1–13

Borzy M S, Ridgway D, Noya F J, Shearer W T 1989 Successful bone marrow transplantation with split lymphoid chimerism in Di George syndrome. Journal of Clinical Immunology 9: 386–392

Boyd R L, Hugo B 1991 Towards an integrated view of thymopoiesis. Immunology Today 12: 71–79. (Major parts of this issue are devoted to T-cell development)

Brandtzaeg P 1987 Translocation of immunoglobulins across human epithelia: review of the development of a transport model. Acta Histochemistry 34: 9–32

Brandtzaeg P, Valnes, Scott H, Rognum T O, Bjerke K, Baklien K 1985 The human gastrointestinal secretory immune system in health and disease. Scandinavian Journal of Gastroenterology 20 (suppl. 114): 17–38

Bruton O C 1952 Agammaglobulinemia. Pediatrics 9: 722–728

Buckley R H, Schiff S E, Sampson H A et al 1986 Development of immunity in human severe primary T cell deficiency following haploidentical bone marrow stem cell transplantation. Journal of Immunology 136: 2398–2407

Buckley R H, Wray B B, Belmaker E Z 1972 Extreme hyperimmunoglobulinaemia E and undue susceptibility to infection. Pediatrics 49: 59–64

Cederbaum S D, Kaitila I, Rimoin D L, Stiehm E R 1976 The chondro-osseous dysplasia of adenosine deaminase deficiency. Journal of Pediatrics 89: 737–742

Centre for Disease Control 1990 Public health service statement on management of occupational exposure of human immunodeficiency virus, including considerations regarding zidovudine post exposure use. Morbidity Mortality Weekly Reports 39: RR1

Chatila T, Wong R, Young M, Miller R, Terhorst C, Geha R S 1989 An immunodeficiency characterized by defective signal transduction in T lymphocytes. New England Journal of Medicine 320: 696–702

Cleveland W W, Fogel B J, Brown W T, Kay H E M 1968 Foetal thymic transplant in a case of Di George's syndrome. Lancet 2: 1211–1214

Communicable Disease Report 1992 AIDS and HIV-I infection in the United Kingdom 2(4): 17–20

Conley M E, Beckwith J B, Mancer J G K, Tenckhoff L 1979 The spectrum of the Di George syndrome. Journal of Pediatrics 94: 883–890

Conley M E, Buckley R H, Hong R et al 1990 X-linked severe combined immunodeficiency: diagnosis in males with sporadic severe combined immunodeficiency and clarification of clinical findings. Journal of Clinical Investigation 85: 1548–1554

Conley M E, Park C L, Douglas S D 1986 Childhood common variable immunodeficiency with autoimmune disease. Journal of Pediatrics 108: 915–919

Cooper D A, Gold J, Maclean P et al 1985 Acute AIDS retrovirus infection: definition of a clinical illness associated with seroconversion. Lancet 1: 537–540

Cunningham-Rundles C 1989 Clinical and immunologic analysis of 103 patients with common variable immunodeficiency. Journal of Clinical Immunology 9: 22–33

Dalakas M C, Pezeshkpour G H 1988 Neuromuscular disease associated with human immunodeficiency virus infection. Annals of Neurology, 23: S38-48

Davis S D, Schaller J, Wedgwood R 1966 Job's syndrome: recurrent 'cold' staphylococcal abscesses. Lancet 1: 1013–1015

De Vaal O M, Seynhaeve V 1959 Reticular dysgenesia. Lancet 2: 1123–1125

de Saint Basile G, Arveiler B, Oberle I et al 1987 Close linkage of the locus for X-chromosome-linked severe combined immunodeficiency to polymorphic DNA markers in Xq11–q13. Proceedings National Academy of Sciences USA 84: 7576–7579

Deeg H J, Lum L G, Sanders J et al 1986 Severe aplastic anemia associated with chronic mucocutaneous candidiasis. Immunologic and hematologic reconstitution after allogeneic bone marrow transplantation. Transplantation 41: 583–586

Di George A M 1965 A new concept of the cellular basis of immunity (discussion). Journal of Pediatrics 67: 907–908

Duffy L F, Daum F, Kahn E 1986 Hepatitis in children with acquired immune deficiency syndrome: histopathologic and immunocytologic features. Gastroenterology 90: 173–181

Ellaurie M, Burns E, Bernstein L, Shah K, Rubinstein A 1988 Thrombocytopenia and human immunodeficiency virus in children. Pediatrics 82: 905–908

European Collaborative Study Group 1991 Children born to women with HIV-1 infection: natural history and risk of transmission. Lancet 337: 253–260

Falloon J, Eddy J, Wiener L, Pizzo P A 1989 Human immunodeficiency virus infection in children. Journal of Pediatrics 114: 1–30

Fauci A S 1988 The human immunodeficiency virus: infectivity and mechanisms of pathogenesis. Science 239: 617–639

Fischer A, Landais P, Friedrich W et al 1990 European experience of bone-marrow transplantation for severe combined immunodeficiency. Lancet 336: 850–854

Friedman J M, Fialkow P J, Davis S D, Ochs H D, Wedgwood R J 1977 Autoimmunity in relatives of patients with immunodeficiency diseases. Clinical Experimental Immunology 28: 375–388

Gagnon S, Boota A M, Fishl M A, Baier H, Kirksey O W, La Voie L 1990 Corticosteroids as adjunctive therapy for severe Pneumocystis carinii pneumonia in in the acquired immunodeficiency syndrome. New England Journal of Medicine 323: 1444–1450

Gatti R A, Berkel I, Boder E et al 1988 Localization of an ataxia-telangiectasia gene to chromosome 11q22–23. Nature 336: 577–580

Geha R S, Leung D Y M 1989 Hyperimmunuglobulin E syndrome. Immunodeficiency Reviews 1: 155–172

Giblett E R, Ammann A J, Wara D W, Sandman R, Diamond L K 1972 Nucleoside-phosphorylase deficiency in a child with severely defective T-cell immunity and normal B-cell immunity. Lancet 1: 1010–1013

Goldblatt D, Morgan G, Seymour N D, Strobel S, Turner M W, Levinsky R J 1989 The clinical manifestations of IgG subclass deficiency. In: Levinsky J R (ed) IgG subclass deficiencies. Royal Society of Medicine Services International Congress and Symposium Series No. 143: 19–26

Good R A 1954 Agammaglobulinemia – a provocative experiment of nature. Bulletin of the University of Minnesota Medical Foundation 26: 1–19

Gray G F, Gutowski W T III 1979 Thymoma. A clinicopathologic study of 54 cases. American Journal of Surgical Pathology 3: 235–249

Greene W C 1991 Mechanisms of disease: the molecular biology of human immunodeficiency type 1 infection. New England of Medicine 324: 308–316

Griscelli C, Durandy A, Virelizier J L, Ballet J J, D'Aguillard F 1978 Selective defect of precursor T-cells with apparently normal B lymphocytes in severe combined

immunodeficiency disease. Journal of Pediatrics
93: 404–411

Griscelli C, Fischer A Lisowska-Grospierre B et al 1985
Defective synthesis of HLA class I and II molecules
associated with a combined immunodeficiency. In: Aiuti R,
Rosen F, Cooper M D (eds) Recent advances in primary
and acquired Immunodeficiencies, vol. 28 Serono
Symposia, Raven Press, New York, p 176–183

Griscelli C, Lisowska G B, Mach B 1989 Combined
immunodeficiency with defective expression in MHC class
II genes. Immunodeficiency Review 1: 135–154

Haas W, Kaufman S, Martinez-A C 1990 The development
and function of γ,δ T cells. Immunology Today
10: 344–343

Hadam M R, Dopfer R, Peter H H, Niethammer D 1984
Congenital agammaglobulinemia associated with lack of
expression of HLA D-region antigens. In: Griscelli C,
Vossen J (eds), Progress in immunodeficiency research and
therapy, Excerpta Medica, Amsterdam, p 19–24

Hayward A R, Paolucci P, Webster A D B, Kohler P 1982
Pre-B cell suppression by thymoma patient lymphocytes.
Clinical Experimental Immunology 48: 437–442

Herrod H G 1990 Chronic mucocutaneous candidiasis in
childhood and complications of non-candida infection: a
report of the Pediatric Immunodeficiency Collaborative
Study Group. Journal of Pediatrics 116: 337–82

Heyderman R S, Levinsky R J, Strobel S 1991 Successful
bone marrow transplantation and treatment of BCG
infection in two patients with severe combined
immunodeficiency. European Journal of Paediatrics
150: 477–80

Hirschhorn R 1977 Defects of purine metabolism in
immunodeficiency diseases. Progress in Clinical
Immunology 3: 67–83

Hitzig W H, Landot R, Muller G, Bodmer P 1971
Heterogeneity of phenotypic expression in a family with
Swiss-type agammaglobulinemia: Observations on the
acquisition of agammaglobulinemia. Journal of Pediatrics
78: 968–980

Jacobson M A, Hahn S M, Gerberding J L, Sande M A 1989
Ciprofloxacin for salmonella bacteremia in the acquired
immunodeficiency syndrome (AIDS). Annals of Internal
Medicine 110: 1027–1029

Jeannet M, Sztajzel R, Carpentier N, Hirschel B, Tiercy J M
1989 HLA antigens are risk factors for development of
AIDS. Journal of Acquired Immunodeficiency Syndrome
2: 28–32

Joshi V V, Oleske J M, Connor E M 1990 Morphologic
findings in children with AIDS. Pathogenesis and clinical
implications. Pediatric Pathology 10: 155–165

Jouan H, LeDeist F, Nezelof C 1987 Omenn's syndrome –
pathologic arguments in favour of graft versus host disease.
Human Pathology 18: 1101–1108

Katz F, Malcolm S, Strobel S, Finn A, Morgan G, Levinsky
R J 1990 The use of locus-specific minisatellite probes to
investigate engraftment following bone marrow
transplantation for severe combined immunodeficiency.
Bone Marrow Transplantation 5: 199–204

Kelley R I, Zaclao E H, Emmanuel B S, Kistenmacher M,
Greenberg F, Punnett H H 1982 The association of the Di
George anomaly with partial monosomy of chromosome
22. Journal of Pediatrics 101: 197–200

Kestelyn P, Lepage P, Van de Perre P 1985 Perivasculitis of
the retinal vessels as an important sign in children with
AIDS related complex. American Journal of Diseases of

Ophthalmology 100: 614–615

Krasinski K, Borkowski W, Bank S, Lawrence R, Chandwani
S 1988 Bacterial infections in human immunodeficiency
virus infected children. Pediatric Infectious Diseases
Journal 7: 323–328

Lane H C, Masur H, Edgar L C, Whalen G, Rook A H,
Fauci A S 1983 Abnormalities of B cell activation and
immunoregulation in patients with the acquired
immunodeficiency syndrome. New England Journal of
Medicine 309: 453–458

LeDeist F, Blanche S, Keable H et al 1989 Successful HLA
non-identical bone marrow transplantation in three
patients with the leukocyte adhesion deficiency. Blood
74: 512–516

Lederman H M, Winkelstein J A 1985 X-linked
agammaglobulinaemia: an analysis of 96 patients. Medicine
64: 145–156

Levy Y, Hershfield M S, Fernandez-Mejla C, Polmar S H,
Scudiery D, Berger M, Sorensen R U 1988 Adenosine
deaminase deficiency with late onset of recurrent infections:
response to treatment with polyethylene glycol-modified
adenosine deaminase. Journal of Pediatrics 117: 312–317

Mayer L 1986 Evidence for a defect in switch T-cells in
patients with immunodeficiency and
hyperimmunoglobulinaemia. New England Journal of
Medicine 314: 409–413

Mease P J, Ochs H D, Wedgwood R J 1981 Successful
treatment of echovirus miningoencephalitis and myositis-
fasciitis with intravenous immune globulin therapy in a
patient with X-linked agammaglobulineamia. New England
Journal of Medicine 304: 1278–1281

Mensink E J B M, Thompson A, Sandkuyl L A et al 1987 X-
linked agammaglobulinemia with hyperimmunoglubulinemia
M appears to be linked to the DXS 42 restriction fragment
length polymorphism locus. Human Genetics 76: 96–99

Meyers J D, Reed E C, Shepp D H 1988 Acyclovir for
prevention of cytomegalovirus infection and disease after
allogeneic bone marrow transplantation. New England
Journal of Medicine 318: 70–75

Miller J F A P 1991 Immunology yesterday: the discovery of
the immunological function of the thymus. Immunology
Today 12: 42–45

Müller W, Peter H H, Wilken M et al 1988 The Di George
syndrome I. Clinical evaluation and course of partial and
complete forms of the syndrome. European Journal of
Pediatrics 147: 496–502

Müller W, Peter H H, Kallfelz H C, Franz A, Rieger C H
1989 The Di George sequence. Immunologic findings in
partial and complete forms of the disorder. European
Journal of Pediatrics 149: 96–103

Nadal D, Hunziker U A, Schupbach J et al 1989
Immunological evaluation in the early diagnosis of prenatal
or perinatal HIV infection. Archives of Diseases of
Childhood 64: 662–9

The National Institute of Child Health and Human
Development Intravenous Immunoglobulin Study Group
1991 Intravenous immune globulin for the prevention of
bacterial infections in children with symptomatic human
immunodeficiency virus syndrome. New England Journal
of Medicine 325: 73–80

Nezelof C, Jammet M I, Lortholary P, Labrune B, Lamy M
1964 L'hypoplasie héréditaire du thymus. Sa place et sa
résponsabilite dans une observation d'aplasie
lymphocytaire, normoplasmocytaire et
normoglobulinémique du nourrisson. Archives Francaises

de Pediatrie 21: 897–920

O'Reilly R J, Keever C A, Small T N, Brochstein J 1989 The use of HLA-non-identical T-cell depleted marrow transplants for correction of severe combined immunodeficiency disease. Immunodeficiency Reviews 4: 273–310

Ochs H D 1987 Intravenous immunoglobulin in the treatment of human immunodeficiency virus infection. Pediatric Infectious Diseases 6: 509–511

Omenn G S 1965 Familial reticuloendotheliosis and eosinophilia. New England Journal of Medicine 273: 427–432

Ownby D R, Pizzo S, Blackmon L, Gall S A, Buckley R H 1976 Severe combined immunodeficiency with leukopenia (reticular dysgenesis) in siblings: immunologic and histopathologic findings. Journal of Pediatrics 89: 384–387

Oxelius V A 1974 Chronic infections in a family with hereditary deficiency of IgG2 and IgG4. Clinical and Experimental Immunology 17: 19–27

Pahwa R, Good R A, Pahwa S 1987 Prematurity, hypogammaglobulineamia, and neuropathology with human immunodeficiency virus (HIV) infection. Proceedings of the National Academy of Sciences USA 84: 3826–3830

Penn I 1988 Tumours of the immunocompromised patient. Annual Reviews of Medicine 39: 63–73

Pizzo P A 1990 Paediatric AIDS: Problems within problems. Journal of Infectious Diseases 161: 315–325

Pizzo P A, Eddy J, Falloon J 1988 Effect of continuous intravenous infusion of zidovudine (AZT) in children with symptomatic HIV infection. New England Journal of Medicine 319: 889–896

Prose N 1990 Paediatric human immunodeficiency virus infection in childhood: the disease and its cutaneous manifestations. Advances in Dermatology 5: 113–130

Puck J M, Nussbaum R L, Conley M E 1987 Carrier detection in X-linked severe combined immunodeficiency based on patterns of X chromosome inactivation. Journal of Clinical Investigation 79: 1395–1400

Purtilo D T, Cassel C K, Yang J P S, Harper R 1975 X-linked recessive progressive combined variable immunodeficiency (Duncan's disease). Lancet 1: 935–940

Purtilo D T, Sakmoto K, Barnabei V et al 1982 Epstein-Barr-virus-induced diseases in boys with X-linked lymphoproliferative syndrome (XLP). American Journal of Medicine 73: 49–56

Rao T K S, Friedman E A, Nicastri A D 1987 The types of renal disease in the acquired immunodeficiency syndrome. New England Journal of Medicine 316: 1062–1068

Reisner Y, Kapoor N, Kirkpatrick D et al 1983 Transplantation for severe combined immunodeficiency with HLA-A, B, D, DR incompatible parenteral marrow cells fractioned by soybean agglutinin and sheep red blood cells. Blood 61: 341–348

Reisner Y, Kapoor N, Kirkpatrick D, Pollack M S, Dupont B, Good R A, O'Reilly R J 1981 Transplantation for acute leukemia with HLA-A and B non-identical parental marrow cells fractioned with soybean agglutinin and sheep red cells. Lancet ii 327–331

Reith W, Satola S, Sanchez C H, et al 1988 Congenital immunodeficiency with a regulatory defect in MHC class II gene expression lacks a specific HLA-DR promoter binding protein, RF-X. Cell 53: 897–906

Remold O'Donnell E, Rosen F S 1990 Sialophorin (CD43)

and the Wiskott-Aldrich syndrome. Immunodeficiency Reviews 2: 151–174

Rockey J H, Hanson L Å, Heremans J F, Kunkel H G 1964 Beta 2A aglobulinemia in two healthy men. Journal of Laboratory and Clinical Medicine 63: 205–212

Roifman C M, Levison H, Gelfand E W 1987 High-dose versus low-dose intravenous immunoglobulin in hypogammaglobulinaemia and chronic lung disease. Lancet 1: 1075–1077

Rosen F S, Kevy S V, Merler E, Janeway C A, Gitlin D 1961 Recurrent bacterial infections and dysgammaglobulinemia: Deficiency of 7S gammaglobulins in the presence of elevated 19S gammaglobulins. Pediatrics 28: 1982–195

Rubinstein A 1986 Pediatric AIDS. Current Problems in Pediatrics 16: 361–401

Rubinstein A, Morecki R, Silverman R et al 1986 Pulmonary disease in children with acquired immune deficiency syndrome and AIDS related complex. Journal of Pediatrics 108: 498–503

Rubinstein A, Sicklick M, Gupta A et al 1983 Acquired immunodeficiency with reserved T4/T8 ratio in infants born to promiscuous and drug-addicted mothers. Journal of the American Medical Association 249: 2350–2356

Schaffer F M, Palermos J, Zhu Z B, Barger B O, Cooper M D, Volanakis J E 1989 Individuals with IgA deficiency and common variable immunodeficiency share polymorphisms of major histocompatibility complex class III genes. Proceedings National Academy of Sciences USA 86: 8015–8019

Schur P H, Borel H, Gelfand E W, Alper C A, Rosen F S 1970 Selective gamma-G globulin deficiencies in patients with recurrent pyogenic infections. New England Journal of Medicine 283: 631–635

Schuurman R K B, Van Rood J J, Vossen J M et al 1979 Failure of lymphocyte-membrane HLA-A and B expression in two siblings with combined immunodeficiency. Clinical Immunology and Immunopathology 14: 418–434

Scott G B, Hutho C, Makruk R W et al 1989 Survival in children with perinatally acquired human immunodeficiency virus type 1 infection. New England Journal of Medicine 321: 1791–1796

Seeger R, Galle J, Wildfeuer A, Frater-Schröder M, Linnell J, Hitzig W H 1980 Impaired functions of lymphocytes and granulocytes in transcobalamin 2 deficiency and their response to treatment. In: Seligmann M, Hitzig W H (eds) Primary Immunodeficiencies. Elsevier/North-Holland, Amsterdam, p 353–362

Seeger R C, Robins R A, Stevens R H et al 1976 Severe combined immunodeficiency with B lymphocytes: in vitro correction of defective immunoglobulin production by the addition of normal T lymphocytes. Clinical and Experimental Immunology 26: 1–10

Sonigo P, Montagnier L, Tiollais P, Girad M 1989 Aids vaccines: concepts and first trials. Immunodeficiency Reviews 1: 349–366

Sorensen R U, Polmar S H 1984 Efficacy and safety of high-dose intravenous immune globulin therapy for antibody deficiency syndromes. American Journal of Medicine 76: 83–90

Spector B D, Perry G S III, Kersey J H 1978 Genetically determined immunodeficiency disease (GDID) and malignancy: Report from the Immunodeficiency-Cancer Registry. Clinical Immunology and Immunopathology 11: 12–29

Spencer J, Isaacson P G, Diss T C, MacDonald T T 1989

Expression of disulfide-linked and non-disulfide-linked forms of the T-cell receptor gamma/delta heterodimer in human intestinal intraepithelial lymphocytes. European Journal of Immunology 19: 1335–8

Springer T A 1990 Adhesion receptors of the immune system. Nature 346: 425–434

Steinherz L J, Brochstein J A, Robins J 1986 Cardiac involvement in congenital acquired immunodeficiency syndrome. American Journal of Diseases in Children 140: 1241–1244

Strobel S, Morgan G, Levinsky R J 1989 Fatal GVHD after platelet transfusion in a child with SCID due to PNP deficiency. European Journal of Pediatrics 148: 315–317

Sullivan J L, Byron K S, Brewster F E, Baker S M, Ochs H A 1983 X-linked lymphoproliferative syndrome: natural history of the immunodeficiency. Journal of Clinical Investigation 71: 1765–1778

Sullivan K E, Woda B A 1989 X-linked lymphoproliferative syndrome. Immunodeficiency Reviews 1: 325–348

Sullivan K M, Kopecky K J, Jocom J et al 1990 Immunomodulatory and antimicrobial efficacy of intravenous immunoglobulin in bone marrow transplantation. New England Journal of Medicine 323: 705–711

Tiller T L, Buckley R H 1978 Transient hypogammaglobulinaemia of infancy: review of the literature, clinical and immunological features of 11 new cases and long term follow-up. Journal of Paediatrics 92: 347–353

Torre D, Montanari M, Fiorio G P, Dietz A, Sampietro C 1987 HIV and the pancreas. Lancet 2: 1212

Touraine J 1981 The bare-lymphocyte syndrome: Report on the registry. Lancet 1: 319–320

Touraine J L, Betuel H, Souillet G 1978 Combined immunodeficiency disease associated with absence of cell-surface HLA-A and B antigens. Journal of Pediatrics 93: 47–51

Varmis H 1988 Retroviruses. Science 240: 1427–1435

Waldman H 1989 Manipulation of T-cell responses with monoclonal antibodies. Annual Review of Immunology 7: 407–444

Walsh T J, Butler K M 1990 Fungal infections complicating pediatric AIDS. In: Pizzo P A, Wilfert C M (eds) Pediatric Aids. Williams and Wilkins, Baltimore, p 225–244

Wedgwood R J, Ochs H D, Davis S D 1975 The recognition and classification of immunodeficiency disease with bacteriophage 174. In: Bergsma D (ed) Immunodeficiency in Man and Animals. Birth defects. Original article series, Vol. XI, No 1. Sinauer Associates, Sunderland, Mass, p 331–338

WHO Report 1989 Primary immunodeficiency diseases. Immunodeficiency Reviews 1: 173–205

Wiskott A 1937 Familiärer, angeborener Morbus Werlhofii ? Monatsschrift Kinderheilkunde 68: 2212–2216

Wong-Staal F, Gallo R C 1985 Human T-lymphotropic retroviruses. Nature 317: 395–403

Yanase Y, Tango T, Okumura K, Tada T, Kawasaki T 1986 Lymphocyte subsets identified by monoclonal antibodies in healthy children. Pediatric Res 20: 1147–1151

Young L S, 1987 Treatable aspects of infection due to human immunodeficiency virus. Lancet 2: 1503-1506

Zagury D, Bernard J, Cheynier R et al 1988 A group specific anamnestic immune reaction against HIV-1 induced by a candidate vaccine against AIDS. Nature 332: 728–731

12. Malignant disorders of lymphocytes

O. B. Eden

ACUTE LYMPHOBLASTIC LEUKAEMIA

Acute lymphoblastic leukaemia (ALL) is the single most common form of childhood cancer seen in the Western world. Thirty years ago, the majority of children presenting with ALL were expected to die within 4–6 months; today, over 50% of patients are living long term, with complete cure the prospect for the majority. However, neither incidence nor improved prognosis is uniform throughout the world.

Incidence, aetiology and epidemiological factors

Acute leukaemia accounts for approximately one-third of all childhood cancers in the UK, with ALL making up approximately 75–80% of these (Parkin et al 1988). During the first 10 years of life, the risk of a child developing ALL is approximately 1 in 3500. Worldwide variation (Tables 12.1 and 12.2) can be explained by genetic or environmental aetiological factors, by early death rates from other causes, and by under-reporting or recording of actual cases. In the UK, a peak age incidence between 2 and 6 years (median 4 years) emerged in the 1920s and has subsequently been seen in the majority of developed, but not developing, countries. Other demographic features which are associated with an apparent increased risk of developing ALL include male sex, advanced maternal age, prior maternal fetal loss, and increased birth weight.

The interesting peak has led to one of the current aetiological hypotheses, namely that the emergence of ALL represents an abnormal immune response to an as yet unidentified virus or group of viruses (Greaves 1988). Children who are well nourished, fully vaccinated and more protected from antigenic exposure will have reduced or delayed exposure to many common pathogens. The peak incidence corresponds with start of nursery or preschool education. The B-cell lymphoid lineage shows a veritable explosion of activity at this age, and the overwhelming type of ALL at this age is of a B-cell precursor (common ALL). There is further evidence that this common ALL occurs more frequently in new towns or new housing estates, either because the

Table 12.1 Relative incidence figures for childhood leukaemias and lymphomas (%)

	England & Wales*	Eastern Nigeria[†]	USA* White	USA* Black
Leukaemias	33.6	12.9	31.0	23.1
Lymphomas:				
NHL Burkitts	0.3	26.5	1.5	0.4
NHL all others	5.8	6.2	5.7	4.4
Hodgkin's disease	4.3	6.6	5.6	4.9

*Data derived from Parkin D M et al 1988 Means of male and female incidence England & Wales 1971–80, n = 11 479. USA S.E.E.R. data on white children 1973–82, n = 5142; black children 1973–82, n = 610.
[†]Data from Obioha FI, Kaine WN, Ikerionwu SE et al. Annals of Tropical Paediatrics 1989, n = 257.

Table 12.2 Crude rates per million children aged 0–15 of childhood leukaemia and lymphoma by sex

	England & Wales M	F	USA White M	F	USA Black M	F
Leukaemias	38.7	30.5	44.2	35.9	22.9	25.6
Lymphomas	16.0	7.4	21.7	12.7	15.0	6.2
NHL Burkitts	0.3	0.2	3.6	0.4	0.7	(–)
NHL all other	8.5	3.7	9.6	4.1	5.5	3.1
Hodgkin's disease	6.3	2.7	7.5	5.9	8.2	2.1

Data derived from Parkin D M et al 1988

children of incoming families are at increased risk having not been exposed previously to specific antigens, or because incoming families bring in the antigen, exposing residents who are not immune (Kinlen et al 1990). However, this hypothesis is proving extremely difficult to confirm. In some series, the finding of a higher risk for common ALL in higher socioeconomic groups has been cited as supportive evidence.

In contrast, the peak age of ALL is not seen, for example, in tropical Africa and other developing countries. In equatorial Africa, the combination of early antigenic stimulation, malnutrition and chronic malarial infection is associated with a high incidence of Burkitt's B-cell lymphoma and leukaemia, and proliferative Epstein-Barr virus (EBV) infection. There is also a very high incidence of lymphoma compared with leukaemia (both B- and T-cell disease) in such areas. A similar high lymphoma-to-leukaemia ratio was once seen amongst Arab children living in the Gaza strip, but following major changes in this area during the 1970s, with improved social circumstances, the ratio was reversed and a peak of ALL has emerged (Ramot & Magrath 1982). Interestingly, to date, black American children have not shown the peak age incidence but have an overall lower incidence of ALL.

Genetic factors may explain some of this variation. Siblings of an affected child have a somewhat higher risk, and consequently incidence rate, than the general population (1 in 700). This could represent shared environmental as well as genetic factors. However, an identical twin of a child with ALL is reported to have a 14–20% chance of developing the leukaemia before the age of 10 years, and there are reports identifying the same gene rearrangements in both affected children even when the leukaemia in the second twin develops after a considerable interval (Chaganti et al 1979). This evidence strongly supports a common clonal origin of the leukaemia. However, although congenital, the leukaemia may not be truly genetic, but represent a very early embryonic event secondary to as yet unknown mitogens (Greaves & Chan 1986). Rarely, multiple ALL cases have been born to consanguineous parents (Kurita et al 1974), and there is further evidence for genetic factors with an ever increasing list of genetically

determined conditions associated with a high risk of developing ALL and other tumours (Table 12.3). In some of these, there is clearly genetic instability, immune surveillance problems, lack of normal capability to respond to antigenic onslaught or, increasingly, biochemical disturbances, whose link with the leukaemia is not yet fully understood.

Environmental factors which have been under particularly close scrutiny of late are viruses, chemicals, ionizing radiation and electromagnetic fields.

Viruses

The only proven virus association with childhood leukaemia involves postnatal exposure to EBV. In endemic malarial areas of tropical Africa, there is almost universal exposure to the virus, before 3 years of age, with high blood titres and a high incidence of Burkitt's lymphoma, with viral DNA within the tumour in 95% of cases; the most

Table 12.3 Genetic and familial factors predisposing to leukaemia and lymphomas in childhood

Condition	Estimated risk
Familial	
Twin of leukaemic patient (age dependent)	14–20% in first 10 years
Sibling of leukaemic patient	1 in 700 (4 × normal)
Congenital immunodeficiency disorders:	
X-linked lymphoproliferative (NHL)	?
Bruton's aggammaglobulinaemia (Leukaemia & NHL)	?
SCID (Leukaemia & NHL)	?
Wiskott-Aldrich (Leukaemia & NHL)	?
IgA deficiency (Leukaemia & NHL)	?
Chromosomal abnormality	
Down's syndrome	1 in 74 (15 × normal)
(ALL most common, but more ANLL than in general population)	
Turner's syndrome	?
Klinefelter's syndrome (ALL & ANLL)	?
XYY + XYY mosaics	?
Trisomy 13	?
Genetic instability syndromes	
Fanconi's anaemia (most often ANLL)	1 in 12
Bloom's syndrome (Leukaemias)	1 in 8
Ataxia telangiectasia (defective DNA repair – lymphoma and leukaemia	1 in 8
Others	
Neurofibromatosis I (ANLL, NHL, juvenile CML)	?
Schwachman syndrome (usually ANLL)	?

consistent antigen is EB surface capsid antigen (Burkitt 1958, Magrath 1990). Infection early in life is thought to enlarge the size of certain pre-B- and B-cell populations and maintain them in a proliferative state, making them more likely to genetic change. An alternative suggestion is that EBV produces an immortal cell clone with genetic translocation already present. With repeated infections, especially of malaria (a T-cell suppressor and B-cell mitogen), and malnutrition there follows T-cell immunosuppression and B-cell hyperplasia. What is not known is whether the initial infection with EBV or subsequent events lead to the very characteristic translocation of DNA from chromosome 8 into the immunoglobulin coding sites on chromosomes 14, 2 or 22. The breakpoint on chromosome 8 corresponds to the proto oncogene c-myc, and that on 14 to the immunoglobulin heavy chain gene. The 8:14 translocation is the commonest abnormality found. In a few cases, a part of the light chain gene (either the kappa light chain locus on chromosome 2 or the lambda light chain locus on chromosome 22) is translocated to chromosome 8 distal to the c-myc gene. Thus, in all cases, the c-myc gene lies adjacent to the immunoglobulin constant region sequences. The c-myc gene appears necessary for proliferation, and when activated, cell proliferation occurs. It is also known that the q24 band on chromosome 8 is a fragile site, but what specifically initiates the translocation is not yet clear. Again, the interaction of genetic and environmental factors are highlighted, as some workers have postulated that patients who develop Burkitt's lymphoma have inherent DNA repair defects. The final lesson to be learnt from Burkitt's lymphoma is that, although most childhood lymphoblastic leukaemias and lymphomas are of precursor cells, this tumour is of EBV virus memory B-cells. B-cell lymphoma and ALL occur outwith equatorial Africa; some (10–15%) have identifiable capsid antigen (as compared to the 90% incidence seen in Africa), but most have the characteristic chromosome translocation seen in Burkitt's lymphoma. The specific role of all the factors – EBV, immune status, malnutrition and malaria – in the malignant process have not yet been clarified. EBV has recently been implicated in other immunoregulatory and lymphoproliferative disorders.

There has been considerable interest recently in retroviruses which alter growth and differentiation of cells of various haemopoietic lineages. Abelson murine leukaemia virus can induce nonthymic lymphoma in mice, whilst feline leukaemia is associated with another retrovirus. Yoshida et al (1982) demonstrated the relationship between human T lymphotropic virus (HTLV) I and adult T cell leukaemia and lymphoma, but no case has yet been fully documented in a child.

Human immunodeficiency virus (HIV) infection, presumably as a result of profound helper T-cell depression, predisposes to a variety of lymphoid malignancies, some of which are now being shown to be polyclonal B-cell proliferations, although few have yet been described in children.

Chemicals and drugs

Most drugs implicated as causative of leukaemia produce marrow hypoplasia and subsequent acute nonlymphoblastic leukaemia (ANLL), and occur in adults. Recently hydrocarbons, organic solvents and pesticides have all been incriminated in the causation of childhood cancers, but principally for tumours of the brain and kidney. What is not known is whether prolonged parental (especially paternal) exposure could induce subsequent germ cell damage and leukaemia. In-utero or postnatal exposure risks also require investigation. An ever increasing list of occupations associated with an increased incidence of leukaemia and non-Hodgkin's lymphoma (NHL) are reported for adults, but only time will tell whether these risks also involve their offspring. Some associations have been made with hydrocarbons, motor vehicle jobs and solvents (Mills & Miller 1990). Stjernfeldt et al (1986) suggested a dose response between maternal smoking during pregnancy and an increased risk of ALL in their children (10 or more cigarettes per day doubled the risk), but this has not been confirmed. Early life exposure to parental smoking has also been implicated. Prenatal drug exposure has not yet been firmly incriminated in the causation of ALL or lymphoma, but postnatal immunosuppression in, for example, those receiving kidney transplants is associated with a 20–40-fold increased risk of lymphoma development. Modern intensive tumour therapy may carry such a risk. The Late Effects International Study Group has demonstrated an 8% 20-year incidence of second tumours for children treated for cancer between 1936 and 1979, i.e. 15 times the general population risk (Meadows 1988). The second largest group of second malignancies was leukaemia, principally ANLL and predominantly related to the use of alkylating agents. Some non-Hodgkin's lymphomas are being reported after intensive therapy for ALL, but they may represent localized nodal relapse of the original leukaemia. Postnatal exposure to phenytoin can induce benign lymphadenopathy, a self-limiting pseudo-lymphoma condition but also, rarely, a true lymphoma.

Ionizing irradiation

Prenatal exposure. Stewart et al (1958) reported an approximately 1.5-fold increased risk of childhood cancer developing after fetuses were exposed to X-rays performed on the maternal abdomen and pelvis during the first trimester of pregnancy. This apparent dose-related phenomenon has not been corroborated in any subsequent studies, and no such effect was reported for the progeny of mothers exposed to the atomic bombs at Hiroshima and Nagasaki (Jablon & Kato 1970). However, there was some effect on fetal head size among the Hiroshima bomb survivors (Miller & Mulvihill 1976).

In addition, Gardner et al (1990) have recently demonstrated an apparently increased risk for children of fathers working in the nuclear reprocessing plant at Sellafield in the UK. There appeared to be a relationship with a whole-life dose exposure of 100 mSv, or an excessive single 6-month preconception exposure of more than 10 mSv. There was speculation that there might be a paternal preconception germ cell DNA rearrangement or mutation. If this hypothesis can be proved, the consequences are immense. Until now, the influence of irradiation for those living around such plants – where an excess incidence of childhood leukaemia has been demonstrated – has always been considered one of environmental pollution, but known environmental nuclide levels have not explained the observed increased incidence.

Postnatal exposure. Survivors who were within one kilometre of the epicentre of the Hiroshima nuclear explosion had a marked increased risk of developing leukaemia (1 in 60). ALL was most common in children, occurring 3–10 years after exposure (peak 8 years). In adults, ANLL was more common, but ALL and chronic myeloid leukaemia (CML) were also seen. Even now, more than 40 years later, survivors are developing new thyroid and other adult cancers. Reassessment of dosage received suggests a lower exposure than previously calculated. Radionuclide fall-out ingestion (from atmospheric nuclear detonation) was reported by Lyon et al (1979) to be associated with an excess of childhood ALL in Utah, USA. Relatively low-dose therapeutic external beam irradiation for such minor conditions as scalp tinea capitis or for 'thymic enlargement' has been associated with increased risk of the development of leukaemia, brain tumours and thyroid cancer (Modan 1977, Upton 1986). Furthermore, external beam irradiation is also associated with a considerably increased incidence of second tumours, predominantly sarcomas, in those with a genetic predisposition, such as retinoblastoma patients. The combination of therapeutic irradiation and some chemotherapeutic agents, particularly alkylating agents, appears to generate an additive risk factor for second tumour formation.

Concerted efforts are being made to try to understand all the factors which influence the effects of irradiation, including age of exposure, sex, genetic susceptibility, and the means of inhalation, ingestion, or other mode of absorption of radionuclides.

Electromagnetic fields

Both proximity to high-voltage electricity cabling and the effect of electromagnetic field exposure have recently come under investigation as factors possibly contributing to childhood cancer; so far, the results are equivocal. Children living near low-power magnetic fields (< 2 mG) may have an increased risk of developing leukaemia (Savitz et al 1988). Wertheimer & Leeper (1979) showed that such fields can be produced by home appliances and the overhead household power lines common in the USA.

Conclusions

Leukaemia resulting from an inherited predisposition or known exogenous leukaemogen account for no more than 1% of ALL cases in the UK, (Greaves & Chan 1986). Much more research is required to clarify the cause of the majority of cases.

Clinical features

Children with ALL usually present with a constellation of symptoms and signs, none of which in isolation is diagnostic or specific, but which together indicate a need for further investigation (Miller & Miller 1990). Fever, easy bruising (or, less commonly, frank bleeding), tiredness, pallor and pains, especially of the limbs and abdomen, are the most common complaints which bring the child to medical attention. Anorexia and generalized malaise are common, but significant weight loss is rare at presentation. Some 60–80% of children presenting with ALL have fever, which may be secondary to infection (neutropenia and disturbed lymphoid function) or to the disease process itself (Ishii et al 1990). Parents may have noted increasing bruising or petechiae and purpura. Overt bleeding is less common in children than in adults, since they have more elastic tissues and good vessel support. Epistaxes can be a presenting feature secondary to thrombocytopenia and local nasal mucosal irritation. Since the disease process has almost certainly been present for months, it is surprising that most histories are of short duration – often days, at most weeks. This phenomenon is almost certainly due to the iceberg effect of the malignant clone slowly building up. As the tumour bulk expands, normal cell production is progressively impaired. Neutrophils with a high turnover requirement and a short half-life fall first, followed by platelets and, finally, red cell numbers. This sequence explains why those leukaemias with a primary nonmedullary origin (such as T- and B-cell ALL) have preserved neutrophils and haemoglobin levels (late marrow involvement).

Pallor is frequently not noticed by parents until a late stage (it is a slow, progressive process and may make close acquaintances blind to its development). The pains of ALL are frequently severe,

diffuse and associated with a limp or refusal to walk. All such complaints in young children should be treated seriously and investigated. The pain is due to involvement of the periosteum and bone itself, and may precipitate early referral. Major bony lesions have been reported to be associated with an improved prognosis, maybe due in part to earlier referral, but also because they appear to occur more frequently in 'common' ALL, which has the most favourable prognosis.

Apart from identification of pallor, bruising and purpura, the other commonly occurring signs are of lymphadenopathy and hepatosplenomegaly. Presentation with gross lymphadenopathy appears to be decreasing in the UK, with only 10–15% of patients now displaying visible node enlargement. The extent of organomegaly (liver, spleen or node size) correlates closely with peripheral blood white cell count (WBC) and thus overall tumour bulk. It also reflects on the subtype of ALL. Both T and B cell ALL are associated with a high WBC and striking organomegaly. Although such masses may be detected early, the higher growth fraction of these specific leukaemias means that there is, nevertheless, a high initial tumour load at presentation. An anterior mediastinal mass is present in 5–10% of childhood leukaemias and correlates very closely with T-cell disease. Occasional patients with such a mass have 'common' ALL, but very rarely have B-cell disease.

Approximately 2.5% of all patients will present with overt CNS disease at diagnosis. This usually manifests itself as headache and vomiting or focal signs especially involving the cranial nerves (VIIth, IIIrd, Vth and VIth). Another 2.5% of patients will have detectable leukaemic blast cells in their lumbar CSF, but without clinical signs or symptoms.

The differential diagnosis of a child presenting with fatigue, pallor, fever and bruising includes glandular fever, other serious viral infections (such as cytomegalovirus), idiopathic thrombocytopenia (ITP), aplastic anaemia (pancytopenia) and other malignancies, especially neuroblastoma and lymphomas. The presence of severe joint or limb pains often raises the possibility of juvenile rheumatoid arthritis or of osteomyelitis or neuroblastoma. The latter tumour frequently produces marked periosteal reactions in several bones, but since 70% of patients have metastases at diagnosis, they frequently have a history very similar to that of leukaemic children at presentation. ALL can present initially as aplastic anaemia, with slow evolution to frank leukaemia over weeks or months. Rarely, it can present with a hypereosinophilic syndrome.

Laboratory findings

Thrombocytopenia is present in over 70% of patients with ALL at presentation and is often profound. There is no direct correlation with prognosis, but the lower the initial platelet count, the higher the apparent risk of subsequent CNS and testicular relapse.

The white cell count is raised in at least half of all new patients, and is greater than $50 \times 10^9/l$ in 15–20% of cases. The elevation is a reflection of numbers of circulating leukaemic cells. In those with low white counts (below $10 \times 10^9/l$), and especially in the inappropriately named 'aleukaemic leukaemia', where no circulating blasts are seen, the WBC may be very low, (below $2–3 \times 10^9/l$). Almost all patients have neutropenia (below $1 \times 10^9/l$ at diagnosis) with the exception of some patients with a very high WBC and a primary extramedullary disease (such as T-cell disease) where bone marrow involvement is late and preservation of myeloid production coincides with a high tumour burden. The WBC at diagnosis is the single most important prognostic indicator (see below).

Although blast cells may be easily identifiable in the peripheral blood, morphologically they may little resemble those in the bone marrow, and conclusions regarding morphological subtype should not be drawn from peripheral blood smears. All patients require a bone marrow aspirate for this purpose.

Anaemia of variable degree is present in about two-thirds of all cases. A presenting haemoglobin *above* 10 g/dl is associated with late marrow involvement, as in primary extramedullary disease (T-cell or B-cell), and is associated with a worse prognosis.

Bone marrow

Although there may be no circulating peripheral blood blasts, to make a diagnosis of leukaemia the bone marrow has to be infiltrated by primitive cells. Usually, such cells comprise 90–100% of those present, although by arbitrary convention only 25% is required in order to confirm the diagnosis and distinguish leukaemia from lymphoma. To classify leukaemias and lymphomas on such a biologically irrelevant criterion is clinically unhelpful and currently being reconsidered.

For cytomorphological purposes, anterior or posterior iliac crest aspirates, smeared in the same way as blood films (not squash or cover slip preparations) are ideal. Sometimes aspiration, even from multiple sites, fails to yield adequate material, especially in children with a low initial WBC who may have associated secondary myelofibrosis, then marrow trephines are necessary. Trephines can be rolled on slides, although detailed morphological cytology on such material is often not possible.

Smears should be stained with a Romanowsky stain, together with periodic acid-Schiff (PAS), Sudan black (SB) or myeloperoxidase, nonspecific esterase (NSE) and acid phosphatase. These stains will enable the rapid distinction between ALL and ANLL in the vast majority of cases (Poplack 1988).

The cells should also be immunophenotyped and examined for specific biochemical markers (such as TdT and 5' nucleotidase). Cytogenetic analysis is also helpful. For future studies of molecular genetics, it may be useful to extract DNA from leukaemic blasts at diagnosis and store it for future analysis. Recent studies have suggested that the estimation of p-glycoprotein expression in the leukaemic cells at diagnosis may be of value in predicting drug resistance and consequent poor response to standard therapy. Several other biochemical markers have been explored, some of which have occasionally proved useful when standard methods have failed to distinguish the type of leukaemia (Eden et al 1985).

Other investigation and abnormalities at diagnosis

Table 12.4 summarizes the basic investigations required at diagnosis in childhood ALL. A chest X-ray to identify any mediastinal widening, pleural effusions or cardiomegaly must be performed

Table 12.4 Basic investigations required at diagnosis of childhood ALL

Blood tests
Full blood count + film
Immunophenotyping of peripheral blood
Cytogenetics
Renal and liver function (urea and electrolytes, Ca, Mg, phosphate, urate, albumen, LFT's, lactate dehydrogenase)
Viral serology (especially baseline immunity for measles, chickenpox, CMV, herpes simplex)
Immunoglobulin levels
Blood cultures and infection screen

Bone marrow
Morphology
Immunophenotyping
Cytogenetics

Lumbar puncture
CSF cell count and cytospin
Protein and glucose

Radiology
Chest X-ray
Ultrasound of abdomen for liver, spleen and kidney size

Cardiology
ECG + echocardiography especially in T-cell disease

---

prior to any anaesthetic procedure needed to obtain bone marrow or cerebrospinal fluid (CSF) samples. Abdominal ultrasonography is the most useful way of measuring organomegaly. It is especially important to identify large kidneys prior to commencement of treatment in those with bulky disease, because such children may be particularly liable to the tumour lysis syndrome. A diagnostic lumbar puncture for CSF examination (cell count and cytospin) is required. The presence of circulating CSF blasts (under 5% of cases) is not an adverse prognostic feature if treatment is suitably modified to include early therapy which penetrates the CNS.

Biochemical tests must include a pretreatment check on plasma urea, sodium, potassium, calcium, phosphate, uric acid, albumen and liver enzymes. Pretreatment elevation of urea, urate, potassium and phosphate requires appropriate treatment to prevent the tumour lysis syndrome (see below).

Blood can also be studied for cytogenetic analysis, estimation of immunoglobulin and lactate dehydrogenase levels (all of which may be of possible prognostic usefulness), for baseline viral serology (especially immune status for measles and chickenpox), and can be cultured if fever is present. Most centres perform some sort of diagnostic infection screen since the majority of patients are febrile at presentation, or certainly within the first 4–5 days of treatment.

Prognostic factors

Table 12.5 shows an unstratified and stratified analysis of prognostic features in the Medical Research Council (MRC) UKALL VIII protocol for a total of 829 patients (Eden et al 1990a).

Table 12.5 Prognostic indicators for disease-free survival in the Medical Research Council UKALL VIII Study and Trial 1980–84

Variable*	Total analyzed	Unstratified	Stratified by: WBC	sex	age
WBC	829	< .00005	–	–	–
Age*	829	.001	.05	.03	–
Sex	829	.0001	< .0005	–	–
FAB (L3 excluded)	733	.06	.08	.1	.2
Mediastinal mass	814	.008	.09		
Spleen size	827	.0002	.04	.04	.06
Liver size	829	.003	.08		
Cell type (C,T,N)*	611	< .00005	.08	.2	
Cell type (C,T)*	584	.0001	.01	.04	.2
Haemoglobin	813	.02	.04	.06	.2
Ph¹ chromosome	552	.0007	.007	.008	.006
Chromosomes*	281	.05	.3		
High hyper v other**	281	.004	.03	.03	.04
Pseudo v other**	281	.03	.1		
Day 14 BM % blasts	577	.0002	.0009	.0005	.003

*p-value for heterogeneity
**refers to state of diploidy. See p. 338

The variable numbers analyzed for specific features reflect the present difficulty in completely documenting some features, particularly immunophenotyping and cytogenetics, but it is apparently useful to perform these tests on all patients wherever possible. It must not, of course, be forgotten that prognostic factors vary considerably with the treatment given and that the single most important prognostic factor is the therapeutic schedule employed. The features listed in Table 12.5 are very similar to those reported by Kalwinsky et al (1985) from 236 children, and by Hammond et al (1986) based on a series of 1490 patients.

White cell count (WBC)

In every series so far described, the single most important prognostic indicator in childhood ALL is the initial WBC (Chessells 1982, Kalwinsky et al 1985, Hammond et al 1986). There has been considerable variation between collaborative groups as to where the arbitrary cut-off point is made for the analysis of WBC (10, 20, 50 or 100 × 10^9/l), but a consensus is emerging that all those with WBC above 50 × 10^9/l have a substantially worsened prognosis, particularly so if the count is above 100 × 10^9/l. Children with WBC less than 50 × 10^9/l given current therapy may have a more uniform outlook.

Age

Age appears to be of some prognostic significance, but not independently of WBC. It has long been accepted that those aged 2–10 years fare better than those younger or older (Simone et al 1975, Miller et al 1980). The worst prognosis is seen in those under one year of age at diagnosis (Leiper & Chessells 1986). However, in the UKALL VIII Study (an unselected series), 85% of such infants had a WBC over 50 × 10^9/l and none had a count below 10 × 10^9/l; furthermore nearly 50% had 'null' cell ALL, compared with only 2% with 'null' ALL in those older than 2 years (Eden et al 1990b).

Table 12.6 shows the features for those under 2 years of age compared with those more than 2 years in UKALL VIII. Those aged 18 months or older with an initial WBC of 10–50 × 10^9/l fared

no worse than older children; those with a WBC less than 10 × 10^9/l and aged under 2 years had an intermediate prognosis; whilst the greatest risk was for those under 6 months, all of whom had a high WBC (over 50 × 10^9/l) at diagnosis. Only 2 out of 8 such patients survive. The predominant form of relapse for these very young children, as can be seen in the Table, is recurrent marrow disease, but with a doubling of CNS relapses and excessive infection-related mortality. For those aged 1–2 years, the CNS was the most likely site of relapse, underlining the need for improved CNS treatment at this young age.

It is less clear whether children in their early teens genuinely have a worse prognosis, but there is an excess of teenage boys with high white counts and T-cell disease. Young adults also have a greater incidence of Philadelphia-positive ALL, which responds less well to treatment.

Sex

There is a slight excess incidence of ALL in boys compared with girls in most series (1.2:1), and in

Table 12.6 Medical Research Council UKALL VIII Study and Trial. Children under 2 years (n = 80) – comparison of features and events with those of older children

Feature/event	Age at diagnosis (%)		
	Under 1 year	1–2 years	Over 2 years
WBC			
> 50	85	45	13
10–50	15	34	32
< 10	0	21	55
Sex			
Male	60	54	55
Cell type			
Common	14	51	73
Null	48	22.5	2
T-cell	0	10	7.6
B-cell	9.5	2.5	0.4
? (includes difficult to type + inadequate sample)	29	14	18
Induction deaths	10	6.2	4.6
Remission deaths (especially high early pneumonitis)	10	7.5	5
Relapses (% of remitters)			
Marrow	24	12.5	14.5
CNS	9.5	17.5	5.9
Testicular	0	2.5	4.5
Combined	5	8.8	5.9

many series there is a more favourable prognosis for girls which becomes increasingly obvious at 2 years and later after diagnosis. This is in contrast to other prognostic indicators, the significance of which diminish with time (Sather et al 1981). In the early UK MRC UKALL Trials II and III, the sex difference in prognosis was associated with a simultaneously observed increasing incidence of overt testicular relapse (Medical Research Council 1978). Prophylactic testicular irradiation failed to eradicate the sex difference in outlook, however, and it is now thought to be an early marker of residual disease rather than a true 'sanctuary' (Nesbit et al 1982, Eden et al 1990c). In other words, there must be other sex-related features which worsens the prognosis for boys. It can also not be fully explained by the excess of T-cell disease in teenage boys, as the difference is still apparent in non-T disease.

Morphology

The morphology of leukaemic blast cells has been refined by the use of the French-American-British (FAB) classification, which divides ALL into L_1 (small microlymphoblastic), L_2 (larger, more undifferentiated) and L_3 (Burkitt-like). Occasionally, there can be problems in assigning an individual case to the L_1 or L_2 category, and the exercise is best carried out by a panel who reach a consensus view (Bennet et al 1981). The proportions in each group are roughly 80–85% L_1, 10–15% L_2 and 2–3% L_3. If the original methodology is followed precisely, patients with L_2 disease are found to be somewhat less likely to remit and have a higher relapse rate than those with L_1 blasts (Hann et al 1979, Miller et al 1981). When L_1 patients relapse, they can change to L_2 disease (Lilleyman et al 1986). L_2 cells are thought to show evidence of more rapid DNA and protein synthesis and to have a higher proliferative rate.

There is no correlation between immunophenotype and L_1 and L_2 morphology, but L_3 appearances correlate closely with B-cell ALL. Perhaps an equally important morphological feature is the presence of cytoplasmic vacuoles in L_1 and L_2 disease (they are a defined feature in L_3 cells). Vacuoles in more than 10% of blasts correlates

quite closely with PAS positivity. Lilleyman et al (1986) also reported a very close relationship with a diagnostic WBC under $50 \times 10^9/l$ and the 'common' ALL immunophenotype. In that series, patients with vacuolated cells had a significantly improved disease-free survival compared with those without vacuoles. The significance remained when stratified by FAB type but was lost when stratified by WBC.

Organomegaly

The presence of a mediastinal mass on chest X-ray does not appear to be of independent prognostic significance. Although closely associated with T-cell ALL and a high WBC, when present with a low WBC it does not adversely affect outcome (Chilcote et al 1984).

Spleen, node and liver size also appear to correlate closely with a high WBC. The North American Children's Cancer Study Group (CCSG) define a poor-prognosis leukaemia/lymphoma syndrome with nodal or mediastinal enlargement, organomegaly and a high haemoglobin, but what significance organomegaly per se has remains unclear (Miller et al 1985).

Immunophenotype

Although considerable effort has been made over the last 10 years to type leukaemia immunologically, there is less correlation with prognosis than originally thought when white count is taken into account. Table 12.7 shows subcategories of ALL, and their defining monoclonal antibodies and biochemical markers. Approximately 70% of childhood ALL cases have CD10 (cALLA)-positive leukaemia, but it is important to remember that CD10-positive cells are found in small proportions within normal bone marrow and that the antigen can be found in a small percentage of adult T-cell ALL (Ia^+, CD9-positive). Immunologically defined disease which appears to be resistant to conventional therapy includes Group VI, B-cell ALL (Flandrin et al 1975), Group V, pre-B ALL (Crist et al 1980), null ALL in infants and T-cell ALL with a high WBC. Immunological recognition of mature B-cell ALL, and the use of different therapeutic strategies, has been rewarded

Table 12.7   Classification of childhood ALL by immunophenotyping and biochemical markers*

A. B-cell lineage

Group	% of patients	Tdt	Ia	CD19 (B4)	CD10 (cALLA)	CD20 (B1)	Cytoplasmic IgM	Surface IgM
I	5	Maybe –	+/–	–	–	–	–	–
II	15	+	+	+	–	–	–	–
III	33	+	+	+	+	–	–	–
IV	30	+	+	+	+	+	–	–
V	15	+	+	+	+	+	+	–
VI	2	–	+	+	+/–	+	–	+

Most are Tdt-positive and contain rearranged Ig genes

B. T-cell lineage

Group	Class II Ag	Leu 9	T1 (CD5)	T11 (CD2)	T3 (CD3)	T4 (CD4)	T8 (CD8)	T6 (CD1)
I	–	+	+	+	–	–	–	–
II	–	+	+	+	+	+	+	+
III	–	+	+	+	+	+/–	+/–	–

Most are Tdt-positive and express T-cell receptor genes

*Modified from Foon & Todd 1986 with permission.

by a dramatic improvement in disease-free survival (Hann et al 1990). Too few laboratories search for intracytoplasmic IgM, which defines pre-B ALL and separates it from common ALL. Pre-B disease may have an unfavourable prognosis irrespective of WBC (Crist et al 1984), though recent evidence suggests that this may depend on the presence of an associated 1:19 chromosomal translocation (Crist et al 1990). In short, it seems that the further a leukaemia appears to have differentiated along the B-cell pathway, the worse the prognosis. Attempts to similarly subdivide T-cell ALL have proved less helpful. Nadler et al (1980) considered that T NHL might arise in more mature T cells than does T ALL, but this has not been confirmed.

Campana et al (1990) have used double-marker immunofluorescence assays to detect combinations of differentiation antigen expressed on leukaemic cells but absent from regenerating marrow cells (e.g. CD3/Tdt) in order to detect low levels of residual disease ($<10^{-4}$ cells) not apparent morphologically. This approach depends on subjecting the initial bone marrow to a battery of markers to identify known combinations in the search for minimal residual disease.

Molecular genetics, especially the detection of DNA gene rearrangements and T-cell receptor genes, will further subdivide childhood ALL and help in the detection of late minimal residual disease. For example, Yamada et al (1990) have used the polymerase chain reaction to amplify unique CDRIII sequences within B-cell lineage leukaemic cells associated with the heavy chain immunoglobulin locus.

Haemoglobin and platelets

Blood haemoglobin concentration may be relatively spared if the primary disease is nonmedullary and late bone marrow infiltration occurs. Paradoxically, a high haemoglobin appears to be an adverse prognostic feature (Chessels 1982). Low platelet counts at diagnosis do appear to correlate with subsequent increased risk of testicular (Nesbit et al 1980, MRC 1978) and CNS disease (West et al 1972). A possible reason for this is increased tissue microhaemorrhages and greater deposition of leukaemic cells.

Immunoglobulin

Serum immunoglobulin levels are low in about 30% of cases at diagnosis but the prognostic importance of this, if any, is not clear (Leiken et al 1981).

Cytogenetics

Crudely, ALL can be divided into five categories

Table 12.8 Commonly identified chromosomal translocations and deletions in lymphoblasts

Translocation	Oncogene or associated growth factor	Immunophenotype	Prognosis
t 9;22 (q34, q11) (Philadelphia)	abl, bcr	B-cell precursor T-cell	difficult to induce may be poor
t 1;19 (q23, p13)	Insulin receptor	pre-B	Poor
t 4;11 (q21, q23)	ets 1	Very early B-cell lineage or null (monocytic)	Very poor
t 8;14 (q24, q32)	c myc IgH	B-cell	Poor with conventional treatment
(t 2;8, t 8:22)	(c myc IgK c myc IgL)	B-cell	
t 11;14 (p13, q11.2)	Int 2 T-cell receptor A	T-cell II	Poor unless aggressive treatment

Data modified from Miller & Miller 1990

based on the number of chromosomes within the blast cells: high hyperdiploid (over 50), hyperdiploid (47–50), normal, hypodiploid and pseudodiploid (Secker-Walker 1984, Williams et al 1982). Those with pseudodiploidy appear to have the worst prognosis, those with high hyperdiploidy the best (being associated with low-WBC 'common' ALL). However, mere chromosome numbers are less important than identification of translocations, most easily seen in pseudodiploidy (Williams et al 1985). Table 12.8 shows the most regularly seen nonrandom translocations and their associated clinical features. It is important to identify such cytogenetic abnormalities, since their presence may signify unfavourable prognosis not identified by other means. This is particularly important for pre-B ALL and Ph[1]-positive disease.

Cell proliferation

Although rarely routine, flow cytometric analysis and measurements of cell proliferation rates and other features can be used in the classification and prediction of response to therapy of ALL (Scarfe et al 1980). Both B- and T-cell ALL have high proliferative rates, and had a uniformly poor outlook until intensive, sustained chemotherapy was introduced. Increased DNA content of blasts, identified by flow cytometry, echoes hyperdiploidy and correlates with 'common' ALL. Such cells have a longer-lasting S phase and are more sensitive to cell-cycle-specific agents. They are

also more terminally differentiated and more likely to respond to glucocorticosteroids.

Treatment

When no treatment was available for ALL, all patients died, but over the last 30 years effective combination therapy has been developed which potentially avoids development of drug resistance. A sustained whole-body approach is now preferred, which may remove the necessity to concentrate separately on specific 'sanctuary' sites.

The rate of cell kill may be extremely important. Jacquillat et al (1973) and Miller et al (1989) showed that marrow clearance in the early days of treatment is a highly significant prognostic indicator for long-term disease-free survival. Remission achieved at day 14, and possibly even at day 7 (Gaynon et al 1990), bodes well. Conversely, failure to achieve remission by days 28–30 is an adverse prognostic indicator (Sallan et al 1978). The West German BFM Group (Riehm et al 1987) have used blast cell kill in response to steroids at the beginning of therapy in order to classify patients into risk groups. They have used an absolute level below which the blast cell count should have fallen in order to qualify for a more favourable prognostic category.

Induction of remission

The three traditional agents for reducing the initial cell bulk and inducing remission in ALL are vincristine, prednisolone and L-asparaginase. The combination of oral prednisolone (40 mg/m^2 per day for 28 days) and vincristine (1.5 mg/m^2 i.v. weekly × 5 doses) induces remission in 85–90% of cases, whilst the addition of L-asparaginase raises this to 95% and appears also to prolong remission duration (Ortego et al 1977). As a single agent, the most effective dose of L-asparaginase appears to be 12 000 units/m^2 given 3 times a week for 12 doses (Ertel et al 1979). In combination therapy, lower dosages are usually employed, such as the 6 000 units/m^2 3 times a week for 9 doses used in the CCG 160 series and MRC UKALL VIII, although more recently there has been a trend towards higher doses again. This escalation has usually been as part of consolidation therapy rather than during induction, to avoid the combined toxic effects of steroids and asparaginase. Both can induce hyperglycaemia and pancreatic dysfunction. High-dose asparaginase, with its prolonged plasma half-life, is also best avoided if possible during periods of profound thrombocytopenia, due to a greater risk from acquired coagulopathies which the drug can produce.

Concerning the route of administration, there is evidence of equal efficacy and a considerable reduction in anaphylactic risk if the drug is given intramuscularly rather than intravenously (Nesbit et al 1979, Eden et al 1990d). Perhaps surprisingly, bruising and bleeding are seldom a problem in thrombocytopenic patients receiving i.m. asparaginase.

The addition of other systemic drugs during induction has not been shown definitely to improve remission rate or duration. Sallan et al (1978) did observe some probable late benefit for the addition of an anthracycline, but in the MRC UKALL VIII Trial (Eden et al 1990a) there is no statistically significant difference in event-free survival to date between those who did and those who did not receive 2 doses of daunorubicin in a dose of 45 mg/m^2 on days 1 and 2 of induction. Those receiving the drug had an almost doubling of deaths early in treatment due to infection associated with more protracted myelosuppression, but to balance this, there was reduction in subsequent haematological relapses. In future, control of the risk of early infection might unmask a true benefit for the addition of an anthracycline induction agent.

The 5% or so of patients who are not in remission within a month tend to fare poorly, and if a remission can subsequently be achieved (usually by 2 further weeks of prednisolone and vincristine) and consolidated, such children become candidates for early allogeneic bone marrow transplantation or 'megatherapy' and autologous bone marrow rescue. They most commonly present with a high initial white cell count (Ortega et al 1977), null cell ALL (especially with 4:11 translocation), B-cell ALL treated in a conventional fashion; or Ph- chromosome-positive ALL (Chessells et al 1979, Secker-Walker et al 1985). Some centres electively withdraw such categories of patients from standard therapy and use more aggressive protocols for them. The use of cyclophosphamide, adriamycin and vincristine interspersed with high-dose systemic methotrexate and cytosine arabinoside (to have both a systemic and CNS effect) has resulted in dramatic improvement in survival for B-cell leukaemia (Hann et al 1990). Historically, such patients seldom survived more than 6 months. In contrast, there is presently little evidence that different induction regimens are worthwhile for T-cell ALL.

Intensification

In the 1970s, the West German BFM Group started to explore the use of an intensive 4-week induction followed by a further 4-week consolidation phase using a combination of cyclophosphamide, cytosine arabinoside, L-asparaginase, adriamycin and thioguanine (Riehm et al 1980). Their aggressive approach was rewarded with the best results described at that time (approximately 70% 5-year survival). The group developed a 'risk index' method of stratifying patients and introduced further intensive therapy modules for higher risk patients, together with, latterly, a very intensive new regimen for the highest risk group (WBC over 100 × 10^9/l, Ph[1]-chromosome-positive, and initial poor responders). All of their patients receive a standard induction protocol.

Noting the good response in the nonrandomized single-arm BFM studies, in 1985 the MRC established the UKALL X Trial, where patients were randomized to receive: (A) no consolidation treatment; (B) a course of early consolidation therapy (cytarabine, thioguanine, prednisolone, vincristine, daunorubicin and etoposide for 5 days) immediately after induction; (C) late consolidation (the same module at 5 months from diagnosis); and (D) both early and late consolidation. Initially, all girls with an initial WBC under $20 \times 10^9/l$ were put into the no-consolidation arm, whilst high-count patients with a WBC over $100 \times 10^9/l$ all went into arm D. Subsequent experience with the consolidation phase reassured participants of its safety, and after 2 years the 'good risk' girls were also randomized.

In both the BFM and UK series, although low-WBC patients, especially girls, currently fare well with over 70% showing 5-year event free survival, too many still relapse to justify therapeutic complacency.

At the time of writing, it is premature to report on the results of the UKALL X trial as it only closed to new entrants in 1990, but early signs suggest a benefit for arms which include late consolidation. Unpublished data from the CCSG and the BFM group are also suggestive of a similar possible benefit for late consolidation. This is in contrast to a whole range of previous studies where early consolidation pulses with a variety of drugs, or the use of extra agents during maintenance therapy, gave no benefit or, indeed, conveyed a positive disadvantage (MRC 1986).

CNS minimal disease therapy

The use of specifically directed CNS treatment has been considered a prerequisite for long-term survival since the early studies of Pinkel and his colleagues at the St Jude Children's Research Hospital (Aur et al 1971, Hustu et al 1973). Before its introduction, at least 50% of children developed overt meningeal disease whilst in systemic remission. Most of such relapsing patients subsequently developed marrow disease and died. Similar results were seen in more recent studies, including an MRC series between 1977 and 1987, where only 23 out of 116 patients with primary CNS relapse were alive following retreatment. The majority had a degree of neuropsychological impairment (Darbyshire et al 1990). Only relatively rare isolated CNS relapses arising a long time after cessation of treatment are associated

with a better survival. The need for targeted CNS treatment has been challenged in one series where it was doubted whether CNS relapse really influenced survival or systemic remission duration in 'standard risk' patients (Nesbit et al 1981a); however, the consensus view is that some CNS disease control is necessary.

Pinkel and his group pioneered symptomatic CNS irradiation, initially craniospinal and then subsequently just cranial irradiation with adjunctive intrathecal (IT) methotrexate. This dramatically reduced overt CNS relapses to under 10% Their standard therapy consisted of 24-Gy cranial irradiation in 14 or 15 fractions over 17–18 days, coupled with 5 IT injections of methotrexate in a dose of 12 mg/m^2 every 3–4 days (Hustu et al 1973). A number of modifications have been made to this regimen since, including adjustment of IT methotrexate dosage by age, rather than surface area (this correlates better with CSF volume) so that patients under one year receive 5 mg, those aged 1–2 years 7.5 mg, those aged 2–3 years 10 mg, and all the rest 12.5 mg (Bleyer et al 1983). There is also acceptance of a reduction in cranial irradiation dosage to 18 Gy for those with an initial WBC under $50 \times 10^9/l$. The CCSG have shown that this dose is as effective as 24 Gy for this group of patients (Nesbit et al 1981b). For those with higher WBCs, there is a suggestion of better CNS disease control with 24 Gy compared with 18 Gy, but the difference is not statistically significant. Moreover, preliminary evidence suggests that 18 Gy may be no less neurotoxic in the long term than 24 Gy (Chessells et al 1987). Two dilemmas have arisen with regard to CNS therapy; first, current regimens for patients with an initial WBC of $>50 \times 10^9/l$ or higher are associated with unacceptably high (15–20%) CNS relapse rates; and second, for the lower risk patients, there is worry about long-term toxicity. Long-term toxicity includes impairment of learning and of growth, and disturbed puberty (see below). From a meta-analysis of published studies, late toxicity appears to be of greater degree where cranial irradiation is included in therapy, and least when IT methotrexate is used alone.

In the CCSG 101 Study, craniospinal irradiation with extended-field sanctuary irradiation to the liver, spleen and gonads was compared with (1) craniospinal irradiation alone and (2) IT methotrexate alone (Nesbit et al 1982). An excess of CNS relapses was seen with the IT-only arm, and patients were eventually recalled for delayed irradiation, but there was no significant difference in terms of overall haematological relapses. In more recent studies, 'low risk' patients received IT methotrexate not only during induction but also during the maintenance phase, and this has shown no significant excess of CNS relapses. The Paediatric Oncology Group AlinC 11 protocol incorporated triple-IT chemotherapy during both induction and continuing therapy, with a 5% CNS relapse rate. This was equivalent to the rate they had obtained in previous studies using cranial radiotherapy and 5 IT injections of methotrexate (Sullivan et al 1982). They did find that patients with high initial WBC or a lymphoma/leukaemia syndrome had higher CNS relapse rates.

Green et al (1980) retrospectively reviewed a number of studies, comparing those employing 'standard' irradiation and IT methotrexate with those based on prolonged courses of triple IT chemotherapy only and those where intermediate-dose systemic methotrexate plus IT methotrexate was used. (The systemic methotrexate dose was fairly low by current standards, at 500 mg/m^2). The lowest CNS relapse rates in both standard and high-risk patient categories were seen in children given irradiation. The lowest marrow relapse rate for standard-risk patients was in those given systemic intermediate-dose methotrexate. In high-risk patients, the best relapse-free and overall survival was observed in those given cranial irradiation. A high CNS relapse rate was associated with poor overall survival, but the converse did not apply. This was a type of 'meta-analysis', a review of a series of studies, rather than a randomized prospective trial, but it provided some evidence to suggest that systemic methotrexate could be used instead of cranial irradiation for CNS control.

Abromovitch et al (1988) compared systemic methotrexate given in a dose of 1 gm/m^2 together with IT methotrexate both during the early phase of therapy and repeated during the first 18 months, with cranial irradiation (18 Gy) plus IT methotrexate also continued for 18 months. No patients with a WBC over 100 × 10^9/l were in-

cluded, nor were any with overt CNS disease at diagnosis. In both arms, the CNS relapse rate was approximately 10%, but remission duration and disease-free survival were superior in the group of patients given systemic methotrexate (67% 4-year disease-free survival compared with 56% in the irradiated arm).

Moe et al (1981) achieved very similar results – 74% 5-year disease-free survival for standard-risk, and 50% for high-WBC patients using 500 mg/m^2 of systemic methotrexate.

Methotrexate has limited lipid solubility, which reduces its ability to cross into the CSF, so traditionally it has been injected directly into the CSF at either lumbar or ventricular level. When injected into the ventricles, there is a very variable half-life (range of 3.9–20 hours), whilst lumbar injection leads to less than 10% of the drug reaching the ventricles. In contrast, when injected systemically, methotrexate has a uniform distribution throughout the different CNS compartments (Shapiro et al 1975). CSF:serum ratio depends on dose, duration of infusion and serum concentration reached. Borsi et al (1987) demonstrated that at a systemic dose of 500 mg/m^2 a third of patients did not achieve CSF levels of 10^{-6}M which is considered to be essential for a useful therapeutic effect. Even at a dose of 1 gm/m^2, 22% of patients did not reach this CSF concentration. However, once methotrexate dosages were escalated to the range 6–8 g/m^2, adequate cytocidal concentrations were uniformly achieved. Paradoxically, perhaps, children under 4 years of age appear to need higher doses. This is due to their more rapid clearance of the drug, and doses up to 33 g/m^2 have been attempted.

In a joint study between the CCSG and the National Cancer Institute in America, randomization between cranial irradiation (24 Gy plus 5 IT methotrexate injections) and very high-dose systemic methotrexate showed no differences in CNS relapse rates between the two arms (Poplack et al 1984). The protocol was for intermediate- and poor-risk patients only. Of particular interest was the difference in recorded toxicity. Those receiving conventional radiotherapy and IT methotrexate were shown to have the well-recognized fall in full-scale IQ, and also underachieved in reading, spelling and arithmetic tests. Unlike most other studies, these children also had some deterioration in verbal IQ. In contrast, those receiving systemic high-dose methotrexate had no fall in full-scale IQ, had a small rise in verbal IQ, and just a modest fall in arithmetic skills. The findings are preliminary, and the patients require much longer follow-up for the full pattern of differential toxicity to emerge. The incidence of neurological sequelae with high-dose methotrexate has been reported as 5–15%, but most problems seem to be transient (Jaffe et al 1985). There appears to be a much lower incidence of learning difficulties than with irradiation, at least in the short term. A potential advantage of high-dose systemic methotrexate is that it is well distributed throughout the body, including the CNS; and that it may overcome cell resistance mechanisms by a sheer concentration effect. Such doses are possible because of the ability to 'rescue' patients from lethal toxicity by the use of folinic acid (leukovorin). Given 6–8 g/m² of methotrexate i.v. (one-tenth of the dose as an initial first hour prime and the rest over 23 hours) the CSF concentration falls below 10^{-6} M at about 36 hours post-initiation of the 24-hour infusion, and at this point intravenous folinic acid is started. With doses of methotrexate as high as 33 mg/m², the addition of adjunctive IT therapy may not be needed, but it is still recommended when the systemic dose is in the range of 6–8 g/m² (Bleyer 1989). Properly managed (which includes monitoring the fall in serum drug concentration and tailoring the regimen of folinic acid accordingly), high-dose methotrexate does not produce any important myelosuppression.

The UK Medical Research Council (MRC) have embarked on a new trial which randomizes patients with a WBC under $50 \times 10^9/l$ between IT methotrexate alone (the standard 6 IT injections during the early phase of therapy and continuing less frequently during maintenance therapy), and high-dose systemic methotrexate with adjunctive IT treatment. For higher WBC patients, there is a randomization between high-dose methotrexate, and cranial irradiation (24 Gy) with 6 IT methotrexate injections. So far, it is not clear which patients can be successfully treated with IT therapy only, but none are completely immune from CNS relapse (Table 12.9). Apart from girls

aged 3–6 years with a WBC below $10 \times 10^9/l$, there is remarkable uniformity in CNS relapse rates for patients with a WBC under $50 \times 10^9/l$.

Lack of myelosuppression seen with high-dose methotrexate and rescue has enabled both the French LMB Group and the UK Children's Cancer Study Group (UKCCSG) to interpose high-dose systemic methotrexate at the nadir of counts following myelosuppressive therapy for patients with B-cell leukaemia (Patte et al 1986, Hann et al 1990). These protocols also incorporate high-dose cytarabine, which appears to be effective against B-cell leukaemia, but which does not have an established place in the treatment of other types of ALL in childhood.

Continuing therapy (maintenance)

Unlike most other malignant diseases, there does appear to be a need to give long continuing maintenance therapy (for approximately 2 years) in children with ALL. Early studies, where no extended therapy was given after remission induction, were associated with rapid relapse (MRC 1971). Furthermore, continuing therapy should be uninterrupted. Intermittent pulses, aimed at reducing the immunosuppressive effect of maintenance treatment, have proved inferior in terms of disease control when subjected to a prospective trial (MRC 1986).

The 'standard' approach has therefore become the use of continuous oral drugs, given on an outpatient basis. There has been no improvement over the use of oral daily 6-mercaptopurine (commonly 75 mg/m² per day) and weekly oral methotrexate (commonly 20 mg/m² per week). 6-mercaptopurine (6-MP), a purine analogue, and methotrexate, a folate antagonist, work through

Table 12.9 MRC UKALL VIII Study and Trial isolated CNS relapses

	%Relapses in each patient category (no. of relapses/no. in category)		
	Low	Average	High
Girls	2.8% (2/71)	7.7% (17/221)	9.1% (6/66)
Boys	6.4% (8/125)	7.0% (17/244)	12.5% (8/64)

Low	=	Aged 3–6 years, initial WBC $< 10 \times 10^9/l$
Average	=	all patients with WBC $0–50 \times 10^9/l$ except 'Low' group
High	=	all with WBC $> 50 \times 10^9/l$

different mechanisms but are both myelotoxic and immunosuppressive. Methotrexate can cause mouth ulceration, whilst mercaptopurine occasionally causes hepatic dysfunction. Most protocols currently include intermittent pulses of prednisolone and vincristine in addition to the oral therapy, and these are usually given at 4-weekly intervals. Their addition has been thought to reduce marrow relapses (Bleyer et al 1985). The addition of other myelotoxic agents during maintenance treatment may be counterproductive, by necessitating reduction of the doses of 6-MP and methotrexate.

Increasingly, it is also recognized that the dosage of 6-MP and methotrexate should be titrated against the blood counts for each patient, with escalation of dosage if there is no evident myelosuppression. Emphasis is usually placed on neutrophil counts, but a closer correlation with the antileukaemic effect of therapy may be demonstrated by the lymphocyte count (Hayder et al 1990). Several factors influence the therapeutic effect of oral maintenance agents, including drug absorption, which appears to be especially variable for methotrexate, depending on such variables as the time of taking medication (Pinkerton et al 1980), and metabolism, as has been described for 6-MP (Lennard & Lilleyman 1987). The addition of long-term oral cotrimoxazole to reduce the risk of *Pneumocystis carinii* pneumonitis complicates the picture through an unpredictable effect of the drug on folate metabolism, though it is doubtful if there is an important effect on the antileukaemic action of the other agents (Hughes et al 1977).

Many early American studies used 5 or even 7 years of continuing therapy, but there has been a downward trend in recent years. The CCSG showed no advantage of 5 years of therapy compared with 3 years (Nesbit et al 1983), and in the UKALL VIII Study and Trial there was a trend for less relapses in those patients receiving 3 years of therapy, which was balanced by an increase in infective remission deaths during the third year (Eden et al 1990a). The BFM group tried to reduce duration of therapy to 18 months, but found this to be less effective than 2 years. Thus, it does appear that patients require at least 2 years of continuing therapy given current induction and consolidation schedules. Since such continuing

therapy is perhaps a mopping up exercise to eradicate leukaemic cells left after the induction cell kill, duration of therapy may be dependent on the intensity and/or efficacy of early treatment.

Complications of treatment

Table 12.10 shows some of the side-effects of the commonly used antileukaemic drugs. The chief worries for most patients are painful procedures and the development of nausea, retching and vomiting. Older children fret about alopecia, but for physicians secondary marrow failure and the consequent risk of haemorrhage and infection is the main problem.

Fever and infection

During induction. In a recent review, 74% of ALL patients were febrile at or before the time of diagnosis, but in 65% of these the start of antileukaemic therapy alone led to resolution of the fever (Ishii et al 1990). In the author's own hospital, 33 of 55 patients had early fever but only 2 had positive blood cultures, so such fever is common and probably due to the disease itself. Because of the associated neutropenia, however, treatment with intravenous broad-spectrum antibiotics is commonly given until the patient's temperature subsides.

Wiley et al (1990) went further and recommended antibiotics until the neutrophil count reaches $0.5 \times 10^9/l$ or more, but 16% of their patients acquired invasive fungal disease, presumably as a result of such protracted antibiotic therapy. Shorter courses of antibiotics appear adequate for controlling both unexplained fever and demonstrable sepsis.

Up to 85% of patients can be expected to develop fever later during the induction period whilst neutropenic. The commonest organisms isolated are Gram-positive skin flora (in MRC UKALL VIII, 57% of positive blood cultures in induction grew Gram-positive cocci, chiefly *Staphylococcus epidermidis* and *staphylococcus aureus*), but the greatest threat to life comes from Gram-negative organisms, including *Escherichia coli*, *Proteus*, *Klebsiella* and *Pseudomonas*. Vigilance, coupled with early vigorous use of broad-spectrum i.v. antibiotics (usually an aminoglycoside

Table 12.10 Toxic effects of drugs used in the therapy of childhood ALL

Drug	Myelosuppression	Immunosuppression	Tissue irritant	Nausea & vomiting	Cystitis	Nephrotoxicity	Cardiotoxicity	Neuropathic	Hepatotoxicity
Steroids	–	+++	High-dose i.v.-painful	–	–	–	–	–	–
Vincristine	+/–	++	+++	–	–	–	–	+++ (+IADH)	–
Asparaginase	+	++	–	+/–	–	–	–	Encephalopathy	++
Anthracyclines									
adriamycin	++	+	+++	++	–	–	+++	–	Radiation recall effect
daunomycin	+								
Antimetabolites									
Methotrexate (oral, i.v., i.m. IT)	++*	++	–	Mucositis ++ (esp. high dose)	–	++ (High dose potential)	–	++ (high dose + chronic i.m. + IT)	++
6-mercaptopurine (+ thioguanine)	+	+	–	Rarely	–	–	–	–	+
Cytosine arabinoside (i.v., i.m., IT)	++	++	–	++ (diarrhoea with infusions)	–	–	–	Cerebellar in high dose	–
Alkylating agents									
Cyclophosphamide	++	++	++	+++	++	+	+ (High)dose	+ (IADH)	–
Epipodophyllo-toxins (e.g. etoposide)	++	+	+	+/– (mucositis)	–	–	± (hypotension)	+ (mild peripheral)	+ (enzymes)

1. + to +++ denotes varying degree of toxicity; – denotes no recorded toxicity.
2. Etoposide, asparaginase and (rarely) cytosine can induce severe hypersensitivity reactions.
3. *High-dose systemic methotrexate with folinic acid rescue has no important myelosuppressive effect.

and a third-generation cephalosporin or ureido-penicillin) can reduce mortality. In UKALL VIII, during the first year, infective induction deaths approached 5%, but using the same cytotoxic drugs in UKALL X the induction death rate due to sepsis fell to under 1% (Chessells & Bailey 1990). The more intensive the induction regimen and the more prolonged the period of neutropenia, the greater the risk of life-threatening sepsis.

Other preventative measures may also decrease risks of infection, including good oral hygiene, regular oral antifungals (usually nystatin or amphotericin lozenges) the use of topical nasal antibiotics (if the nose is irritated or dry) and the use of meticulous techniques when any invasive procedures are carried out. The increasing use of central venous catheters (Hickman or Broviac) does appear to have increased the risk of septicaemia, particularly due to Gram-positive organisms, principally due to poor handling techniques (Russell et al 1990). Ideally, such lines should not be inserted during periods of myelosuppression. To avoid precipitating a bacteraemia, all rectal procedures should be discouraged in neutropenic patients, including rectal temperature recording, the use of suppositories, enemas and rectal examinations. It is unclear whether nonabsorbable or other antibiotic regimens designed to 'sterilize' the bowel have any part to play in the routine treatment of ALL, though there may be a place for such an approach in patients undergoing bone marrow transplantation.

It should be standard policy to give blind i.v. antibiotics to all patients who have neutrophil counts under $1 \times 10^9/l$ and who have fever of 38.5°C or more for more than 2–4 hours. If the fever fails to resolve within 48 hours, or if any worsening of clinical condition occurs, the antibiotics should be changed (even if blood cultures are negative), and 72 hours later systemic antifungal treatment should be given if the fever persists and the patient is unwell.

The most widely used antifungal is amphotericin. It is safe enough provided careful review of renal function and potassium levels are maintained. The drug is normally started at a dose of 0.25 mg/kg with an escalation daily by 0.25 mg/kg per day up to a maximum of 1 mg/kg per day, provided no evidence of renal toxicity or uncorrectable hypokalaemia are developing. Fluconazole, well-absorbed orally, appears to be effective as a possible alternative to amphotericin, although further studies are required to compare the effectiveness of the two drugs.

The presence of abdominal pain and diarrhoea is taken by some to indicate the use of metronidazole in addition to standard antibiotics. Also increasingly used is vancomycin, either for Gram-positive systemic sepsis (i.v.) or gut infection with *Clostridium difficile* (orally).

During remission. With the evolution of more aggressive and prolonged induction regimens, especially during the period of profound lymphopenia seen after cranial irradiation, a subsequent high risk of *Pneumocystis carinii* pneumonitis became apparent (Hughes et al 1975, Siegel et al 1980). Affected patients presented with a high swinging fever, tachypnoea, progressive hypoxaemia and eventual complete respiratory failure. Frequently, there were few other abnormal physical signs, but the chest X-ray usually showed bilateral peribronchial infiltrates, progressing to diffuse shadowing, with an associated air bronchogram. In the MRC UKALL VIII Trial, 20% of patients developed this problem in the first 6 months after the introduction of the protocol, and 20% of these died (Darbyshire et al 1985). The subsequent introduction of prophylactic long-term cotrimoxazole (calculated on the basis of the dosage of trimethoprim in the mixture of 150 mg/m^2 per day given 3 times per week) has prevented any further patients developing the problem whilst taking the drug. However, the risk of pneumocystis appears to continue after withdrawal of chemotherapy until the regeneration of adequate immune surveillance has occurred (up to 6 months off treatment). If pneumonitis actually develops, higher doses of i.v. cotrimoxazole (calculated on the basis of 20 mg/kg per day of trimethoprim and 100 mg/kg per day of sulphamethoxazole) given in 2 divided doses is effective in about 80% of cases. In a few patients, the response is greatly improved if steroids are added to the cotrimoxazole, possibly by suppressing the inflammatory response to the antigen. Unresponsive patients may fare better on i.m. pentamidine, but this drug is nephrotoxic and can also produce

Table 12.11   MRC UKALL VIII Trial – deaths in first remission (n = 53)

Pneumonitis	10	Other viral:	
Measles	9	chickenpox	3
Pneumonia	5	herpes encephalitis	2
Septicaemia	5	flu	1
Other sepsis (meningitis)	3	other	1
		Encephalitis/	2
Bleeding (incl. one post liver biopsy)	5	encephalopathy	
		Post BMT	2
		Fibrosing alveolitis	2
		Road traffic accident	1
		Unknown	2

Data from Eden et al 1990a

profound hypoglycaemia. Dual infections with both *Pneumocystis carinii* and cytomegalovirus may be the reason for the poor response in some patients.

For patients with pneumonitis, Darbyshire et al (1985) reported that only half had evidence of pneumocystis by antibody detection, but new methods have been developed which detect the antigen in nasopharyngeal aspirates by immunofluorescence. Inhalation of nebulized pentamidine has been developed as a prophylactic measure for patients with HIV infection, but preliminary results in ALL patients do not suggest that it should replace oral prophylaxis with co-trimoxazole.

Table 12.11 shows deaths that occurred during remission in the MRC UKALL VIII Study. In the early part of remission until complete marrow recovery has occurred, bacterial infections remain a problem, but as immunosuppressive therapy continues the emphasis shifts towards viral infections, especially measles and chickenpox.

Measles. Although preventable by effective immunization programmes, measles remains the single most common cause of death in remission for children with ALL in the UK. With increasing vaccine uptake this risk may decline. Children with leukaemia who develop measles may initially have a mild illness without a noticeable rash. They can then develop either encephalitis (weeks or months after infection) or the more immediate giant cell pneumonitis, apparently out of the blue. Both have a near 100% mortality (Gray et al 1987). Human immunoglobulin in a dose of 1 g/m^2 i.m. given within 48–72 hours of a known contact may reduce the risk of a patient developing the disease, but the benefit of such therapy has never been shown in a controlled trial. Use of high-titre measles-specific immunoglobulin has also been used, as has interferon, in attempted therapy of established or presumed infection, but clear evidence of benefit is lacking (Simpson & Eden 1984).

Varicella. Children with cancer who contracted chickenpox or had reactivated zoster infections used to have a 10% mortality, but the introduction of the antiviral agent acyclovir, used either prophylactically or therapeutically, has dramatically reduced that risk. The usual doses are 400 mg 4 times daily for prophylaxis, and 10 mg/kg (5 mg/kg for herpes simplex) i.v. 8-hourly for the therapy of overt disease. The i.v. preparation must be given over an hour in at least 50 ml of normal saline. The drug is extremely well tolerated. Prophylaxis after contact should be for the full incubation period of 21 days, whilst therapy of overt infection should be i.v. for at least 5 days. Recent evidence suggests that protracted low-dose therapy may be required for several weeks to prevent recrudescence. Trials are currently in progress to assess the efficacy of i.v. acyclovir compared with 1 g/m^2 high-titre zoster-specific immunoglobulin given i.m. within 72 hours of contact with a case of chickenpox.

Other viruses. Other viruses, chiefly respiratory tract pathogens, can cause problems due to a failure of the immunosuppressed child to clear the infective agent, leading to its prolonged presence in nasopharyngeal secretions (Craft et al 1979). For such respiratory viruses there are few effective treatments, though nebulized ribavirin may prove useful for some patients during winter to prevent respiratory syncytial virus infection.

Haemorrhage

Children with ALL tend to bleed only when their platelet counts are very low (below $10 \times 10^9/l$), except in the presence of concomitant infection. There is no evidence to support the use of prophylactic platelet transfusions below any arbitrary platelet count; reasonable indications for such transfusions include epistaxes or other mucosal bleeding and/or a florid petechial rash. Cover may be needed for invasive procedures, such as the insertion of central venous catheters, where the aim should be to keep counts above $50 \times 10^9/l$ for 24 hours afterwards. The frequent use of platelet transfusions increases the risk of allo-antibody development and subsequent poor response. All children with newly diagnosed leukaemia or lymphoma should have their CMV immune status assessed, and only CMV-negative donors used for those with no immunity.

Biochemical disturbances

The most important biochemical problem seen in children with leukaemia is the tumour lysis syndrome. This is most frequently seen in T- and B-cell leukaemia (and lymphoma) where there is a high initial tumour load and rapid cell lysis at the start of treatment. Uric acid and oxypurines resulting from DNA and RNA breakdown precipitate in the renal tubules leading to renal failure. Potassium is released from the lysed cells leading to hyperkalaemia which can be exacerbated by secondary renal insufficiency. All of this can be complicated by tumour infiltration of the kidney or intrarenal haemorrhage (Tsokos et al 1981).

In addition, lymphoblasts have a high intracellular phosphate content which, when suddenly released into the circulation, can produce hyperphosphataemia and a compensatory hypocalcaemia. The combination of a high potassium and low calcium generates a risk of cardiac arrhythmias and cardiac arrest.

The tumour lysis syndrome can be controlled or avoided by a 'gentle' start to therapy in high-risk patients, the rapid control of infection, a high fluid intake (3 l/m^2 per day) to induce a diuresis, prior allopurinol (10 g/kg per day given in 2 or 3 divided doses) to lower uric acid levels, and urinary alkalinization to maintain a urine pH between 6 and 7. This requires some 3–6 milliequivalents of sodium bicarbonate/kg per day. Phosphate is not very soluble in alkaline urine, but at pH 7 uric acid is some 10–12 times more soluble, and xanthine more than twice as soluble as at pH 5. If the pH is pushed much above 7, there will be phosphate deposition in the urine and potentially in the tubules. Serum albumin concentration should be checked at diagnosis, as if it is low it will further affect calcium metabolism. Intravenous calcium should be avoided if possible since it is likely to be deposited in the tissues. For the symptoms of hypocalcaemia, especially tetany, systemic magnesium given either i.m. or slowly i.v. will be effective. Thiazide diuretics should be used only with extreme caution, since they can potentially exacerbate problems with uric acid. Undoubtedly the most important measure is to maintain a good diuresis. Occasional patients do require dialysis, but most develop a high urine output failure from which they will recover given adequate support. Hypercalcaemia has been reported in childhood leukaemia only very rarely.

Local tissue toxicity

Vincristine, adriamycin, daunomycin, cyclophosphamide and etoposide are toxic to tissues if they are allowed to extravasate during injection. Immediate intensive flushing with or without topical hyaluronidase, may ameliorate the problem.

Nausea and vomiting

Anthracyclines can cause severe but fairly short-lived nausea and vomiting, but the majority of antileukaemic agents, particularly those used during induction, are not emetogenic. However, with the increasing use of drug combinations during consolidation therapy, emesis is becoming more of a problem. The new range of 5'HT3 antagonists are showing great promise in alleviating the problem for patients with short sharp courses of emetogenic chemotherapy (Lancet 1987). Alternative regimens centre mostly round phenothiazines (with or without anxiolytics such as diazepam) or dexamethasone.

Mucositis

Both anthracyclines and methotrexate can cause oral and oesophageal mucositis which can become secondarily infected. For those developing oral ulceration on continuing therapy with oral methotrexate, the use of folinic acid mouthwash (3 mg/100 ml) has been claimed to ameliorate symptoms.

Other gastrointestinal disturbances

During induction therapy, the commonly produced vincristine constipation resulting from an autonomic neuropathy can occasionally progress to a full ileus. This may lead in turn to absorption of Gram-negative organisms across a static bowel with secondary enterocolitis and septicaemia. Consequently, regular use of stool softeners, such as lactulose, with attention to regular evacuation of the bowels is advisable during the induction period.

Asparaginase frequently produces loss of appetite and is also associated with a rise in blood urea secondary to disturbances of protein metabolism. More rarely, the drug can produce both hyperglycaemia (exacerbated by steroids) and other pancreatic dysfunction occasionally amounting to acute pancreatitis. Elevated serum amylase levels are frequently seen.

Renal tract toxicity

When cyclophosphamide is given, a good diuresis must be maintained for at least 24 hours afterwards to avoid haemorrhagic cystitis. The use of mesna (2-mercapto ethane sulphonate sodium) to reduce the risk is advisable when high doses are given.

Cardiac toxicity

The increasing use of anthracyclines in ALL protocols has inevitably been associated with an increased incidence of cardiac toxicity. Occasionally idiosyncratic, the problem is usually dose-dependent. Problems are unusual below a total cumulative dose of 450 mg/m^2 of adriamycin or daunomycin. Until recently, with less efficient ways of assessing cardiac function, there has been emphasis only upon ventricular systolic activity. New ultrasonography techniques suggest that the toxicity generates increased afterload due to endocardial muscle damage. Diastolic changes are detectable at lower cumulative dosage (Hausdorf et al 1988). Toxicity may be related more to peak drug concentrations rather than to total dosage given, and increasingly these agents are being given either as continuous infusions or as multiple small-dose pulses (Bielack et al 1989). The development of anthracycline analogues with possibly less cardiotoxicity, such as idarubicin and epirubicin, has helped, and such drugs may be preferred in the future. For patients receiving anthracyclines, careful echocardiographic monitoring of both ventricular and diastolic function is advisable, with cessation of the drug at the first sign of any dysfunction. Patients who have had a combination of anthracyclines with any chest or mediastinal irradiation appear to be at special risk. Congestive cardiac failure due to anthracycline-induced cardiomyopathy can be treated by diuretics and digoxin in some cases, but the long-term outlook for such patients appears to be poor. Transplantation may help a few.

Neurotoxicity

Vincristine is neurotoxic. The commonest manifestations are symmetrical peripheral neuropathy including loss of ankle jerks (over 90%), foot drop (5%) or wrist drop (2%), slapping gait, parasthesiae of the extremities and even convulsions and encephalopathy (rare). In young children, the drug can also produce an inappropriate antidiuretic hormone-like effect and a consequent dilutional hyponatraemia. Encephalopathy noted during induction therapy has frequently been blamed upon vincristine, but is more likely to be due to asparaginase, also known to be neurotoxic. Asparaginase elevates blood ammonia levels and depletes the brain of asparagine (an essential amino acid) occasionally leading to seizures and coma (Eden et al 1990d).

Vincristine may also cause severe pains, especially in the jaw, limbs or abdomen, but whether or not this is a neurological effect remains unclear. Abdominal pain may be associated with constipation secondary to an autonomic neuropathy.

Rarely, high-dose systemic methotrexate can produce an encephalopathy. More commonly, a combination of cranial irradiation with IT methotrexate, or IT methotrexate combined with systemic methotrexate, produces a slowly progressive leukoencephalopathy. The more therapeutic modalities that are used, the higher the risk of such a leucoencephalopathy. IT methotrexate alone seems to be the safest CNS treatment in this respect (Weiss et al 1975, Price & Jamieson 1975).

Hepatotoxicity

Chronic low-dose therapy with methotrexate can cause eventual cirrhosis, and oral mercaptopurine occasionally produces a cholestatic jaundice. High-dose systemic methotrexate can cause acute hepatitis along with mucositis and severe myelosuppression if folinic acid rescue is inadequate. The problem is exacerbated if the drug is administered with other agents, such as anthracyclines, which are normally metabolised by the liver.

Relapses

Bone marrow

The bone marrow is the commonest site of disease recurrence in ALL, and although second remissions can usually be obtained quite easily, the chance of long-term survival after relapse is poor, especially if the relapse has occurred whilst the patient is still on therapy (Cornbleet & Chessells 1978). In the MRC UKALL VIII Trial which closed in 1984, 115 marrow relapses (14% of entrants) had occurred at the time of writing, but only 22% of those patients remain alive in second remission. For the 54 who relapsed whilst on treatment, only 3 (5.7%) are still alive, (2 having had bone marrow allografts and one being treated with both induction and two pulses of intensive consolidation therapy). Relapses on treatment are indicative of tumour cell resistance to therapy. In contrast, for those relapsing off treatment, 24 out of 61 (39%) are alive in second remission, while those relapsing after more than a year off treatment do best of all (61% in second remission). Those with a low initial WBC at first presentation (below $10 \times 10^9/l$) who relapsed were more likely to do so off treatment. What percentage of those still in second remission will survive in the long term is not yet known. For on-treatment relapses there is clearly a need for a different approach to treatment, probably including marrow ablation and allogeneic or autologous bone marrow rescue. Patients relapsing within a year of stopping therapy may need similar new therapies. As treatment becomes more intensive, it is likely that the numbers of patients who relapse on treatment will decrease, but for those who do so, treatment is going to be even more difficult. It should also be noted that any successful second line treatment must include further CNS therapy (Rivera et al 1976).

CNS relapse

Between 1 and 3% of children with ALL will

present with overt CNS disease at diagnosis (Sullivan et al 1969, Eden et al 1990a) and up to 10% of patients will relapse in the CNS at some stage, despite treatment to prevent it (Table 12.10). Features which may predict an increased risk of CNS relapse include a high initial WBC (over $50 \times 10^9/l$), age under one year (and possibly over 10 years), a low initial platelet count, and a T- or B-cell immunophenotype. Paradoxically, if treated aggressively using initial IT methotrexate and subsequent craniospinal irradiation, patients with CSF blasts at diagnosis who have no actual neurological signs do not appear to have a worse prognosis. It is important to note that no-one has yet identified any specific subgroup of ALL with no risk of developing CNS disease, although girls age 3–6 years with a diagnostic WBC below $10 \times 10^9/l$ do appear to have a very low risk (Table 12.10).

Signs and symptoms. Meningeal leukaemia usually presents with features of raised intracranial pressure (Haghbin & Zeulzer 1965, Hardisty & Norman 1967). Disturbance of the arachnoid tissues interferes with CSF flow and absorption. Usually, all the ventricles are dilated and basal obstruction may be present. Headache, nausea, vomiting, lethargy and irritability are to be expected. Subtle personality changes are sometimes the first sign of developing CNS disease, with some patients developing anorexia, vertigo and ataxia, and experiencing visual disturbance (especially diplopia). Less commonly, patients present with convulsions or coma. Insatiable appetite and gross weight gain is a worrying symptom in the absence of steroid therapy, but is much more likely after repeated CNS relapse with advancing parenchymal infiltration of the hypothalamus (the so-called 'hypothalamic syndrome').

The most frequent signs are papilloedema (reported in 40–70% of cases; Hardisty & Norman 1967), nuchal rigidity, cranial nerve palsies (most commonly IIIrd, IVth, VIth and VIIth), weight gain and, in the young child, separation of cranial sutures. The absence of papilloedema does not exclude the diagnosis. Any patient presenting with headache and vomiting must be suspected of having meningeal disease until proved otherwise. Rarely, abdominal pain can occur and resolves with IT medication though the reason for this is not known (Koch et al 1966). Fever is uncommon but has been described. Within the CSF there is a monomorphic cytosis (with cell counts up to 60–$70 \times 10^9/l$), but occasionally the number of cells is low and presents diagnostic difficulties. Improved cytological preparations from sedimentation or cytocentrifugation permit more accurate morphological identification of lymphoblasts, and provide material for cytochemistry, immunophenotyping and even cytogenetic studies (Mastrangelo et al 1970).

The initial CSF cell count does not closely correlate with the subsequent response to treatment, but where there is greater than $1 \times 10^9/l$ blasts in the CSF, early recurrence can be expected (Hardisty & Norman 1967). In up to half the patients, the protein is elevated and glucose decreased, but neither are consistent findings (Sullivan et al 1969, Hyman et al 1965). The majority of patients have raised intrathecal pressure, with the median in one study being 335 ml of water (Hyman et al 1965). There is no correlation between IT pressure and CSF cell count. If a lumbar puncture (LP) is performed under general anaesthetic, the operator should be aware that most anaesthetic induction agents elevate the CSF pressure still further, but probably not as much as if the patient is crying and awake (Evans et al 1965). Despite high pressures, presumably because of the diffuse nature of the infiltration, lumbar puncture does not appear to be dangerous, and the risk of coning is low. On the other hand, if there is any suspicion of lateralizing signs, it is wise to perform a CT scan first to exclude the rare possibility of localized deposit or cerebral abscess where there is a much higher risk of uncal herniation.

Electroencephalogram (EEG) changes are frequently present, and include diffuse dysrrythmias with nonspecific alpha- and delta- wave activity, but these are not diagnostically helpful (Hyman et al 1965). There has been speculation that an LP performed early in the course of ALL, when cytopenia is combined with circulating leukaemic blast cells, might increase the risk of CNS leukaemia due to intrathecal bleeding and consequent cell seeding. There is no supportive evidence for such a hypothesis, but the possibility cannot be completely excluded, so IT methotrexate should always be given. Overt bleeding is very rare, but extensive spinal subarachnoid haemorrhage with local haematoma has been described with platelets below $10 \times 10^9/l$ (Sullivan and Windmiller 1966). Some physicians choose to cover patients for their initial LP with a platelet transfusion, but most feel this to be unnecessary.

The best way of treating overt CNS disease remains uncertain. To develop rational therapy it is necessary to understand the pathology of neuroleukaemia. Circulating blast cells are deposited in multiple sites when microhaemorrhages occur, including in the walls of the superficial arachnoid veins (Price & Johnson 1973). The cells migrate into the surrounding adventitia, destroying the arachnoid trabeculae with access to CSF channels over the brain surface (Thomas 1965). Further expansion impinges on the grey and white matter, disrupts the pia-glial membrane and finally, at a very late stage, directly infiltrates neural tissue. True parenchymal infiltration is rare and only seen after multiple relapses, and the very rare multifocal parenchymal disease cannot easily be explained by any understood pathogenic mechanisms (Moore et al 1960). It is assumed that nearly all children with ALL will have leukaemic cells in the walls of the arachnoid veins at diagnosis, forming the basis of the rationale for CNS-directed therapy. When such therapy fails, it suggests either drug or radiotherapy resistance or, more probably, that the therapy has been inadequate by failing to penetrate the tissue around arachnoid veins or to deal with the initial cell bulk where this is unusually large.

It appears to be quite easy to clear the CSF of blasts by using weekly IT injections of either methotrexate alone or a combination of methotrexate, cytarabine and hydrocortisone (Murphy 1959, Sullivan et al 1971). The triple-drug approach has been reported to increase CNS remission duration, but is more toxic. In early studies of CNS relapse, nearly all patients died of marrow relapse which soon followed, not of the neurological problems (Evans 1964, Hyman at al 1965, Hardisty 1969). In a more recent series in the UK, 23 of 116 children who had a CNS relapse were alive up to 10 years later but, worryingly, 50% were severely limited neurologically or educationally (Darbyshire 1990). Most received IT methotrexate to clear the CSF and then craniospinal irradiation (24 Gy to the cranium, 12 Gy to the spine). This approach produced reasonable CNS disease control but proved very damaging for the survivors. The use of intraventricular reservoirs and regular intraventricular methotrexate injections is equally neurotoxic in those who have had previous CNS irradiation, but may give longer remissions (Haghbin & Galicich 1979). The damaging effect of retreatment of the CNS may be mitigated in future, since cranial irradiation is becoming progressively less used as primary CNS-directed therapy. Future patients with CNS relapse will most often previously have received IT methotrexate alone or in combination with systemic high-dose methotrexate, and will be more able to tolerate radiotherapy at the time of their relapse. It appears that a double dose of radiotherapy, which some now receive for CNS relapse, is too toxic. There appears to be less risk of subsequent leukoencephalopathy if high-dose methotrexate is followed by radiotherapy (particularly if the two are well separated in time), rather than the other way round which is very toxic.

Since systemic relapse is the main problem in terms of life expectancy, even after multiple CNS relapses, a recent pilot study has offered an alternative way of dealing with isolated CNS relapse (Mandell et al 1990). Clearance of CSF blasts is achieved with either IT or intraventricular medication (methotrexate and cytosine), and this is coupled with intensive systemic chemotherapy. Consolidation of CNS remission using craniospinal irradiation (18 Gy to the cranium, 12 Gy to the spine) is delayed for some 12 months from time of relapse. As most systemic relapses following CNS disease occur at about 6–8 months, this approach enables the major risk period of systemic relapse to be passed and prevents the need for repeated CNS-directed therapy, particularly in those patients who have not previously received cranial irradiation. If systemic relapse *does* occur, it can be treated with high-dose IT methotrexate together with a full programme of other systemic therapy. If such children subsequently stay in remission for a year or more, then they can be given irradiation. None of the patients controlled in this way has had a subsequent CNS relapse. Five out of the 9 patients in the series are now off treatment in remission at a range of 31–46 months from diagnosis. This is a small, but promising, study and supports the idea that a good approach to CNS disease, particularly when it arises on treatment, should be reinduction, marrow ablation, total body irradiation and bone marrow transplantation. This will be an easier option to pursue if patients have not previously received irradiation.

Testicular relapse

Boys with a high initial WBC and low platelet counts can have a testicular relapse during treatment, or even present with testicular swelling (Nesbit et al 1980, MRC 1978). Gonadal involvement of this type is simply an indicator of extensive disease and is associated with a poor prognosis. For such patients, salvage rates are low, even with aggressive reinduction, consolidation, local irradiation and bone marrow transplantation. Of the UK MRC children enrolled in the first three UKALL Trials (522 in all) 9 patients had an isolated testicular relapse on treatment and all died (MRC 1978). More relapses occurred after stopping treatment, and 29 out of 60 were apparently isolated without obvious CNS or bone marrow disease. Infiltration is usually present bilaterally, but clinically the picture is usually one of unilateral, painless swelling (MRC 1978, Stoffel et al 1975). Baum et al (1979) demonstrated that by more invasive investigation evidence of disease at sites other than the marrow and CSF can often be found. This is important, because so-called 'isolated' testicular relapse is probably merely indicative of residual disease rather than of relapse in a 'sanctuary' site like the CNS. For this reason, treatment must not be directed simply towards local control but should include a full programme of systemic treatment for 2 years. Tiedemann et al (1982) demonstrated long-term control in nearly all patients with such an aggressive approach, whereas when the emphasis is placed on local 'sanctuary' therapy, as in the early UK MRC children, less than one-third subsequently achieved long-term remission.

Assuming that the testis is a site of residual disease rather than a sanctuary, there have been attempts to predict 'at-risk' boys by elective biopsy before stopping treatment. This does not appear to be helpful. There are too many false negatives, too many equivocal biopsies (even when bilateral wedges are taken), and even occasional false positives (Eden & Rankin 1980). Attempts to improve identification of lymphoblasts using immunofluorescence to detect cells containing Tdt have not been successful. In the series reported by Thomas et al (1982), two biopsies were histologically negative and Tdt-positive, but no subsequent relapse of any sort has occurred in either patient.

Prophylactic testicular irradiation has been used, either alone (Eden et al 1990) or in combination with more extensive abdominal field irradiation (Nesbit et al 1982). Irradiation of the testes given at the same time as CNS prophylaxis appears to prevent subsequent testicular relapse, but affords no overall benefit in terms of disease-free survival in those receiving it as compared with those who do not (Eden et al 1990c). Testicular radiotherapy has the disadvantage of virtually ensuring subsequent sterility, and frequently has an effect on Leydig cell function as well – particularly in very young children (Shalet et al 1977). For these reasons, prophylactic testicular irradiation is no longer recommended.

Relapse at other sites

In early studies, multiple organ involvement was commonly found at post mortem examination and an equal incidence of ovarian and testicular involvement (Nesbit et al 1965). However, clinically presenting ovarian disease is rare. Children with B-ALL do occasionally present with massive ovarian disease, and girls off treatment can present with large pelvic masses as the main site of recurrence. This usually heralds subsequent systemic relapse.

Cardiac, pulmonary, bowel and renal disease, although reported in early studies, have very rarely presented as isolated recurrence sites in recent years (Nies et al 1965). There have been some isolated ocular deposits, particularly in the anterior chamber, where there may be a degree of sanctuary from normal drug concentrations and where the site is protected from standard cranial radiotherapy fields (Ninane 1980). However, in the 5 patients described by Hustu & Aur (1978) there was a strong suggestion that the problem was associated with previous or subsequent CNS relapse. The treatment should probably be similar.

Bone marrow transplantation (BMT) in ALL

At present, the most aggressive therapy for ALL is bone marrow ablation and reconstitution with donor marrow from a matched sibling, matched unrelated donor, or with the patient's own, previously harvested, either purged or nonpurged marrow.

Current conventional indications for bone marrow transplantation (BMT) in first remission would appear to be patients with initial WBC greater than $100 \times 10^9/l$ and, more controversially, those with specific cytogenetic translocations (such as the Philadelphia chromosome) in whom achieving complete remission and maintaining it has appeared to be very difficult in the past. Infants with null cell ALL and B-cell leukaemia with CNS involvement may also benefit. Since only approximately 1 in 4 have fully matched siblings, the possibility of allogeneic transplantation from a family member is limited. Whether there is a place for autologous BMT in those without a matched donor, as is now being tested in acute myeloid leukaemia, remains unclear. The techniques of matched unrelated donor BMT and haploidentical transplantation are not yet well enough established to justify widespread use, but there may be a place for such procedures in the future (Gale & Champlin 1986).

Following relapse, the indications for BMT change, but as with conventional chemotherapy, success depends on the timing of the relapse. Those relapsing on treatment apparently do as poorly following transplantation as those receiving chemotherapy alone (Chessells et al 1986). Overall, however, if a second remission can be achieved and maintained, then BMT does appear to offer better results than chemotherapy in the longer term (Woods et al 1983). There has, perhaps, been a tendency to transplant too early before the achievement of a sustainable remission. Patients who appear to benefit most from transplantation are those who relapse off treatment.

'Bad' players

The main therapeutic challenge at present is to identify reliably high-risk patients with ALL and devise new strategies for their management. However, numerically, the majority of relapses still occur in the presence of features which are not recognized as being unfavourable. There is much to be done to understand the true nature of the disease in such patients or how they as individuals differ in their response to antineoplastic drugs.

Tumour cell resistance

Much interest has recently arisen in tumour cell drug resistance and how to circumvent it. There are a number of known mechanisms which enable tumour cells to survive (Erttman 1989). Drugs may not actually be reaching tumour cells in adequate concentrations and this mechanism may well apply to minimal CNS disease around arachnoid vessels. Apparent resistance may arise because of poor bio-availability of a drug, rapid metabolism of that drug, or its rapid elimination.

Secondary, rather than primary, resistance is the most common problem, with relapse occurring after an initial response. Resistance can develop against a single agent or against a battery of cytotoxic drugs. It was to avoid the development of such resistance that combination chemotherapy was developed. The rationale is to expose tumour cells to a range of agents in as short a time as possible, hoping that the drugs will have complementary or synergistic effects. This approach forms the basis of the Goldie-Coldman hypothesis (Goldie et al 1982).

A number of different mechanisms are recognized whereby tumour cells intrinsically develop drug resistance. Overamplification of the gene for dihydrofolate reductase has been demonstrated, for example (Curt et al 1983), as has enhanced transcription of that gene (Simonsen & Levison 1983). As the enzyme is the target for methotrexate, this drug will be less effective in the presence of high enzyme levels. An enzyme with low affinity for methotrexate has also been described.

Reduced transport of drugs into cells and their enhanced removal is now well documented. Again for methotrexate, there is evidence of inhibition of folate-specific transmembranal transportation, inhibition of methotrexate polyglutamation (essential for effective action), and also activation of thymidine salvage pathways to counteract the methotrexate effect. Enhanced drug elimination from cells has been demonstrated with many drugs ranging from vinca alkaloids to the anthracyclines. Juliano & Ling (1976) and Roninson et al (1984) demonstrated activation of what has now become known as the multiple-drug-resistant (MDR) gene, which codes for P-glycoprotein, a complex molecule which facilitates the removal of drugs from cells. P-glycoprotein overexpression does appear to be the principle mechanism causing pleiotropic resistance and, although only present in a small percentage of patients at diagnosis, is seen in many more at the time of relapse (Kartner et al 1985, Fojo et al 1987). Other cells appear to develop enhanced biochemical detoxification. A number of agents, including the anthracyclines and alkylating agents, as well as irradiation, produce active metabolites which the glutathione redox system renders harmless (Kramer et al 1988). Overproduction of glutathione by cells inactivates these metabolites and resistance can develop. Enhanced glutathione redox activity may coexist with overexpression of the MDR gene. Compensatory hypertrophy of DNA repair systems has also been shown following exposure to alkylating agents and anthracyclines, and some patients have developed apparent resistance to those agents due to enhanced DNA repair.

To some extent, resistance can be overcome by application of the Goldie-Coldman model and giving rapidly alternating drug therapy in as short a time as possible. An alternative is to use high-dose chemotherapy, such as methotrexate (with the ability to reverse potential toxicity with folinic acid) or other drugs (using some sort of marrow replacement as a rescue technique).

Evidence is accumulating to indicate that the effect of P-glycoprotein can be inhibited by agents such as verapamil and cyclosporin which block the outward pumping of cytotoxic drugs (Tsuruo 1983). Such drugs have their own side-effects, particularly verapamil, which is cardiotoxic. Similarly, glutathione production can be inhibited by buthione sulphoximine and is under investigation for use with alkylating agents.

Table 12.12 Potential long-term sequelae of childhood leukaemia and lymphoma

Late reccurence
Secondary neoplasia
Growth impairment
Endocrine dysfunction
Infertility
Education and psychological dysfunction
Other organ toxicity, e.g. cardiopulmonary
Problems with obtaining jobs and insurance and acceptance as adopters

Long-term sequelae

Table 12.12 shows some of the potential long-term sequelae for children treated for ALL and lymphoma.

Late recurrence

Hawkins et al (1989) showed in an historical series of ALL patients that only 60% of patients who survived 3 years from diagnosis were still alive at 10 years. There was an excess death rate in these long-term survivors (1 in 100), principally due to boys having late relapses. There have been reports of boys relapsing up to 18 years from diagnosis, but very few girls have relapsed beyond 6 years in their first remission.

Second tumours

A survivor of any childhood cancer has a risk of developing a second neoplasm which has been estimated to be in the range of 4–8% at 20 years (Meadows 1988). Despite ALL being the single most common childhood cancer, it is well down on the list of tumours associated with the development of secondary neoplasms. Where second tumours have arisen, the most common types have been brain tumours and secondary acute myeloid leukaemia.

Growth impairment

Most children with ALL, in common with all children with cancer, show a slowing of growth during the early stages of treatment with later catch-up, but cranial and spinal irradiation have a measurable impact on eventual height reached. Old protocols using spinal irradiation produced a considerable shortening effect on spinal length. Cranial irradiation at the dosages usually used for leukaemia (18–24 Gy) affects growth hormone release, and later also gonadotrophin and adrenocorticotrophic hormones. Most children given standard therapy during the l970s and 1980s have some evidence of impairment of overall height achieved (Shalet et al 1988); this is of the order of -1 standard deviation from the expected. There also appears to be more marked growth impairment with more intensive chemotherapy regimens, and some drugs may have an additive effect with that of cranial irradiation, though longer follow-up is required to clarify this. Some patients, usually girls, show premature onset of puberty with rapid progress through the various stages. This also influences the ability to achieve full growth potential. For children who have shown normal prepubertal growth but appear unable to produce adequate growth hormone release during puberty, some physicians now delay puberty and give additional growth hormone. In patients receiving total body irradiation for marrow transplantation, growth impairment is to be expected. Response to replacement therapy may be disappointing as a result of spinal shortening, thyroid deficiency, impaired direct bone growth from epiphysial damage, chronic graft-versus-host reaction and chronic malnutrition. Such patients may also have pituitary damage resulting in failure of growth hormone production rather than its release.

Premature puberty and failure to reach full growth potential may be associated with obesity. It is presently unclear whether this is a true reflection of hypothalamic dysfunction leading to dietary excess. Long-term accurate monitoring of growth is essential for any long-term leukaemia survivor (Leiper 1990).

Other endocrine dysfunction

Occasionally children who previously received spinal irradiation develop thyroid dysfunction. Any lymphoma patient who has received neck irradiation is likely to have impairment of thyroid function, manifest initially as a rise in TSH with subsequent thyroid failure.

Other endocrine problems in children with ALL are very uncommon, except in those receiving whole body irradiation prior to transplantation, where ovarian failure and infertility in girls is seen. Gonadal dysfunction in boys who have had total body irradiation is less predictable, but those who receive 20–24 Gy for the treatment of overt testicular relapse (or even lower prophylactic doses) show almost complete ablation of the germinal epithelium. Very young boys are likely to have associated Leydig cell dysfunction as well (Shalet 1989).

As far as drug effects on gonadal function are concerned, both cyclophosphamide and cytosine have been shown to have an effect on testicular germinal epithelium, although some recovery of spermatogenesis has been reported following the end of treatment. Leydig cell function appears to be undamaged.

Long-term fertility of children treated in a conventional way without spinal or total body irradiation remains unclear. Many girls have had children following a full programme of therapy and a few boys have successfully fathered children, but some will be infertile. Infertility may increase following more recent intensive therapy schedules.

Educational and psychological dysfunction

Any serious illness with much time lost from school will retard educational achievement, albeit temporarily. Most attempts to measure this have been performed on patients where additional factors complicate the situation. The peak age for the presentation of leukaemia is between 3 and 6 years, which is the time of maximum learning for basic literacy and numeracy. Time lost at this stage may be crucial. Additionally, CNS therapy produces neuropsychological sequelae, with the youngest children (below 3 years) most affected (Jannoun 1983). Cognitive function is impaired, with short-term memory defects and difficulty in problem solving (Eiser 1978, Moss et al 1981). Although overall IQ may remain within the normal range, performance will be disproportionately impaired compared with verbal IQ. Some defects can be overcome by remedial help and repetitive learning. It is hoped that current strategies to try to avoid cranial irradiation with the use of high-dose systemic methotrexate and IT therapy will produce less damaging effects.

Surveys of long-term survivors show them often to have a rather relaxed approach to life, with some underachievement of their potential. Questionnaires indicate that they place considerable emphasis on maintaining good health and avoiding hazards such as smoking, but frequently, even up to 20 years later, express worries about the possible recurrence of their disease.

Other organ toxicity

Late cardiac toxicity due to anthracylines has been described. Pulmonary function has also recently been studied in a cohort of long survivors (at least 5 years off therapy), and 65% had one or more of the following defects: low vital capacity, total lung capacity, residual volume or transfer factor (Shaw et al 1990). Few patients were symptomatic, but the most likely explanation of these changes is impairment of lung growth which could have clinical importance in later life, especially for anyone who is a smoker.

Life prospects

The vast majority of those treated in childhood for leukaemia complete normal education (Allen et al 1990), and may even have slightly higher employment prospects than their peers, although they tend to prefer jobs which are perhaps beneath their true capabilities (Malpas 1988).

Some employers, and some insurance and pension companies penalize long survivors, so it is important to gather data to reassure their actuaries.

NON-HODGKIN'S LYMPHOMA

Tables 12.1 and 12.2 (p. 329) show the worldwide variation in incidence of childhood non-Hodgkin's lymphomas (NHL). The heterogeneity is mostly due to the great geographical variation in the incidence of B-cell lymphoma, but partly also to that of T-cell tumours. Childhood NHL is twice as common in boys as in girls. Compared with adults, the range of types found in childhood is very narrow. Histologically, nearly all are diffuse rather than nodular, overwhelmingly dissemi-

nated, and their pattern of dissemination follows the disposition of the lymphoid immune system.

Aetiology

The childhood immune system consists of many different end stage functional cells as well as a wide array of precursor and stem cells. Malignancy can occur at any stage in lymphocyte ontogeny, and monoclonal antibodies have helped to define the differentiation process of both normal and malignant lymphocytes. Like adults, young children are constantly exposed to antigens, but unlike adults they do not have a large immune memory bank to help them to recognize and repel them. As a result, a large proportion of lymphoid cells during childhood are in a very active state, undergoing molecular rearrangements to produce specific immunoglobulins and other factors required for the normal immune response. For B-cells to function, the genes which regulate the different components of immunoglobulin production have to be brought together or rearranged. In T-cells, the genes which control T-cell antigen receptor molecules similarly need to be organized. The immunoglobulin heavy chain genes are on chromosome 14 (q24), the lambda light chain genes on chromosome 22 (q11), and the kappa light chain genes on chromosome 2 (p11). For B-cells to function properly, the rearrangments must occur in an ordered sequence.

The T-cell receptor genes are on chromosome 14 (q35–6; beta locus). A complete molecule requires two chains; an alpha from chromosome 14 and a beta from chromosome 7. In normal health, the rearrangement process to produce the product of the receptor gene is very similar to that for immunoglobulin gene rearrangements.

Malignant change can occur when genetic defects arise secondary to deletion, mutation or translocation. This can interrupt the normal orderly process, but what actually initiates the disorganization is not clear.

Accumulating evidence incriminates viruses, at least in some lymphomas. The products from retroviruses HTLVl and HTLV2 rearrange genes within the host cell, thus stimulating production of interleukin 2 and its receptor which can activate T cell proliferation. Clonal or polyclonal proliferation provides the opportunity for a second 'strike' which may be necessary to produce a malignant clone. Adult T-cell leukaemia or lymphoma can be produced in such a fashion. The involvement of EBV in the aetiology of Burkitt's lymphoma has been described earlier, but the rearrangements seen in that particular condition all involve the translocation of c-myc gene close to immunoglobulin constant region sequences. This oncogene appears to be necessary for proliferation, and its translocation appears to activate it (Magrath 1990). For other lymphomas, translocations have not been so consistently found.

The enzyme Tdt appears to be intimately involved in T-cell gene rearrangements; it persists in cells from lymphoblastic lymphomas and ALL, but is not found in mature B-cell ALL or lymphoma. It serves as a useful marker to distinguish T- from B-cell disease. Both T-ALL and NHL occur in precursor T-cells, commonly of a thymic origin. The suggestion that they represent malignancy of different stages of T-cell development has not been borne out consistently. B-cell tumours arise from B-cell precursors and tend to appear in the gut or associated lymph nodes.

In adults, NHL is more commonly nodal and arises from more mature cells. In children this is not the case, apart from Burkitt's lymphoma which appears to be a malignancy of EBV memory B-cells (Murphy 1980).

Aetiological factors other than viruses associated with the development of lymphoma have been discussed in the preceding section on leukaemia (see Table 12.3). Attention should be drawn to NHL associated with acquired or congenital immune deficiency syndromes and secondary lymphomas following treatment for other childhood tumours (Meadows 1988).

Classification of NHL

A confusing array of classifications exists for NHL, but in childhood none bears much relationship to present understanding of the cell of origin or the pattern of behaviour of an individual tumour.

Since Burkitt (1958) first described the geographical distribution of the characteristic jaw tumour which bears his name, it has been classi-

fied as lymphoid malignancy of undifferentiated type according to the Rappaport system (Rappaport & Braylon 1975), and as a small noncleaved follicular centre cell tumour according to Lukes & Collins (1975). Lukes & Collins described a T-cell lymphoma of convoluted lymphocytes, but Nathwani (1976) called this a lymphoblastic lymphoma to distinguish it from poorly differentiated lymphocytic lymphoma, which is much more frequently seen in adults. To avoid confusion in childhood NHL, it is perhaps best to classify tumours according to the following National Cancer Institute Working Formulation:

1. Lymphoblastic lymphomas, including both convoluted and nonconvoluted types, are mostly of T-cell origin though some are derived from early B-cells. They are diffuse and of high-grade malignancy. The histology is indistinguishable from the cells seen in ALL, and both T-ALL and NHL arise from early thymocytes. T-NHL, however, is more frequently of intermediate or late T-cell type. All T-cell tumours have a high propensity for marrow infiltration and CNS involvement as the disease evolves.

2. All small-cell non-cleaved types of lymphoma, including Burkitt's and non-Burkitt's type, are also diffuse and of high grade, and are mature B-cell tumours.

3. Large cell lymphomas comprise about 15–20% of all childhood NHL and include both large noncleaved and cleaved cells. About half are of intermediate-grade malignancy, the rest are diffuse and high grade. Again, most are of B-cell origin but a few arise from T-cells. There are a few large cell lymphomas (with surface expression of the Ki-1 antigen) which are classified as immunoblastic (Offit et al 1990). Characteristically they involve lymph node sinuses, and often present with skin lesions and lymphadenopathy. They tend to be associated with better survival than other large cell lymphomas. A few large-cell lymphomas are truly histiocytic and not lymphoid malignancies at all.

The increasing use of immunophenotyping has led to some reclassification, including identification of some lymphoblastic lymphomas with natural killer cell characteristics. Where lymphomas infiltrate the bone marrow, they are still classified as lymphomas, provided there is less than 25% marrow infiltration. Above that level, blood changes may start to appear and the patient is then deemed to have leukaemia, but this threshold is quite arbitrary and currently under review. For some of the B-cell lymphomas there may be extensive marrow infiltration (up to 60–70%) without excessive nodal disease, and such patients without peripheral blasts do better than those with massive nodal disease.

A problem with published studies of childhood NHL is that there has been disagreement between pathologists when reviewing the histology. Particular problems appear to be the distinction between small noncleaved and large-cell lymphomas, and separating Burkitt's from non-Burkitt's type. Perhaps for this reason, no consistent correlation between histology and survival has been recorded. Clinical management is based more on the cell of origin than on histological appearances.

Growth fraction

The majority of childhood lymphomas are rapidly growing tumours with a high growth fraction. They also have a high natural cell death rate, so there is the potential for a tumour lysis syndrome to arise even without therapy. Tumour doubling time may be only 2–3 days.

Clinical features

Childhood NHL presents in a huge variety of ways depending on the site of the primary lymphoid mass and the degree of dissemination. Some characteristic broad clinical patterns are seen in the various subtypes of disease:

Lymphoblastic lymphoma. Up to two-thirds of patients present with a mediastinal mass with or without pleural effusion. Frequently, there are signs of superior vena caval obstruction with dysphagia, dyspnoea and pericardial effusion. Lymphadenopathy is usually confined to the neck and axillae. Abdominal node enlargement is rare, but hepatosplenomegaly is common, as is bone marrow involvement (in more than 50% of cases) and CNS infiltration. Occasionally, lymphoblastic lymphomas present peripherally, with primary skin involvement or bone disease. Such atypical

types are frequently found to have a more mature T-cell phenotype.

Small noncleaved tumours. In Europe, these present most frequently as large abdominal tumours with pain and swelling.

There are two commonly recognized types: Type 1 are localized tumours of the bowel wall, most commonly in the terminal ileum (thought to arise in the Peyer's patches), which can lead to intussusception or bleeding with or without perforation of the bowel. Patients most often present with a right iliac fossa mass and are sometimes thought to have appendicitis or an appendix abscess.

Type 2 are diffuse abdominal tumours with involvement throughout the omentum and mesentery, often including infiltration into the kidney, the liver and the spleen. In such tumours, bone marrow and CNS disease are common. A few cases can present with jaw involvement (whereas in the African type of Burkitt's tumour this is almost universal). In equatorial Africa, jaw disease most frequently involves multiple quadrants, but orbital tumours involving the maxillary bone also occur. Abdominal involvement is present in about 50% of African jaw tumour cases. There is a lower incidence of bone marrow involvement in African, compared with non-African, Burkitt's disease (Magrath 1987).

Localized disease. Lymphoid swelling can occur anywhere, but most commonly arises in the neck, and can be of any cell type. There appears to be a fairly low risk in these localized tumours of CNS spread, despite their primary origin in the neck.

Pharyngeal involvement. Primary pharyngeal lymphomas occasionally arise and are usually of B-cell origin.

Isolated testicular disease. Primary testicular lymphomas are rare and usually of lymphoblastic type with a tendency to rapid dissemination. Lymphomas at unusual sites often have large cell histology.

CNS involvement. This is most often secondary spread from disease elsewhere and is seen particularly in lymphoblastic and Burkitt's B-cell lymphoma of the small, cleaved cell type. It leads to headache, vomiting, papilloedema, cranial nerve dysfunction and seizures. It is much more common at diagnosis if the bone marrow is also infiltrated, but is occasionally seen in patients with localized disease and those with large cell histology. Primary cerebral lymphomas arise very rarely.

Diagnostic investigations

The aim of investigation is to confirm the diagnosis as quickly as possible and determine the extent of disease. Chest X-ray is required initially to assess any mediastinal mass and/or pericardial and pleural effusions.

Biopsy

Excision biopsy is indicated in the presence of accessible localized disease. Immunophenotyping, cytogenetics and routine histology can be carried out on the fresh tissue. In more extensive disease, material should be obtained from the most accessible tumour. It is usually preferable to obtain specimens by open biopsy, since there is a risk of an unrepresentative sample from fine needle aspiration.

Table 12.13 St Jude modified staging system for non-Hodgkin's lymphoma

Stage		Approximate % by stage seen in UK
I	Single tumour (extranodal) or single anatomic area (nodal) Not mediastinum or abdomen	5
II	Single tumour (extranodal) with regional node involvement. Primary GI tumour with or without involvement of associated mesenteric nodes only. On the same side of diaphragm: a. Two or more nodal areas b. Two single (extranodal) tumours with or without regional node involvement.	20
III	On both sides of the diaphragm: a. Two single tumours (extranodal) b. Two or more nodal areas. All primary intrathoracic tumours (mediastinal, pleural, thymic); all extensive primary intraabdominal disease; all primary paraspinal or epidural tumours regardless of other sites.	50
IV	Any of the above with initial CNS or bone marrow involvement ($<25\%$)	25

Bone marrow aspiration

Bone marrow needs to be examined from at least two sites, preferably four, with the ideal of two aspirates and two trephines from different sites. Marrow should be examined cytogenetically and immunologically as well as cytomorphologically.

Lumbar puncture

Provided there is no evidence of raised intracranial pressure, CSF should be examined. If there are signs of the intracranial pressure being high, a CT or NMR scan should be carried out before an LP is performed to ensure that there is no focal deposit with consequent risk of brain shift.

Ultrasonography

Abdominal ultrasonography is often the most effective and rapid way to define liver, spleen and kidney involvement. It can often be carried out without sedation, whereas general anaesthesia is often required in young children for CT scanning or other lengthy imaging techniques.

Other imaging procedures

Bones scans are only indicated if there is focal bone pain. Gallium and thallium scans have been used to detect occult disease, but they are not specific and require further evaluation. Small, noncleaved cell lymphomas take up gallium very avidly. CT or NMR scanning may be useful to define the extent of unusual tumours and for the exclusion of nodal intracerebral deposits.

Blood tests

Initial investigations should include a full blood count, liver and renal function studies, lactate dehydrogenase levels, and serum urate, calcium, potassium and urea levels. Recent evidence suggests that serum levels of interleukin 2R may correlate well with prognosis, at least in some forms of childhood NHL, but this requires further evaluation (Magrath 1990).

Staging

Table 12.13 shows the most commonly used staging system for childhood NHL (Murphy 1980). All primary mediastinal and diffuse abdominal tumours are considered to be at least stage III. Spread in NHL, unlike in Hodgkin's disease, is not orderly and is not contiguous from node to node. There does not appear to be a place for routine staging laparotomy or lymphangiography.

Prognostic factors

The most important prognostic factor appears to be the tumour load at diagnosis. There may be some correlation of stage with interleukin 2R levels and also, in B-cell lymphomas, with antibody titres to early EBV antigen. Historically, the worst prognosis used to be seen in patients with advanced stage B-cell disease, particularly those with a large abdominal mass, bone marrow involvement and CNS disease, but new approaches to therapy may have changed the outlook (Patte et al 1986, Hann et al 1990).

Treatment

In the past, clinical excision of localized disease with adjuvant radiotherapy appeared to offer the only cure for any form of NHL. Such therapy was standard until the mid 1970s. Single-drug therapy, particularly cyclophosphamide, produced some benefit for patients with radioresistant disease, such as Burkitt's lymphoma. The introduction of multi-agent therapy, particularly the combination of cyclophosphamide, methotrexate and vincristine, showed improved results over single-drug therapy for patients with B-cell lymphomas. In the mid 1970s, the realization that even apparently localized T-cell lymphoma very closely resembled T-cell ALL led to the use of ALL therapy for lymphoma patients, with a dramatic improvement in their survival (Wollner et al 1976). Since the majority of lymphomas are disseminated high-grade tumours, chemotherapy is now the preferred option for all stages. Even for apparently localized disease, surgery followed by adjuvant chemotherapy appears to have an advantage over irradiation, and radiotherapy now has a very limited role. In an emergency, it is occasionally used to relieve mediastinal compression or renal obstruction, although even in these cir-

cumstances chemotherapy appears to be equally effective (Kingston 1987). Surgery is used for biopsy and occasionally for the removal of any localized lymphoid masses, particularly those interfering with intestinal function. Whether attempts to debulk diffuse abdominal disease surgically is of any value remains unclear, but the morbidity probably outweighs the advantages. Current chemotherapy has developed along the following lines:

Lymphoblastic lymphomas. Intensive multi-agent chemotherapy has produced a good response in 60–80% of patients with disseminated lymphoblastic lymphomas, and over 90% with localized tumours (Wollner 1976, Muller-Weihrich 1985). For stage 3 and 4 disease, 2 years of ALL-type treatment appears best, together with some form of CNS-directed therapy (either cranial irradiation or high-dose systemic methotrexate). It is a mistake in patients with T-lymphoblastic lymphoma to consider surgical debulking in order to relieve pressure on the superior vena cava from a mediastinal mass. Mediastinal shrinkage will occur very rapidly with steroids alone in most cases.

General anaesthesia is contraindicated if there is any suggestion of superior vena caval or airway compression or any large pericardial effusion. Occasionally, a mediastinal mass is the only evidence of disease and biopsy is necessary, but material can be obtained through a small parasternal incision or even by mediastinoscopy without the need to open the chest itself. Most often, however, such patients have peripheral nodes which can be biopsied, or bone marrow involvement.

Patients with bulky disease have a high risk of spontaneous or treatment-precipitated tumour lysis syndrome (Tsokos et al 1981). Occasionally, the pleural or pericardial effusions which occur in this type of lymphoma may require to be tapped to relieve symptoms, but in general such effusions disappear rapidly after the start of treatment. CNS disease at diagnosis requires IT methotrexate to clear the CSF and relieve symptoms. High doses of systemic steroids may reduce intracranial pressure and in about 50% of patients will also reduce the CSF blast cell concentration. Occasionally there may be infiltration of the facial or optic nerves, or even a direct extension into the brain.

For such patients urgent radiotherapy is required. Most centres now treat stage 3 and 4 T-cell lymphomas in exactly the same way as they would T-cell ALL.

Localized lymphoma. Localized disease is generally associated with an excellent prognosis and over 90% long-term disease-free survival. The treatment of choice is excision biopsy, followed by adjuvant chemotherapy of much shorter duration than that for disseminated lymphoblastic lymphoma. The chemotherapy does not have to be as intensive as that used for ALL or stage 3 lymphoma (Wollner et al 1976). The second series of UKCCSG NHL studies for localized lymphomas recruited 57 patients who were treated for a 6-month chemotherapy protocol for stage 1 and 2 disease of all types. At the time of writing, only three have relapsed and all three had lymphoblastic disease (Gerrard & Mott 1990). It appears that nonlymphoblastic localized lymphomas can be successfully treated with short-course chemotherapy and attention is now being focused on ways to reduce the long-term sequelae of therapy. Cyclophosphamide and anthracyclines produce late toxicity, which should be avoided, and current studies are exploring which agents are needed for successful disease control. Lymphoblastic disease, even localized, should be treated in the more aggressive fashion used for advanced disease and ALL.

B-cell lymphomas. After the initial success experienced using cyclophosphamide, methotrexate and vincristine, most B-cell regimens have tended to use intensive alkylating agent therapy, particularly cyclophosphamide. Latterly, particularly for stage 3 and 4 disease, treatment has become even more intensive, with minimal interruption between pulses of chemotherapy to prevent tumour regrowth. Treatment is also needed to control or prevent CNS infiltration, so current protocols use high-dose systemic methotrexate with folinic acid rescue, intensive IT therapy, high-dose cytarabine and other systemic drugs, including cyclophosphamide, adriamycin and vincristine (Patte et al 1986, Hann et al 1990). High-dose methotrexate and folinic acid rescue is not myelotoxic provided renal function is normal, and can be given at the nadir of counts without delaying marrow recovery. In this way, a much more continuous systemic antitumour effect can be maintained with the bonus of penetration into the CNS.

B-cell lymphoma patients have a high risk of tumour lysis syndrome even before therapy is started (Tsokos et al 1981). Forced alkaline diuresis and allopurinol need to be started before any other therapy is given. Haemodialysis is occasionally necessary, but usually the renal failure which develops is of high output type with minimal tubular reabsorption (see above). Provided urine flow can be maintained, the problem usually resolves spontaneously. Patients who present with large kidneys and gross bilateral tumour infiltration may occasionally need pre-emptive haemodialysis. Such patients need very careful monitoring of fluid balance and of their potassium, calcium, urate and urea levels. An added problem in maintaining good fluid balance is the presence of large serous effusions where fluid can accumulate. It is therefore important to maintain good oncotic pressure by keeping albumen levels high with, if necessary, the infusion of salt-poor albumen and the judicious use of diuretics to attract fluid out of the tissues. Central venous pressure monitoring is essential in these circumstances.

Both Wollner et al (1976) and Mott et al (1984) demonstrated that about two-thirds of abdominal lymphomas without bone marrow or CNS disease can be cured. The main problem seems to be to define the true high-risk patients, particularly those with diffuse abdominal disease, and to use more intensive regimens for them (Patte et al 1986, Hann et al 1990). Following resection, localized B-cell abdominal lymphomas appear to require only short courses of chemotherapy and probably do not require CNS therapy.

It has been much more difficult to draw up specific protocols for patients with large cell lymphomas since they are such a heterogeneous group. Many are of B-cell origin and perhaps should be treated as the other B-cell tumours, but some centres have used ALL type treatment with good results (Muller-Weihrich et al 1985). True histiocytic disease may respond better to the sort of therapy used in acute myeloid leukaemia, particularly those regimens incorporating etoposide.

REFERENCES

Abromovitch M, Ochs J, Pui C H et al 1988 High dose methotrexate improved clinical outcome in children with acute lymphoblastic leukaemia. Medical and Pediatric Oncology 16: 297–303

Allen A, Malpas J S, Kingston J E 1990 Educational achievement of survivors of childhood cancer. Pediatric Hematology and Oncology 7(4): 339–46

Aur R J, Simone J, Hustu et al, 1971. CNS therapy and combination chemotherapy of childhood lymphocytic leukaemia. Blood 37: 272–81

Baum E, Nesbit M Tilford D et al 1979 Extent of disease in pediatric patients with ALL experiencing an apparent isolated testicular relapse. Proceedings of the American Association of Cancer Research 20: 435

Bennet J M, Catovsky D, Daniel M T et al 1981 The French-American-British (FAB) Cooperative Group. The morphological classification of acute lymphoblastic leukaemia concordance among observers and clinical correlations. British Journal of Haematology 47: 553–61

Bielack S, Erttman R, Winkler K, Landbeck G 1989 Doxorubicin: effect of different schedules on toxicity and antitumour efficacy. European Journal of Cancer, Clinical Oncology 25: 873–882

Bleyer W A, Coccia P F, Sather H N 1983 Reduction in central nervous system leukaemia with a pharmacokinetically derived intrathecal methotrexate dosage regimen. Journal of Clinical Oncology 1: 317–25

Bleyer W A, Nickerson J M, Coccia P et al 1985 Monthly pulses of vincristine and prednisolone prevent marrow and testicular relapse in childhood ALL: one conclusion of the CCG 161 Study. Proceedings of the American Society of Clinical Oncology 4: 160

Bleyer W A 1989 High dose methotrexate in childhood ALL – How high should the dose be? In: Borsi J D (ed) The role of pharmacology. Proceedings of the International Society of Paediatric Oncology Workshop. Prague p 19–31

Borsi J D, Moe P J 1987 A comparative study on the pharmacokinetics of methotrexate in a dose range of 0.5 g to 33.6 g/m² in children with ALL. Cancer 60: 513

Burkitt D 1958 A sarcoma involving the jaws in African children. British Journal of Surgery 46: 218–23

Campana D, Couston-Smith E, Janossy G 1990 The immunologic detection of minimal residual disease in acute leukaemia. Blood 76(1): 163–71

Chaganti R S K, Miller D R, Meyers P A, German J 1979 Cytogenetic evidence of the intrauterine origin of acute leukaemia in monozygotic twins. New England Journal of Medicine 300: 1032

Chessells J M, Janossy G, Lawler S D, Secker-Walker L M, 1979 The Ph' chromosome in childhood leukaemia. British Journal of Haematology 41: 25–41

Chessells J M 1982 Acute lymphoblastic leukaemia. Seminars in Haematology 19: 155–71

Chessells J M, Rogers D W, Leiper A D et al 1986 Bone marrow transplantation has a limited role in prolonging second marrow remission in childhood lymphoblastic leukaemia. Lancet i: 1239–41

Chessells J M, Cox T, Cavanagh N et al 1987 Methotrexate, cranial irradiation and neurotoxicity in childhood ALL. Proceedings of International Society of Paediatric Oncology. Medical and Pediatric Oncology 16: 102–3

Chessells J, Bailey C 1990 Personal communication

Chilcote R R, Coccia P, Sather H N et al 1984 Mediastinal mass in acute lymphoblastic leukaemia. Medical and Pediatric Oncology 12: 9–16

Cornbleet M A, Chessells J M 1978 Bone marrow relapse in ALL in childhood. British Medical Journal 2: 104–6

Craft A W, Reid M, Gardner P 1979 Virus infections in children with ALL. Archives of Disease in Childhood 54: 755–9

Crist W, Boyett J, Roper M et al 1984 Pre-B-cell leukaemia responds poorly to treatment – A Pediatric Oncology Group Study. Blood 63: 407–14

Crist W M, Carroll A J, Shuster J J et al 1990 Poor prognosis of children with pre-B acute lymphoblastic leukaemia is associated with the t(1;19(q23,p13) – a Pediatric Oncology Group Study. Blood 76(1): 117–22

Curt G A, Carney D N, Cowan K H et al 1983 Unstable methotrexate resistance in human small cell carcinoma associated with double minute chromosomes. New England Journal of Medicine 308: 199–202

Darbyshire P, Eden O B, Jameson B et al 1985 Pneumonitis in lymphoblastic leukaemia of childhood. European Journal of Paediatric Haematology and Oncology 2: 141–7

Darbyshire P J 1990 Personal communication

Eden O B, Rankin A, 1982 Testicular biopsies in childhood ALL. In: Willoughby M, Siegel S E (eds) Butterworth International Medical Review ch 4: 47–79

Eden O B, Rankin A, Kay H 1983 Isolated testicular relapse in acute lymphoblastic leukaemia of childhood. Archives of Disease in Childhood 58 (2): 128–32

Eden O B, Darbyshire P, Simpson R McD et al 1985 Lysosomal iso-enzyme profiles used to classify cases of acute undifferentiated leukaemia. British Journal of Haematology 59: 109–114

Eden O B, Lilleyman J, Richards S et al 1990a Report to the Medical Research Council on behalf of the Working Party on Leukaemia in Childhood – results of MRC UKALL VIII. British Journal of Haematology - 78(2): 187–196

Eden O B, Shaw M P, Lilleyman J, Richards S 1990b Results of the Medical Research Council UKALL VIII study and trial for children aged under 2 years at diagnosis. British Journal of Cancer (supplement) - in press.

Eden O B, Lilleyman J S, Richards S 1990c Testicular irradiation in childhood lymphoblastic leukaemia. British Journal of Haematology 75: 496–8

Eden O B, Shaw M P, Lilleyman J S, Richards S 1990d A non-randomised sequential study comparing *Escherichia coli* and *Erwinia asparaginase* in MRC UKALL VIII study and trial. Medical and Pediatric Oncology 18: 497–502

Eiser C 1978 Intellectual abilities among survivors of childhood leukaemia as a function of CNS irradiation. Archives of Disease in Childhood 53: 391–5

Ertel I J, Nesbit M E, Hammond D et al 1979 Effective dose of L-asparaginase for induction of remission in previously treated children with ALL: a report from the Children's Cancer Study Group. Cancer Research 39: 3893–6

Erttmann R 1989 Tumour cell resistance against cytostatic drugs. Biological mechanisms and clinical implications. In: Borsi J D (ed) The role of clinical pharmacology. Proceedings of the International Society of Paediatric Oncology Workshop. SIOP, Prague, p 84–96

Evans A 1963 The cerebrospinal fluid of leukaemic children without CNS manifestation. Pediatrics 31: 1024

Evans A E 1964 Central nervous system involvement in children with acute leukaemia: a study of 921 patients. Cancer 17: 256–8

Flandrin G, Bruoet J C, Daniel M T Preud'homme J L 1975

Acute leukaemia with Burkitt's tumour cells. Blood 45: 183–8

Fojo A T, Ueda K, Slamon D J et al 1987 Expression of a multi drug resistance gene in human tumours and tissues. Proceedings of the National Academical Society USA 84: 265–9

Foon K A, Todd R F III 1986 Immunological classification of leukaemia and lymphoma. Blood 68: 1

Gale R P, Champlin R E 1986 Bone marrow transplantation in acute leukaemia. Clinics in Haematology 15 (3): 851–72

Gardner M J, Snee M P, Hall A J, Pavell C A, Downes S, Terrell J D 1990 Results of a case control study of leukaemia and lymphoma among young people near Sellafield nuclear plant in West Cumbria. British Medical Journal 300: 423–34

Gaynon P, Bleyer W A, Steinherz P G et al 1990 Day 7 marrow response and outcome for children with acute lymphoblastic leukaemia and unfavourable presenting features. Medical and Pediatric Oncology 18: 273–9

Gerrard M, Mott M G 1990 Personal communication (on results of UKCCSG second series of NHL studies)

Goldie J H, Coldman A J, Gudauskas G S 1982 Rationale for the use of alternating non cross-resistant chemotherapy. Cancer Treatment Reports 66: 439–49

Gray M, Hann I, Glass S et al 1987 Mortality and morbidity caused by measles in children with malignant disease attending four major treatment centres: a retrospective review. British Medical Journal 295: 19–22

Greaves M F, Chan L C 1986 Is spontaneous mutation the 'cause' of childhood acute lymphoblastic leukaemia? British Journal of Haematology 41: 1

Greaves M F 1988 Speculations on the cause of childhood acute lymphoblastic leukaemia. Leukaemia 2: 120–125

Green D M, Freeman A L, Sather H et al 1980 Comparison of three methods of central nervous system prophylaxis in childhood ALL. Lancet i: 1398–1403

Haghbin M, Zeulzer W W 1965 A long term study of cerebrospinal leukaemia. Journal of Pediatrics 67: 23

Haghbin M, Galicich J 1979 Use of the Ommaya reservoir in the prevention and treatment of CNS leukaemia. American Journal of Pediatric Hematology and Oncology 1: 111

Hammond D, Sather H, Nesbit M et al 1986 Analysis of prognostic factors in acute lymphoblastic leukaemia. Medical and Paediatric Oncology 14: 124–34

Hann I M, Evans D I K, Palmer M K, Morris Jones P H, Haworth C 1979 The prognostic significance of morphological features in childhood acute lymphoblastic leukaemia. Clinical and Laboratory Haematology 1: 215–6

Hann I M, Eden O B, Barnes J, Pinkerton C R (on behalf of the United Kingdom Children's Cancer Study Group) 1990 'MACHO' chemotherapy for Stage IV B cell lymphoma and B cell ALL of childhood. British Journal of Haematology 76: 359–60

Hardisty R M, Norman P 1967 Meningeal leukaemia. Archives of Disease of Childhood 42: 411

Hausdorf G, Morf G, Beron G et al 1988 Long term doxorubicin cardiotoxicity in childhood non-invasive evaluation of the contractile state and diastolic filling. British Heart Journal 60: 309–315

Hawkins M M 1989 Long term survival and cure after childhood cancer. Archives of Disease in Childhood 64: 798–807

Hayder S, Bjork O, Lafolie P 1990 The course of biological parameters and 6-mercaptopurine pharmacokinetics during maintenance treatment of children with ALL. Acta

Paediatrica Scandinavica 79: 832–837

Hughes W T, Feldman S, Aur R J et al 1975 Intensity of immunosuppressive therapy and the incidence of Pneumocystis carinii pneumonitis. Cancer 36: 2004–9

Hughes W T, Kuhn S, Chaudhary S et al 1977 Successful chemoprophylaxis for Pneumocysti carinii pneumonitis. New England Journal of Medicine 297: 1419–26

Hustu H O, Aur R J A, Verzosa M S et al 1973 Prevention of CNS leukaemia by irradiation. Cancer 32: 585

Hustu H, Aur R, 1978 Extramedullary leukaemia. Clinics in Haematology 7: 313–337

Hyman C, Bogle J, Brubaker C, Williams K, Hammond D 1965 CNS involvement by leukaemia in children: relationship to systemic leukaemia and description of clinical and laboratory manifestations. Blood 25: 1

Ishii E, Euda K, Adazasw K et al 1990 Fever in children with acute leukaemia: cause and role of febrile episode at initial diagnosis. Pediatric Hematology and Oncology 7: 109–112

Jablon S, Kato M 1970 Childhood cancer in relation to prenatal exposure to atomic bomb radiation. Lancet ii: 1000–3

Jacquillat C, Weil M, Gemon M F et al 1973 Combination therapy in 130 patients with acute lymphoblastic leukaemia. Cancer Research 33: 3278–84

Jaffe N, Takaue Y, Anzai et al 1985 Transient neurological disturbance induced by high dose methotrexate treatment. Cancer 56: 1356–60

Jannoun L 1983 Are cognitive and educational development affected by age at which prophylactic therapy is given in ALL? Archives of Disease in Childhood 58: 953–8

Juliano R L, Ling V, 1976 A surface glycoprotein modulating drug permeability in Chinese hamster ovary cell mutants. Biochemical, Biophysical Acta 455: 152–62

Kalwinsky D K, Robertson P, Dahl G et al 1985 Clinical relevance of lymphoblastic biological features in children with acute lymphoblastic leukaemia. Journal of Clinical Oncology 3(4): 477–84

Kartner N, Evernden-Porelle D, Bradley G, Ling V 1985 Detection of p-glucoprotein in multidrug resistant cell lines by monoclonal antibodies. Nature 316: 820–3

Kingston J E 1987 Special aspects of treatment of paediatric lymphomas. In: McElwain T, Lister T A (eds) Clinical haematology. The lymphoma. Bailliere Tindall, London, p 223–33

Kinlen L J, Clarke K, Hudson C 1990 Evidence from population mixing in British new towns 1946–85 of an infective basis for childhood leukaemia. Lancet 336: 577–82

Koch K, Reiquam C W, Beatty E C 1966 Acute childhood leukaemia: unusual complications. Rocky Mountain Medical Journal 63: 50

Kramer R A, Zakker J, Kim G 1988 Role of the glutathione redox cycle in acquired and de novo multidrug resistance. Science 241: 694–7

Kurita S, Kamei Y, Ota K 1974 Genetic studies on familial leukaemia. Cancer 34: 1089–1109

Lancet editorial 1987 5HT3 receptor antagonists: a new class of antiemetics. Lancet i: 1470–1

Leikin S, Miller D R, Sather H et al 1981 Immunologic evaluation in the prognosis of acute lymphoblastic leukaemia: a report from the Children's Cancer Study Group. Blood 58: 5601

Leiper A D, Chessells J M 1986 Acute lymphoblastic leukaemia under two. Archives of Disease in Childhood 61(12): 1007

Leiper A D 1990 Management of growth failure in the treatment of malignant disease. Pediatric Hematology and Oncology 7(4): 365–72

Lennard L, Lilleyman J S 1987 Are children with lymphoblastic leukaemia given enough 6-mercaptopurine? Lancet ii: 785–7

Lilleyman J, Hann I M, Stevens R F et al 1986 French American British (FAB) morphological classification of childhood lymphoblastic leukaemia and its clinical importance. Journal of Clinical Pathology 39: 998–1002

Lukes R J, Collins R D 1975 New approaches to the classification of the lymphomata. British Journal of Cancer 31: 1–28

Lyon J L, Klauber M R, Gardner J W et al 1979 Childhood leukaemias associated with fallout from nuclear testing. New England Journal of Medicine 300: 397–402

Magrath I T 1987 Malignant non-Hodgkin's lymphomas in children. Hematology and Oncology Clinics of North America 1: 577–602

Magrath I T (ed) 1990 The non-Hodgkin's lymphomas. Edward Arnold, London

Malpas J S 1988 Cancer: the consequences of cure. Clinical Radiology 39: 166–72

Mandell L R, Steinherz P, Fuks Z, 1990 Delayed central nervous system (CNS) radiation in childhood CNS acute lymphoblastic leukaemia. Cancer 66: 447–450

Mastrangelo R, Zeuler W, Eckland P, Thompson R 1970 Chromosomes in the spinal fluid: evidence for metastatic origin of meningeal leukaemia. Blood 35: 227

Meadows A T 1988 Risk factors for second malignant neoplasms: report from the Late Effect Study Group. Bulletin of Cancer 75: 125–30

Medical Research Council 1971 Treatment of ALL: Comparison of BCG, intermittent methotrexate and no therapy after a two-month intensive cytotoxic regime. British Medical Journal 4: 189–94

Medical Research Council 1978 Testicular disease in acute lymphoblastic leukaemia in childhood. British Medical Journal 1: 334–8

Medical Research Council 1986 Improvement in outlook for children with lymphoblastic leukaemia in the British Isles: the MRC trial 1972–85. Lancet i: 408–11

Miller D R, Leikin S, Albo V et al 1980 Use of prognostic factors in improving the design and efficiency of clinical trials in childhood leukaemia: Children's Cancer Study Group report. Cancer Treatment Reports 64: 381–92

Miller D R, Leikin S, Albo V et al 1981 Prognostic importance of morphology (FAB classification) in childhood acute lymphoblastic leukaemia (ALL). British Journal of Haematology 48: 199–206

Miller D R, Leikin S, Albo V et al 1985 Prognostic factors and therapy in acute lymphoblastic leukaemia of childhood CCG - 141. Cancer 51: 1041–49

Miller D R, Coccia P F, Bleyer W A et al 1989 Early response to induction therapy as a predictor of disease-free survival and late recurrence of childhood acute lymphoblastic leukaemia: a report to the Children's Cancer Study group. Journal of Clinical Oncology: 1807–15

Miller D R, Miller L P 1990 Acute lymphoblastic leukaemia in children: an update of clinical, biological and therapeutic aspects. Critical Reviews in Oncology Haematology 10(2): 131–64

Miller R W, Mulvihill J J 1976 Small head size after atomic irradiation. Teratology 14: 355–7

Modan B, Ron E, Verner A 1977 Thyroid cancer following scalp irradiation. Radiology 123: 741–4

Moe P J, Seip M, Finne P 1981 Intermediate dose methotrexate in childhood acute lymphocytic leukaemia in Norway. Haematologica 14: 257–63

Moore E W, Thomas L P, Shaw R K, Freireich E J 1960. The CNS in acute leukaemia: a PM study of 117 consecutive cases with particular reference to haemorrhage, leukaemic infiltration, and the syndrome of meningeal leukaemia. Archives of Internal Medicine 105: 451

Moss H A, Nannis E D, Poplack D G 1981 The effects of prophylactic treatment of the central nervous system on the intellectual functioning of children with acute lymphocytic leukaemia. American Journal of Medicine 71: 47–52

Mott M G, Palmer M K, Eden O B 1984 Adjuvant low dose radiation in childhood non-Hodgkin's lymphoma. British Journal of Cancer 50: 463–9

Muller-Weihrich S, Henze G, Odenwald E et al 1985 BFM trials for childhood non-Hodgkin's lymphoma. In: Cavalli F, Bonadonna G, Rosensweig M (eds) Malignant lymphomas and Hodgkin's disease. Martinuus Nighoff, Boston p 633

Murphy S 1980 Classification, staging and end results of the treatment of non-Hodgkin's lymphoma: dissimilarities from lymphomas in adults. Seminars in Oncology 7: 332–9

Nadler L M, Reinherz E L, Weinstein H J et al 1980 Heterogeneity of T cell lymphoblastic malignancies. Blood 55: 806–10

Nathwani B W, Kim H, Rappaport H 1976 Malignant lymphoma, lymphoblastic. Cancer 38: 964–83

Neglia J P, Robison L 1988 Epidemiology of the childhood acute leukaemias. Pediatric Clinics of North America 35(4): 675–92

Nesbit M E, Chard R M, Evans A et al 1979 Evaluation of intramuscular versus intravenous administration of L-asparaginase in childhood leukaemias. American Journal of Pediatric Hematology/Oncology 1(1): 9–13

Nesbit M E, Robison L, Ortega J A et al 1980 Testicular relapse in childhood acute lymphoblastic leukaemia; association with pretreatment patients characteristics and treatment. Cancer 45: 2009–16

Nesbit M E, D'Angio G J, Sather et al 1981a Effect of isolated CNS leukaemia on bone marrow remission and survival in childhood ALL. Lancet: 1386–9

Nesbit M, Sather H, Robison L et al 1981b Presymptomatic central nervous system therapy in previously untreated childhood acute lymphoblastic leukaemia: comparison of 1800 rads and 2400 rads. A report from the Children's Cancer Study Group. Lancet i: 461–6

Nesbit M, Sather H, Robison L et al 1982 Sanctuary therapy: a randomised trial of 724 children with previously untreated acute lymphoblastic leukaemia. A report of CCSG. Cancer Research 42: 674–80

Nesbit M E, Sather H, Robison L et al 1983 Randomised study of 3 years versus 5 years of chemotherapy in childhood ALL. Journal of Clinical Oncology 1: 308–16

Nies B A, Bodey G, Thomas L B et al 1965 The persistence of extra medullary leukaemia infiltrates during bone marrow remission of acute lymphoblastic leukaemia. Blood 26: 133–41

Ninane J 1980 The eye as a sanctuary in acute lymphoblastic leukaemia. Lancet 1: 452–3

Obioha F, Kaine W, Ikerionwu S et al 1989 The pattern of childhood malignancy in Eastern Nigeria. Annals of Tropical Paediactrics 9: 261–265

Offit K, Ladangi M, Gangi M E et al 1990 Ki-1 antigen

expression defines a favourable clinical subset of non-B cell non-Hodgkin's lymphoma. Leukaemia 4(9): 625–30

Ortego J A, Nesbit M E, Donaldson M H et al 1977 L-asparaginase, vincristine and prednisone for indication of first remission in acute lymphocytic leukaemia. Cancer Research 37: 535–40

Parkin D M, Stiller C A, Draper G J et al 1988 International childhood cancer incidence. IARC Scientific Publications 87

Patte C, Philip T, Rodary C et al 1986 Improved survival rate in children with Stage III and IV B cell NHL and leukaemia using multiagent chemotherapy: results of a study of 114 children from the French Paediatric Oncology Society. Journal of Clinical Oncology 8: 1219–26

Pinkerton C R, Welshman S G, Glasgow J, Bridges J 1980 Can food influence the absorption of methotrexate in children with ALL? Lancet ii: 944–6

Poplack D G, Reaman G, Bleyer W A et al 1984 Central nervous system preventative therapy with high dose methotrexate in ALL. Proceeding of the American Society of Clinical Oncology 3: 294

Poplack D G 1988 Acute lymphoblastic leukaemia. In: Pizza P A, Poplack D G (ed) Principles of pediatric oncology. J B Lippincott, Philadelphia

Price R A, Johnson W W 1973 The central nervous system in childhood lymphocytic leukaemia: the arachnoid. Cancer 31: 520

Price R A, Jamieson P A 1975 The central nervous system in childhood leukaemia II: subacute leukoencephalopathy. Cancer 35: 306

Ramot B, Magrath I 1982 Hypothesis: the environment is a major determinant of the immunologic subtype of lymphoma and acute lymphoblastic leukaemia in children. British Journal of Haematology 52: 183–9

Rappaport H, Braylan R C 1975 Changing concepts in the classification of malignant neoplasms of the haemopoietic system. International Academy of Pathology Monographs 16: 1–19

Riehm H, Gadner H, Henze G et al 1980 The Berlin childhood acute lymphoblastic leukaemia therapy studies 1970–1976. American Journal of Hematology/Oncology 2: 299–306

Riehm H, Feickert H-J, Schrappe M et al for the BFM Study Group 1987 Therapy results in five ALL-BFM studies since 1970: implications of risk factors for prognosis. Haematology and Blood Transfusion 30: 139–46

Rivera G, Pratt C B, Aur R J et al 1976 Recurrent childhood lymphocytic leukaemia following cessation of therapy. Cancer 37: 1679–86

Roninson I B, Ablerson H T, Housman D E et al 1984 Amplification of specific DNA sequences correlates with multi-drug resistance in Chinese hamster cells. Nature 309: 626–8

Russell L, Craig J, MacKinlay G, Eden O B 1990 The use of central venous catheters in paediatric oncology – a cautionary tale. Scottish Medical Journal 35: 11–4

Sather H, Miller D, Nesbit M, Heyn R, Hammond D 1981 Differences in prognosis of boys and girls with acute lymphoblastic leukaemia. Lancet i: 739–43

Sallan S E, Camitta B, Cassady J R et al 1978 Intermittent combination chemotherapy with adriamycin for childhood acute lymphoblastic leukaemia: clinical results. Blood 51: 425–33

Savitz D A, Wachtel H, Barnes F A et al 1988 Case control study of childhood cancer and exposure to 60-Hertz electric and magnetic fields. American Journal of Epidemiology 128: 21

Scarfe J H, Hann I M, Evans D K 1980 The relationship between the pre-treatment proliferative activity of bone marrow blast cells measured by flow cytometry and prognosis of ALL. British Journal of Cancer 41: 764–71

Secker-Walker L M 1984 The prognostic implications of chromosomal findings in ALL. Cancer Genetics and Cytogenetics 11: 233–248

Secker-Walker L M, Stewart E L, Chan L et al 1985 The 4;11 translocation in acute leukaemia of childhood: the importance of additional chromosomal aberrations. British Journal of Haematology 61: 101–11

Shalet S M, Beardwell D G, Turomey J A et al 1977 Endocrine function following the treatment of acute leukaemia in childhood. Journal of Pediatrics 90: 920–3

Shalet S M, Clayton P, Price D 1988 Growth and pituitary function in children treated for brain tumours or acute lymphoblastic leukaemia. Hormone Research 30: 53–61

Shalet S M 1989 Endocrine consequences of the treatment of malignant disease. Archives of Disease in Childhood 64: 1635–41

Shapiro W R, Young D F, Mehta B M 1975 Methotrexate distribution in cerebrospinal fluid after intravenous, ventricular and lumbar injection. New England Journal of Medicine 293: 161–6

Shaw M P 1990 Personal communication

Shaw N J, Tweeddale P M, Eden O B 1990 Pulmonary function in childhood leukaemia survivors. Medical and Pediatric Oncology 17: 149–54

Siegel S, Nesbit M, Baehner R et al 1980 Pneumonia during therapy for childhood acute lymphoblastic leukaemia. American Journal of Diseases of Childhood 134: 28–30

Simone J V, Verzosa M S, Rudy J A 1975 Initial features and prognosis in 363 children with acute lymphocytic leukaemia. Cancer 36: 2099–108

Simonsen C C, Levison A D 1983 Isolation and expression of an altered mouse dihydrofolate reductase cDNA. Proceedings of the Academy of Sciences, USA 80: 2495–2499

Simpson R McD, Eden O B 1984 Possible interferon response in a child with measles encephalitis during immunosuppression. Scandanavian Journal of Infectious Disease 16: 315–9

Stewart A, Webb J, Hewett D 1958 A survey of childhood malignancies. British Medical Journal 1: 1495

Stjernfeldt M, Berglund K, Lindsten J, Ludwigsson J 1986 Maternal smoking during pregnancy and risk of childhood cancer. Lancet i: 1350

Stoffel T J, Nesbit M E, Levitt S M 1975 Extramedullary involvement of the testes in childhood leukaemia. Cancer 35: 1203–1211

Sullivan M P, Windmiller J 1966 Side effects of amethopterin administered intrathecally in the treatment of meningeal leukaemia. Medical Record and Annals 50: 92

Sullivan M, Vietti T, Fernbach D J et al 1969 Clinical investigations in the treatment of meningeal leukaemia radiation therapy regimens versus conventional intrathecal methotrexate. Blood 34: 301–19

Sullivan M P, Sutow W W, Taylor H, Wilbur J R 1971 Intrathecal (IT) combination chemotherapy for meningeal leukaemia using methotrexate (MTX), cytosine arabinoside (CA) and hydrocortisone (HDC). Proceedings of the American Association for Cancer Research 12: 45

Sullivan M P, Chen T, Dyment P K et al 1982 Equivalence

of intrathecal chemotherapy and radiotherapy as central nervous system prophylaxis in children with ALL. A Pediatric Oncology Group Study. Blood 60: 948–58

Thomas J, Janossy G, Eden O B, Bollum F 1982 Nuclear terminal deoxynucleotidyl transferase in leukaemic infiltrates of testicular tissue. British Journal of Cancer 45: 709–17

Thomas L B 1965 Pathology of leukaemia in brain and meninges. PM studies of patients with acute leukaemia and of mice given inocculations of L1210 leukaemia. Cancer Research 25: 1555

Tiedmann K, Chessells J M, Sandland R 1982 Isolated testicular relapse in boys with acute lymphoblastic leukaemia: treatment and outcome. British Medical Journal 285: 1614–16

Tsokos G E, Balow J E, Spiegel R J, Magrath I T 1981 Renal and metabolic complications of undifferentiated and lymphoblastic lymphoma. Medicine 60: 218

Tsuruo T 1983 Reversal of acquired resistance to vinca alkaloids and anthracycline antibiotics. Cancer Treatment Reports 67: 889–94

Upton A C, Albert R E, Burns F J, Shore E 1986 Radiation carcinogenesis. Elsevier Publications, New York

Weiss H D, Walker M D, Wiernik P H 1975 Neurotoxicity of commonly used antineoplastic agents. New England Journal of Medicine 291: 75–127

Wertheimer H, Leeper E 1979 Electrical wiring configurations and childhood cancer. American Journal of Epidemiology 109: 273

West R J, Graham-Pole J, Hardisty P M, Pike M C 1972 Factors in pathogenesis of CNS leukaemia. British Medical Journal 3: 311–4

Wiley J M, Smith N, Leventhal B G et al 1990 Invasive fungal disease in pediatric acute leukaemia patients with fever and neutropenia during induction chemotherapy: A multivariate analysis of risk factors. Journal of Clinical Oncology 8: 280–6

Williams D L, Tsiatis A, Brodeur G M et al 1982 Prognostic importance of chromosome number in 136 untreated children with ALL. Blood 60: 864–71

Williams D L, Raimondi, Rivera G et al 1985 Presence of clonal chromosome abnormalities in virtually all cases of ALL. New England Journal of Medicine 313: 640–1

Wolcott G J, Grunnet M, Lakey M 1970 Spinal subdural haematoma in a leukaemic child. Journal of Pediatrics 77: 1060

Wollner N, Burchenal J H, Lieberman P H et al 1976 Non Hodgkin's lymphoma in children. A comparative study of two modalities of therapy. Cancer 37: 123–34

Woods W G, Nesbit M E, Ramsay N K et al 1983 Intensive therapy followed by bone marrow transplantation for patients with ALL in second or subsequent remission: determination of prognostic factors. Blood 61: 1182–9

Yamada M, Wasserman R, Lange B et al 1990 Minimal residual disease in childhood B-lineage lymphoblastic leukaemia. New England Journal of Medicine 323: 448–54

Yoshida M, Miyoshi I, Hinuma Y 1982 Isolation and characterisation of retrovirus from cell lines of human adult T cell leukaemia and its implication in the disease. Proceedings of the National Academy of Sciences, USA 79: 2031–5

13. Disorders of haemostasis

B. E. S. Gibson

PHYSIOLOGY OF NORMAL HAEMOSTASIS AND ITS REGULATION

Normal haemostasis is dependent upon the integrity of complex interactions between platelets, the vessel wall and the plasma factors involved in the coagulation and fibrinolytic systems. It is convenient to describe haemostasis under the following headings:

1. the platelet–vessel interaction
2. the coagulation system
3. the inhibitors of coagulation
4. fibrinolysis.

However, in vivo these pathways do not act in isolation, but interact in a complex manner to activate the procoagulant system (generate thrombin), localize its effects to the site of damage and maintain vascular patency.

1. The platelet–vessel interaction

Platelets can be activated by a range of substances, and their response to activation divided into adhesion, aggregation, granular secretion and surface expression of procoagulant activities. The vascular endothelium synthesizes a number of important components of haemostasis, in particular collagen, von Willebrand factor (vWF) and prostacyclin (PGI_2). Collagen is exposed when the vascular endothelial surface is damaged (Fig. 13.1). Circulating vWF is absorbed to the collagen and binds to the platelet glycoprotein membrane receptor sites (GPIb), causing platelet adhesion. Platelets adhering to collagen are activated, change in shape from disc to sphere, and release adenosine diphosphonate (ADP) and serotonin from their dense bodies, resulting in platelet aggregation. Fibrino-

gen is the most important substance released from α granules and binds to specific platelet glycoprotein membrane receptors (GPIIb and GPIIIa), facilitating further aggregation. Platelet activation makes available platelet phospholipid (platelet factor 3) on the platelet surface, which interacts with coagulation factors, accelerating the local formation of thrombin. Thrombin causes irreversible platelet aggregation and fibrin formation. Finally, platelets adhere to fibrin via the receptors GPIIb

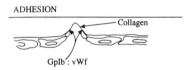

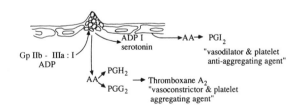

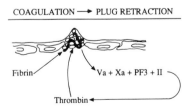

Fig. 13.1 Events in the formation of a haemostatic plug. Adapted from Hathaway & Bonnar 1987, with permission of Elsevier Science Publishing Co, Inc.

367

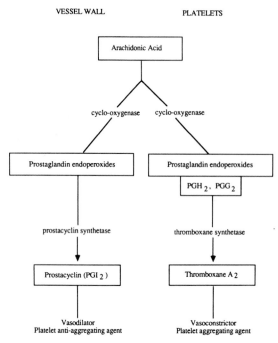

Fig. 13.2   Prostaglandin metabolism.

and GPIIIa, forming a stable platelet-fibrin plug.

The prostaglandin pathway provides an additional route for platelet aggregation and is initiated when platelet arachidonic acid is released from phospholipids under the influence of membrane phospholipase. Cyclo-oxygenase converts the arachidonic acid to the prostaglandin endoperoxides, PGG_2 and PGH_2. These in turn are converted to thromboxane A_2 (TXA_2), a potent aggregating agent and vasoconstrictor, by thromboxane synthetase. Thromboxane B_2 (TXB_2) is the stable metabolite of TXA_2. Prostacyclin (PGI_2) is a prostaglandin synthesized by blood vessels, and is a powerful vasodilator and potent inhibitor of platelet aggregation. In health, the production of PGI_2 by the vessel wall, and TXA_2 by platelets is balanced (Fig. 13.2).

2. The coagulation system

Through the serial interactions of enzymes and substrates, the coagulation cascade produces a stable fibrin clot at the site of injury (Fig. 13.3, Table 13.1). It is useful to consider this clotting mechanism as following two pathways: the 'intrinsic' and the 'extrinsic' pathways.

Intrinsic system

Factor XII (Hageman factor) circulates in the blood as an inactive zymogen. The contact system

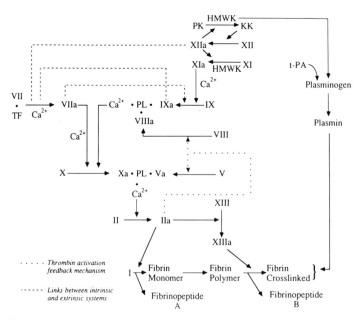

Fig. 13.3   The factors involved in the formation of a stable fibrin clot and their interactions.

Table 13.1 Concentrations and half-life of coagulation factors

Factor	Synonym	Half-life of transfused factor	Concentration
I	Fibrinogen	2–4 days	3 g/l
II	Prothrombin	2–3 days	100 µg/ml
III	Tissue factor	–	–
IV	Calcium ions	–	–
V	Proaccelerin	12–36 hours	10 µg/ml
VII	Proconvertin	4–6 hours	0.13–1.0 µg/ml
VIII:C	Antihaemophilic factor (AHF)	8–12 hours	0.2 µg/ml
vWF:Ag	von Willebrand's factor	–	5–10 µg/ml
IX	Christmas factor	18–24 hours	4 µg/ml
X	Stuart-Power factor	2 days	10 µg/ml
XI	Plasma thromboplastin antecedent	60–80 hours	2–7 µg/ml
XII	Hageman factor	40–50 hours	30 µg/ml
XIII	Fibrin stabilizing factor	6–8 days	15 µg/ml
PK	Fletcher factor	–	50 µg/ml
HMWK	Williams-Fitzgerald-Flaujeac factor	–	70–90 µg/ml
ATIII	Heparin cofactor I	2–5 days	150 µg/ml
Protein C –		4–6 hours	4 µg/ml
Protein S –		–	35 µg/ml

is initiated when FXII binds to a negatively charged surface (damaged endothelium), where it is converted to FXIIa by autoactivation. FXII may also initiate the extrinsic pathway, fibrinolysis, kinin generation and complement activation. Surface bound FXIIa activates prekallikrein (PK) to kallikrein, which reciprocates by accelerating the activation of FXII to FXIIa. The former reaction is enhanced by high molecular weight kininogen (HMWK), which also acts as a cofactor for the activation of FXI by FXIIa. FXIa activates FIX in a calcium-dependent reaction. FIX (like II, VII and X) is rich in glutamic acid residues, which are transcarboxylated by vitamin K to form γ-carboxyglutamic acid. The modified vitamin K-dependent protein is then able to bind calcium ions, which in turn act as bridges binding the FIX molecule to phospholipid. FX is next activated to FXa by a reaction which takes place on the cell surface and involves a complex (the 'tenase complex') of FIXa, thrombin-activated FVIII:C, calcium ions and phospholipid.

Extrinsic system

The conversion of FX to FXa via the extrinsic system involves tissue factor (TF or thromboplastin), FVII and calcium ions. The active component of tissue factor released from damaged cells is thought to be a lipoprotein complex, which acts as a cell surface receptor for FVII, activating it to FVIIa in the presence of calcium ions. The lipid of the tissue factor plays an additional role by adsorbing FX onto its surface and thereby enhancing the reaction between factors VIIa, X and calcium ions. FVII can also be activated by FIXa and FXII fragments (XIIf).

Common pathway

The common pathway involves conversion of prothrombin (II) to thrombin (IIa), clotting fibrinogen (I) to fibrin and stabilization of the fibrin clot. FXa, formed by either the intrinsic or extrinsic system, forms a cell surface complex (the prothombinase complex) with phospholipid, calcium ions and thrombin-activated Va. This complex cleaves prothrombin into thrombin and prothrombin fragments 1 and 2. Thrombin converts fibrinogen to fibrin and also activates factors VIII, V and (by positive feedback) XIII. Conversion of soluble fibrinogen to insoluble fibrin involves the thrombin-mediated cleavage of peptides A and B from the amino-terminal ends of the α and β chains of fibrinogen, liberating fibrinopeptides A and B and producing fibrin monomers, which polymerize into a meshwork of fibrin. FXIII (previously activated to FXIIIa by thrombin) stabilizes the fibrin clot by cross-linking adjacent fibrin strands. Activated factor XIII is able to crosslink other proteins to fibrin, including α_2 antiplasmin (α_2AP) and fibronectin; the latter is also crosslinked to collagen, and provides a possible means of anchoring the fibrin clot to connective tissue, which may be important in wound repair .

Two positive-feedback systems should be noted in the coagulation cascade, which can result in explosive thrombin generation. Firstly, FIXa activates FVII, linking the intrinsic and extrinsic systems and demonstrating the tenuous distinction between these pathways. It has been suggested that, in vivo, there is only one pathway of coagulation and different mechanisms of activation. Secondly, thrombin promotes its own formation by activating factor V and VIII. The importance of an activation complex (prothrombinase complex and tenase complex) involving a serine protease, a zymogen substrate, a cofactor and an organizing surface are several fold. Firstly, kinetic studies show that the relative rate of thrombin formation by the prothrombinase complex is 20,000-fold that of physiological concentrations of FXa and prothrombin alone. An additional feature of the activation complex is that it appears to protect the components from inhibition.

3. The inhibitors of coagulation

Antithrombin III (ATIII) and activated protein C are the major natural inhibitors of coagulation and play an important role in localizing fibrin formation to the site of injury. ATIII is a potent inhibitor of thrombin and FXa, but also has inhibiting action against factors IXa, XIa, XIIa, kallikrein and plasmin. The reaction is greatly enhanced by the presence of heparin (or vessel wall heparin sulphate) which produces a conformational change in the molecule resulting in the rapid inactivation of thrombin. Heparin cofactor II (HCII) is the second most important antithrombin, with limited specificity, inhibiting thrombin, but with no activity against FXa. α_2 macroglobulin and α_1 antitrypsin have broad-spectrum inhibitory activity and can inactivate thrombin, but are physiologically less important than ATIII and HCII.

Protein C and its cofactor, protein S, are vitamin K-dependant factors. Thrombin binds to a cofactor, thrombomodulin, an endothelial cell surface glycoprotein, and the complex activates protein C to form activated protein C (APC) at a 1000-fold increased rate. Protein S circulates in two forms, a free active form which comprises approximately 40% of the total, and as a complex with C4b-binding protein. Protein S only functions while it is in its free form. APC inactivates cofactor Va and VIII:C, and enhances fibrinolysis by the inhibition of plasminogen activator inhibitor (PAI). Thrombomodulin, by binding thrombin, plays an important role in regulating haemostasis, as complexed thrombin is no longer able to activate FV or convert fibrinogen to fibrin. The high density of thrombomodulin in the microcirculation may be an important defence mechanism against disseminated intravascular coagulation (DIC).

The vascular endothelium maintains vessel patency and limits thrombus formation by localizing reactions to its surface by synthesizing and binding key molecules in the anticoagulant and profibrinolytic reactions (Fig. 13.4) as described below. The thromboresistance of the luminal surface is further regulated by metabolites of the prostaglandin pathway.

Inactivation of thrombin. The sulphated proteoglycans are synthesized by endothelial cells and incorporated into extracellular matrix. Endothe-

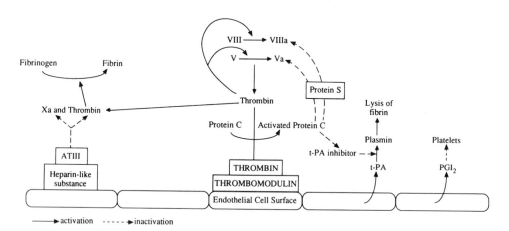

Fig. 13.4   The various mechanisms involved in the inhibition of thrombus formation and the maintenance of vascular patency. Adapted from: Bloom A L, Thomas D P 1987 Hemostasis and Thrombosis, 2nd edn. Churchill Livingstone, Edinburgh, with permission.

lial cell-bound heparin sulphate binds ATIII and greatly increases its capacity to neutralize thrombin generated on or in the vicinity of the luminal surface. Thrombomodulin also mops up thrombin.

The protein C pathway. The activation of protein C by the thrombin/thrombomodulin complex to APC limits thrombin generation by inactivating Va and VIIIa.

Tissue-type plasminogen activator and PAI synthesis. Both tissue-type plasminogen activator (t-PA) and its inhibitor PAI-1 are synthesized and released from the vascular endothelium. However, in the presence of fibrin the net effect of a number of interactions results in the greater local availability of functional t-PA, which can activate plasminogen and digest clot.

Cyclo-oxygenase metabolites. PGI_2 is a potent inhibitor in vitro of platelet aggregation.

4. Fibrinolysis

Fibrinolysis, the lysis of fibrin or fibrinogen by plasmin, is an important physiological mechanism limiting thrombus formation. It is dependent on the presence of plasminogen activators and the conversion of plasminogen to plasmin. Plasminogen may be activated to plasmin by surface contact (via kallikrein) which activates urokinase-type plasminogen activator (u-PA) or by t-PA. t-PA is the most important activator of plasminogen, and is synthesized and released from endothelial cells after their stimulation or damage. Inhibitors of the fibrinolytic system include antiplasmins (e.g. α_2AP) and PAIs. α_2AP binds to fibrin and is rapidly crosslinked to new fibrin clots by FXIII, thereby ensuring the initial stability of the haemostatic plug, by neutralizing any free plasmin. There are a number of plasminogen activator inhibitors (PAI-1, PAI-2, PAI-3). PAI-1 is released from the endothelium along with t-PA, preventing excessive t-PA activity. However, in the presence of fibrin there is a preferential binding of t-PA to fibrin rather than to PAI-1. The complex of t-PA, plasminogen and fibrin facilitates the conversion of clot-bound plasminogen to plasmin, which is then protected from the action of α_2AP. The protein C system has a direct potentiating effect on fibrinolysis. APC can increase t-PA synthesis and release from the endothelium, and decrease PAI-1

activity. Platelets also contain PAI-1, which may prevent lysis of fibrin-stabilized platelet aggregates in haemostasis. PAI-2 is measured in the plasma only during pregnancy. PAI-3 is not yet fully characterized. When fibrinogen or fibrin is broken down by plasmin, a series of fibrin(ogen) degradation products (FDPs) are produced (fragments X, Y, D and E). These can modify the thrombin/fibrinogen interaction; fragment X delays the clotting time, fragments Y and D have potent antipolymerizing effects, and fibrin mops up and neutralizes large amounts of thrombin.

THE DEVELOPMENT OF HAEMOSTASIS IN THE NEWBORN

Coagulation factors do not cross the placental barrier to any significant degree. Many of the procoagulants, anticoagulants and proteins involved in fibrinolysis are gestation-dependent and do not reach adult values until 6 months of age. This probably causes no clinical problem for the healthy newborn, but may contribute to morbidity in the sick and preterm infant.

Procoagulants

The information available suggests that factors I, V, VIII:C and vWF are within the normal adult range from the beginning of the third trimester onwards. All other procoagulants are reduced at birth to variable levels and are dependent on gestational age (Fig. 13.5, Table 13.2). A fibrinogen level of 1.5 g/l at birth should be regarded as the lower limit of normal in both the term and preterm infant. A number of observations suggest the existence of a fetal fibrinogen structurally distinct from the 'adult' molecule. Firstly, thrombin and reptilase times are generally prolonged in the newborn, even in the presence of both normal fibrinogen and FDP levels and this can best be explained by a dysfibrinogenaemia. Secondly, fibrinogen levels based on heat precipitation or protein estimations are often higher than those obtained by clotting assays. Fetal fibrinogen is relatively insensitive to thrombin-induced proteolysis (Mills & Karpatkin 1972). Fetal fibrinogen has an increased sialic acid content compared to adult fibrinogen, and this varies with the degree of

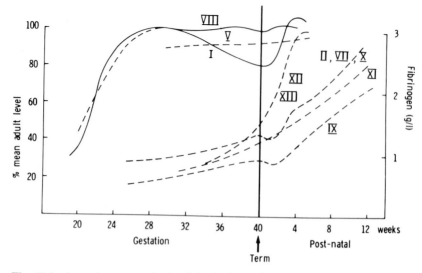

Fig. 13.5 Approximate mean levels of clotting factors in preterm and fullterm infants related to gestation. From: Hardisty R M, Weatherall D J 1982 Blood and its disorders, 2nd edn. Blackwell Scientific Publications, Oxford, with permission.

prematurity and correlates with the prolongation of the thrombin clotting time. Although the role of sialic acid in the conversion of fibrinogen to fibrin is controversial, its removal from the fibrinogen molecule enhances clot formation by thrombin. There is, however, no firm evidence that fetal fibrinogen is structurally distinct from adult fibrinogen and, as such, comparable to fetal haemoglobin and coded for by a specific gene. Similar abnormalities of fibrin formation are found in liver disease in adult patients, and fetal fibrinogen may represent a post-synthetic modification of a basic

fibrinogen protein in which hypersialation occurs in the fetal liver.

At birth, factor V levels are within the normal adult range in both term and preterm infants and are only slightly lower during the second trimester (Sell & Corrigan 1973, Holmberg et al 1974, Mibashan & Millar 1983).

At birth, the term infant has a FVIII:C level above the normal adult value whilst that of the preterm infant is within the normal adult range. There is no correlation between maternal and infant FVIII:C concentrations. Both term and

Table 13.2   Values for the procoagulants in the fetus and newborn infant

	Cofactors (U/ml)				Vitamin K-dependent factors (U/ml)				Contact factors (U/ml)				
	I (g/L)	V	VIII:C	vWF:Ag	II	VII	IX	X	XI	XII	PK	HMWK	XIII
Adult	3.4	1.00	1.00	1.00	1.00	1.00	1.00	1.00	1.00	1.00	1.00	1.00	1.00
Term newborn (37–41 wks)	2.4	1.00	1.50	1.60	0.52	0.57	0.35	0.45	0.42	0.44	0.35	0.64	0.61
Preterm newborn (33–36 wks)	3.0	0.82	0.93	1.66	0.45	0.59	0.41	0.44	–	0.25	0.33	–	–
(25–32 wks)	2.5	0.80	0.75	1.50	0.32	0.37	0.22	0.38	0.20	0.22	0.26	0.28	0.11–0.40
Fetus (approx 20 wks)	0.96	0.70	0.50	0.65	0.16	0.21	0.10	0.19	–	–	–	–	≈ 0.30

One unit is the amount of factor in 1 ml of normal plasma; means are given.
All values are venous and for the first 24 hours of life.
All subjects received vitamin K at birth.
Adapted from Hathaway & Bonnar, 1987 with permission of Elsevier Science Publishing Company, Inc.

premature infants have raised vWF:Ag values. Neonatal and fetal plasma contains unusually large vWF multimers (ULvWFM), not present in normal adult plasma, and similarly elevated proportions of high molecular weight (HMW) multimers (Weinstein et al 1989). The testing of infants for von Willebrand's disease (vWD) subtypes may be more complicated than at present appreciated.

Levels of the vitamin K-dependent factors (II, VII, IX and X) are gestation-dependent, and are approximately 50% of the normal adult value at term and about half of that value at 24 weeks' gestation.

All factors involved in the initial contact-activated phase of the intrinsic coagulation pathway (XI, XII, PK and HMWK) are reduced in both the term and preterm infant. The levels are dependent on gestational age, with ranges of 20–30% and 30–50% reported in the preterm and term infant respectively (Gordon et al 1980, Barnard et al 1979). A deficiency of these factors usually results in a greater prolongation of the APTT than occurs with a corresponding deficiency of FVIII:C or FIX:C.

Levels of FXIII in the term infant are about 70% of adult values. As only small quantities are required for clot stabilization, this minor decrease in activity has no clinical significance.

Anticoagulants

ATIII, HCII, protein C and protein S are all reduced at birth and are dependent on gestational age; α_2 macroglobulin concentrations are above adult values at birth (Table 13.3). Although levels of the inhibitors ATIII, HCII, protein C and protein S are in the range at which thrombotic disorders occur in the heterozygously affected adult, healthy infants do not develop spontaneous thrombosis.

ATIII levels in the term infant are 50–60% of adult values, and are further reduced in the preterm infant, paralleling the reduction in levels of its substrates, factors II and X. HCII activity is approximately 30% of adult values in the preterm infant and 50% in the term infant (Andersson et al 1988). Normal children attain adult values around 5–7 months of age (Chuansumrit et al 1989). Protein C and its cofactor, protein S, are reduced to levels similar to those of the other vitamin K-dependent proteins in the term and preterm infant: their substrates, factors Va and VIIIa are not reduced at birth. Mean day 1 protein C values of 0.39 and 0.35 U/ml, and protein S values of 0.36 U/ml, have been reported in term infants (Schettini et al 1985, Andrew et al 1987). However, newborns show a marked discrepancy between protein S activity and antigen, due to very low levels of C4b-binding protein which result in the presence of most, if not all, protein S existing in its free and active form (Schwartz et al 1988, Malm et al 1988). Sthoeger found the level of total protein S in the term infant to be in the adult range by 10 months of age. In contrast, the mean level of free protein S is similar to adult values by 2–4 months of age (Sthoeger et al 1989).

The elevated level of α_2 macroglobulin at birth may play a protective role against thrombosis at

Table 13.3 Values for the anticoagulants in the fetus and newborn infant

	ATIII (U/ml)	α_2-antiplasmin (U/ml)	C1-esterase inhibitor (U/ml)	α_2 macroglobulin (U/ml)	Plasminogen (U/ml)	Protein C:Ag (U/ml)	Protein S:Ag (U/ml)
Adult	1.00	1.00	1.00	1.00	1.00	1.00	1.00
Term newborn (37–41 wks)	0.56	0.83	1.00	1.80	0.49	0.50*	0.24*
Preterm newborn (33–36 wks)	0.40	0.73	–	1.29	0.38	0.38	
(25–32 wks)	0.35	0.74	–	1.58	0.35	0.29	
Fetus (approx. 20 wks)	0.23	–	–	–	–	0.10	

One unit is the amount of factor in 1 ml of normal plasma; means stated.
*Cord, all other values are venous and for the first 24 hours of life.
All subjects received vitamin K at birth.
Source: McDonald MM, Hathaway WE (1983). Perinatal hematology/oncology. Seminars in Perinatology 7:213 and Hathaway & Bonnar, 1987 with permission of Elsevier Publishing Company, Inc.

a time when other major anticoagulants are deficient. It inhibits significantly more thrombin, and ATIII less thrombin, in the newborn compared with the adult (Schmidt et al 1988). Similarly, the relatively high level of active protein S in infants may enhance the potential of the protein C pathway and partially compensate for deficiencies of the other inhibitors.

Fibrinolysis

Increased fibrinolytic activity, as reflected in a short euglobulin lysis time, has been reported from as early as 16 weeks' gestation onwards (Ekelund et al 1970). Plasminogen concentrations are gestation-dependent and are about 50% in the term infant, reaching adult levels at about 6 months of age. tPA and PAI are both high at term, whilst the major inhibitor of plasmin, $\alpha_2 AP$ is within the normal adult range (Barnard 1984).

Postnatal values for most components of the coagulation system are given in Figure 13.6 (Andrew et al 1987a). (See also Chapter 1.) All 118 healthy full-term infants had received 1 mg vitamin K intramuscularly at birth, at least 12 hours prior to the first blood sample being drawn. The study confirmed the following previously known facts:

1. coagulation tests vary with postnatal age
2. different coagulation factors show different postnatal patterns of maturation
3. most coagulation factors achieve near adult values by 6 months of age.

Reference ranges are now available from the study of 137 healthy premature infants evenly distributed in age between 30 and 36 weeks (Andrew et al 1988); these show their maturation towards adult levels to be accelerated, such that they too achieve mean adult values for most components of the coagulation system by 6 months of age. One of the more important purposes of reference ranges is to aid the correct diagnosis of specific congenital or acquired coagulopathies, and these studies have established several interesting facts:

1. Mild, moderate and severe haemophilia A can be confidently diagnosed in both term and preterm infants.

2. Mean values for FIX suggest that severe haemophilia B can be diagnosed with confidence in the newborn period in term and premature infants, but that mild or moderate haemophilia B cannot.

3. Diagnosis of the more common forms of vWD are difficult in the first months of life, because vWF behaves as an acute phase reactant and is markedly elevated in the early postnatal period in term and preterm infants.

4. Accurate diagnosis of the heterozygote state for specific inhibitors (e.g. AT-III, protein C and protein S) is difficult, although homozygosity has been and should be diagnosed at birth.

5. Acquired disorders, e.g. DIC and liver disease, should be easily diagnosed in view of the adult levels for fibrinogen and factors V and VIII in the term and premature newborn.

6. Vitamin K deficiency is difficult to diagnose in the newborn, particularly in the premature infant, because of the very low levels of the four vitamin K-dependent factors. Assays that measure discrepancies between the amount of existing protein and its activity may be more helpful.

7. Mean values for protein C are still low at 6 months of age. α_2 macroglobulin is elevated at birth and Cl esterase inhibitor (C_1E-INH) and HCII become elevated during the first 6 months of life, compared with adult values. The significance is unknown, but a compensatory mechanism may be in play.

8. It must be remembered that only healthy preterm and full-term infants were included in these studies. Some coagulation parameters have lower values in sick infants and rise more slowly. ATIII is a particularly well-recognized example of this, and values are significantly lower in neonates with respiratory distress syndrome (RDS) than in healthy term infants.

THE INVESTIGATION AND DIAGNOSIS OF DISORDERS OF HAEMOSTASIS

The cause of bleeding and/or thrombosis in childhood is usually obvious and acquired secondary to infection or indwelling catheters. However, this is also the age at which inherited disorders present. The assessment of a patient with a bleeding disorder begins with a detailed history and physical examination.

APTT, PT, FIBRINOGEN LEVEL AND TCT IN 118 HEALTHY FULL-TERM
INFANTS THROUGHOUT THE FIRST 6 MONTHS OF LIFE

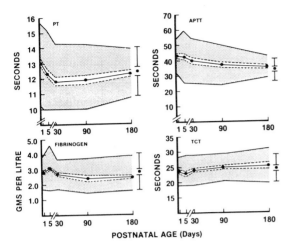

The inner line represents the mean values, the inner clear
area the 95% confidence interval, and the shaded area 95%
of all values (±2SD)

Adult values are indicated ●

A

THE VITAMIN K-DEPENDENT FACTORS (II, VII, IX, X) IN 118 HEALTHY
FULL-TERM INFANTS THROUGHOUT THE FIRST 6 MONTHS OF LIFE

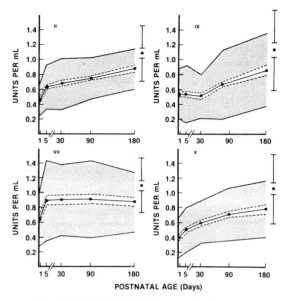

The inner line represents the mean values, the inner clear
area the 95% confidence interval, and the shaded area 95%
of all values (±2SD)

Adult values are indicated ●

B

FACTORS V, VIII AND vWF IN 118 HEALTHY FULL-TERM
INFANTS THROUGHOUT THE FIRST 6 MONTHS OF LIFE

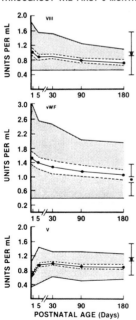

The inner line represents the mean values, the inner clear
area the 95% confidence interval, and the shaded area 95%
of all values (±2SD)

Adult values are indicated ●

C

THE CONTACT FACTORS (XI, XII, PK, HMWK) IN 118 HEALTHY
FULL-TERM INFANTS THROUGHOUT THE FIRST 6 MONTHS OF LIFE

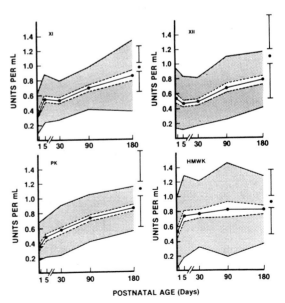

The inner line represents the mean values, the inner clear
area the 95% confidence interval, and the shaded area 95%
of all values (±2SD)

Adult values are indicated ●

D

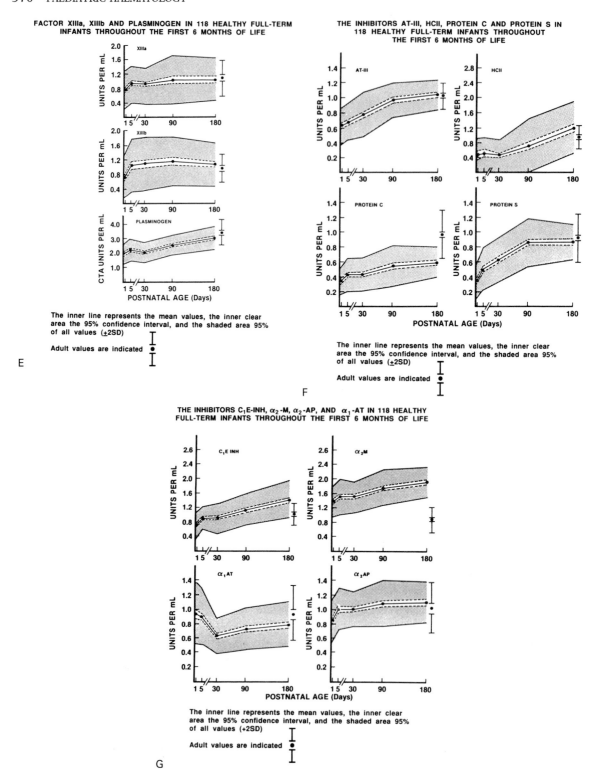

Fig. 13.6 Development of the human coagulation system in the full-term infant. From: Andrew et al 1987a, with permission of Grune & Stratton, Inc.

History

A comprehensive history of bleeding problems in both the child and his or her family is critical. Previous surgery or dental extraction uncomplicated by haemorrhage is strong evidence against an underlying inherited bleeding disorder, whilst haemorrhage of a degree requiring transfusion is highly significant. Bleeding problems manifested only after surgery or trauma may be a hallmark of mild haemophilia or vWD. It is, therefore very important, when taking a family history, to establish the sex affected. Points worthy of specific enquiry in the neonatal period include bleeding post-circumcision, delayed bleeding from the umbilical stump (particularly characteristic of FXIII deficiency), haematoma formation after infantile immunizations given intramuscularly, or bleeding from the site of the Guthrie test. In older children and adolescents, a history of easy bruising, epistaxis, prolonged bleeding after lacerations, menorrhagia, haematuria, gastrointestinal bleeding and postoperative haemorrhage (including dental) should be sought. The nature of the bleeding may help to distinguish the underlying problem. For example, haemorrhage from the skin and mucous membranes are usually associated with platelet disorders, whilst deep-seated haematomas and haemarthrosis are characteristic of severe clotting factor deficiencies. Bruising and nose bleeds are common complaints in childhood and unlikely to be significant, if the only manifestations of a bleeding problem. A drug history is also important, with particular reference to aspirin ingestion; not only might drugs cause haemorrhagic problems, but they will also cause difficulty with interpretation of coagulation studies.

Examination

Physical examination should pay particular reference to evidence of abnormal bleeding, e.g. petechiae, ecchymosis, joint abnormalities, haematomas, and to physical signs such as hepatosplenomegaly which might suggest an underlying haematological disorder.

Laboratory investigations

This section is not intended to be a comprehensive review of laboratory coagulation tests, but merely a brief overview of the indications for the commoner studies. Investigation of a patient with a suspected bleeding disorder starts with a number of screening tests which are designed to detect the presence of an abnormality but fall short of specific identification. Screening tests do not identify all coagulation problems and may be normal in the presence of a mild disorder. Therefore, if the history is strongly suggestive of a bleeding disorder, more specific testing is indicated.

Screening tests

Platelet count. A low platelet count may be acquired, as in DIC, or inherited, as in Bernard Soulier syndrome. Examination of a blood smear may be helpful, as disorders such as Bernard Soulier syndrome are characterized by megathrombocytes.

Bleeding time. Most laboratories now employ a standardized template bleeding time which is a good test of platelet function. The bleeding time will be prolonged, with significant thrombocytopenia or defective platelet function. An abnormal bleeding time in the presence of a normal platelet count suggests a platelet function abnormality and merits more specific investigation.

Prothrombin time. The prothrombin time (PT) is used to test the extrinsic coagulation pathway (fibrinogen and factors II, V, VII and X). The PT is reported in seconds and an abnormal value is a clotting time more than 2 seconds above the range for that laboratory. It is usual for a control value to be reported along with the test PT. It is important to remember that a control test is merely carried out to ensure that the reagents etc. are working, and is not a 'mean' value or the upper limit of normal for that laboratory. It should not be used to determine whether or not the test is within the normal range.

Activated partial thromboplastin time. The activated partial thromboplastin time (APPT) is used to test the intrinsic coagulation pathway (fibrinogen and factors II, V, VIII, IX, X, XI, XII, PK and HMWK). The APTT value is reported in seconds, and is abnormal if 5 seconds or more above the normal range for the laboratory. The APTT should be sensitive to a FVIII:C level of less than 30 iu/dl, so that haemophilia A will not go undiagnosed. In the author's laboratory, if the APTT is prolonged without an obvious reason, the test is repeated using a 1:1 mixture with normal pool plasma. This will correct the APTT if due to a factor deficiency, but not if due to a circulating anticoagulant. Incubation of the test plasma will significantly further prolong the APTT in the presence of a specific inhibitor (e.g. FVIII:C inhibitor) but not of a nonspecific inhibitor (e.g. lupus anticoagulant).

Thrombin clotting time. The thrombin clotting time (TCT) measures the conversion of fibrinogen to fibrin only. It is reported in seconds and will be prolonged in hypofibrinogenaemia, dysfibrinogenaemia or by an inhibitor to thrombin, e.g. heparin or FDPs.

Specific tests

Further investigations are generally indicated by an abnormality of one or more of the screening tests or by a history strongly suggestive of an underlying haemorrhagic disorder, even in the presence of normal screening tests.

Fibrinogen concentration. The fibrinogen level should be determined, if DIC or an inherited deficiency of fibrinogen are suspected. A discrepancy between the immunological and coagulant assay suggests dysfibrinogenaemia rather than hypofibrinogenaemia, in which both values are usually similarly reduced.

Fibrinogen degradation products (FDPs and D-dimer). Fragment DD or D-dimer is generated when crosslinked fibrin clots are lysed by plasmin; this is in contrast to FDPs, which are generated by the lysis of fibrinogen and non-crosslinked fibrin. Both are elevated in the presence of DIC. D-dimer is more specific and FDP a more sensitive indicator.

Coagulation factor assays. Specific factor assays usually employ a variation of the APTT or PT. Very small quantities of plasma are required, and these assays are generally performed to identify a specific factor deficiency. Results are expressed as unit/ml or unit/dl, although previously as % activity of normal. One unit is the amount of activity found in 1 ml of fresh plasma, and a factor assay of 100% is equivalent to 1 unit/ml or 100 units/dl. FXIII is not, measured by either the PT or the APTT. It can be screened by using 5M urea or 1% monochloracetic acid, and

clot from plasma deficient in FXIII dissolves more rapidly than the control. Specific assays confirm the diagnosis and are necessary to detect the heterozygous state.

vWF:Ag and ristocetin cofactor activity. FVIII:C, vWF:Ag and the ristocetin cofactor activity are determined in patients suspected of having vWD. vWF:Ag is measured by precipitating heterogenous antibodies made against human FVIII in the rabbit. The ristocetin cofactor activity is a quantitative assay of ristocetin-induced aggregation of platelet-rich plasma. The diagnosis of vWD is usually completed by plasma and platelet multimeric analysis.

Platelet aggregation studies. The response of platelet-rich plasma to a number of agonists (ADP, thrombin, collagen, adrenaline and ristocetin) can detect and classify platelet defects. These studies employ relatively large quantities of plasma. Monoclonal antibody techniques can detect GPIb and GPIIb/IIIa on the platelet surface, making the diagnosis of Bernard Soulier syndrome and Glanzmann's thrombasthenia possible on small volumes of whole blood.

Tests of fibrinolysis. Tests of fibrinolysis may include a global test of fibrinolytic function, the euglobulin clot lysis time, or specific assays of plasminogen, α_2 antiplasmin and plasminogen activator levels.

Tests of natural anticoagulants. Although clinical thrombosis in children is rare, children may be referred for diagnosis because of a positive family history. ATIII, protein C, protein S and HCII can all be measured by activity or immunological methods or both.

THE EVALUATION OF COAGULATION DISORDERS IN THE NEONATE

The interpretation of coagulation parameters in the newborn is complicated by the physiological gestation-dependent low values and the difficulty in obtaining uncontaminated plasma in sufficient volumes for testing. All laboratories providing a service to neonatal units should establish microtechniques for routine coagulation screening. One to two millilitres of blood are sufficient to perform a coagulation screen and full range of factor assays (Andrews et al 1987a). As little as 20 µl of plasma suffice for each of the screening tests (PT, APTT, PTT and TCT). Factor assays employing dilutions of 1:10 (10 µl plasma diluted in 90 µl buffer), rising to 1:100, require very small quantities of plasma. Once a dilution has been prepared, this can theoretically be used for more than one factor assay. Although coagulation tests are generally performed in duplicate, this may not be possible in the neonate. It is essential that all clinical information is available to the haematologist, so that the most appropriate tests are carried out first, and precious plasma is not wasted.

It is important to test a venous sample which is not contaminated by intravenous solutions, has flowed freely and has neither activated nor clotted in the process of sampling. Activation of the specimen characteristically shortens the APTT. Specimens should always be checked for fibrin strands or clots, as such artefacts are particularly common in samples taken from very small babies. The development of immunological assays has helped to overcome some of the problems of contaminated or partially activated specimens, as they measure total and not just functional protein. However, at the present time we rely heavily on functional assays, particularly for screening tests which can only be measured in this way. Heparin contamination of specimens obtained from arterial or venous catheters, through which heparin is being infused to prevent thrombosis, is a common problem. At least 4 ml of blood must be withdrawn prior to sampling to prevent contamination. A blood sample which might potentially be contaminated with heparin should always be checked for the presence of a circulating anticoagulant. An abnormal result which is not in keeping with the clinical picture should be repeated in the first instance. However, the problems of repeatedly taking blood from the neonate may make this difficult or impossible.

The anticoagulant ratio should be based on the plasma volume and not on the total volume of whole blood. The volume of anticoagulant should be reduced proportionately to the increased haematocrit value (Table 13.4). This is particularly important for infants with very high haematocrits.

A modified template bleeding time can be used to assess platelet function, as unacceptably large volumes of plasma are required for formal platelet aggregation studies. Newer aggregometers have been modified for small volumes, but many still require about 150 µl of platelet-rich plasma per aggregating agent. Andrews reported a shortened bleeding time in neonates, compared to adults, using a modified template bleeding time developed for infants. The mean bleeding time of 61 non-thrombocytopenic infants was 142 + 37 seconds {mean + SD} (Andrew et al 1987b). Other workers have also reported the newborn's bleeding time to be shorter than that of the adult, despite their impaired platelet function (Feusner 1980). Andrew postulated that the short bleeding time may be related to the high haematocrit or elevated vWF in the infant. Stuart gives an alternative suggestion for a normal bleeding time in the presence of impairment of platelet aggregation (Stuart 1981). She reported the neonate to have a markedly reduced ability to regenerate PGI_2 compared to the adult. The PGI_2-like regenerating activity normalizes by 3–5 months of age, at a time when platelet function is no longer impaired.

Table 13.4 Volume of anticoagulant for 9 volumes of whole blood (used in newborns to correct volume of anticoagulant for a high haematocrit)

Haematocrit (%)	Vol. of anticoagulant (ml)
45	1.0
50	0.9
51	0.9
53	0.85
55	0.8
57	0.8
59	0.75
60	0.7
63	0.65
65	0.65
67	0.6
69	0.55
70	0.55
71	0.5
73	0.5
75	0.45
77	0.4
79	0.4
80	0.35
81	0.35
83	0.3
85	0.3
87	0.25
89	0.2
90	0.2

From Corrigan Jr J J 1989 Neonatal coagulation disorders. In: Alter B P (ed) Perinatal haematology. Churchill Livingstone, Edinburgh, p 167, with permission of the publisher.

Table 13.5   Reference values for screening tests in the healthy full-term infant during the first 6 months of life*

Tests	Day 1	Day 5	Day 30	Day 90	Day 180	Adult
PT (s)	13.0 ± 1.43	12.4 ± 1.46	11.8 ± 1.25	11.9 ± 1.15	12.3 ± 0.79	12.4 ± 0.78
APTT (s)	42.9 ± 5.80	42.6 ± 8.62	40.4 ± 7.42	37.1 ± 6.52	35.5 ± 3.71	33.5 ± 3.44
TCT (s)	23.5 ± 2.38	23.1 ± 3.07	24.3 ± 2.44	25.1 ± 2.32	25.5 ± 2.86	25.0 ± 2.66

All values are expressed as mean ± 1 SD
Adapted from Andrew et al 1987a, with permission of Grune & Stratton Inc.
*See also Ch. 1, Table 1.26

Table 13.6   Reference values for screening tests in health premature infants (30–36 weeks gestation) during the first 6 months of life*

Tests	Day 1 M	B	Day 5 M	B	Day 30 M	B	Day 90 M	B	Day 180 M	B	Adult M	B
PT (s)	13.0	(10.6–16.2)	12.5	(10.0–15.3)	11.8	(10.0–13.6)	12.3	(10.0–14.6)	12.5	(10.0–15.0)	12.4	(10.8–13.9)
APTT (s)	53.6	(27.5–79.4)	50.5	(26.9–74.1)	44.7	(26.9–62.5)	37.5	(28.3–50.7)	37.5	(21.7–53.3)	33.5	(26.6–40.3)
TCT (s)	24.8	(19.2–30.4)	24.1	(18.8–29.4)	24.4	(18.8–29.9)	25.1	(19.4–30.8)	25.2	(18.9–31.5)	25.0	(19.7–30.3)

M = mean; B = lower and upper boundary encompassing 95% of the population.
Adapted from Andrew et al 1988, with permission of Grune and Stratton Inc.
*See also Ch. 1, Table 1.27

Stuart suggests that the physiological impairment in platelet function provides a safety mechanism to counteract the prothrombotic state induced by a deficiency of PGI_2.

Tables 13.5 and 13.6 give values for the PT, APTT and TCT based on a large number of healthy full-term and preterm infants studied longitudinally over a 6-month period (Andrew et al 1987a, Andrew et al 1988). Venous samples only were tested, and all infants had received 1 mg of vitamin K at birth. This comprehensive study showed that, although the variability of the PT was greater in the preterm and term newborn infant, the mean values were not significantly different from the adult. The PT shortened during the first month of life. Low levels of the contact factors in infants may greatly prolong the APTT such that the test becomes of little diagnostic value. Andrew used a reagent containing ellagic acid rather than kaolin as an activating agent, which narrowed the normal range, thereby increasing the usefulness of the APTT as a screening test. She reported the APTT to be prolonged at birth, and to reach adult values by 3 months of age, in the full-term infant. The APTT was further prolonged in the preterm infant at birth and remained significantly statistically longer than the adult value until 6 months of age. The TCT performed with calcium present in the buffering system to overcome the relative thrombin insensitivity of fetal fibrinogen was in the adult range at birth and a narrow normal range delineated.

HEREDITARY COAGULATION DISORDERS

Haemophilia A and B and von Willebrand's disease account for more than 90% of inherited clotting factor deficiencies. Haemophilia A is the commonest, with a frequency of approximately 1 per 10 000 in the general population (Levine 1987). Haemophilia B (Christmas disease) is less common, accounting for only 15–20% of all cases of haemophilia (Department of Health, Education and Welfare 1972, Ramgren 1962). Both types of haemophilia occur with similar incidence in all areas of the world. Estimates for vWD of 3–4 per 100 000 population have been reported in the UK (Bloom 1980), but other studies have differed widely. All other inherited coagulation disorders are rare.

Haemophilia A

Haemophilia A is an X-linked recessive bleeding disorder attributable to decreased plasma levels of the procoagulant activity (FVIII:C) of the FVIII molecule. FVIII:C circulates in plasma with vWF as a noncovalently linked protein complex, and its importance in normal coagulation is evident from the severe haemorrhagic disorder which results from its functional deficiency.

Human FVIII has now been purified from a number of plasma products. It is synthesized as a single-chain polypeptide and subsequently converted to the two chain molecule which circulates in plasma. A heavy chain of 92–210 kDa circulates with a light chain of 80 kDa, presumably associated via a calcium linkage. The cloning of the human FVIII gene and the expression of active recombinant FVIII have provided important information about the structure of the molecule. The heavy and light chains are both required for procoagulant function but the binding site for vWF is believed to be on the light chain. Specific thrombin, activated protein C and FXa cleavage sites have been identified. Those interested should consult the reviews on the structure-function relationships of the FVIII molecule by Foster & Zimmerman (1989) and White & Shoemaker, (1989). Along with our expanded understanding of the molecular nature of FVIII and vWF, has come new recommendations for the nomenclature of each protein (Table 13.7). The gene that codes for FVIII:C has been assigned to band q28 of the

Table 13.7 Proposed abbreviations for Factor VIII and von Willebrand factor from the Subcommittee on Factor VIII and von Willebrand Factor* of the International Committee on Thrombosis and Haemostasis

Attribute	Abbreviations	
	Proposed	Outmoded
Factor VIII		
Protein	VIII	VIII:C
Antigen	VIII:Ag	VIIIC:Ag
Function	VIII:C	–
von Willebrand factor		
Protein	vWF	VIIIR:Ag. VIII/vWF AHF-like protein
Antigen	vWF:Ag	VIIIR:Ag AHF-like antigen
Function	–	**VIIIR:RCo. VIIIR:vWF

*The two proteins form a bimolecular complex which can be abbreviated as 'VIII/vWF'.
**These abbreviations have been used to indicate the ristocetin cofactor activity of von Willebrand factor. Since neither this test nor any other in-vitro test completely reflects vWF activity, no abbreviation is recommended as representative of its function.
From Marder et al 1985, with permission of publishers, FK Schattauer Verlag GmbH, Stuttgart

long arm of the X chromosome. It is a large gene of nearly 186,000 base pairs (bp) and constitutes 0.1% of the X chromosome.

Inheritance and genetic defects

Phenotypically, patients with haemophilia A are deficient in FVIII procoagulant activity and fall into two main groups; (1) those in whom the FVIII protein is present in approximately normal amounts but is nonfunctional; and (2) those in whom the protein concentration is greatly reduced, due to a defect of expression or secretion of FVIII or to the production of a defective molecule which is not recognized by alloantibodies against the FVIII protein (VIII:Ag). It is clear from DNA analysis that diverse defects give rise to the same clinical disorder recognized as haemophilia A. Both deletions and point mutations have been identified.

Haemophilia is expressed in males who inherit a haemophilia gene (X^h) from their mother, and a male chromosome (Y) from their father. Haemophilia is carried by females who inherit a haemophilia gene (X^h) from one parent and a normal gene (X) from the other parent. The sons of a female carrier have a 50/50 chance of being affected, and the daughters a 50/50 chance of being a carrier. A father with haemophilia cannot transmit the disease to his sons, but all his daughters will be carriers. The severity of the deficiency is consistent within members of the same family. About 30% of cases have no family history and arise from new mutations in the mother or a grandparent, or from familial transmission through female members.

The identification of female carriers is important for genetic counselling. A female carrier possesses two X chromosomes (X^hX), only one of which is expressed in a given somatic cell. Inactivation of the second chromosome (lyonization) is a random event. Thus, FVIII-producing cells with an active X chromosome will express normal amounts of FVIII:C, and those with an inactive, X^h, chromosome will not do so. On average, FVIII:C levels in a carrier will be one-half of the normal value of females. Normal individuals have roughly equal amounts of FVIII:C and vWF:Ag. vWF:Ag has an autosomal inheritance, and levels are normal or increased in males with haemophilia

A and in obligate carriers, who should have relatively less FVIII:C. One can thus distinguish over 80% of carriers by determining the ratio of FVIII:C and vWF:Ag using both assays and statistical refinements. The advent of DNA analysis by gene probing has increased the accuracy of carrier detection. Two approaches are available. The first depends on direct recognition of the specific genomic defect and has the advantage of not requiring pedigree information if the precise defect has already been established in the family under study. The second approach employs restriction fragment length polymorphisms (RFLPs) linked to the FVIII gene, and the DNA probes identify independently segregating restriction polymorphisms close to or in the FVIII gene. The specific genomic defect does not need to be known, but this approach requires an affected male to establish the allele present on the mutant X-chromosome and requires that the mother be heterozygous for the polymorphism. Carrier detection can be enhanced by using multiple DNA probes, and the new technique of gene amplification using the polymerase chain reaction may prove useful. Because there is a significant risk of recombination between extragenic RFLPs and the FVIII gene, diagnosis of carrier status should be based on intragenic RFLPs wherever possible; if this is not possible, results obtained by extragenic RFLPs alone must be analyzed in combination with conventional biological assays and pedigree analysis.

Prenatal testing

The majority of haemophiliacs have a family history, and many women now seek prenatal diagnosis. In the past, women who knew themselves to be carriers of haemophilia A often would not risk the birth of a haemophiliac son and elected to terminate all male pregnancies, many of which would in fact be unaffected. The advent of prenatal diagnosis offers a rational approach to family planning for obligate or possible carriers. Unfortunately, termination of affected pregnancies will not eradicate haemophilia, because 30% of cases arise from new mutations and many obligate carriers will not consider termination and decline prenatal diagnosis. Again, prenatal diagnosis can be based on DNA analysis or immunological assays of FVIII:Ag and vWF:Ag on fetal blood. Prenatal diagnosis should only be offered to women who would proceed with termination of the pregnancy of an affected fetus. To make this decision, she must understand the problems and expectations for a haemophiliac and be counselled on the risks and limitations of the diagnostic procedures used. The next step in prenatal diagnosis is to establish the sex of the fetus. DNA can be obtained by amniocentesis or chorionic villus sampling. Fetal blood sampling will be necessary if DNA analysis is noninformative, and can be done at about 20 weeks' gestation. It is important to use immunological assays, because of the small volume of blood and the risk of contamination.

The female carrier will not generally exhibit a clinical bleeding tendency, but extreme lyonization of the normal X chromosome may result in carriers with clinical bleeding problems. This is more commonly seen in Christmas disease. Homozygous female haemophiliacs, the offspring of a male haemophiliac with a carrier female, are occasionally encountered.

Clinical features

The clinical severity of haemophilia A varies considerably, and patients are classified into mild, moderate or severely affected according to their level of FVIII:C. Severely affected males have a FVIII:C level of less than 2% and will bleed spontaneously without trauma. Moderately affected males have a FVIII:C level of 2–10% and bleed following minor trauma. Those individuals with FVIII:C levels of 10% and above are considered mildly affected and bleed only after trauma or surgery. The relationship between activity level and clinical severity is not as straightforward as this classification implies. At least 50% of haemophiliacs have FVIII:C levels below 2% and are severely affected. The severity of the deficiency is consistent within members of the same family and dictates the type and frequency of clinical problems.

Less than 10% of haemophiliac infants present with bleeding problems in the newborn period and they will be severely affected. Haematoma following an intramuscular vitamin K injection, oozing after heel prick screening for PKU, or haematoma formation at the site of infantile vaccinations may draw attention to the underlying coagulopathy. Bleeding may occur from the cord or from a circumcision site, if this has been performed on an undiagnosed haemophiliac. Intracranial bleeding is rare (Olson et al 1985, Yonker et al 1985) although cephalhaematoma is seen. Splenic and adrenal haemorrhage have also been described (Jannaccone & Pasquino 1981, Schmidt & Zipursky 1986). Caesarian section is only indicated for documented cephalopelvic disproportion, or causes which would indicate caesarian section in a normal infant. Forceps delivery should be avoided. The majority of affected males will have no problems in the neonatal period and will not present until they begin crawling and bumping into objects, or attempt standing and fall.

Severe haemophilia A (FVIII:C less than 2%). Abnormal bleeding may occur at any site of the body, but severe haemophilia is characterized by recurrent episodes of bleeding into joints, muscles and soft tissues. Although haemorrhagic episodes may appear spontaneous, they are probably the consequence of physiological trauma to muscles and joints. Haemophiliacs do not have exsanguinating haemorrhage but, rather, a slow continuous ooze which is difficult to stop without specific therapy. Superficial cuts usually stop bleeding normally if the initial clot is undisturbed, but cuts on moist mucosal surfaces, such as inside the mouth and tongue, may be troublesome and continue to ooze because the clot is constantly disturbed by movement of the tongue and saliva. This is a common site of injury in infants who have a tendency to put toys in their mouths. By the second year of life, most severely and moderately affected haemophiliacs will have shown an abnormal bleeding tendency, with easy bruising and subcutaneous haematoma formation. Infants with no family history may be diagnosed because of referral by the Social Work Department for investigation of a suspected nonaccidental injury (Johnson et al 1988).

Any joint may be the site of haemorrhage, but weight-bearing joints are the most vulnerable. In young children, ankles are most commonly affected, and in the older child, knees, followed by ankles and elbows. Following injury, the synovial vessels rupture and blood accumulates in the joint. Repeated haemorrhage results in hypertrophy and increased vascularity of the joint capsule predisposing to further haemorrhage. There is an initial stage of synovial reaction and a later stage of cartilage degeneration and joint destruction. The degree of haemophilic arthropathy can be classified radiologically according to recommendations of the World Federation of Haemophilia (Pettersson et al 1987), by the existence and severity of osteopenia, enlargement of the epiphysis, irregularity of the subchondral surface, narrowing of the joint space, subchondral cyst formation, erosion at the joint margins, gross incongruence of the articulating bone ends and joint deformity. It is now hoped that early and effective replacement therapy will prevent these typical changes of haemophilic arthropathy occurring. Newer techniques, such as magnetic resonance imaging, may add to our understanding of the more subtle early damage of arthropathy (Pettersson et al 1987). Pain, swelling, increased heat, local tenderness and limitation of movement are the principle findings of an acute haemarthrosis, but are dependent on the severity of haemorrhage. The joint will assume the position of minimal discomfort. The hip joint, for example, will be held in a position of flexion, abduction and lateral rotation, and the knee joint in flexion. The intense pain subsides and the swelling resolves rapidly with replacement therapy. However, a joint which has been the site of repeated bleeding episodes may never return to normal but remains slightly swollen and boggy because of synovial thickening. Soft-tissue swelling due to distention of the joint capsule characterizes the radiological findings of an acute haemarthrosis. Many severely affected haemophiliacs experience 'targeting' of one joint, with relative sparing of the others.

Deep intramuscular haematomas affect the lower limb more commonly than the upper; the quadriceps and other muscles of the thigh are frequently involved, although calf bleeds are not uncommon. Physical findings consist of pain and swelling, with limitation of movement of the adjacent joints. If large enough, haematomas may compress blood vessels or nerves; involvement of the femoral nerve in iliopsoas haematoma is particularly characteristic. An iliopsoas or retroperitoneal haematoma may mimic a variety of surgical or medical emergencies, such as appendicitis or renal colic. Ultrasound examination may be diagnostically helpful in detecting these deep-seated haematomas. A particularly serious complication is the development of Volkmann's ischaemic contracture of the hand, due to bleeding into the muscles of the forearm.

Intracranial haemorrhage following minor trauma is a small but constant hazard and a potential life-threatening complication which can be associated with significant neurological sequelae in survivors. Haematoma can occur at any site in the body, and the possibility of pressure upon vital structures, including nerves, blood vessels and air passages, should always be borne in mind. Superficial bruising of the lower limbs is very common in children. Gastrointestinal haemorrhage and haematuria are unusual in early childhood, although bleeding from the urinary tract is relatively common in adolescence. Epistaxis usually results from local injury.

Moderate (FVIII:C 2–10%) and mild (FVIII:C > 10%) haemophilia A. Boys with mild haemophilia only bleed after significant trauma or after dental extraction or surgery. These patients may not be diagnosed until later in life when they meet an appropriate challenge. Boys who are moderately affected may experience haemarthrosis or soft-tissue haematomas after mild trauma, although not spontaneously.

Diagnosis

Two-thirds of the boys will have a family history and will present for diagnosis in the immediate neonatal period, as even families who have decided to risk a haemophiliac child are anxious to have their worse fears allayed. Diagnosis can easily be made in the newborn, as FVIII:C levels are within the adult range at birth and FVIII:C does not cross the placenta and therefore is fetal in origin. However, one-third of haemophiliacs have no family history and are investigated because of a clinical bleeding problem. Laboratory investigation should start with a coagulation screen and a FVIII:C level. In haemophilia, the APTT will be prolonged in proportion to the reduction of FVIII:C. vWF:Ag and ristocetin cofactor activity are generally performed to exclude vWD, if the suspected diagnosis is not already known from the family history. The bleeding time is normal in haemophilia but prolonged in vWD. However, a prolonged template BT has been reported in a small percentage of patients with haemophilia A and this is attributed to a defect in vascular function associated with the presence of circulating immune complexes (Stuart et al 1986). These tests are adequate to confirm the diagnosis and classify the severity. The FVIII:C level should be done on at least two occasions, because of the significance of such a serious diagnosis. Ancillary tests include: (1) a FBC to exclude anaemia, resulting from bleeding episodes; (2) determination of the blood group so that this is available should transfusion be necessary at some stage; (3) a FVIII:C inhibitor assay; and (4) LFTs and hepatitis serology as baseline evaluations prior to replacement therapy and hepatitis B vaccination.

Management

The management of haemophilia can be considered under two major headings. (1) the treatment of bleeding episodes and their complications; and (2) the education and psychosocial support of the boys and their families. Firstly, some general points will be considered. After diagnosis has been confirmed, the parents should be interviewed and given an outline of likely problems associated with haemophilia, tailored to the severity of the defect in their son. This should be positive and optimistic, but must include sensible guidelines and necessary restrictions on activities.

All new patients should be registered and issued with a Haemophilia Card stating the level of their deficient factor, their inhibitor status and their blood group. Details of their local heamophilia centre should be included, so that the family or other medical personnel can make immediate contact, if necessary.

The pattern of inheritance should be explained to the parents, including the statistical likelihood of future siblings being affected or carriers, and genetic counselling offered.

Several points need emphasizing to parents, family doctors and junior medical staff alike:

1. Children with bleeding disorders should never be given intramuscular injections. This must be remembered in the context of premedication for anaesthesia. However, they should be immunized like any other child, using the deep subcutaneous route with a small-gauge needle (25 size) with

pressure on the site for several minutes. In many haemophilia centres, the haemophilia sister will carry out and assume responsibility for vaccinations. Most importantly, all recipients or potential recipients of pooled-blood products should be immunized against hepatitis B and their immunity regularly monitored.

2. Aspirin, with its antiplatelet effect, should never be given to patients with an inherited bleeding problem, as this will add to the likelihood of bleeding. Paracetamol is a safe alternative. Case-records should bear a hazard warning label stating that the patient should not receive intramuscular injections or aspirin-containing products.

3. Prophylactic dental care is essential and should be provided by regular attendance at a dental surgeon experienced in the management of haemophilia.

4. Treatment should be given at the first sign of pain or swelling in a joint, day or night. Particular attention must be given to head injuries or gastro-intestinal bleeding.

5. The risks associated with the use of blood products must be honestly discussed. However, it is now fair to state that presently recommended factor concentrates are free from the risk of HIV transmission. Any other risks they harbour are small compared with the morbidity and mortality associated with not treating bleeding episodes appropriately.

6. The importance of a good education should be stressed.

7. In addition to outpatient attendances for the treatment of acute bleeding episodes, the boys must be seen at an outpatient clinic on a regular basis to monitor the frequency of bleeds and any treatment-related side-effects, for assessment of musculoskeletal problems by a physiotherapist and orthopaedic surgeon, and for dental review.

8. The care of patients with inherited coagulation disorders necessitates a multidisciplinary team approach because of the range of problems encountered. All patients should have ready access to a treatment centre which can provide the following services:

a. Open access treatment available 24 hours for acute bleeds for both inpatients and outpatients. Advice and organisation of home therapy and prophylactic treatment programmes.

b. Special consultant services with regular medical, surgical, orthopaedic, rheumatological, dental and infectious diseases review of patients. Provision of haemostatic cover for surgery and physiotherapy.

c. Maintenance of a register of all patients, including a pedigree on each family. This is essential for carrier detection and prenatal diagnosis.

d. Laboratory service for diagnosis of hereditary and acquired disorders, including genetic analysis.

e. Provision of social work support and counselling in relation to haemophilia, carrier status, HIV, education and employment.

Treatment of bleeding episodes and their complications

The principle of treatment of bleeding episodes in haemophilia is the infusion of an appropriate blood product in sufficient quantities to raise the deficient factor to a haemostatic level. Patients who can be managed without blood products should be. Mild haemophilia should be treated with desmopressin (DDAVP) whenever possible. DDAVP acts by releasing endogenously synthesized FVIII from its stores. It is given in a dose of 0.3 µg/kg dissolved in about 10–20 ml N saline and infused over 20 minutes, and will raise the FVIII:C level by 2–4 times its basal level. If it is anticipated that such a rise will bring the FVIII:C value into a haemostatic range, DDAVP is the treatment of choice and avoids the use of blood products. However, if treatment is required on a regular daily basis, a diminished response is usually seen by the third or fourth day due to depletion of FVIII:C stores, though not inevitably (Isola et al 1984). For this reason even mildly affected haemophiliacs may require factor FVIII:C concentrates for surgical procedures necessitating the maintenance of relatively high levels of FVIII:C for longer than 3–4 days. There are advantages in doing an elective therapeutic trial of DDAVP and monitoring the FVIII:C rise some time before a planned procedure. All other patients with haemophilia A are now treated with FVIII concentrates, and those with haemophilia B with factor IX concentrates. The precise number of units of FVIII:C or FIX are stated on the bottle of concentrate, making calculation of the required dose simple. One unit of FVIII:C or FIX is defined as the activity present in 1 ml of fresh pooled normal plasma. A recipient's plasma volume is 40–50 ml/kg body weight; therefore 1 unit of FVIII:C/kg body weight raises the FVIII:C level by approximately 2%. The in vivo recovery is less than expected in patients with continuing haemorrhage or circulating antibodies to FVIII:C. The half-life of FVIII:C is around 8–12 hours. After calculating the dose, concentrate is prescribed in numbers of bottles, and not absolute numbers of units, to avoid any wastage of an expensive and scarce commodity.

Management of specific problems

Most severely affected haemophiliacs will average 2–4 bleeding episodes per month. The level of FVIII required for adequate haemostasis depends upon the clinical situation (Table 13.8). In gen-

eral, the minimum haemostatic level for relatively mild haemorrhage in haemophilia A is 30% (30 iu/dl). More major bleeding episodes including advanced joint and muscle haematomas require a FVIII:C level of about 50%, and it may be necessary to treat on a number of consecutive days. A FVIII:C level of 80–100% is required for life-threatening haemorrhage or for surgery. In such circumstances, the FVIII:C level must be kept above 30–50% by means of appropriate doses of FVIII concentrate at 8 to 12-hourly intervals for 10–14 days.

Oral bleeding. Superficial cuts tend to stop bleeding in the normal time. It is usually cuts in the mouth and tongue which cause problems. Although FVIII concentrate at a dose of 15 units/kg will result in clot formation and temporarily stop bleeding, it is difficult to prevent the clot dissolving, especially in very young children. Tranexamic acid should be given to help stabilize

Table 13.8 Suggested initial doses of replacement products for haemophilia A and B

Indications for replacement	Haemophilia A Infusate (units of FVIII:C/kg)	Desired FVIII:C level (%)	Haemophilia B Infusate (units of FIX:C/kg)	Desired FIX:C level (%)
Mild haemorrhage Early haemarthrosis Subcutaneous haematoma Epistaxis Haematuria Gum and dental bleeding unresponsive to tranexamic acid	15	30	20	20
Major haemorrhage Established haemarthrosis Haematomas with pain and swelling Retroperitoneal bleeding Haematomas with the potential to cause pressure on blood vessels or nerves Head trauma without neurological deficit Severe physical trauma without evidence of bleeding Severe abdominal pain Gastrointestinal haemorrhage	25	50	40	40
Life-threatening lesions Intracranial haemorrhage Major trauma with bleeding Surgery Potential airway obstruction	40–50	80–100	60	60

For major haemorrhage, subsequent doses are usually required; for life-threatening lesions, one to several weeks of maintenance of minimum levels is mandatory.
Adapted from Levine 1987, with permission of J B Lippincott Co, Philadelphia, USA

the clot and prevent rebleeding, but it is often necessary to give repeated doses of FVIII concentrate on consecutive days. Boys with oral bleeds which might track posteriorly and obstruct the airway should be hospitalized for observation, and a higher level of FVIII:C maintained.

Soft-tissue bleeding. The severity and the anatomical site of bleeding dictates the level at which FVIII:C must be maintained. Subcutaneous haematomas can be treated with FVIII 15 units/kg until symptoms resolve. More major soft-tissue bleeding episodes require a FVIII level in the region of about 50% and a larger dose of 25–30 units/kg. The response, site and severity therefore determines the frequency of administration, which may have to be twice a day and for several days. More serious bleeding episodes requiring more aggressive treatment include those with the potential to cause pressure problems on nerves or vessels or obstruction of the airway, or excessively large bleeds such as into the thigh or psoas muscles or retroperitoneal space. In many instances, bedrest or immobilization, followed by physiotherapy will speed recovery.

Haemarthrosis. A haemarthrosis requires a FVIII:C level in the region of 30% or even 50%. The earlier a joint bleed is treated, the less damage results and, usually, the less FVIII is required. Most patients describe an aura of vague warmth or a tingling sensation which may precede swelling and pain by a few hours and this is the optimal time to treat. If treated early, 15 units/kg FVIII will usually suffice and immobilization not be necessary, although it is advisable to minimize weightbearing, if the lower limb is involved. Joint bleeds, which are not treated until swelling and pain have occurred, need 25 units/kg FVIII, immobilization and daily treatment until the signs have resolved and a full range of movement returned at the joint. When immobilization is necessary, it should be used for the minimum necessary period, because muscle atrophy develops quickly. Splinting, with a light-weight splint or back-slab should be in the position of maximum comfort, and reviewed with change to a more functional position as the degree of swelling allows.

Following severe bleeding episodes which have required several days treatment and immobilization, physiotherapy will be necessary to mobilize the joint and should be started once the pain has resolved. Initial isometric muscle exercises are followed by gentle active assisted exercises, firstly with gravity eliminated and then against gravity, before weight-bearing is attempted, if the lower limb is involved. Physiotherapy and the first days of weight-bearing are usually covered with replacement therapy. The quadriceps are particularly vulnerable to atrophy which leaves the joint unstable and prone to recurrent haemarthrosis. Swimming is strongly recommended for improving and maintaining muscle tone. For young children with recurrent ankle bleeds, high-top padded boots provide ankle stability.

In children, recurrent spontaneous haemarthrosis in a target joint often results in chronic synovial hypertrophy. The joint is persistently swollen and boggy due to proliferation of the highly vascular synovium, which encourages further haemarthrosis. The ankle joint is most commonly involved in small children, and the knee and elbow in older children. The anticipated course is one of progressive joint destruction, although several months of intensive prophylactic replacement therapy is often given in the hope of resolving the lesion and preventing further joint changes. Miser et al (1986) reported the outcome of administering 20–30 units/kg of FVIII two or 2–3 times weekly for 3–8 months to 12 children with chronic synovitis affecting 19 joints. Physiotherapy was used in conjunction with factor replacement. Prophylaxis given 3 times weekly eliminated clinical bleeding episodes, and twice-weekly infusions did so in the majority of cases. Fourteen of 19 joints with chronic synovitis treated with 1–3 courses of vigorous factor replacement had no clinical evidence of synovitis at a median of 31 months after stopping prophylaxis. Radiological changes of progressive joint deterioration were seen in the majority of joints with either uncontrolled or relapsing chronic synovitis. Synovectomy may have to be considered in children who have continued haemarthrosis because of incomplete clinical resolution or relapses of synovitis despite intensive prophylaxis. Synovectomy decreases the incidence of recurrent bleeding, but usually also results in some loss of joint motion and may not alter the course of joint destruction, especially if done late (Canale et al 1988).

At present, demand therapy is utilized by most haemophilia centres around the world. However, in Europe, studies are underway in children to determine the benefits in the prevention of joint disease of regular infusions of FVIII, independent of any symptoms. It remains to be proven if prophylaxis will prove superior to demand treatment, especially when the complications of therapy are added to the equation.

Haematuria. Haematuria is a relatively common problem in older boys and generally occurs spontaneously, although it can follow trauma. Extensive urological evaluation is not necessary, although a renal ultrasound is helpful to exclude renal calculi or a hydronephrosis behind an obstructed ureter in boys with recurrent or persistent haematuria. A high fluid intake alone might suffice, but otherwise FVIII concentrate should be tried. Antifibrinolytic agents, such as tranexamic acid, are contraindicated because of the risk of producing unlysable clots in the renal tract and resultant hydronephrosis.

Gastrointestinal bleeding. This is relatively rare in children, although, in general, patients with haemophilia are more likely to have problematic bleeding from a concurrent gastrointestinal problem than are individuals with intact haemostasis. Such bleeding requires the usual resuscitative measures, in addition to FVIII replacement given at a sufficient dose and frequency to maintain a FVIII:C level of about 50% until the bleeding has stopped and for a number of days thereafter. Radiological investigation or endoscopy is indicated to identify any underlying cause, if the problem is recurrent.

Head injury and CNS bleeding. Prior to AIDS, intracranial haemorrhage (ICH) was the commonest cause of death in patients with haemophilia. Head injuries are very common in small children, although many are relatively trivial. However, the severity of injury is not prognostically helpful in predicting the risk of ICH, and early FVIII replacement appears important in preventing ICH post-trauma. Andes (1984), reporting 47 episodes of head injury, found that no patient given replacement therapy within 6 hours of trauma experienced ICH, and that both mild and severe injury preceded definite bleeding. Boys on a home therapy programme should be infused with FVIII concentrate before they are brought to hospital, and all others should receive replacement treatment on arrival. CT scanning is a helpful diagnostic tool in identifying episodes of ICH, but in the author's unit, head injury is such a common occurrence that it is not practical to scan every boy who attends with a minor head injury. Hennes (1987) retrospectively studied 28 episodes of head injury in which a CT scan had been carried out within 24 hours of injury. The severity of head injury was classified according to objective clinical findings:

1. severe–presence of altered conscious level and/or evidence of increased intracranial pressure
2. moderate – presence of facial or scalp haematoma, contusion or laceration
3. minor – none of the above present.

Normal CT scans were found in all 24 episodes of moderate or minor head trauma, but 3 of 4 patients with severe head injuries had CT scan evidence of intracranial haemorrhage. In the author's unit all boys receive factor VIII concentrate sufficient to raise their FVIII:C to 50–100% (dependent on the degree of injury), as soon as possible after the event. All but minor injuries are hospitalized for observation overnight and treated prophylactically for 3 days. This can be completed as an outpatient if the parents are considered capable of recognizing important symptoms and immediately returning to hospital. Worrying symptoms include lethargy, headache, vomiting and a loss of consciousness after the injury. Boys with any of these symptoms should have an immediate CT scan. It should be remembered that there may be a latent period of 24 hours or more before symptoms or signs of intracranial bleeding develop. Boys with documented evidence of intracranial haemorrhage should receive intensive replacement therapy. Their FVIII:C level should be raised initially to 80–100% and maintained at 50% by twice-daily infusions of concentrate for at least 14 days. If these boys do not show a rapid response to replacement therapy, or develop symptoms with adequate FVIII levels, early neurosurgical intervention is indicated.

Dental treatment. Preventative dental care should be started at an early age and should include tooth brushing after meals, fluoride tablets and regular dental review. Bleeding is not usually associated with the loss of baby teeth, provided that they are not deliberately loosened. Dental fillings may be performed as an outpatient. Local anaesthesia may be given by papillary infiltration or nerve block (Ah Pin 1987), but if the latter is used, adequate replacement therapy must be given to prevent bleeding into the neck or floor of the mouth and the author's unit avoids this route. The extraction of permanent teeth usually requires a short hospital admission. A single dose of FVIII concentrate is given 1 hour before the procedure, along with tranexamic acid at 25 mg/kg every 8 hours for 5 days; the first dose is given preoperatively. It is good practice to test the urine for RBCs before giving antifibrinolytic drugs. The recommended dose of FVIII is 20–25 units/kg if general anaesthesia is used, and 40–50 units/kg for a deep mandibular block.

Surgery. Prior to any surgery, an inhibitor screen which will detect the presence of circulating antibodies to FVIII:C should always be performed and, if possible, a test dose given to determine the half-life of infused concentrate, which is the most sensitive means of detecting low levels of inhibitor. Replacement therapy should be given 1 hour preoperatively in a dose sufficient to raise the FVIII:C level to 80–100%. FVIII concentrate is given for 10–14 days to maintain FVIII:C levels of 50% for the first 4–5 days, and thereafter above 30%. FVIII:C levels are measured pre and post treatment and determine subsequent therapy, which may initially have to be given 8-hourly and thereafter 12-hourly.

Pain relief. Paracetamol is the safest drug and is usually effective in children. DF118 may be substituted if stronger analgesia is required.

Regular prophylaxis. Regular prophylactic treatment may be given to severely affected boys who suffer frequent haemorrhage. This is perhaps most appropriately used when targeting of one specific joint is problematic. In such circumstances, prophylaxis may be used for a period of time to assess its effect on the frequency and severity of bleeding episodes. A dose of 15–20 units/kg is generally employed and given twice weekly. Prophylaxis is based on the rationale that spontaneous haemorrhage only occurs when the FVIII:C level is below 1–2%, and it is intended

that regular infusions will maintain a level above this for much of the time.

Home therapy. The availability of lyophilized concentrates has made home treatment possible, because this material can be stored at 4°C. Home therapy allows prompt replacement therapy and the potential for limiting or, indeed, preventing chronic joint problems. The families' dependance on hospital personnel is decreased and the boys become more independent with less school absenteeism. Parents, usually the mother, are trained to reconstitute and infuse the concentrate before their son starts regular school, by which age venous access should be reasonable. Older boys should be encouraged to prepare their own treatment and be able to inject themselves by adolescence. The family must be taught when to treat, how to calculate the dose and the techniques of reconstituting and infusing the material. Most mothers quickly learn to cannulate their son's veins, but must be aware of the importance of good venepuncture technique, including the need to press firmly on the site for several minutes after injection. The families are supplied with all the necessary equipment for preparation and injection, and the means of disposing of the used needles and syringes. In the author's unit, parents administering FVIII concentrate are advised that they themselves be vaccinated against hepatitis B. It is equally important that families know when to call the haemophilia centre for guidance (e.g. head injuries or bleeds which have not responded promptly to treatment). Medical personnel must monitor the use of home treatment and insist that treatment sheets are completed and handed in for examination regularly. Recorded details must include the date and site of bleed, type, batch number and dose of concentrate given, its effectiveness and any side-effects experienced.

Psychosocial support of the boys and their families

The haemophilia sister and the social worker attached to the haemophilia centre can give invaluable support to families. This is particularly necessary in the absence of a family history and the experience of other affected family members. Parents must be encouraged to allow their sons to lead as normal a life as possible, although sporting activities have to be restricted to those which would not be predicted to cause injury, which usually means the exclusion of contact sports. Advice and practical aids, such as the wearing of soft leather crash helmets, may help in preventing injury. Many parents are helped by meeting families in a similar situation, and this can be achieved by parent groups or meetings organized by the local branch of the Haemophilia Society. Many boys wear medical alert medallions or bracelets, and if requested these should be provided. The use of long-distance radio pagers give mothers independence by allowing them to go shopping or socializing in the knowledge that they can be contacted quickly by their boy's school if necessary. The social worker can guide the family in the application for mobility and attendance allowances. All boys should attend toddler groups and nursery school prior to their normal school, just like their nonhaemophiliac friends. It is helpful for the haemophilia sister to pay a visit to the school prior to, or just after, the boy has started, to allay any fears that the teacher may have and to give appropriate advice. This may enable potential problems to be dealt with before they develop.

The above guidelines on therapy apply more specifically to patients with severe haemophilia. However, the same level of FVIII:C is required for haemostasis after surgery or trauma or with any bleeding episode, irrespective of the severity of haemophilia, although dosages of FVIII concentrate to achieve these levels will differ. Most importantly, a haemostatic level of FVIII:C can often be achieved with DDAVP alone, avoiding the use of blood products, in patients with mild or moderate haemophilia. Carriers of haemophilia A may have problems with postoperative bleeding, and their bleeding tendency is related to their FVIII:C activity (Mauser Bunschoten et al 1988). When the clotting activity is less than 30%, it may be necessary to increase the FVIII:C level to cover surgery or dental extraction by using DDAVP or FVIII concentrate. It is advisable to vaccinate carriers with a FVIII:C activity of less than 30% against hepatitis B in order to prevent post-transfusion hepatitis.

Non-haemorrhagic problems in haemophilia

The improved treatment of acute haemarthroses has reduced chronic arthropathy and deformity,

but other problems remain, namely FVIII inhibitors, chronic liver disease and HIV infection.

Factor VIII inhibitors. Inhibitors (alloantibodies to factor VIII) develop in approximately 6–10% of patients with haemophilia A. Their appearance is a very serious development, because they rapidly neutralize the infused FVIII and make bleeding more difficult to control. These inhibitors are IgG antibodies and act against the procoagulant part of the FVIII complex (FVIII:C) and have some degree of species specificity. Over 90% of inhibitors occur in patients with severe haemophilia, and do not appear to be related to the type or frequency of replacement therapy (McMillan et al 1988). Rarely, patients with mild haemophilia develop inhibitors, but these tend to be of low titre and disappear spontaneously (Bovill et al, 1985, Capel et al 1986). Some haemophiliacs develop inhibitors after a very short period of exposure, whilst others do so after many years. Nearly one-third of inhibitors are detected by 5 years of age, and two-thirds by age 20 (McMillan et al 1988). However, most patients do not develop inhibitors, and treatment should never be withheld for fear of precipitating their development.

Genetic predisposition appears to play a role in the development of inhibitors. There is a higher incidence in brother pairs and amongst black haemophiliacs. More than half of patients with haemophilia B and inhibitors to FIX have gene deletions. Studies seeking to correlate gene deletion and inhibitors of FVIII in haemophilia A have given conflicting results. FVIII is a large molecule and as such may be very antigenic. Studies of histocompatibility antigens as genetic markers predicting the development of antibodies to FVIII have been inconclusive.

The plasma level of the inhibitor and its response to FVIII therapy vary considerably between patients, who can be categorized as 'high' or 'low' responders, depending on the degree of anamnestic response that they exhibit. Most (75%) are high responders, producing a brisk amnestic response 4–7 days after therapy, with a dramatic increase in antibody titre; in low responders (25%), the antibody level seldom rises above 10 Bethesda units (BU), even after repeated antigenic challenge (Feinstein 1987). A Bethesda unit is the current accepted measurement of inhibitor activity and is the activity in 1 ml of inhibitor plasma that reduces 1 unit of FVIII:C in 1 ml of normal plasma to 0.5 units of FVIII:C after 2 hours of incubation of the mixture under standard conditions. In low responders, the inhibitor may disappear spontaneously, but this rarely occurs in patients with high-titre antibodies. The disappearance of high-response inhibitors coinciding with the development of AIDS has recently been reported (Leyva et al 1988). The presence of inhibitors should be suspected in any patient who fails to respond adequately to replacement therapy, especially if assay and other coagulant tests fail to show the expected rise in factor level.

The management of bleeding episodes in haemophiliacs with inhibitors is still a major problem, because the antibodies make them more or less resistant to FVIII replacement therapy, although the frequency of bleeding is not increased. Many therapeutic approaches have been tried and can be divided into those used for treatment of acute bleeding episodes and those aimed at eradicating the antibody. The treatment of bleeding episodes must be tailored to the type (i.e. low or high responder) and level of the antibody. Patients who are low responders and have a low level of inhibitor (less than 10 BU) may respond to repeated infusions of human FVIII concentrate (at 2–3 times the dose given to patients without inhibitors, i.e. 50 units/kg), either with a rise in plasma FVIII:C or clinically, without a measurable increase in FVIII:C. Many experienced haematologists will in fact treat all patients with inhibitors irrespective of their titre or anamnestic response with human FVIII concentrate, provided they have an acceptable clinical response, because they are uncomfortable with the use of alternative therapies whose mode of action and safety remains undetermined. Others prefer to reserve human FVIII concentrates for serious haemaorrhage, and for noncritical haemorrhage use treatment which will not result in anamnestic response. This hopefully allows the titre of antibodies to human FVIII to decline to a level where human FVIII concentrate might be effective in a life-threatening situation. For this reason, many recommend the use of prothrombin complex concentrates (PCCs) or, particularly, activated concentrates (APCCs) such as Feiba or Autoplex for treatment of noncritical haemorrhage, to avoid needless anamnesis in all high responders irrespective of the level of inhibitor. The mechanism of action of these products is unknown, but their efficacy may be related to their content of activated clotting factors (e.g. FXa or FVIIa). A single dose of PCC is subjectively effective in approximately 50% of bleeds. APCCs are not significantly better. More recently, haemostasis has been secured in patients with inhibitors by the infusion of plasma-derived and recombinant FVIIa (Hedner et al 1988). This material combines with tissue factor to activate FX directly, so bypassing the FVIII-dependent step in the coagulation cascade.

In the event of serious haemorrhage, it is necessary to achieve a FVIII level of at least 30 iu/dl, and preferably higher. In patients who are high responders but currently have a low inhibitor level, this can usually be achieved with a large dose of human FVIII concentrate. Alternatively, porcine FVIII (Hyate-C) may be used if cross-reactivity is low. However, with repeated infusions, antibody specificity may change, resulting in a rise in antibody to porcine material, making subsequent infusions less effective. If there is no response to FVIII concentrates, PCC or APCCs should be tried. The real challenge lies in the treatment of serious haemorrhage in a patient who is a high responder and currently has a high inhibitor titre. If the anti-porcine FVIII inhibitor level is low, porcine FVIII may effect haemostasis. It may, however, be necessary to reduce the inhibitor titre by exchange plasmapheresis and thereafter infuse human or porcine FVIII concentrate. PCC or APCCs may be given in the interim. Elective surgery should never be considered in patients with inhibitors, and all patients with haemophilia should be screened for antibodies prior to any surgery. This is done by an incubated APTT screening test, but the most sensitive test for an unsuspected, weak inhibitor is an in-vivo FVIII recovery and survival study. All patients with inhibitors should have both anti-human and anti-porcine FVIII antibody titres measured at regular intervals, in order to determine in advance which patients might be candidates for porcine FVIII. DDAVP has been used with success in mild hae-mophiliacs who develop inhibitors, as the endogenous FVIII released is less immunogenic than exogenous FVIII. As our knowledge of structure–function relationship of the FVIII molecule advances, and the production of FVIII via recombinant DNA technology becomes a reality, it may be possible to engineer molecules which lack antigenic sites for inhibitors and retain procoagulant activity.

Several approaches to eradicate FVIII:C antibodies have been tried. Immune tolerance may be induced by the regular administration of human FVIII concentrate. Variable doses (high, intermediate and low) and frequency of administration (mainly daily or alternate days) have been used. Adherence to such an intensive regimen is difficult with children. The success rate is high, but is less so for high responders than for those patients with low level inhibitors. Immune tolerance may be more easy to achieve when the inhibitor has recently developed. FVIII recovery normalized within a few months in 3 of 4 young patients in whom FVIII prophylactic therapy was started or continued as soon as there was evidence of FVIII:C antibody activity (van Leeuwen et al 1986). Plasmapheresis and extracorporeal passage of plasma over a Sepharose A Column have been used to reduce the antibody level in patients with severe haemorrhage or before surgery (Bona et al 1986). Other approaches have included the use of immunosuppressive agents such as cyclophosphamide or high-dose intravenous immunoglobulin, but neither has been very effective when used alone. In the many patients with haemophilia A who are already immunocompromized from HIV infection, further immunosuppression would be contraindicated. Several good reviews of this topic are recommended to the reader (Lusher 1987, Bloom 1981, Kasper 1989).

Chronic liver disease in haemophilia

The rush to produce factor concentrates which will not transmit virus is due not just to the AIDS epidemic, but also to a growing awareness that substantial numbers of haemophiliacs are developing chronic progressive liver disease secondary to non-A, non-B hepatitis (NANBH). Hepatitis C is considered largely responsible and nearly all patients become infected after their first exposure to non-viricidally treated FVIII concentrate. Although many patients have a transient elevation of hepatic transaminases, which probably reflects acute self-limiting hepatitis, in a substantial proportion these biochemical abnormalities persist. The prevalence of abnormal liver function tests in haemophiliacs increased rapidly with the widespread introduction of factor VIII and IX concentrates in the mid 1970s. Hay, in 1985, reported 70% (50/79) of recipients of factor concentrates to have persistently abnormal liver function tests, and 17 of 34 patients biopsied had histological evidence of chronic progressive liver disease – 9 cirrhosis, 8 chronic active hepatitis (CAH). The frequency of cirrhosis for the whole group was 11.5%. Symptoms and abnormal physical signs were uncommon in these patients, and there was no correlation between the elevation of liver transaminases and the underlying liver pathology, which in turn did not correlate with FVIII usage. Schimpf (1986) reported a 20% incidence of progressive liver disease (10% CAH, 13% cirrhosis), and Aledort (1985), in a large multicentre retrospective study of biopsy material, found an incidence of 15% and 7% for CAH and cirrhosis respectively. By contrast, Mannucci (1982) reported no evidence of progression of chronic persistent hepatitis to CAH or cirrhosis in 11 patients, with a mean age of 12 years, studied by serial biopsy over a period of 6 years. The degree of liver damage may be inversely related to the age at which patients become infected with the virus (Mannucci & Colombo 1985).

End-stage liver failure is now recognized to be a major cause of morbidity and mortality in haemophilia. The incidence of hepatitis C (HCV), the likeliest causative agent, was difficult to estimate, in the absence of a serological marker. A marker is now available, and the incidence of anti-HCV has been variably reported from Spain (70%; Esteban et al 1989), France (67%; Noel et al 1989), West Germany (78%; Roggendorf et al 1989), the UK (59%; Makris et al 1990) and the USA (76%; Brettler et al 1990). Second generation tests for HCV have recently been evaluated and may improve our diagnostic accuracy. There is no association between HCV positivity and age, but a positive correlation with FVIII consumption has been reported (Makris et al 1990). The same investigators also found a correlation between anti-HCV and anti-HIV and markers of hepatitis B infection (88% v 39%, and 75% v 46% respectively). Of their patients with persistently raised serum ALT concentrations, 78% were anti-HCV positive. Factor concentrates are viral-inactivated and this will hopefully reduce the incidence of NANBH due to HCV and other agents implicated in transfusion-associated hepatitis. It is unlikely that this will completely eradicate the problem but the information to date is encouraging. Sixteen children were anti-HCV negative after receiving, for at least two years, factor concentrate treated by a solvent/detergent process to eliminate virus, compared with 137 of 400 who had received unmodified product (Noel et al 1989). Likewise, Ludlam found all of 7 patients who had received only heat-treated product to be anti-HCV negative, compared with only 7 of 48 who had received non-heat-treated product (Ludlam et al, 1989). The role of interferon in patients with haemophilia and chronic liver disease is under evaluation.

HIV infection in haemophilia

Although lyophilized factor VIII concentrates have revolutionalized the treatment of haemophilia, this has been at a price. Transfusion-associated HIV infection has had a devastating effect on the haemophilia community. The first case of transfusion-induced acquired immune deficiency syndrome (AIDS) was diagnosed in a patient with haemophilia who died of *Pneumocystis carinii* pneumonia in 1982 (Centres for Disease Control 1982). The majority of haemophiliacs seroconverted between 1981 and 1983. A survey of prevalence of antibody to HIV in patients with haemophilia A, B or vWD in the UK found 41% of haemophilia A patients and 6% of haemophilia B patients to be anti-HIV positive. The prevalence in severely affected patients is greater; 59% in haemophilia A, and 11% in haemophilia B patients. This reflects the intensity of treatment received by severely affected patients. Of patients tested with vWD, 3.5% were found to have antibody to HIV (AIDS Group of the UK Haemophilia Centre Directors 1988).

The proportion of people positive for HIV who proceed to develop AIDS is still uncertain. Many believe that progression is inevitable. Bachetti (1988) reported a 3-year survival rate from the time of diagnosis of AIDS of 11%, and Rothenberg (1987) a 5-year survival rate of 15%. A recent survey of patients with haemophilia in the UK reported the progression of AIDS to be strongly age-dependent. The cumulative incidence of AIDS 5 years after seroconversion was 4% among patients aged less than 25 years at first positive test for HIV, 6% among those aged 25–44 years and 19% among those aged over 45 years (Darby et al 1989). The rate of progression to AIDS once seroconversion has taken place is not influenced by the severity or type of haemophilia, or the type of concentrate which has transmitted the infection (Darby et al 1989, Darby et al 1990). The risk of progression to AIDS probably increases smoothly with age, and even years after seroconversion is estimated at 6% of patients aged under 25 years, 20% of those aged 25–44 years and 34% of those older than 45 years at seroconversion (Fig. 13.7; Darby et al 1990). Possible endogenous age-related factors which might play a role in the rate of progression of HIV infection include the size of the pool of mature CD4 lymphocytes, and the mass and activity of the thymus. Of concern is a significant increase in the mortality observed in antibody-positive individuals, who do not fulfil the criteria for the diagnosis of AIDS, especially patients with AIDS related complex (Darby et al 1989). Doctors should be aware of this risk when treating infections in all anti-HIV positive patients with haemophilia. The progression to AIDS as presently defined may well be delayed by therapeutic interventions, including the early use of Zidovudine and prophylaxis against *Pneumocystis carinii* pneumonia.

HIV infection produces impaired cellular immunity by destroying CD4 helper lymphocytes, thus predisposing individuals to opportunistic infections and malignancies. There is now evidence that defective helper, and elevated suppressor, function of T-cells in HIV-infected patients are caused not only by a change in the CD4/CD8 cell counts, but also by functional abnormalities of the CD4+ T-cell subset (Weimer et al 1989). Clinical manifestations do not usually occur until several years after the initial infection. A number of serological and cellular immune parameters have been studied for their predictive value for the

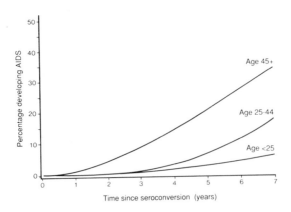

Fig. 13.7   Estimated percentage of haemophiliacs developing AIDS by time since seroconversion and by age at the time of the first seropositive test. From: Darby et al 1990.

development of AIDS. Useful predictors include falling absolute CD4+ lymphocyte numbers, increased levels of β_2 microglobulin and neopterin (Kramer et al 1990), increased levels of β_2 microglobulin (Smith et al 1989, Rugman et al 1989), HIV antigenaemia and decline of p24 antibody (Allain et al 1987), and absolute CD4+ lymphocyte numbers below 200/mm^3 (Lee et al 1990) and below 100/mm^3 (Ragni et al 1986). It has been suggested that viruses such as herpes simplex and cytomegalovirus might act as cofactors in the progression of HIV infection to AIDS. An association between CMV infection and a rapid progression to HIV disease was reported by Webster et al (1989), but was not confirmed by Rugman (1989). However, many viruses induce immunosuppression, and viral illness may have a deleterious effect.

Immunological screening of seronegative individuals with haemophilia A has shown abnormalities of T-cell dependent immunity, and this also is age-related, with increasing age being associated with a gradually decreasing trend in CD4/CD8 ratios (Kessler et al 1984) and a progressive increase in the degree of IgG hypergammaglobulinemia (Shannon et al 1986). A similarly age-related impaired lymphocyte proliferative response to PHA and concanavalin A has been reported (Mahir et al 1988, Kessler et al 1984). These and other data suggest that intensive treatment with lyophilized factor VIII concentrates of low purity may impair cellular immunity. A similar disturbance of the

normal CD4/CD8 ratio has not been observed in recipients of factor IX concentrate, but this requires confirmation, as age-related abnormalities of immune function have been reported in patients treated exclusively with cryoprecipitate and who are anti-HIV negative (Pollack at al 1985).

Controversy surrounds the significance of the immune abnormalities observed in seronegative individuals. These boys do not appear to have an increased susceptibility to opportunistic infections. However, Beddall reported six cases of primary pulmonary tuberculosis in two boys with positive skin reactions amongst 30 children with bleeding disorders exposed to an index tuberculosis case. The incidence for inpatients was similar to that of the immunocompromised children receiving chemotherapy. Only two of the boys had antibodies to HIV. There was a significant correlation between the amount of replacement therapy received and the development of evidence of tuberculous infection (Beddall et al 1985).

The diversity of symptoms of HIV infection demand a multidisciplinary approach. Patients with haemophilia are developing both opportunistic infections and malignancies, mainly non-Hodgkins lymphoma (Howard & McVerry 1987). However, because progression to AIDS is slow in children, many boys either have nonspecific symptoms or remain reasonably well. The commonest nonspecific symptoms include poor appetite, failure to gain weight, minimal or moderate lymphadenopathy (Wang et al 1987), intermittent oral candidiasis and skin rashes. Atopic manifestations have been reported with established AIDS (Parkin et al 1987), and boys with haemophilia who have no evidence of clinical progression to AIDS have developed atopic eczema for the first time, or had a recurrence of previously quiescent eczema, soon after recorded seroconversion (Ball and Harper 1987). Septic arthritis is an unusual complication of haemarthrosis in patients with haemophilia, but is now being increasingly recognized in sero-positive boys, and should be considered if a hae-marthrosis is associated with fever or the response to replacement therapy unsatisfactory (Ragni & Hanley 1989).

Confidentiality is very important to the parents of children with haemophilia who fear the hostility of neighbours and other children at school. This remains a concern despite the knowledge that no family member or social contact has contracted the virus without sexual intercourse. Many parents also agonize over what to tell their infected sons. A very important group is that of the adolescent boys who may be sexually active and capable of infecting partners (Aronstam 1987).

Zidovudine, an analogue of thymidine, inhibits the viral enzyme reverse transcriptase, and therefore is a potent inhibitor of HIV replication in vitro. In 1986, a double-blind placebo-controlled trial showed Zidovudine to decrease the mortality rate in patients with advanced HIV infection (Creagh-Kirk et al 1988). However, treatment was associated with substantial toxicity, mainly haematological, including macrocytosis, anaemia and neutropenia. More recently it has been claimed that Zidovudine delays the development of AIDS in patients with mild symptomatic illness and a CD4+ cell count between 200 and 499/mm^3 (Fischl et al 1990). A second study has shown that Zidovudine in asymptomatic patients with fewer than 500 CD4+ cells/mm^3 significantly delayed the progression to symptomatic illness (Volberding et al 1990). Patients showed a transient improvement followed by a delay in the loss of CD4+ cells, which could be attributed to Zidovudine. The drug is better tolerated in asymptomatic patients than in those with more advanced disease. Volberding also found that a dose of 500 mg/day was equally efficacious and less toxic than a dose of 1500 mg/day in adults (Friedland, 1990). It is

not known whether the early use of Zidovudine treatment will encourage the selection of Zido-vudine-resistant isolates and deny patients the benefits of the drug when clinical illness occurs. Most physicians would now recommend treatment with Zidovudine when CD4+ cell counts fall to 200/mm^3. The relative merit of the early use of Zidovudine in patients with CD4+ cell counts close to 500 cells/mm^3 as compared with a strategy of clinical and laboratory monitoring and delaying the initiation of Zidovudine until CD4+ cell counts have declined close to 200/mm^3 is not known. Most studies indicate that clinical disease occurs mostly when the CD4+ cell counts become very depressed. There is obviously a time when CD4+ cell counts are between 200 and 500/mm^3 and the maximum benefit with the minimum toxicity can be obtained from the drug. We cannot yet identify this time and neither do we know if early treatment will ultimately improve survival for persons infected with HIV.

It is equally difficult to assess independently the successful impact of prophylaxis against *Pneumocystis carinii* with nebulized pentamidine or cotrimoxazole in reducing progression to AIDS, as this pneumonia was previously often the development on which the diagnosis of AIDS was made. A number of new anti-viral agents with activity against the HIV virus are undergoing clinical evaluation and may soon be available to boys who either cannot tolerate Zidovudine or continue to deteriorate on this drug.

Choice of factor concentrate

Brettler & Levine (1989) recently reviewed this topic comprehensively. The treatment of severe haemophilia was revolutionized in the mid 70s by the ready availability of lyophilized concentrates, which brought the expectations of a relatively normal life and lifespan, until the AIDS era. These concentrates are prepared from plasma obtained from 2 000–30 000 donors, and infectious complications from transfusion-transmitted viruses have been apparent since the mid to late 1970s. These products also appear to impair cellular immunity, secondary to the large amounts of contaminating foreign protein. Enormous energies are now concentrated on producing lyophilized concentrates of high purity, which have undergone viricidal processes to eliminate the risk of viral transmission.

Viral complications of concentrate infusion. Hepatitis B (HBV), hepatitis C (HCV) and HIV are the major viruses transmitted by factor concentrates.

Hepatitis B. About 90% of haemophiliacs who have received non-heat-treated concentrate are HBsAb positive, indicating past exposure, and about 5–10% become chronic carriers (HBsAg positive). Infection with hepatitis B still occurs even in recipients of heat-treated product. Therefore, all newly diagnosed infants and older children who are not already immune should be immunized. Their HBsAb titres should be monitored regularly, and booster doses of vaccine given as required. It is well recognized that many HIV antibody positive boys fail to respond, or have a reduced anti-HBs response to immunization (Zanetti et al 1986).

Hepatitis C. Almost all (90–100%) of haemophiliacs who have received non-heat-treated concentrates have either persistently or intermittently elevated liver enzymes, which probably reflect hepatitis C. A significant percentage (25–40%) may go on to develop chronic active hepatitis.

HIV infection. In the UK, 41% of haemophiliacs have antibody to HIV (AIDS Group of the UK Haemophilic Centre Directors 1988). They include patients who were treated before 1985, when heat-treated product became available, and a small number of patients treated with non-heat-treated cryoprecipitate.

Non-viral complications of concentrate infusion. It is now recognized that conventional factor concentrates may cause alterations in the immune system. Clinical observations and laboratory data of immunosuppression have been responsible for pressing forward the development of concentrates of high purity. Allergic reactions to factor concentrate are uncommon, and anaphylaxis rare.

Viricidal treatments of concentrates. Both donor screening and viral inactivation procedures should decrease the incidence of viral transmission. All units of blood are now screened for HIV antibodies, although HIV may be transmitted by anti HIV negative blood if the donor is in the process of seroconversion. All units of blood are also screened for HBsAg but, again, the test is not foolproof. The best protection is afforded by immunization. Surrogate testing for HCV by screening for ALT elevation and hepatitis B core antibody (anti-HBc) is practised in some parts of the world and by some commercial companies, but is not in routine use in the UK. The screening of donor units of blood for anti-HCV was introduced in the UK in September 1991, but the test is probably subject to the same limitations as that for HBV and HIV. It is likely that agents other than HIV, HCV and HBV contribute to transfusion-associated hepatitis and clear that the screening of donor units for these viruses alone will not eradicate the problem.

Current accepted safe viricidal procedures include super-dry-heat treatment (80°C for 72 hours) in the lyophilized state, wet-heat treatment in suspension or solution (pasteurization), viral attenuation using solvent/detergent methods, or high purification by affinity chromatography with a mouse monoclonal antibody (MoAb) for either FVIII/vWF or FVIII:C, or conventional chromatographic techniques without MoAbs plus viral inactivation. HIV is more easily inactivated than HBV or HCV. Human parvovirus appears to be less susceptible to inactivation than hepatitis viruses and, as such, may act as a useful marker of process efficacy.

In addition to viral safety, the other requirement of concentrates are that they are of high purity to reduce the load of foreign protein. These concentrates should reduce allergic reactions and are certainly indicated for patients who have reacted to conventional concentrates. Concern has been expressed that high purity concentrates may be associated with an increased development of inhibitors, but at present this in unproven. Whether they stabilize the immune system remains to be established. A high-purity factor IX concentrate devoid of factors II, VII and X may have a reduced thrombotic risk.

The choice of factor VIII concentrate is now complex and much influenced by litigation surrounding HIV transmission. Physicians wish to administer an efficacious and safe product which would stand up to peer review. Only fully licensed commercial products and NHS products used on a 'crown immunity' basis should be used for regular treatment. All products are now viral-inactivated, and clinical trials and product review will identify the best methods, although it is unlikely that any one method of viral inactivation will be completely foolproof. However, the best viral-attenuated product should be administered to all patients, whether they are HIV-infected or not. A concentrate of high purity free of viral contamination may be especially beneficial to HIV-positive haemophiliacs by preventing further immune suppression. Intense viral inactivation and purification procedures result in a lower yield of factor VIII from plasma, reducing supply and increasing cost, but highly purified products offer theoretical benefit to all haemophiliacs. If we believe this to be true, then it is impossible to select out groups who should be preferentially treated with these products.

Recent EEC regulations outlaw the use of paid donors and recommend self-sufficiency for all member countries by 1992. Adequate supplies of an acceptably safe product should be a prime government concern.

The availability of factor VIII concentrate made by recombinant technology could revolutionize the treatment of haemophilia, by producing large quantities of factor VIII at low cost and free of human virus. Cloning of the genes for factor VIII and IX and recombinant genetic technology may allow cure by 'gene therapy'. More dramatically, liver transplant for end-stage liver disease has normalized the factor VIII level in survivors (Scharrer et al 1988, Lewis et al 1985).

Haemophilia B

Haemophilia B is characterized by a deficiency of FIX activity. It is clinically indistinguishable from haemophilia A and similarly has an X-linked recessive mode of inheritance. In the UK, only 0.8% of patients with haemophilia B have antibodies to FIX, compared to 6% of patients with haemophilia A who have antibodies to FVIII, and many have in common a large deletion of the FIX gene (Giannelli et al 1983, Hassan et al 1985).

The clinical manifestations of haemophilia B are, in general, identical to these of haemophilia A. Diagnosis in the neonatal period is, however, more complicated, because FIX is a vitamin K-dependent factor and gestationally-reduced at birth. As a result, it is difficult to diagnose mild haemophilia B in the newborn infant because of potential overlap with the normal range, although severely affected neonates should be easily identified (Andrew et al 1988).

Haemophilia B should be treated with FIX concentrates which have undergone viricidal treatment. FIX is a relatively small molecule, which diffuses extravascularly and has an in-vivo recovery of only 25–50% of the administered dose. One unit of FIX:C/kg body weight will raise the plasma FIX:C level by approximately 1%. The half-life is approximately 24 hours. A minimum level of FIX:C of 10–20% is needed for the early treatment of acute bleeding episodes into joints or muscles, and a FIX:C level of 40% for more advanced joint or muscle bleeding and for major haemorrhage. For life-threatening haemorrhage, or surgery, an initial FIX:C level of 60% should be achieved, followed by a level of 40% for several days and then above 20% for a total of 7–10 days. Because of the relatively long half-life of FIX:C compared with FVIII:C, repeat doses are less often necessary and if so at a lesser frequency. Recommended dosage of FIX concentrate for intensive prophylaxis for the management of chronic synovitis is 20–30 units 2–3 times weekly (Miser et al 1986). Factor IX concentrates are stable at 4°C and are suitable for home treatment programmes.

Presumably because of contamination with tiny amounts of activated clotting factors, FIX concentrates, especially when infused in large repeated quantities, have been associated with thrombotic episodes. Heparin prophylaxis is usually recommended to cover surgical procedures. Monoclonally produced FIX concentrate may be free of thrombogenicity. It is usually recommended that antifibrinolytic agents are not used concurrently with FIX concentrates, but that 6 hours are allowed to elapse after the last dose of concentrate to avoid thromboembolic complications. In the UK, the incidence of treatment-related HIV seropositivity is lower in patients with haemophilia B than haemophilia A which is thought to be due to the frequent exclusive use of non-commercially produced material in the former group. Patients with FIX deficiency have also been reported to have a lesser degree of immune dysfunction. This is not because FIX concentrate itself is less immunosuppressive, but because immunosuppression is related to the intensity of treatment, and patients with haemophilia B use less replacement treatment per annum than do haemophilia A patients (Brettler et al 1987). Cloning of the FIX gene has made treatment by gene therapy a possibility for the future (Anson et al 1987), and FIX deficiency has been corrected in a patient with haemophilia B by liver transplantation (Merion et al 1988).

The deficiency of FIX activity in haemophilia B can result from a failure to synthesize the molecule or from the synthesis of a nonfunctional variant of the FIX molecule. Such patients have a discrepancy between their FIX activity (FIX:C) and FIX antigen (FIX:Ag). Carriers of haemophilia B tend to have lower levels of FIX:C and are more often symptomatic than are carriers of haemophilia A, so FIX:C levels alone may have some predictive value in carrier detection. Measurement of both procoagulant and antigen levels may increase the predictive accuracy in those families whose haemophilia B is due to synthesis of a non-functional molecule. The accuracy of carrier detection and prenatal diagnosis has been improved by the use of linkage analysis with intragenic restriction fragment length polymorphisms (Hassan et al 1985, Hay et al 1986, Winship & Brownlee 1986, Lillicrap et al 1986). The use of polymerase chain reaction techniques is likely to make carrier detection and prenatal diagnosis available to increased numbers of families (Siguret et al 1988, Winship et al 1989, Bottema et al 1989). Genetic defects responsible for haemophilia B include several different mutations (Ware et al 1988, Taylor 1990, Reitsma et al, 1988, Liddell et al 1989, Siguret et al 1988, Bottema et al 1990), many of which are single-molecule substitutions and partial gene deletions. Clinical severity may correlate better with the presence of a given mutation than with the FIX coagulant activity.

von Willebrand's Disease

von Willebrand factor (vWF) is a large and highly complex molecule with important functions in haemostasis, and is the plasma protein which is deficient and/or defective in vWD. The vWF gene is located at the tip of the short arm of chromosome 12, but homologous sequences have also been localized to chromosome 22. vWF is synthesized by endothelial cells and megakaryocytes, and then secreted or stored in the Weibel-Palade bodies in the endothelial cells or the α granules of platelets. In plasma, vWF circulates as a series of polymers ranging in MW from $1–20 \times 10^6$ at a concentration of about 10 µg/ml; FVIII:C is present at a concentration of about 0.2 µg/ml. von Willebrand factor has two main roles. Firstly, it mediates platelet adhesion to the damaged endothelium; the size of the vWF multimers is important, because the largest possess the greatest affinity for the vWF receptors on platelets. The second function for vWF is that of a carrier protein for FVIII:C, protecting it from degradation. Thus, patients with severe vWD, who lack vWF, have very low levels of FVIII:C. Factor VIII is released from vWF upon activation by thrombin. vWD is probably the most common of the inherited disorders of haemostasis, but the incidence is difficult to determine because mild cases often go undiagnosed. The prevalence may be as high as 1% (Rodeghiero et al 1987). Most patients have reduced amounts of apparently normal vWF, and others a vWF with aberrant structure and function. As vWF is the carrier protein for FVIII:C, reduced levels of vWF:Ag are usually accompanied by a corresponding decrease in FVIII:C. vWF normally facilitates platelet adhesion to sub-endothelium, and its absence is demonstrated in the laboratory by a prolonged bleeding time (BT), defective ristocetin-induced platelet aggregation and reduced vWF activity (measured by the ristocetin cofactor assay). The disorder is very heterogenous and is classified according to the multimeric structure of vWF.

Diagnosis of vWD

The investigation of a patient suspected of suffering from vWD can be divided into those tests which establish the diagnosis and those which classify the type of vWD.

Routine diagnostic testing of a patient suspected of suffering from vWD.

1. A template bleeding time. This is the test which best correlates with clinical symptoms. It is

always prolonged in severe disease, but in mildly affected individuals may be normal or have to be repeated on a number of occasions to document prolongation.

2. APTT. Although this screening test is generally included in the investigation of vWD, it merely reflects the level of FVIII:C and will be generally prolonged if the FVIII:C is less than 30%.

3. FVIII:C. The vast majority of patients with vWD have FVIII:C levels below the normal range, but mildly affected patients and those with variants of vWD may have normal levels of FVIII:C.

4. vWF:Ag. Quantification of vWF:Ag may be performed by a number of different techniques, most of which give abnormal results in the majority of patients, although some are more sensitive than others to specific types and subtypes of vWD.

5. Ristocetin-induced platelet aggregation. The addition of ristocetin to platelet-rich plasma results in aggregation which is dependent at least in part on the level of vWF; it is decreased or absent in most patients with vWD, except for patients with type IIb who have increased aggregation at low concentrations of ristocetin.

6. Ristocetin cofactor activity. This is a quantitative assay of ristocetin-induced aggregation of platelet-rich plasma which compares the ability of dilutions of normal or test plasma to restore the aggregation of vWD platelet-rich plasma. This is the best in-vitro assay for the diagnosis of vWD, correlating most closely with the bleeding time.

Tests to classify the type of vWD. vWF multimers in plasma and platelets can be precisely characterized by electropheresing through SDS agarose gel and then identifying the multimeric forms with radiolabelled monospecific anti-vWF antibodies.

vWD is an extremely heterogenous condition and in some individuals it may be difficult to make (or to exclude) the diagnosis on the basis of laboratory testing done on one or two occasions. There is considerable variation in clinical and laboratory manifestations not only among families but also among affected members of the same family, and some individuals vary considerably when tested at different times. Thus, once the diagnosis of vWD has been entertained, it cannot

be excluded on the basis of a single set of normal coagulation studies. However, such diagnostically difficult cases generally involve very mild disease.

Clinical features

Types I and II vWD (see below) are characterized by mucocutaneous bleeding. Affected individuals bruise easily and bleed abnormally from cuts. Gum bleeding and epistaxis are characteristic. In the absence of replacement therapy, haemorrhage post dental extraction and surgery occurs. Menorrhagia is common in older girls. Type III vWD is characterized by mucocutaneous bleeding and sometimes problems typically associated with very low levels of FVIII:C, i.e. haemarthrosis and haematomas.

New types of vWD continue to be described, in terms of structural and functional abnormalities of the protein. Broadly, three types can be identified (Table 13.9). Type I (classical) vWD is transmitted by an autosomal dominant gene with variable penetrance in some families (Miller et al 1979). Levels of all components of the FVIII-vWF complex are reduced, i.e. FVIII:C, vWF:Ag and ristocetin cofactor activity. Plasma vWF multimers are normal in pattern although reduced; the highest MW forms are still detectable. Platelet vWF content is either decreased or normal, and several subvarieties have been distinguished based on the

Table 13.9 Main subtypes of von Willebrand's disease and variants

	I	IIa	IIb	III
Genetics	Autosomal Dominant	Autosomal Dominant	Autosomal Dominant	Autosomal Recessive
Bleeding time	Prolonged or Normal	Prolonged	Prolonged	Very Prolonged
VIII:C	Reduced	Reduced or Normal	Reduced or Normal	Absent
vWF:RiCo	Reduced or Normal	Absent or Reduced	Increased	Absent
vWF:Ag:				
EIA	Reduced	Normal	Normal	Absent
ELISA	Reduced	Reduced	Reduced	Absent
Multimer:				
plasma	Reduced	Large Absent	Large Absent	Absent
platelet	Reduced or Normal	Large Absent	Normal	Absent

Adapted from Han 1988, with permission.

multimer analysis and vWF content of platelets (Mannucci et al 1985). The bleeding tendency is due to the low vWF and FVIII:C levels, and the bleeding time is normal or moderately prolonged. Bleeding problems are usually mild, particularly so in patients with normal platelet vWF, the subgroup with the best response to DDAVP.

Type II vWD, with its many subvariants, is characterized by a loss of the highest MW vWF multimers in all cases, and of intermediate MW vWF multimers in some. Types IIa–IIh have been described and differentiated on the multimeric pattern of vWF in plasma and platelets. vWF activity (ristocetin cofactor activity) is reduced further than either FVIII:C or vWF:Ag. Large and intermediate multimers are absent from both plasma and platelets in type IIa (the commonest subtype), whilst large multimers are absent from plasma but present in normal amounts in the platelets of individuals with type IIb. This latter subtype is distinguished by enhanced platelet aggregation with low concentrations of ristocetin. In vivo, the abnormal vWF has increased affinity for platelets, and enhanced interaction with platelet GPIb, such that it can bind to platelets causing aggregation in the absence of collagen. These patients often have moderate thrombocytopenia presumed to be due to intravascular platelet aggregation induced by their abnormal vWF. DDAVP, by releasing endogenous vWF, can result in a fall in the platelet count. Subtypes IIc–IIh, reported in a few individuals, are characterized by aberrant multimeric patterns. The bleeding tendency in type II variants is generally more marked than in type I, due to the lack of the large multimers and low FVIII:C, if present. Clinical problems are more frequent, and bleeding times tend to be more prolonged, especially in type IIa. Inheritance is autosomal dominant, except for type IIc in which compound heterozygosity is usual. However, three children from two families have been reported, who exhibited all the laboratory characteristics of type IIb vWD and severe thrombocytopenia in infancy, in whom autosomal recessive inheritance was thought more likely (Donnér et al 1987).

Type III vWD has an autosomal inheritance and represents homozygous or doubly heterozygous vWD. Consanguineous marriage is common amongst the parents of affected children. All components of the FVIII-vWF complex, including FVIII:C, vWF:Ag and ristocetin cofactor activity, are present in minute amounts only. FVIII:C levels may be as low as 2% of normal. Symptoms may include haemarthrosis or muscle haematomas resembling haemophilia, in addition to mucous membrane bleeding characteristic of vWD. This severe form is the most likely to present in infancy.

Among 116 patients from the UK, Hoyer (1983) reported type I vWD in 71%, type II vWD in 23%, and type III vWD in 6%. Lenk found a higher incidence of type III vWD at 12% in a German study, with type I vWD in 76% and type II vWD in the remaining 12% (Lenk et al 1988).

The molecular defects in families with vWD have been identified in only a few patients so far. Gene tracking by RFLP analysis (Fig. 13.8) has become an important procedure for carrier de-

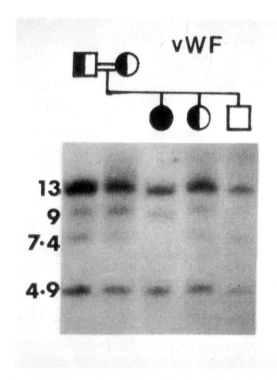

Fig. 13.8 Autoradiograph from a Southern blot in a family with vWD. The polymorphic bands shown by the vWF probe are 9 and 7.4 kilobases (kb) in size. The parents and the second child, who are heterozygotes for vWD are heterozygotes for this RFLP. The affected child is homozygous for the 9-kb fragment, so the vWF gene is tracking with the 9-kb fragment in this family.

tection and prenatal diagnosis of severe double heterozygous and homozygous forms of vWD (Bahnak et al 1988). The newer technique of polymerase chain reaction (PCR) amplification has been successfully employed in the prenatal diagnosis of a fetus at risk of severe type III vWD (Peake et al 1990a). Large, probably complete, deletions have been reported in the vWF gene in patients with type III vWD who have developed antibodies to infused vWF, but not in type III vWD patients who have not developed antibodies (Shelton-Inloes et al 1987, Ngo K-Y et al 1988). A patient with severe type III vWD and an allo-antibody to vWF has been reported with a partial deletion of the vWF gene, and the defect was traced by DNA analysis to seven members of the kindred, who were shown to be heterozygous carriers (Peake et al 1990b). Point mutations have been identified in two patients with type IIa vWD (Ginsburg et al 1988). No point mutations or gene deletions have been reported to date in patients with type I vWD.

Treatment

Treatment, which may be with desmopressin (DDAVP), factor VIII concentrate, cryoprecipitate or specific vWF concentrates, depends on the severity and type of vWD. Wherever possible, DDAVP is used in preference to plasma-derived products because of the concern of viral transmission. DDAVP is a synthetic agent which releases endogenous FVIII-vWF complex, including high molecular weight vWF, from its storage site. DDAVP is the treatment of choice for type I vWD, and produces a rapid rise of all components of the FVIII-vWF complex and transient correction of the bleeding time. DDAVP may be clinically ineffective in type II vWD because only structurally and functionally abnormal FVIII-vWF components will be released, which do not correct the bleeding time or improve haemostasis, although FVIII:C rises satisfactorily. However, type IIa is characterized by variable amounts of large multimers, and in some patients DDAVP will produce a release of large vWF multimers and correction of vWF activity and bleeding, whereas others who cannot respond in this fashion will have no correction of their bleeding time. DDAVP is ineffective

in type III vWD, and contraindicated in type IIb vWD, because the abnormal forms released have an increased affinity for platelets, resulting in in-vivo platelet aggregation and a transient drop in the platelet count. DDAVP should be given with tranexamic acid to block the effect of the concomitant release of tissue plasminogen activator induced by the former. Individuals with type III vWD, and those with type II vWD and type I vWD with no response to DDAVP or more serious bleeding episodes, should be treated with factor VIII concentrate rich in HMW multimers. Many lyophilized factor VIII concentrates are deficient in the HMW forms of vWF, but these are important in haemostasis because they possess the greatest affinity for the vWF receptors on platelets. However, a number of concentrates have been reported to give satisfactory haemostasis in vWD patients (Köhler et al 1985, Fukui et al 1988, Schimf et al 1987, Pasi et al 1990, Cumming et al 1990) and many were recently evaluated (Fricke et al 1989). Cryoprecipitate contains the entire FVIII-vWF complex, with little or no alteration in vWF:Ag multimeric structure and distribution, and may secure haemostasis in patients when FVIII concentrates have been unsuccessful: however, cryoprecipitate which has not undergone viricidal attenuation carries the risks of HCV and HIV infection. It has the advantage of being a single donor product, but its safety is entirely dependent on donor screening procedures, which are not foolproof. With the recent development of specific vWF concentrates, cryoprecipitate should rarely be needed for the treatment of vWD. The infusion of any product rich in HMW multimers will correct the bleeding time for only a few hours, probably because the larger forms of vWF are cleared more rapidly from the circulation. The frequency of treatment is guided by clinical bleeding, ristocetin-cofactor activity and the bleeding time.

Other hereditary coagulation disorders

All hereditary coagulation disorders other than haemophilia A, B and vWD are rare and have an autosomal recessive mode of inheritance. Some are not associated with a bleeding tendency (e.g. deficiencies of FXII or prekallikrein), others are associated with mild bleeding and are only un-masked after dental extraction or surgery, whilst others (e.g. FXIII deficiency) may be associated with a significant bleeding problem and present symptomatically in the newborn period. Most deficiencies cause a defect in the intrinsic coagulation pathway with prolongation of the APTT, except for FVII which prolongs the PT. FXIII and α_2 antiplasmin are not detected by routine screening tests and have to be specifically sought. A definitive diagnosis is made by demonstrating an absence or disporportionate reduction of an isolated factor.

Disorders of fibrinogen

Inherited disorders of fibrinogen synthesis include afibrinogenaemia, hypofibrinogenaemia and dysfibrinogenaemia. Congenital afibrinogenaemia is a rare inherited bleeding disorder characterized by complete absence of fibrinogen in the plasma. Inheritance is by an autosomal recessive gene resulting in afibrinogenaemia in the homozygote, and normal or reduced fibrinogen levels in the heterozygote. Homozygotes have a mild-to-moderate bleeding tendency, whilst heterozygotes are asymptomatic. In the homozygous state, neonatal presentation is common, and symptoms range in severity from bruising to intracranial haemorrhage. Mucous membrane bleeding presenting as melaena or haematemesis, haematomas secondary to trauma at delivery and bleeding from the umbilical cord are particularly common. In childhood the disorder is characterised by easy bruising and bleeding after trauma, although spontaneous haemarthrosis can occur. In homozygotes, the results of all screening tests based on fibrin formation – i.e. PT, APTT and TCT – are prolonged. Fibrinogen is completely absent when measured by clotting techniques, but immunological assays may detect trace amounts.

Patients with dysfibrinogenaemia may have a mild-to-moderate bleeding diathesis, have a tendency to thrombosis or may be asymptomatic, depending on the variant inherited. The disorder is inherited as an autosomal trait, and the clinical manifestations are dependent on the function inhibited by the specific molecular defect. The PT, APTT and TCT are all prolonged in the homozygous state, but only the TCT in heterozygotes. In addition, the reptilase time is prolonged. Fibrinogen activity levels are reduced, but antigen levels are normal.

Bleeding episodes can be controlled by replacement of fibrinogen with FFP or cryoprecipitate. Fibrinogen has a long half-life and therefore treatment need be given only every 4–5 days.

Congenital factor XI deficiency

Congenital FXI deficiency is a mild bleeding disorder. Most cases have been reported in Jewish patients, and the inheritance is autosomal and incompletely recessive. The bleeding tendency is extremely variable, and some homozygotes have no bleeding problems and have undergone surgery uneventfully. The level of haemostatic challenge may correlate with the likelihood of bleeding. Even in the most severely affected (homozygotes) the bleeding problem is usually mild, but does not necessarily correlate with the FXI coagulant activity, and may include postoperative bleeding and, occasionally, easy bruising, epistaxis and menorrhagia. The PT is normal and the APTT prolonged. A specific FXI coagulant assay is necessary to confirm the diagnosis. The amount of FXI protein, measured immunologically, parallels the coagulant level. Tests of contact activation factors may be influenced by freezing and thawing and should therefore be performed on fresh plasma. Diagnosis in the neonatal period is difficult because of the physiological depression, and may have to be delayed until 3–6 months of age. However, diagnosis should be possible for homozygotes with FXI levels of less than 1 iu/dl. FFP is the best source of FXI and, if replacement therapy is necessary, should be given at 10–15 ml/kg to maintain a FXI level of 20% or above.

Congenital factor XII deficiency

This disorder, with an autosomal recessive inheritance, is not associated with haemorrhagic manifestations and therefore diagnosis is by chance rather than by the investigation of a clinical problem. The APTT is markedly prolonged, and a specific FXII assay is required for definitive diagnosis.

Other contact factors

Congenital deficiencies of prekallikrein (Fletcher factor) and high molecular weight kininogen (Fitzgerald factor) have been reported. The inheritance is autosomal recessive. Although they result in a marked prolongation of the APTT, there are no associated haemorrhagic problems, and diagnosis is by specific assay.

Congenital prothrombin deficiency

This exceedingly rare disorder is inherited in an autosomal recessive manner. Both a true deficiency (hypoprothrombinaemia) and synthesis of an abnormal molecular variant (dysprothrombinaemia) have been described. The deficiency is not complete, and homozygotes produce between 2 and 25 iu/dl of functional prothrombin. The bleeding disorder in homozygotes is usually mild to moderate, and characterized by easy bruising, menorrhagia and prolonged bleeding after trauma, dental extraction or surgery. Umbilical and post-circumcision bleeding have occurred in the neonatal period, and haematemesis and intracranial bleeding reported. Patients with dysprothrombinaemia may be asymptomatic or have problems comparable to those of patients with hypoprothrombinaemia.

The prothrombin time is slightly to moderately prolonged and the APTT likewise variably prolonged. The TCT is normal. In hypoprothrombinaemia, both functional and immunological assays show reduced levels of FII, whilst FII protein is at normal levels in dysprothrombinaemia. Treatment is rarely necessary, but if required, FFP at 10–15 ml/kg should be given. Treatment need only be given every 2–3 days because of the long half-life of the protein. Vitamin K is of no value.

Congenital factor V deficiency

This autosomal recessive disorder is associated with a mild bleeding tendency usually from the mucous membranes or following injury or surgery. It is unlikely to manifest itself in the neonatal period, but if so this is generally by umbilical bleeding. The deficiency is due to failure of production of the protein, with functional and immunological levels being equally reduced; most patients have values ranging from undetectable to 10% of normal. The PT and APTT are prolonged and the diagnosis is confirmed by a specific assay. Both the term and preterm infant have normal levels of FV at birth, and diagnosis can therefore be made in the newborn period. The half-life of the transfused protein is 36 hours, and replacement therapy is with FFP to maintain a haemostatic level of approximately 25 iu/dl.

Congenital factor VII deficiency

This rare clotting disorder is thought to be inherited as an autosomal recessive trait with intermediate expressivity. The severity of the bleeding problem depends on the degree of deficiency. The more mildly affected individuals rarely have bleeding problems, but the severely affected may experience serious mucous membrane bleeding, haemarthrosis and muscle haematomas. Neonates have been reported with fatal bleeding, usually due to intracranial haemorrhage. Other neonatal presentations include oozing from the umbilical cord, bleeding post circumcision, cephalohaematoma, ecchymoses and haematemesis. In older children, bruising, epistaxis, menorrhagia and haemorrhage post dental extraction and surgery may occur. Heterozygotes may have clinical problems. Homozygotes may synthesize no protein or produce a nonfunctional molecule. The PT is abnormally prolonged but the APTT is not affected. The Russell's viper venom time is normal, and diagnosis is with a specific FVII assay. Immunological FVII assays may detect no protein, or reduced or normal levels. The half-life of the protein is 5 hours, and treatment, if required, should be with FFP. Vitamin K is of no value.

Congenital factor X deficiency

This is an extremely rare coagulation disorder inherited as an incompletely recessive trait. The disorder can be due to a deficiency of the factor or synthesis of a nonfunctional protein. The bleeding manifestations are moderate to severe in the homozygote, and include easy bruising, mucous membrane bleeding and haemorrhage post trauma, dental extraction and surgery. Heterozygotes may also bleed after a challenge to the haemostatic system. Infants have been reported with intra-cranial haemorrhage and bleeding from the umbilical cord and gastrointestinal tract. The PT and APTT are prolonged, and the definitive diagnosis is dependent on a specific FX coagulant assay. FX antigen may be normal or reduced, depending on whether the functional deficiency is due to an absence of the protein or the synthesis of an abnormal molecule. The half-life of FX is 24–48 hours, and replacement, if required, should be with FFP. Vitamin K is of no value.

Congenital factor XIII deficiency

This disorder is inherited as an autosomal recessive trait and is characterized by poor wound healing and late wound bleeding. In the absence of FXIII, an unstable friable clot is formed. The molecule is composed of two subunits – A and B (or S). Only subunit A has fibrin-stabilizing activity. Two types of FXIII deficiency exist. In the first type, both subunits A and S are immunologically decreased, whilst in the second form only subunit A is defective, subunit S being normal or near normal. Infants who are homozygotes (usually FXIII activity of less than 1 iu/dl) commonly bleed from the umbilicus. Intracranial bleeding has also been reported. In children wounds heal slowly and, although clotting takes place at the time of surgery, secondary bleeding occurs 24–36 hours later. Easy bruising is characteristic with haematoma formation after trauma. Habitual abortion may be reported in the mothers. In the absence of FXIII, cross-linkage of the fibrin polymer does not take place, resulting in an unstable clot which is more susceptible to digestion by plasmin. The PT, APTT and TCT are normal. Cross-linked fibrin is normally soluble. The diagnosis is confirmed by the urea solubility test, but this does not detect heterozygotes. The FXIII activity can be measured using a chromogenic assay, and the subtypes differentiated by immunological techniques. Only tiny quantities in the region of 2–3% FXIII are necessary for fibrin stabilization. Replacement, if required, should be given with FFP at 5–10 ml/kg. FXIII has a half-life of 6 days.

Combined factor deficiencies

Combined factor deficiencies occurring in the same patient is a rare event. The most common combination is the coexistence of factor V and VIII deficiency (Fischer et al 1988). Some of these cases may be due to a deficiency of protein C inhibitor. Rarer combinations include hereditary deficiency of all vitamin K-dependent procoagulants and anticoagulants (Brenner et al 1990).

Alpha$_2$ antiplasmin deficiency

Alpha$_2$ antiplasmin deficiency causes a severe bleeding disorder and is inherited in an autosomal recessive manner. Alpha$_2$ antiplasmin normally neutralizes plasmin which, in the absence of its inhibitor, is free to lyse normal fibrin clots. Coagulation screening tests are normal and, as with FXIII deficiency, this defect has to be specifically sought. The whole-blood clot lysis, plasma clot lysis and euglobulin clot lysis times are markedly shortened. Alpha$_2$ antiplasmin is absent by both a functional and immunological assay. Antifibrinolytic agents, such as tranexamic acid, may be useful in treatment.

CONGENITAL THROMBOTIC DISORDERS

Any inherited imbalance between the activators and inhibitors of either the coagulation or fibrinolytic mechanisms may predispose towards thrombosis. An arterial thrombosis suggests endothelial change or abnormal platelet aggregation, whereas venous thrombosis may result from a defect in fibrinolysis or the physiological anticoagulant system. The major inhibitors of coagulation (ATIII, HCII, protein C, protein S) are autosomally inherited. Heterozygotes have levels that are approximately half the normal value, and rarely present clinically until adolescence or early adult life. Only homozygous protein C deficiency presents in the newborn period.

Protein C deficiency

Two types of hereditary protein C deficiency are recognized. In type 1, which is the commoner, both protein C antigen and activity are reduced.

Families synthesizing a nonfunctional protein have been reported and this type II deficiency is characterized by normal protein C antigen levels but reduced protein C activity. On the basis of clinical manifestations, hereditary protein C deficiency may possibly be divided into two distinct phenotypes: autosomal recessive and autosomal dominant. In the autosomal dominant phenotype, heterozygotes have recurrent venous thrombosis during adult life. A 50% reduction of protein C appears to be sufficient to predispose the adult to venous thrombosis, although clinical problems in heterozygotes are highly variable and do not occur until early adulthood or later. In the autosomal recessive phenotype, heterozygotes have no symptoms and homozygotes present in the newborn period with a syndrome resembling purpura fulminans. However, caution is recommended in the evaluation of infants with low levels of protein C. A low protein C value alone, in the absence of clinical manifestations and a family history, cannot be considered diagnostic of homozygous protein C deficiency, as physiological levels can be very low (Manco-Johnson et al 1988). In both phenotypes, the protein C deficiency may be type I or type II.

A small number of neonates have been reported with homozygosity for protein C deficiency and a syndrome characterized by fulminant thrombosis, purpura fulminans and disseminated intravascular coagulation (Seligsohn et al 1984, Marciniak et al 1985, Estelles et al 1984).It was once thought that untreated homozygous protein C deficiency might be incompatible with life, but it is now apparent that not all homozygotes present in the immediate newborn period. Two cousins have been reported who presented at 7 months and 10 months respectively with recurrent ecchymotic skin lesions, disseminated intravascular coagulation and venous thrombosis (Tuddenham et al 1989). Branson reported the combination of purpura fulminans and disseminated intravascular coagulation presenting at 11 hours of age in a heterozygote for protein C deficiency (Branson et al 1983). The infant had repeated thrombotic and haemorrhagic episodes. He was latterly treated with coumarin and died 3 months later of a fatal subarachnoid and intracerebral haemorrhage. His protein C level on coumarin was below 6%. The mother and siblings had protein C levels in the heterozygote

range and the father was unaffected. The very low value found in this infant can best be explained by a combination of heterozygous protein C deficiency, coumarin therapy and DIC.

A small number of cases have now been reported where diagnosis was suspected early and treatment instigated. Anticoagulation alone, with heparin, has not been helpful. Initial treatment should always be with FFP (10–15 ml/kg twice daily). However, the half-life of protein C is about 7 hours and treatment has to be given at such regular intervals to maintain adequate levels that this is not a practical long-term solution. Hopefully, protein C concentrates or recombinant protein C will become routinely available in the near future and enable these individuals to receive specific therapy. The recent cloning of DNA encoding protein C makes this a possibility. Vukovich (1988) successfully treated a 10-month-old female infant with homozygous protein C deficiency with a concentrate of human protein C and S and low levels of other coagulation factors. However, replacement therapy had to be given every 48 hours.

At present, two therapeutic approaches are available for long-term management. Firstly, the successful use of factor IX concentrate as a vehicle for administering protein C has been reported (Sills et al 1984). It appears that every-other-day infusions of 50–75 U/kg of protein C are sufficient to stop thrombotic episodes, although levels approach zero by the end of 48 hours. The FIX concentrate should be selected with care to minimize its thrombotic risk, and levels of protein C, FII, FIX and FX monitored carefully to prevent excessive rises (Montgomery et al 1985). Heat-treated concentrates should be used and the risk of transmission of hepatitis not underestimated. Alternatively, warfarin has also been employed with some success and is now recommended by the International Committee on Thrombosis and Haemostasis. They suggest that affected neonates initially be treated with infusions of FFP (10–15 ml/kg every 12 hours) until the infant is 2–3 months old, all symptoms have resolved and the other vitamin K-dependent factors have approached adult levels. Warfarin is then started at a daily dose of 0.15–0.4 mg/kg until a minimum maintenance dose is established to keep the child symptom free. The PT will range from 1.5 to 2 times the control value, and the International Normalized Ratio (INR) will be between 2.5 and 4.4. FFP should be administered for the first 5–7 days of oral anticoagulant therapy as protection against recurring purpuric lesions. FFP should be reinstituted if purpura fulminans recurs on oral anticoagulation (Marlar et al 1989, Report of the Working Party on Homozygous Protein C Deficiency of the Sub-committee on Protein C and Protein S, International Committee on Thrombosis and Haemostasis). The dose of oral anticoagulant and the therapeutic range should be individualized on the basis of a number of factors: (1) minimum dose to remain symptom free; (2) age; (3) weight; (4) drugs the infant may be receiving. It is difficult to achieve a stable therapeutic warfarin dose in neonates, and this therapy does nothing to raise the level of protein C or to correct the imbalance between protein C and its procoagulants. Bone growth and development (followed by bone densitometry) should be monitored every 6–12 months, because the long-term effect of vitamin K antagonist use in childhood is not fully understood. Reconstitution of protein C activity and resolution of the thrombotic condition has followed liver transplantation in a 20-month infant with protein C deficiency (Casella et al 1988). However, such an approach cannot be recommended at present. Antenatal diagnosis by fetal blood sampling can be offered to parents at risk.

Protein S deficiency

Adults deficient in protein S, the cofactor for protein C, are predisposed to recurrent venous thrombotic disease. Protein-S-deficient patients with normal or mildly reduced total protein S antigen, but most of their protein S complexed to C4b-binding protein with little or no free protein and correspondingly low levels of protein S functional activity, are designated as having type I deficiency. A few cases of type II deficiency have been described, characterized by little or no protein S, either bound or free (Comp et al 1986). A two-year-old female infant has been reported with homozygous protein S deficiency and relapsing purpura fulminans since the age of 10 days (Mahasandana et al 1990). A heterozygote with a

protein S antigen level of 49% had a deep-vein thrombosis at the age of 3 years, after a burn involving less than 2% of the skin surface, and another episode at age 14 after appendectomy (Mannucci et al 1986). A high FIX level (182%) may have been an additional risk factor.

Antithrombin III deficiency

Antithrombin III deficiency may result from a quantitative defect (type I) or a qualitative defect (type II). Homozygous ATIII deficiency is probably incompatible with life. Whether some of the recurrent abortions and intrauterine fetal deaths observed in ATIII-deficient women represent homozygous cases is unknown. However, half of the infants born to heterozygous ATIII-deficient mothers will be ATIII-deficient themselves. This, combined with the gestational-dependent reduction in ATIII levels, may predispose the neonate to thrombosis. A small number of infants born to mothers with congenital ATIII deficiency have died in the newborn period with thrombotic complications (Bjarke et al 1974); ATIII deficiency was suspected, but not proven. Brenner (1988) reported an infant born to an ATIII-deficient mother, who himself was subsequently shown to be a heterozygote for ATIII deficiency and presented at the age of 2 weeks with superior sagittal and rectus sinus thrombosis. Two female infants have been reported presenting at age 2 years with cerebral thrombosis considered secondary to ATIII deficiency. In at least one case the deficiency was clearly inherited (Vomberg et al 1987).

Infants born to mothers with ATIII deficiency should have their level measured at birth. An ATIII-deficient infant would be expected to have a cord blood ATIII level of 20–30%. It has been recommended that affected infants should receive prophylactic antithrombin III concentrate or FFP to maintain values appropriate for the newborn (60%) until the infant's own level has risen to around 50% at 3 months of age (Hambley et al 1982). However, these infants have a relatively small risk of thrombosis and such an aggressive therapeutic approach may produce morbidity from transfusion-related viral infections, despite the availability of pasteurized ATIII concentrates. On balance, a more conservative approach seems appropriate, although the neonate's ATIII level may be useful in finally determining the need for prophylaxis.

ACQUIRED COAGULATION DISORDERS

Disseminated intravascular coagulation (DIC)

Disseminated intravascular coagulation (DIC) is a common acquired coagulopathy wherein the physiological balance of clotting and clot lysis is disrupted. It is always associated with an underlying disorder, which triggers the coagulation system by stimulating either the intrinsic clotting cascade via endothelial injury, or the extrinsic cascade via tissue factor. The end product is an excess formation of fibrin which may result in disseminated microthrombi, coincident coagulation factor and platelet consumption and secondary fibrin (ogen) lysis. The consumptive coagulopathy may be compensated and only detectable by in-vivo half-life studies of platelet or fibrinogen, or may be noncompensated and easily diagnosed by routine laboratory testing. In addition, the consumption may be chronic and localized, as in Kasabach-Merritt syndrome, or acute and generalized, as when associated with meningococcal septicaemia. The pattern of intravascular coagulation is influenced by the underlying trigger, reticuloendothelial function, blood flow and levels of naturally occurring anticoagulants.

Bleeding is the main clinical problem associated with DIC, although thrombosis, particularly of the small blood vessels, occurs, this is usually clinically insignificant. The pathophysiology of DIC results from excessive thrombin generation. Coagulation factors are consumed and natural inhibitors overwhelmed. Thrombin activates protein C and results in secondary generation of plasmin by increasing levels of plasminogen activator. Thrombin also causes platelet aggregation and subsequent thrombocytopenia. Plasmin degrades fibrin monomers and fibrinogen, producing fibrinolytic degradation products, fragments X, Y, D and E. Haemorrhage can thus result from a number of mechanisms:

1. consumption of procoagulants – factors I, II, V, VIII
2. thrombocytopenia (see also Ch. 6)
3. inhibition of platelet function and fibrin/fibrinogen by FDPs.

Table 13.10 lists diseases in children known to be associated with disseminated intravascular coagulation; infection is the commonest. Both bacterial and viral infections may be associated with a consumptive coagulopathy.Septic shock is a particularly serious complication of bacterial-related DIC, and is associated with poor tissue perfusion, hypoxia and acidosis which further aggravate consumption. Severe hyaline membrane disease, with its accompanying hypoxia and acidosis, may be complicated by DIC.

Purpura fulminans (see also Ch. 6) is a rare, but serious illness, that most often follows streptococcal infection or chickenpox in children. It is characterized by massive and progressive ecchymotic skin lesions accompanied by widespread thrombosis of capillaries and venules, with subsequent necrosis of affected tissues. Visceral involvement and peripheral gangrene necessitating amputation may occur. The morbidity and mortality are

Table 13.10 Disorders associated with DIC in neonates and children*

Infection
  Bacterial (e.g. meningococcus)
  Parasitic (e.g. malaria)
  Mycotic
  Rickettsial
  Viral (e.g. disseminated varicella)
Neoplasms
  Leukaemia, particularly M3AML
  Metastatic solid tumours
Miscellaneous
  Giant haemangioma (Kasbach-Merritt syndrome)
  Purpura fulminans
  Haemolytic transfusion reaction
  Acute anaphylaxis
  Snake bite
  Burns
  Heat stroke
  Hypothermia
  Massive head injury or trauma
  Haemorrhagic shock
Neonatal (in addition to the above)
  Hypoxia – acidosis (birth asphyxia, respiratory distress syndrome, polycythaemia)
  Infection (bacterial, viral)
  Dead twin fetus
  Small for gestational age
  Abruptio placenta
  Miscellaneous (erythroblastosis fetalis, necrotising enterocolitis, brain injury)

*See also Ch. 6

high. Heparin therapy has not been universally accepted, but may be beneficial (Chenaille et al 1989). Identical lesions occur in infants with homozygous protein C deficiency, and in patients with a heterozygous deficiency of protein C or S during the initial phase of warfarin therapy at a time when protein C levels are much lower than levels of the vitamin K-dependent procoagulants, factors II, VII, IX and X. Acquired deficiencies of protein C and S may contribute to the pathogenesis of purpura fulminans, and FFP may be important adjunctive therapy by replacing many consumed coagulation factors including fibrinogen, ATIII and protein C (Powars et al 1987).

Kasabach-Merritt syndrome is characterized by thrombocytopenia, consumptive coagulopathy and, occasionally, microangiopathic haemolytic anaemia in association with a giant cavernous haemangioma. Treatment is primarily directed at inducing involution of the haemangioma, but the adjuvant use of antifibrinolytic agents may improve haematological parameters where consumption is problematic (Hanna & Bernstein 1989, Shulkin et al 1990).

Acute leukaemia, in particular acute promyelocytic leukaemia, is frequently associated with DIC. The DIC may be induced by activation of the coagulation cascade by procoagulant substances released from leukaemia blast cells, but in addition there is evidence that fibrinogen may be directly activated by blast-cell-derived proteases. Primary fibrinolysis has also been described (Imaoka et al 1986) but would appear to be rare. The main therapeutic strategies for leukaemia-associated DIC include rapid initiation of chemotherapy and vigorous blood product support until the DIC resolves, when the blast cells have cleared from the circulation. Although the role of heparin is controversial, it may reduce the incidence of haemorrhagic death (Hoyle et al 1988, Wilde & Davies 1990).

The diagnosis of DIC is made in most laboratories by carrying out a number of screening tests. The PT, APTT and TCT are usually prolonged, the fibrinogen level and platelet count reduced, and FDPs or D-dimers elevated. DIC can never be ruled out by a single set of normal values. Serial haematological measurements are more informative in making the diagnosis since it is the progressive fall of coagulation components which

demonstrates consumption, if previous levels are not known. The cross-linked fibrin degradation fragment, D-dimer (DD), is detected in the laboratory using monoclonal antibodies. Fragment DD or D-dimer is generated when crosslinked fibrin clots are lysed by plasmin; this is in contrast to FDPs, which are generated by the lysis of fibrinogen and non-crosslinked fibrin. The presence of D-dimer confirms that both thrombin generation (crosslinking of fibrin clot via thrombin activation of FXIII) and plasmin generation (fibrinolysis) have occurred. The detection of D-dimer, which addresses both dimensions of DIC, is strong evidence for its existence. FDP measurement is extremely sensitive but not specific, whilst D-dimer is less sensitive, but highly specific. Carr et al (1989) suggests that D-dimer might be most appropriately used as a confirmatory test for the very sensitive FDP test. Values in preterm infants and those born at full term must be cautiously interpreted, as our study has shown about 50% of infants to have plasma concentrations outwith the accepted adult range in the absence of any other clinical or laboratory evidence of DIC (Hudson et al 1990). Red cell fragmentation is not an early sign of DIC, but only follows the deposition of intravascular fibrin and may not be apparent until 48 hours after the onset. A coagulation screen complemented by a fibrinogen level, platelet count and D-dimer determination is generally sufficient to establish the diagnosis, and these tests are readily available in most laboratories. Levels of the naturally occurring inhibitors and procoagulants, particularly factors I, II, V and VIII, fall as these proteins are consumed and, although specific factor assays are rarely necessary, these may be helpful in certain circumstances where the diagnosis is in doubt. Vitamin K deficiency and liver disease are the conditions most likely to cause confusion. It is helpful to remember that FV, although produced in the liver, is not vitamin K-dependent and therefore will be normal in the latter disorder, although low in liver disease or DIC. FVIII is not vitamin-K-dependent and tends to be normal or elevated in liver disease. DIC is the only acquired coagulopathy in which the FVIII level is reduced.

The most important aspect of management is to treat the underlying disorder, thereby removing the stimulus to further consumption. It is extremely important, where appropriate, to maintain the blood pressure and correct any acidosis or hypoxia. Replacement therapy will depend on laboratory abnormalities and might include the use of platelet concentrates (1 unit of platelets per 5 kg), FFP (10–15 mg/kg), cryoprecipitate as a source of fibrinogen or FVIII (1 bag per 5 kg) or red cell concentrates. In neonates, exchange transfusion may be necessary to avoid volume overload. Antifibrinolytic therapy is contraindicated and may be dangerous. The use of heparin in the treatment of DIC remains controversial, although its role is better established in some situations than in others, such as purpura fulminans. When treatment of the primary condition and replacement therapy have failed to control the ongoing intravascular coagulation, heparin may be used to inhibit a number of procoagulants generated, particularly thrombin. Heparin inhibits the action of thrombin, plasmin, XIIa, IXa, XIa and Xa. Heparin requires ATIII for its action, and this anticoagulant is consumed in DIC. It may, therefore, be necessary to give FFP in conjunction to maintain an adequate level of ATIII for effective heparinization. Indeed, ATIII concentrates have been used in this context (Hanada et al 1985, von Kries et al 1985). However, the possible benefits of heparin must be carefully weighed against the risk of inducing further bleeding.

Hepatocellular disease

The liver is the site of synthesis of fibrinogen, FV and the vitamin-K-dependent factors (II, VII, IX, X), as well as of the major natural anticoagulants and proteins involved in fibrinolysis. Activated coagulation factors and plasminogen activators are cleared from plasma by the liver. Finally, liver disease may be associated with thrombocytopenia secondary to sequestration and hypersplenism, with agents responsible for the liver disease (e.g. toxins, viruses, immune complexes) or with DIC. Platelet dysfunction is not uncommon. A laboratory coagulation abnormality is found in a very high percentage of patients with liver disease, although the incidence of clinical bleeding is much lower, at around 15%. In general, there is correlation between the degree of hepatocellular disease and the resulting coagulation abnormality.

Parenchymal liver disease is characterized by a depression of the vitamin-K-dependent factors in association with prolongation of the PT and APTT and decreased responsiveness to the administration of vitamin K. The prothrombin time remains the most convenient test for monitoring liver function. FVII, with its short half-life, is the most sensitive indicator, but is not as readily available. Vitamin K deficiency and DIC may coexist with hepatocellular dysfunction, and it is not always easy to separate these entities. In certain circumstances, a trial of vitamin K therapy may be diagnostically, as well as therapeutically, helpful.

Fibrinogen levels are usually normal in chronic liver disease, but may be reduced in acute fulminant liver failure, because of concomitant DIC. An increased catabolic rate of labelled fibrinogen has been noted in acute and chronic active hepatitis, despite normal levels of plasma fibrinogen. Fibrinogen is an acute phase reactant, and high levels may occasionally be observed in liver disease, including obstructive jaundice, biliary cirrhosis and hepatoma. A dysfibrinogenaemia has been reported in liver disease, characterized by prolonged reptilase and thrombin clotting times. In common with fetal fibrinogen, the molecule has increased sialiac acid residues.

The treatment of a coagulopathy associated with liver disease should always include the administration of vitamin K. If there is no response or an inadequate response, FFP will correct all of the coagulation factor deficiencies except possibly for fibrinogen, which may require replacement with cryoprecipitate.

Prothrombin complex concentrates do not contain fibrinogen or FV and should be used cautiously, if at all, because of potential thrombogenic complications. Portal vein thrombosis is a substantial cause of mortality in liver transplantation, particularly in children. Deficiencies of protein C and antithrombin III with a concomitant rise in PAI contribute to the genesis of thrombosis (Harper et al 1988) and suggest possible strategies for prophylactic therapy.

Haemorrhagic disease of the newborn

A number of haemorrhagic problems are peculiar

to the neonate because of its physiological immaturity. The term 'haemorrhagic disease of the newborn' was first used in 1894, by Townsend when he reported a series of infants who presented with self-limiting bleeding, usually from the gastrointestinal tract, on the second or third day of life. We now know that this bleeding diathesis is due to very low levels of the vitamin K-dependent procoagulant factors II, VII, IX and X, which in the absence of vitamin K are functionally defective. Vitamin K is required for the post-translational carboxylation of their glutamic acid residues.

The conversion of glutamic acid to γ-carboxyglutamic acid is essential for formation of effective calcium-binding sites, which are necessary for activation of the clotting factors. In the noncarboxylated state, these proteins are unable to bind calcium and are functionally defective. Immaturity of the biosynthetic hepatic enzyme system is responsible for the reduction of the vitamin-K-dependent coagulation factors at birth. However, a further fall is commonly observed in the first three days of life, which can be prevented by the prophylactic administration of vitamin K at birth and is therefore at least in part due to deficiency of this vitamin (Lane & Hathaway 1985). In 1961, the Committee on Nutrition of the American Academy of Pediatrics recommended that prophylactic vitamin K be administered parenterally to all newborn infants at a dose of 0.5–1.0 mg, or orally at a dose of 1–2 mg.

When faced with the clinical problem of a bleeding neonate, it is necessary to differentiate between vitamin K deficiency and an acquired or congenital coagulation problem. It can be particularly difficult to differentiate vitamin K deficiency from hepatic dysfunction. A common presentation is that of generalized haemorrhage in an otherwise healthy term infant with a normal platelet count and fibrinogen level, but a prolonged PT and APTT. A range of laboratory tests are available to help clarify the situation. The PT, APTT and thrombotest are prolonged in vitamin K deficiency, and functional factor assays (II, VII, IX and X) are lower than would be expected for the gestational age, although as the normal range is wide overlap occurs. A shortening of the screening tests (PT, APTT, thrombotest) or a rise in factor levels following the administration of vitamin K

suggests a previous vitamin deficiency. More specific tests measure the abnormal noncarboxylated prothrombin that circulates in vitamin K-deficient patients. The abnormal or precursor prothrombin is antigenically intact, but functionally defective. Initially, the report by Blanchard of small amounts of abnormal prothrombin in the plasma of patients with acquired liver disease challenged the specificity of those assays (Blanchard et al 1981), but assay systems of high specificity have now been developed (Shapiro et al 1986). The PIVKA-II (protein induced in vitamin K's absence: prothrombin) assay involves the absorption of normal carboxylated prothrombin from plasma, using barium carbonate. Any noncarboxylated prothrombin formed in the absence of vitamin K is left behind and is assayed immunologically. Noncarboxylated prothrombin can also be measured by crossed immunoelectrophoresis. Abnormal, noncarboxylated prothrombin migrates further than carboxylated prothrombin in the first dimension in a medium containing calcium, because of decreased calcium binding. If prothrombin antibody is added, the prothrombins will precipitate in the second dimension and a double peak indicates the presence of two species of prothrombin with different calcium binding; one carboxylated and one noncarboxylated.

Using specific assays for noncarboxylated vitamin K, some investigators have found evidence of vitamin K deficiency at birth (Shapiro et al 1986, Motohara et al 1985); others, however, have not (von Kries et al 1985). Part, but not all of the discrepancy, may be explained by differences in the assay methods and in the infants studied. Thus, the true prevalence of vitamin K deficiency in the newborn is poorly defined. Hepatic reserves of vitamin K are low in the neonate and this reflects in part very limited placental transfer of the vitamin. After birth, the diet provides vitamin K_1, which is absorbed in the small intestine and requires the presence of bile salts. Breast milk is particularly deficient in vitamin K_1, with levels as low as 2 μg/l, compared to values greater than 50 μg/l for many commercial formulae (Haroon et al 1982).

In addition to vitamin K_1 provided by diet, vitamin K_2 or fat-soluble menaquinone is produced endogenously by the intestinal flora. Coliforms, which produce vitamin K, flourish in the gut of the bottle-fed baby, whilst bifidobacteria predominate in the breast-fed baby. These flora, through differing capacities for the production of vitamin K, may account in a very small way for the difference in the haemorrhagic tendencies seen between breast- and bottle-fed babies.

Syndromes associated with vitamin K deficiency

Haemorrhagic disease of the newborn has three recognized patterns depending on the time of presentation:

1. early HDN, i.e. within the first 24 hours of life
2. classic HDN, i.e. at 2–5 days of age
3. late HDN, i.e. after the first postnatal month.

Early HDN. Haemorrhagic disease of the newborn presenting within the first 24 hours of life may be associated with severe and sometimes fatal haemorrhage. Symptoms vary from bruising to internal bleeding, intracranial being the most serious. Early haemorrhagic disease is typical of infants, but is not confined to those whose mothers are taking drugs which cross the placenta and affect vitamin K metabolism. The risk of HDN in infants of mothers on anticonvulsants remains undefined. In one survey of 111 such pregnancies, 20 infants had significantly prolonged prothrombin times and 8 infants were symptomatic. Three of these haemorrhagic babies died and one developed neurological sequelae (Deblay at al 1982). The authors recommended that mothers taking anticonvulsant therapy should receive vitamin K prenatally. However, this opinion has recently been challenged by a study of the infants of 23 mothers on chronic anticonvulsant therapy, which showed that 1 mg of vitamin K_1 given intramuscularly immediately after delivery was protective in 22 of the 23 infants (Hulac et al 1986). The antituberculous drugs, rifampicin and isoniazid have also been reported to be associated with early HDN. Warfarin is the classic drug which can cross the placenta and result in serious bleeding problems, and although it is rarely prescribed to pregnant women because of its teratogenicity, it is still indicated for anticoagulation in mothers with artificial heart valves. It is not excreted in breast milk in significant amounts.

Classic HDN presents at 2– is generally manifest by bruisin the gastrointestinal tract or f sion. Intracranial haemorrhag_ Classic HDN can be prevented by the administra tion of vitamin K_1 at birth. Breast feeding is a major risk factor. Not only is breast milk a poor source of vitamin K, but breast-fed babies tend to have a smaller intake of milk in the first days of life than do formula-fed infants, and the volume of milk may be as important as the vitamin K content.

Late HDN. Although one commonly associates vitamin K deficiency with the immediate newborn period, presentation may be delayed until after the first month of life, and it is the prevention of this pattern of disease which is presently the subject of much controversy. Typically, haemorrhage is delayed when an infant (usually breast-fed) has not received vitamin K prophylaxis or when an infant has an underlying condition predisposing to impaired vitamin K absorption. The former generally presents between 1 and 3 months of age, whereas the latter may present at any time during the first year of life. Intracranial haemorrhage is the commonest problem and, if not fatal, may result in severe neurological damage (Motohara et al 1984, Chaou et al 1984). Breast-fed babies are particularly vulnerable. Although diet is important, a pure dietary deficiency alone is unlikely to explain late-onset haemorrhagic disease of the newborn in the breast-fed infant. Mild malabsorption or cholestasis related to infection may play a role (von Kries et al 1985). Vitamin K deficiency can develop in infants with chronic diarrhoea, malabsorption or oral antibiotic therapy, and HDN has been the initial manifestation of cystic fibrosis, biliary atresia, α_1 antitrypsin deficiency and abetalipoproteinaemia. An underlying cause should be sought in all cases of late-onset HDN.

Prevention of haemorrhagic disease of the newborn

Argument still continues as to whether or not all infants should receive vitamin K prophylaxis, and if so, whether this should be given parenterally or orally. Using sensitive assays, some authors have found evidence of vitamin K deficiency at birth and others have not. Furthermore, in the absence concomitant vitamin K levels, evidence that the presence of PIVKA-II represents vitamin K deficiency is circumstantial. Shapiro reported the prevalence of vitamin K deficiency determined with a PIVKA-II test in a prospective study of 934 infants (Shapiro 1986). Of 934 cord blood samples assayed, 2.9% were positive for PIVKA-II. No infant with PIVKA-II in the cord sample subsequently had clinical bleeding and all had been born at term and received prophylactic vitamin K_1. Some 63% of these infants with neonatal vitamin K deficiency were otherwise normal newborns. PIVKA-II detection rates of 50% have been reported in healthy 5-day-old newborns who did not receive prophylactic vitamin K at birth (von Kries 1985). The marginal vitamin K stores at birth may rapidly fall to levels too low to maintain normal haemostasis. It has been suggested that only infants at high risk of developing vitamin K deficiency, i.e. breast-fed babies or recipients of antibiotics etc., need receive prophylaxis. However, vitamin K is a safe drug and virtually no infant in receipt of it develops classic haemorrhagic disease of the newborn. McNinch reported a local recurrence of haemorrhagic disease of the newborn in an area in which prophylactic vitamin K was not routinely given (McNinch et al 1983). In a 17-month period, he encountered 6 cases of HDN, i.e. 1 per 1200 live births. All infants were breast fed and had not received vitamin K at birth. Three of the 6 infants died. Although one infant was born to an epileptic mother receiving phenytoin, bleeding did not occur until day 10 of life, and as with the other infants would undoubtedly have been prevented by prophylactic vitamin K_1. This experience has prompted the authors to reintroduce the administration of vitamin K_1 to all neonates in their hospital. Their example should be followed, as their experience highlights the risk of not adhering to a policy of vitamin K prophylaxis for all newborns, especially in a society where breast feeding is increasingly popular.

Concern about administrating vitamin K_1 orally relates to doubts about optimal absorption and possible regurgitation.There is little available information on the intestinal absorption of vitamin K_1 in neonates. In adults, 70–80% of an orally administered dose is absorbed. Plasma concentrations reach a peak at 2–4 hours, and fall to 10–20% of the peak value by 24 hours. McNinch compared the oral and parenteral administration of 1 mg vitamin K_1 (McNinch et al 1985). The neonates who received oral vitamin K_1 achieved peak median plasma concentrations of 73 ng/ml at 4 hours, compared to 1781 ng/ml at 12 hours for parenteral administration. Although the concentration following oral administration is considerably lower than with parenteral administration, it is still some 300 times the adult median value and represents approximately 8.5 µg of vitamin K_1 in the plasma. No infant in the study developed haemorrhagic disease of the newborn, although in two infants no vitamin K was detected. Oral administration appears an attractive alternative to parenteral administration, but further work is required to determine the percentage of an oral dose absorbed and consequently the optimal dosage. McNinch's study suggests an average absorption of 24%, but the range was wide. The authors recommend oral vitamin K at a dose of 1 mg for routine prophylaxis, and reserve parenteral administration for infants considered at special risk of haemorrhagic disease of the newborn (Tripp & McNinch 1987). Using this policy for 25,000 babies, they have not seen a single case of HDN. However, other experiences with oral prophylaxis have been less satisfactory (Priestley 1987, von Kries et al 1988). In the USA there has never been a case of late-onset HDN where parenteral vitamin K was given, but cases have been reported from other countries (von Kries & Gobel 1988). So, it seems clear that vitamin K prophylaxis should be given to all newborns.

An important additional question is whether or not infants who are exclusively breast fed should receive further vitamin K supplementation after the immediate newborn period. A number of breast-fed infants have been reported who developed late haemorrhagic disease of the newborn despite receiving oral vitamin K at birth, although this appears to be a rare finding. Motohara found a statistically increased incidence of vitamin K deficiency, as defined by PIVKA-II positivity, in infants at one month of age who had been exclusively breast fed and had received 5 mg vitamin K orally at birth, as compared to infants who had received a subsequent dose at 14 days of age (Motohara et al 1986); however, the authors admitted that a larger study was required to deter-mine whether the moderate increase of PIVKA-II carried any risk of bleeding. Although protection in the short term may be afforded by oral vitamin K, the efficacy of a single dose against late-onset HDN must be questioned. It has been suggested that intestinal malabsorption plays a role, and breast-fed infants who develop diarrhoea and in-fants who receive antibiotic therapy are at particu-lar risk of vitamin K deficiency. The American Academy of Pediatrics (Barness 1979) states:

'Breast-fed infants who develop diarrhoea of longer than several days duration should be given one intramuscular injection of vitamin K (1.0 mg). Infants at continued risk of vitamin K deficiency (e.g. malabsorption, biliary atresia) should be given supplements of vitamin K at regular intervals.'

Treatment

1. In the face of life-threatening haemorrhage, vitamin K-dependent factors can immediately be raised by giving FFP 10–15 ml/kg. Otherwise, 1 mg of vitamin K_1 will correct any degree of vitamin K deficiency in the neonate. After pa-renteral administration, correction will occur within a few hours. Vitamin K_1 is a safe drug without side-effects. Only vitamin K_3 (Synkavit) given parenterally has been associated with hae-molytic anaemia and kernicterus.

2. All neonates should receive vitamin K pro-phylaxis as soon after birth as possible. Oral vita-min K appears to prevent classic HDN, but its efficacy in the prevention of late HDN is less well established. In contrast, late HDN is extremely rare in infants who have received parenteral vita-min K at birth; so at present, the best proven prophylaxis is vitamin K 0.5–1 mg parenterally, although this may change with increasing knowl-edge of optimal oral therapy. The parenteral route should always be used for prophylaxis for the following categories of infants:

a. infants of mothers on anticonvulsant therapy
b. premature infants
c. infants admitted to a special care baby unit
d. babies born by traumatic delivery.

The optimal oral dose of vitamin K has not been clearly established. Dosages which are recom-mended range from 1 mg of vitamin K (Tripp &

McNinch 1987) to 5 mg of vitamin K (Hathaway & Bonnar, 1987). The average dose recommended is 1–2 mg.

3. The guidelines of the American Academy of Pediatrics should be followed for breast-fed infants who develop prolonged diarrhoea and for infants at continued risk because of underlying pathology. In the latter group, the interval of optimal supplementation will depend on the route of administration chosen. Several recent reviews of this topic are recommended (von Kries 1988, Hathaway 1987, Shearer 1990, Lane 1985).

Vitamin K deficiency in older children

In older children, the commonest cause of vitamin K deficiency is malabsorption due to coeliac disease, ulcerative colitis, Crohn's disease, cystic fibrosis, biliary atresia, obstructive jaundice, etc. As many as 30% of individuals with chronic gas-trointestinal disease may be vitamin K deficient (Krasinski et al 1985). Although the vitamin-K-dependent-procoagulants may be low, clinical bleeding is rare. However, any child with a sus-pected underlying disorder which might predispose to vitamin K deficiency, and who is to undergo a diagnostic jejunal biopsy or liver biopsy, should have a coagulation screen performed and any abnormality corrected before the procedure. Vitamin K deficiency is also seen in critically ill children with an inadequate diet or in those on unsupplemented parenteral nutrition, particularly if they are also receiving broad-spectrum anti-biotic therapy. Hepatic dysfunction and renal insufficiency are said to accentuate the problem by impeding excretion and impairing metabolism of antibiotics. Children with any underlying condition which could predispose to vitamin K deficiency, whether transient or life-long, should receive appropriate vitamin K prophylactically given parenterally at a dose of 5 mg.

Neonatal intraventricular haemorrhage (IVH)

Intraventricular haemorrhage remains a major cause of morbidity and mortality in premature and low-birth-weight infants, despite a dramatic improvement in their overall survival. The inci-dence has been variably reported to be between 30 and 40% (Volpe 1981, Tarby & Volpe 1982, Beverley et al 1984, McDonald et al 1984).

Intracranial haemorrhage is the commonest manifestation of late-onset haemorrhagic disease of the newborn. As previously emphasized, these infants are almost invariably breast fed and many will not have received vitamin K prophylaxis at birth. Chaou reported late-onset intracranial haemorrhage related to vitamin K deficiency in 32 breast-fed infants, 31 of whom had not received prophylactic vitamin K (Chaou et al 1984). The one infant who had received prophylaxis had Hirshsprung's disease and presented with intracranial haemorrhage at 5 months of age. In each case, the intracranial haemorrhage was proven by CT scanning. The mortality in the series was 9.4%. Lesko reported a 4-fold increase in the risk of intraventricular haemorrhage in low-birth-weight infants receiving low-dose heparin to maintain the patency of vascular catheters (Lesko et al 1986). The association did not extend to the severity of the haemorrhage, dose of heparin or method of administration. Other investigators have similarly reported an association between intraventricular haemorrhage and the use of low-dose heparin to prolong catheter patency, but it must be appreciated that it is the low-birth-weight infant, at the highest risk of intraventricular haemorrhage, who is most likely to require an indwelling catheter for venous access and monitoring.

Intraventricular haemorrhage predominantly affects premature infants of low birth weight. The role of a coagulopathy or physiological immaturity of the preterm's coagulation system remains controversial. Attempts have been made to evaluate this by correcting abnormal coagulation parameters. Beverley reported on 73 premature infants of less than 32 weeks' gestation or less than 1500 g body weight recruited to a prospective controlled trial (Beverley et al 1985). All infants were given vitamin K_1 prophylaxis at birth. The newborns were randomized to receive FFP (10 ml/kg) on admission and at 24 hours of age, or to act as controls and receive no treatment. There was no difference in coagulation parameters (PT, APTT, fibrinogen, FDPs, platelet count) on admission and at 48 hours of age between the treatment and control groups. Fifteen of 37 (41%) control infants sustained an IVH, compared with 5 of 36 (14%)

infants who received FFP; all were diagnosed ultrasonically. FFP therefore appeared to reduce the incidence of IVH, although there was no noticeable effect on mortality and the improvement in the coagulation parameters was short-lived. The authors questioned whether FFP may exert its effect by stabilizing the blood pressure and maintaining cerebral blood flow rather than by improving coagulation. However, the number of babies in their study with an unstable intra-arterial blood pressure tracing was the same in both groups.

Turner made similar observations (Turner et al 1981). He looked at the effect of correcting coagulation parameters on the incidence of IVH in infants of less than 1500 g body weight and 34 weeks' gestation, premature infants with respiratory distress syndrome, and mature infants with asphyxia. Replacement therapy was given to completely correct any coagulation abnormality and maintain correction. Those allocated to the treatment group received either prothrombin complex concentrate, cryoprecipitate or platelet concentration, as appropriate. All infants received vitamin K_1. IVH was not observed in infants who maintained normal haemostasis, (i.e. who did not have abnormal coagulation parameters by the investigators' criteria (PT greater than 28 s, fibrinogen less than 1 g/l, platelet count below 100×10^9/l). Replacement therapy did reduce the incidence of IVH to some extent in the others, but this was not statistically significant and did not result in any improvement in mortality or morbidity.

Vitamin E, which protects endothelial cell membranes from oxidative damage, has been reported to have a protective effect against IVH (Sinha et al 1987, Spear et al 1984). Other studies have shown conflicting results (Phelps 1984). Sinha reported on infants of less than 32 weeks' gestation enrolled into a randomized, controlled trial to assess the efficacy of vitamin E in the prevention of IVH. He found that 210 supplemented babies without haemorrhage on entry to the trial had a lower incidence of IVH than did controls (8.8% v 34.3%), and a lower frequency of combined intraventricular and parenchymal haemorrhage (10.8% v 40.7%), as determined ultrasonically. Vitamin E did not affect mortality, but hopefully reduced neurodevelopmental handicap, due to the lower incidence of combined haemorrhage in surviving supplemented babies. Haemorrhage originates in the subepenchymal region, where it may be confined or rupture into the ventricles or brain parenchyma. Vitamin E did not prevent subepenchymal haemorrhage but appeared to limit its extent. The authors suggest that vitamin E works by scavenging free radicals generated during ischaemic injury of the subepenchymal region and thereby limits tissue damage and the extent of periventricular haemorrhage on reperfusion. Similar results have been reported for ethamsylate (Benson et al 1986).

In 330 infants without evidence of periventricular haemorrhage on entry into the trial, there was little difference between ethamsylate and placebo groups with respect to subepenchymal haemorrhage; however intraventricular and parenchymal haemorrhages developed in 30 of 162 infants (18.5%) in the treated group, compared with 50 of 168 (29.8%) in the control group. The incidence of intraventricular and parenchymal haemorrhage in survivors was 20 of 137 (14.6%) in the ethamsylate group and 37 of 146 (25.3%) in the controls. Ethamsylate treatment limited parenchymal extension but had no effect on mortality. Ethamsylate may reduce capillary bleeding by modifying prostaglandin synthesis although its exact mode of action is unclear. The end result is probably not too dissimilar from the antioxidant action of vitamin E, which reduces the peroxidation of lipids which are the precursors of prostanoids. The precise role of the neonate's hypocoagulable state in the pathogenesis of IVH has not been properly defined, and although coagulation factor replacement appears to reduce the incidence, the means by which this is achieved is unclear, as a measurable improvement in coagulation parameters has not been a consistent finding. However, replacement therapy may act by preventing haemorrhagic extension of an initial ischaemic lesion, a role not dissimilar from that of vitamin E and ethamsylate.

It is therefore appropriate to correct any coagulation abnormalities which are defined as soon as possible. Further controlled studies are required to assess the different therapies available.

Congenital heart disease

Mild-to-moderate thrombocytopenia and impaired platelet function are relatively common in cyanotic heart disease, and some patients show evidence of hyperfibrinolysis (see also Ch. 6). Bleeding is rarely a problem except perhaps at the time of surgery. Minor coagulation abnormalities in keeping with a consumptive coagulopathy have been reported in groups of children with both cyanotic and acyanotic heart disease, but results have been conflicting. The coagulation abnormalities have generally correlated with the degree of polycythaemia, suggesting an in-vitro artefact, although improvement with both heparinization and venesection have been reported. Polycythaemic patients have an elevated haematocrit and decreased plasma volume. If blood from a polycythaemic patient with a haematocrit above 50% is taken into a standard volume of citrate, more anticoagulant per volume of plasma will be present and the clotting tests artefactually prolonged. The volume of citrate should always be adjusted when the haematocrit is greater than 55%. However, hyperviscosity may lead to tissue hypoxia, which could trigger a consumptive process. Some children with acyanotic congenital cardiac lesions may have an acquired abnormality of vWF that is normalized with correction of the abnormal haemodynamic state (Gill et al 1986). Twelve children in a consecutive series with acyanotic congenital cardiac defects were shown to have less of the largest plasma vWF multimers. All had normal or borderline-normal FVIII procoagulant concentrations, and none had laboratory evidence of DIC. Seven had previous histories of mucocutaneous haemorrhage; 10 had a prolonged bleeding time. Four of 5 children restudied after surgical correction of their cardiac lesions had normalization of their vWF multimers, and a fifth child, whose vWF was abnormal postoperatively, had a residual pressure gradient across a previous pulmonary artery banding site. The parents of three of the patients studied did not show multimeric abnormalities (Gill et al 1986).

Cardiac surgical procedures, employing cardiopulmonary bypass, are often complicated by both intraoperative and postoperative haemorrhage. Haemorrhage is more likely to complicate lengthy pump runs, surgery for cyanotic heart disease and surgery in patients with a prior haemostatic defect. Bleeding may be due to:

1. thrombocytopenia or platelet dysfunction
2. primary fibrinolysis
3. incomplete neutralization of heparin by protamine sulphate
4. DIC
5. reduced clotting factors secondary to dilution
6. surgical technique.

Platelet abnormalities and hyperfibrin(ogen) lysis are the commonest sources of problems. Care must be taken to ensure that blood taken for platelet or coagulation studies is free of heparin contamination. Management should be individualized and directed at the likely underlying problem. Treatment is generally directed towards correction of the haemostatic defect with blood product support which may be with platelets, FFP or cryoprecipitate. Protamine sulphate will correct any bleeding secondary to overheparinization. Although hyperfibrinolysis complicates cardiopulmonary bypass, it is short-lived. Antifibrinolytic therapy has had some success in controlling bleeding when blood component therapy has failed, but should only be considered in documented cases of hyperfibrinolysis. The risks of using a fibrinolytic inhibitor in patients with a hypercoagulable state should be carefully quantitated. Desmopressin (DDAVP) has been reported to reduce blood loss during and after cardiopulmonary bypass; the reduction appears most marked in patients with a relatively low concentration of vWF preoperatively. The beneficial effect of DDAVP on haemostasis following cardiopulmonary bypass is more likely to be related to an increase in overall vWF concentration than to an increase in the percentage of vWF HMW multimers specifically (Weinstein et al 1988).

Renal disease

Renal disease can be complicated by both haemorrhagic and thrombotic problems. In patients with uraemia, haemostatic defects responsible for bleeding are still poorly understood. Patients with chronic renal failure have been reported to have a quantitative defect of platelet vWF and a reduction or absence of the largest plasma vWF multimers; the latter abnormality is thought to be responsible for abnormal ristocetin-induced platelet aggregation (Gralnick et al 1988). These defects may play a role in both the prolonged bleeding time and clinical bleeding observed in uraemic patients, and this would be in keeping with the observation that cryoprecipitate and DDAVP infusions have a beneficial effect on the bleeding time in uraemia.

Children with nephrotic syndrome usually have increased levels of fibrinogen and FVIII but reduced plasma concentrations of factors IX, XII, plasminogen and ATIII (Elidrissy & Gader 1985), due to excessive urinary loss. FIX rarely falls below 10% and bleeding is unusual, although in children with heavy proteinuria it is worth checking the level of FIX before renal biopsy or major surgical procedures. Low levels of FXII are not clinically important, because deficiency of this factor is not associated with a bleeding diathesis.

Thromboembolic phenomena complicate renal disease. Urinary loss of naturally occurring inhibitors may play a role. A number of investigators have reported low protein C anticoagulant activity in uraemic patients with both acute and chronic renal failure (Sørensen et al 1987, 1988, 1989). The cause of the decreased protein C activity in uraemia remains unclear. Changes in protein C anticoagulant activity are closely related to fluctuations in renal function, with a significant increase in protein C activity occurring during haemodialysis.

Thrombotic microangiopathies

Haemolytic uraemic syndrome (HUS) is characterized by acute renal failure, microangiopathic haemolytic anaemia and thrombocytopenia (see also Ch. 6). Young children are predominantly affected, with the majority being less than two years of age. The syndrome is usually preceded by a prodromal febrile illness, usually gastrointestinal. Bloody diarrhoea is common, and about one-third of children will have bleeding from the skin, mucous membranes and urinary tract. HUS is believed to result from renal vascular endothelial injury caused by a bacterial or viral illness. Platelet aggregates and fibrin thrombi are deposited in the microvasculature of the glomeruli. The platelet count is reduced during the course of the disorder, with over half of the children having moderate-to-severe thrombocytopenia. Coagulation studies have shown conflicting results, but there is no direct evidence that DIC has a role in the pathogenesis of HUS. HUS may be a heterogenous entity, and possible pathogenic mechanisms include endothelial injury and abnormal endothelial platelet interaction in the renal microvasculature, and prostacyclin deficiency.

Thrombotic thrombocytopenic purpura (TTP) may represent a different clinical expression of the same disease affecting adults, particularly females, although children have been described. Neurological manifestations, which are often fluctuating, are more frequent than in HUS. The thrombocytopenia tends to be more marked and the bleeding manifestations greater. Platelet aggregates and fibrin thrombi are found in the microvasculature of multiple organs. There is no direct evidence of DIC. However, quantitative and qualitative abnormalities of plasma vWF have been reported in patients with TTP and HUS. Both high plasma levels of vWF, particularly during acute disease, and abnormalities of the multimeric structure of the protein have been described. These aberrations of multimeric structure include the appearance in plasma of abnormally large vWF multimers during remission of the chronic relapsing form of TTP (Moake et al 1982) and loss of the larger forms of normal vWF multimers during acute exacerbations of TTP/HUS (Murphy et al 1987). A platelet aggregating factor has also been described, which has been demonstrated to have a consistent relationship with vWF (Murphy et al 1987). During acute exacerbations, the platelet aggregating factor is detected in the patient's serum in association with loss of the larger multimers of vWF (Murphy et al 1987). This platelet aggregating factor, plus large multimers of vWF, may participate in the pathogenesis of TTP/HUS.

With supportive care and renal dialysis, if necessary, the mortality for HUS is low. Plasma exchange and/or plasma infusions have improved the survival rates for TTP, although this remains a serious disorder.

THROMBOSIS

The peak incidence of thrombosis in the paediatric age group is in the neonatal period (Table 13.11), when it is most frequently iatrogenic and associated with indwelling catheters, although not exclusively so. The reviews referenced in Table 13.11 illustrate the increased incidence of spontaneous thrombosis in the first month of life. Thrombosis in the absence of a catheter usually occurs in sick, and often premature, infants with many underlying problems, which in themselves predispose to thrombosis, including sepsis, asphyxia, RDS, dehydration and shock. Any of these associations may result in damage to the endothelium and subsequent activation of the coagulation system and fibrin deposition. Because the pathogenesis of neonatal thrombosis is different

Table 13.11   Thrombotic disease in paediatric age groups: peak incidence in the newborn period and early infancy

Entity	Study design	Reference	Age at diagnosis (%)		
			< 1 month	1 month–1 year	> 1 year
Renal venous thrombosis	a. Literature review of case reports (n = 95)	Kaufman 1958	62%	20%	19%
	b. Clinicopathological survey (n = 113)	Arneil 1973	74%	19%	7%
Pulmonary embolism (no intravascular catheters)	Pathological survey (n = 25)	Emery 1962	20%	52%	28%
Severe arterial thrombosis and embolism in the systemic circulation (no intravascular catheters)	Literature review of case reports (n = 47)	Gross 1945	94%	4%	2%

Adapted from Schmidt & Zipursky 1984, with permission of W B Saunders Co.

from that of older children, the two groups will be considered independently.

Neonatal thrombosis

The triad of factors, first proposed by Virchow, which predispose to thrombosis are:

1. abnormalities of the vessel wall
2. disturbances of blood flow
3. changes in blood coagulability.

Abnormalities of the vessel wall

All intra-arterial and intravenous catheters carry a risk of thrombosis. Indwelling catheters induce thrombosis for a number of reasons. Most importantly, the foreign surface has thrombogenic properties and is a nidus for thrombus formation. Furthermore, the catheter damages the endothelium of the vessel wall predisposing to thrombus formation. Additional contributing factors include mechanical occlusion, vasospasm and alterations in blood flow. Catheter-associated thromboembolism has been reported in association with radial, pulmonary, temporal and femoral arterial lines, as well as with central venous catheters inserted into the jugular and femoral veins. However, in the neonate, umbilical catheters are associated with the majority of catheter-related thrombosis, because of their popularity.

The incidence of umbilical artery catheter-related thrombosis varies widely between studies and is mainly dependent on the criteria employed for diagnosis. Although symptomatic, thrombosis with vessel obstruction is relatively unusual (approximately 1%; O'Neill et al 1981), clinically silent thrombi encasing the catheter are much more common. Autopsy evidence suggests an incidence of thrombosis associated with umbilical artery catheterization as high as 59% (Tyson et al 1976), and angiography has detected thrombi in 20–95% of patients (Neal et al 1972, Goetzman et al 1975). Catheterization of the umbilical vein is also associated with thrombotic lesions but the incidence is unclear. Two factors strongly correlate with the risk of thrombosis at this site: firstly, the incorrect placement of the catheter tip in the portal or hepatic vein; and secondly, the infusion of hyperosmolar solutions. Infants of low birth weight or early gestation, and sick infants appear to be particularly susceptible to catheter-related thrombotic episodes, and are, of course, those infants most likely to be catheterized.

The sequelae of catheter-related arterial thrombosis include renal hypertension, necrotizing enterocolitis, paraplegia, peripheral gangrene, organ infarction and death. Follow-up studies of clinically silent, radiologically diagnosed thrombosis have been limited but have not revealed significant sequelae. Even symptomatic neonates with aortic thrombosis and renovascular hypertension may have a favourable outcome (Caplan et al 1989). Four of 29 patients died in the neonatal period from complications associated with aortic thrombosis. Of 15 children available for follow up, most had normal blood pressure, calculated glomerular filtration rates, urinalyses and plasma renin activities, and also quantitative improvement in their renal blood flow demonstrated by radionuclide renography, at a mean follow up of 26 months. A similar outcome was reported for 12 patients with major aortic thrombus formation in the neonatal period; in two patients, the event occurred antenatally, and four patients had evidence of thrombosis before or without umbilical artery catheterization (Payne et al 1989). Hypertension, oliguria, haematuria and an elevated blood creatinine concentration were present at the time of diagnosis. Seven patients who were haemodynamically stable received supportive care only, and five patients with congestive cardiac failure, shock or both underwent surgical thrombectomy. The five surgically treated patients and six of seven medically treated patients survived. Ultrasound examinations suggested resolution of the thrombus in all survivors in 6–30 days. Sequelae from thrombus formation were present in all patients at the time of discharge, and included hypertension in nine of the 11 survivors and decreased renal function in six of them. Follow-up at 1–3 years revealed normal blood pressure, good growth, and good renal function in 10 of the survivors.

Worthy of special mention is the high incidence of renal vessel thrombosis in the neonatal period. About 70% of cases of renal vein thrombosis have been reported in infants of less than one month of age, and can even be an antenatal event. The small calibre of the renal vessels and the low renal blood flow in the perinatal period are thought to be contributing factors. Haematuria or enlarged kidneys should always alert the physician to the possibility of renal vein thrombosis. Over 90% of cases of hypertension in the neonate are associated with renal vascular disease.

The use of low-dose heparin appears to prolong catheter patency, but does not seem to reduce the incidence of catheter-related thrombosis. Horgan reported the effect of low-dose heparin on the incidence of large vessel thrombosis and serious thrombotic complications in 111 consecutive infants requiring umbilical artery catheterization (Horgan et al 1987). Fifty nine infants were randomized to receive prophylactic heparin, and 52 infants served as controls. The mean dose of heparin was 0.9 U/kg per hour (range 0.46–3.4 U/kg per hour). The number of thrombotic episodes in the two groups were not significantly different – 16 in the heparin group and 18 in the control group. Aortic thrombosis was documented by ultrasonography in 30 infants, by autopsy in two infants, and by clinical criteria in two infants. Twenty four of the 30 infants diagnosed radiologically had sleeve clots and 6 had bulky intraluminal and mural thrombi. Only nine infants (26.4%) with thrombosis were symptomatic, which infers a high incidence of occult thrombus formation. There was no correlation between the length of time that the umbilical arterial catheter (UAC) was in situ and the development of large vessel thrombus. Although low-dose heparin did not appear to reduce the incidence of catheter-related thrombus formation, the number of clotted and nonfunctional umbilical catheters was reduced (10 of 52 in the control group, compared with 2 of 59 in the heparin group). However, the addition of low doses of heparin to UACs did appear to have an effect on thrombotic complications, as the incidence of hypertension, a serious UAC-associated thrombotic complication, was lower in the heparin group (0 of 16, compared with 9 of 18 infants with aortic thrombi). From the available data, it would appear that continuous infusions of low-dose heparin or heparin 'flushes' do little to prevent catheter-related thrombosis, although these measures do prolong catheter patency. Catheters constructed of polyurethane with heparin bonded to the surface may be less

thrombogenic than catheters made of polyvinyl chloride (PVC), but in randomized trials they have not consistently reduced the incidence of UAC-associated thrombus (Jackson et al 1987).

Disturbances of blood flow

In newborns, as in adults, there is a strong correlation between blood viscosity and haematocrit. Submaximal limb blood flow, as measured by strain-gauge plethysmography, decreases in polycythaemic newborns with increasing haematocrit (Bergquist & Zetterstrom 1975). There appears to be a consistent relationship between viscosity and haematocrit within the normal range, but at the relatively high haematocrit values found in the newborn infant, a small rise in the packed cell volume (above or around 70%) produces a considerable rise in blood viscosity. True polycythaemia and dehydration both result in an elevated haematocrit. Additionally, the red cell diameter is important for platelet adherence and the larger diameter of neonatal red blood cells is associated with significantly increased platelet adherence (Piet et al 1983).

Changes in blood coagulation

Any imbalance between the activators and inhibitors of either the coagulation or fibrinolytic mechanisms may predispose towards thrombosis. Hereditary protein C, protein S and antithrombin III (ATIII) deficiency has already been discussed (pp 404–407). There is no real evidence that the physiological reduction of natural anticoagulants in the neonate contributes to thrombosis in the well infant. The lupus anticoagulant, an antiphospholipid antibody, is associated clinically with thrombosis. It is an IgG immunoglobulin and, as such, capable of placental transfer. A preterm infant, born to an affected mother, has been reported with detectable circulating lupus anticoagulant in the plasma, and aortic thrombosis. The infant was preterm, had fetal distress and underwent umbilical vessel instrumentation, all of which are independently associated with thrombosis (Sheridan-Pereira et al 1988).

Treatment of thrombosis in the neonate

In the absence of an obvious identifiable cause

for thrombosis, a congenital deficiency of one of the natural anticoagulants should be considered. Thrombosis should be confirmed by appropriate investigation. If a catheter is in situ it should be removed, but first it may provide a route for radiological confirmation, although ultrasonography is the most popular diagnostic tool at present. The treatment of thrombosis in the neonate is still very controversial. In general, clinically silent thrombosis is not usually treated. Heparin therapy, thrombolytic drugs and surgery have all been employed therapeutically for clinically obvious thrombi. Controlled, multicentre studies with large numbers of patients are required to evaluate the best methods of diagnosis and treatment of neonatal aortic thrombosis (Schmidt & Andrew 1988).

Heparin. Heparin is a prophylactic drug and is used in the primary prevention of thrombosis and thrombus extension. It has a role in prolonging catheter patency and in mild-to-moderate vessel occlusion, but where major vessel obstruction exists, surgery or thrombolytic agents are indicated. The role of heparin is therefore limited. Heparin acts by enhancing ATIII, the major inhibitor of thrombin. The neonate may require a greater amount of heparin than an adult in order to achieve a therapeutic effect because of the low level of ATIII. The initial loading dose required is 50 U/kg. Continuous infusion is the optimal route of administration, beginning with a dose of 20 U/kg per hour for small preterm infants, and 25 U/kg per hour for infants weighing more than 1500 g (McDonald & Hathaway 1982). The monitoring of heparin in the neonate is complicated by their low levels of prothrombin and ATIII; this is particularly so in the preterm infant. Assays dependent upon the endogenous generation of thrombin from prothrombin (APTT) overestimates the amount of heparin circulating in the newborn, because of excess ATIII compared with prothrombin and a decreased ability of neonatal plasma to generate thrombin. In contrast, assays that are based on enhancement of ATIII and subsequent inhibition of exogenous thrombin or FXa will underestimate the amount of heparin in the newborn plasma because of low ATIII levels (Andrew & Schmidt 1988). However, despite this, APTT or heparin assays are most appropriately used for monitoring heparin and avoiding haemorrhagic complication. If the APTT is used, it must incorporate an activating reagent which shortens the newborn APTT to close to the adult control, thereby making the APTT a useful test. A modified PTT incorporating contact product has been suggested as an alternative approach (Andrew & Karpatkin 1982). McDonald recommends the use of the Laidlaw micro whole blood clotting time (McDonald & Hathaway 1982). Low-molecular-weight heparin may be associated with less bleeding problems, and may be particularly indicated in sick preterm newborns with immature coagulation systems who are at particular risk of haemorrhage.

Thrombolytic therapy. Thrombolytic therapy may have a role to play in the treatment of major thrombosis associated with impaired arterial blood flow, especially where surgery is technically difficult and potentially life-threatening. Urokinase is considered the thrombolytic agent of choice in the newborn. Fibrinolytic agents work by converting endogenous plasminogen to plasmin, and the effect may be modified by reduced levels of plasminogen in the newborn, which are approximately 50% of adult values. Again, as with ATIII, plasminogen levels are lowest in the preterm infant, who is the infant most likely to require treatment. Urokinase activates plasminogen directly and, unlike streptokinase, does not require to form a complex with plasminogen to exert its effect. Urokinase is preferable to streptokinase for use in the newborn, as it has a linear dose-effect (Montgomery et al 1985), and is non-antigenic. Thrombolytic agents will lyse all clots, not just those causing vascular occlusion, and cannot be used within 10 days of surgery or if the infant has a pre-existing bleeding problem. This poses a problem for the preterm infant with an immature coagulation system and an increased risk of IVH. A loading dose of 4400 U/kg is given intravenously followed by a continuous infusion of 4400 U/kg per hour (Montgomery et al 1985). This will produce a fall in fibrinogen, and significant levels of FDPs. Some workers advocate the concurrent infusion of FFP to provide plasminogen substrate and natural anticoagulants. Equally controversial is the simultaneous use of heparin. Thrombolytic agents are not given without risk and require careful monitoring. Suggested assays for monitoring include the fibrinogen level, FDPs and euglobulin lysis time.

Warfarin. Oral anticoagulants have little place in the treatment of neonatal thrombotic disease, with the possible exception of homozygous protein C deficiency. In adults, coumarins are not indicated in the immediate treatment of an acute thrombotic episode, but are used later to prevent recurrence. There is no evidence that thrombotic episodes in the neonatal period have a high risk of recurrence.

Surgery. Surgical intervention is indicated for the management of major arterial thrombosis, when occlusion is total. In the adult, surgery is usually the chosen mode of treatment of occlusive vascular disease, because of the high chance of rethrombosis of an atheromatous vessel wall without endarterectomy. This situation is not seen in the neonatal period, and the small calibre of the neonate's vessels reduces the chance of a successful outcome. The role of surgery is therefore limited in this age group, and thrombolytic agents may have a greater part to play than in adults.

Thrombosis beyond the newborn period

After the newborn period, the incidence of thromboembolic disease falls sharply until the second decade of life, when it begins an upward trend to become the major health problem of adult life. In children, a number of inherited and acquired disorders are associated with thrombotic events, but both the natural history and treatment are poorly defined in this age group. Both diagnostic and therapeutic approaches have been adapted from those of the adult and neither have been evaluated properly in children. Arterial thrombosis usually results from endothelial damage and platelet plug formation, whilst venous thrombosis occurs in areas of venous stasis in association with hypercoagulability of the blood and/or endothelial damage.

Inherited conditions predisposing to venous thrombosis have already been discussed (pp 404–407). Thromboembolic problems do not usually occur until the second or third decade of life, and the first event often develops in connection with a precipitating factor, e.g. surgery, pregnancy or after infections. Arterial thrombosis is very rare in association with heterozygous deficiency of any of the natural anticoagulants. Table 13.12 lists the many acquired disorders which may be associated with thrombosis in children. Vessel wall injury is particularly common following venepuncture, the insertion of indwelling catheters, ventriculoatrial shunts, central venous pressure Swan-Ganz catheters, etc. In children with nephrotic syndrome, urinary loss of the natural anticoagulants (ATIII and protein C) predisposes to thrombosis, mainly venous. The use of L-asparaginase in the treatment of acute lymphoblastic leukaemia has been

Table 13.12 Causes of acquired thrombosis and thromboembolic disease in childhood and adolesence*

Venous thrombosis	*Arterial thrombosis*
Dehydration	Vascular injury
Shock	Trauma
Infant of a diabetic	Vascular disease
mother	Infections
Neonatal asphyxia	Takayasu's disease
Vascular injury	Periarteritis nodosa
Oral contraceptives	Systemic lupus
(oestrogen-containing)	erythematosus
Pregnancy; puerperium;	Shock
abortion	Thrombotic
Nephrotic syndrome	thrombocytopenic purpura
Cyanotic congenital heart	Haemolytic-uremic
disease	syndrome
Infections	Nephrotic syndrome
Sickle cell disease	Moyamoya syndrome
Systemic lupus	Cardiac disease
erythematosus	Cardiac prosthesis
L-asparaginase	Kawasaki's disease
Epsilon-aminocaproic acid;	Primary endocardial
Tranexamic acid	fibroelastosis
Prothrombin complex	Enlarged left atrium with
concentrates	atrial fibrillation
Paroxysmal nocturnal	Hypereosinophilic syndrome
hemoglobinuria	Cyanotic congenital heart
Cancer	disease
Liver disease	Drugs
Behçet's syndrome	Epsilon-aminocaproic acid,
Spontaneous	Tranexamic acid
	Prothrombin complex
	concentrates
	Idiopathic
	Aortic thrombosis in the
	neonate
	Neonatal nonbacterial
	thrombotic endocarditis
	Disseminated intravascular
	and cardiac thrombosis
	of the neonate

*List does not include disseminated intravascular coagulation syndromes.
From Corrigan 1985, with permission of Churchill Livingstone

associated with venous thrombosis, secondary to reduced hepatic synthesis of ATIII, protein C and plasminogen. Other workers have suggested that the thrombosis is related to a qualitative abnormality of the vWF (Pui et al 1985). The common use of Hickman central venous catheters in patients with leukaemia may aggravate this problem (Kucuk et al 1985). Hyperviscosity states, such as are seen in children with cyanotic heart disease and a high haematocrit, or children with high white cell count leukaemia, are associated with an increased risk of venous thrombosis. Vasculitic disorders are particularly associated with arterial thrombosis. Mechanical cardiac prosthesies are well-recognized causes of thromboembolic disease, but any cardiac disease characterized by mural thrombus may result in embolic complications. Femoral arterial thrombosis is a known complication of cardiac catheterization in infants and children.

Treatment of thromboembolic disease

The treatment of thromboembolic disease is aimed at either removing existing thrombus or embolus, or preventing thrombus extension or development. Thrombus can be removed surgically (thrombectomy, embolectomy) or medically (thrombolytic agent). Anticoagulants are used to inhibit the formation and propagation of a thrombus.

Heparin. The mode of action of heparin has already been discussed. Heparin is best given by continuous infusion. A bolus dose of 50–75 U/kg is followed by a continuous infusion at 15–25 U/kg per hour (Corrigan 1985). Heparin therapy may be monitored by a heparin assay or APTT, which is the simplest and most commonly used method. The APTT should be maintained at 1.5–2 times the patient's pre-heparin control. Because of varying degrees of sensitivity to heparin in the different commercially available coagulation reagents, it is strongly suggested that each laboratory determine its own therapeutic range for this drug. The main side-effect of heparin is bleeding. Heparin can be neutralized almost immediately by protamine sulphate. However, because of the rapid clearance rate of heparin, most cases can be handled by the cessation of the infusion. Contraindications to the use of heparin include pre-existing coagulation defects or bleeding diathesis, recent CNS haemorrhage, malignant hypertension and recent surgery of the brain or spinal cord. The duration of heparin therapy varies considerably, ranging from 5–10 days, with treatment for PE being given for longer than for DVT.

Coumarin derivatives. Warfarin is the most common oral anticoagulant used, and acts by inhibiting vitamin K-dependent carboxylation of the precursor proteins of factors II, VII, IX and X. Following the administration of warfarin, the levels of the vitamin K-dependent coagulation factors decrease gradually according to the half-life of each clotting factor. There are few guidelines for the use of anticoagulants in children. An initial dose of 0.1 mg/kg per day (not to exceed 10 mg) has been recommended, with dose adjustments made according to the PT or INR (Corrigan 1985). Maintenance doses may range from 1–10 mg/day, and the optimal INR differs for various thrombotic states. As with heparin, the duration of warfarin therapy varies considerably, ranging from 3 weeks to 6 months, again with treatment for PE often being longer than for DVT. In general, the trend is towards shorter duration of anticoagulation in patients without underlying risk factors (Fennerty et al 1987). Warfarin is usually started from the third day of heparin so that it is therapeutically effective before heparin is discontinued.

Haemorrhage is the main complication of warfarin therapy. Many drugs affect the metabolism of warfarin and their addition or subtraction can increase the drug's therapeutic effect. If bleeding develops, the drug should be discontinued and vitamin K given. FFP (10–15 ml/kg) will raise the vitamin-K-dependent factors to haemostatic levels. Hereditary warfarin resistance is recognized but exceedingly rare (Alving et al 1985, Warrier et al 1986).

Warfarin necrosis is an interesting and well-recognized complication which usually occurs between days 2 and 5 after starting warfarin therapy. When warfarin is given, protein C levels fall more rapidly than those of factors II and X, and this relative deficiency of protein C results in a hypercoagulable state. This transitory state is catered for by the common practice of overlapping heparin and warfarin therapy for 5–6 days.

Warfarin crosses the placenta, producing characteristic features in the fetus of stippled epiphyses, punctuate calcifications, saddle nose deformities and other bone abnormalities. Warfarin embryopathy is not as common as was once thought and is usually seen when warfarin has been taken in the first trimester of pregnancy. Even if warfarin is maintained well within the therapeutic range in the mother, the neonate's vitamin-K-dependent procoagulants may be dangerously depressed because of the pre-existing physiological depression, and fetal haemorrhage is a real risk. A young boy has been reported with features identical to those of warfarin embryopathy and an inborn deficiency of vitamin K epoxide reductase (Pauli et al 1987).

Thrombolytic therapy. Both streptokinase and urokinase have been used for occlusive events in children. The mode of action has already been explained. The most common complication of thrombolytic therapy is bleeding, which usually stops if the infusion is discontinued, when the lytic activity ceases promptly. Thrombolytic agents are most likely to be of benefit when plasminogen levels are adequate, the clot is young and small and the vessel is not totally occluded, allowing access to the clot. All fibrin clots are susceptible to lysis. Contraindications include major surgery, organ biopsy, recent serious trauma, invasive procedures, uncorrected haemostatic defects and active internal or CNS bleeding. Lysis of a cardiac mural thrombus may result in embolization. Laboratory tests should show an increase in FDPs (more than 40 µg/ml), moderate change in the TCT (2–5 times the normal control) and fibrinogen assay of around 1 g/L.

Femoral artery thrombosis is a frequent complication after cardiac catheterization. In a prospective study, 45 of 526 (8.6%) consecutive infants and children had a decreased or absent pulse after catheterization. Thirty-two of these 45 patients (71.1%) improved with systemic heparinization only. Thirteen patients (28.9%) had a persistently absent pedal pulse suggesting femoral artery thrombosis, despite continuous heparinization. Eleven patients were successfully treated with thrombolytic therapy, and two required surgical thrombectomy. There were no serious complications, although four patients bled from the groin entry site. Systemic thrombolytic therapy compared well with surgical results (Ino et al 1988).

Acquired inhibitors of coagulation

Inhibitors may be specific and directed against specific coagulation factors such as FVIII:C, or nonspecific and directed against reaction sites in the coagulation cascade. The lupus anticoagulant (LAC) is the commonest example of the latter type of inhibitor. It is an antiphospholipid antibody (IgG, IgM or both), which is directed against the phospholipid component of the prothrombin activator complex, (FXa, FV, phospholipid and Ca^{++}) blocking its generation by inhibiting Ca^{++} dependent binding of prothrombin to phosphatidylserine surfaces, and, to a lesser extent, factor X. The LAC occurs in a variety of autoimmune disorders, and in children often follows a viral illness. It is not associated with a bleeding tendency, but may be associated with an increased tendency to thrombosis. LAC prolongs the phospholipid-dependent coagulation tests (APTT and occasionally the PT). In the laboratory, it is suspected when the APTT is prolonged and not normalized by the addition of an equal part of normal plasma, as would happen with a deficiency of one of the coagulation factors. A number of laboratory tests are sensitive to LAC and distinguish it from other anticoagulants, especially those that are associated with bleeding.

REFERENCES

Ah Pin P J 1987 The use of intraligamental injections in haemophiliacs. British Dental Journal 162:151–52

AIDS group of the United Kingdom haemophilia centre directors with the co-operation of the United Kingdom haemophilia centre directors 1988 Prevalence of antibody to HIV in haemophiliacs in the United Kingdom: a second survey. Clinical and Laboratory Haematology 10: 187–91

Aledort L M, Levine P H, Hilgartner M et al 1985 A study of liver biopsies and liver disease among haemophiliacs. Blood 66(2): 367–372

Allain J P, Laurian Y, Paul D A et al 1987 Long-term evaluation of HIV antigen and antibodies to p24 and gp41 in patients with hemophilia. New England Journal of Medicine 317(18): 1114–1120

Alving B M, Strickler M P, Knight R D et al 1985 Hereditary warfarin resistance. Investigation of a rare phenomenon. Archives of Internal Medicine 145:499–501

Andersson T R, Bangstad H, Larsen M L 1988 Heparin cofactor II, antithrombin and protein C in plasma from term and preterm infants. Acta Paediatrica Scandinavica 77: 485–488

Andes W A, Wulff K, Smith W B 1984 Head trauma in hemophilia. A prospective study. Archives of Internal Medicine 144: 1981–1983

Andrew M, Karpatkin M 1982 A simple screening test for evaluating prolonged partial thromboplastin times in newborn infants. Journal of Pediatrics 101: 610–612

Andrew M, Paes B, Milner R et al 1987a Development of the human coagulation system in the full-term infant. Blood 70: 165–172

Andrew M, Castle V, Saigal S et al 1987b Clinical impact of neonatal thrombocytopenia. Journal of Pediatrics 110: 457–464

Andrew M, Paes B, Milner R et al 1988 Development of the human coagulation system in the healthy premature infant. Blood 72: 1651–1657

Andrew M, Schmidt B 1988 Use of heparin in newborn infants. Seminars in Thrombosis & Hemostasis 14(1): 28–32

Anson D S, Hock R A, Austen D et al 1987 Towards gene therapy for hemophilia B. Molecular Biology and Medicine 4: 11–20

Arneil G C, MacDonald A M, Murphy A V, Sweet E M 1973 Renal venous thrombosis. Clinical Nephrology 1(3): 119–131

Aronstam A 1987 AIDS advice to haemophiliacs. Lancet 8563: 861

Bachelet P, Osmond D, Chaisson R E et al 1988 Survival patterns of the first 500 patients with AIDS in San Francisco. Journal of Infectious Diseases 157(5): 1044–1047

Bahnak B R, Lavergne J-M, Verweij C L et al 1988 Carrier detection in severe (type III) von Willebrand disease using two intragenic restriction fragment length polymorphisms. Thrombosis and Haemostasis 60(2): 178–181

Ball L M, Harper J L 1987 Atopic eczema in HIV seropositive haemophiliacs. Lancet 8559: 627–628

Barnard D R, Simmons M A, Hathaway R E 1979 Coagulation studies in extremely premature infants. Pediatrics 13: 1330–1335

Barnard D 1984 Inherited bleeding disorders in the newborn infant. Clinics in Perinatology 11: 309–337

Barness L A 1979 Vitamins. In: Pediatric Nutrition Handbook Evanson III: American Academy of Pediatrics

Beddall A C, Hill F G H, George R H et al 1985 Unusually high incidence of tuberculosis among boys with haemophilia during an outbreak of the disease in hospital. Journal of Clinical Pathology 38: 1163–1165

Benson J W, Drayton M R, Hayward C et al 1986 Multicentre trial of ethamsylate for prevention of periventricular haemorrhage in very low birthweight infants. Lancet 2: 1297–1300

Bergqvist G, Zetterstrom R 1975 Submaximal blood flow and blood viscosity in newborn infants. Acta Paediatrics Scandinavica 64: 254–256

Beverley D W, Chance G W, Coates C F 1984 Intraventricular haemorrhage — timing of occurrence and relationship to perinatal events. British Journal of Obstetrics and Gynaecology 91: 1007–1013

Beverley D W, Pitts-Tucker T J, Congdon P J et al 1985 Prevention of intraventricular haemorrhage by fresh frozen plasma. Archives of Disease in Childhood 60: 710–713

Bjarke B, Herin P, Blomback M 1974 Neonatal aortic thrombosis: a possible clinical manifestation of congenital antithrombin III deficiency. Acta Paediatrica Scandinavica 63: 297–301

Blanchard R A, Furie B C, Jorgenson M et al 1981 Acquired vitamin k-dependent carboxylation deficiency in liver disease. New England Journal of Medicine 305:242–248

Bloom A L 1980 The von Willebrand syndrome. Seminars in Hematology 17(4): 215–227

Bloom A L 1981 Factor VIII inhibitors revisited. British Journal of Haematology 49: 319–324

Bona R D, Pasquale D N, Kalish R I, Witter B A 1986 Porcine factor VIII and plasmapheresis in the management of hemophiliac patients with inhibitors. American Journal of Hematology 21: 201–207

Bottema C D K, Koeberl D D, Sommer S S 1989 Direct carrier testing in 14 families with haemophilia B. Lancet 8662: 526–529

Bottema C D K, Koeberl D D, Ketterling R P et al 1990 A past mutation at Isoleucine[397] is now a common cause of moderate/mild haemophilia B. British Journal of Haematology 75: 212–216

Bovill E G, Burns S L, Golden E A 1985 Factor VIII antibody in a patient with mild haemophilia. British Journal of Haematology 61: 323–328

Branson H E, Katz J, Marble R, Griffin J H 1983 Inherited protein C deficiency and coumarin-responsive chronic relapsing purpura fulminans in a newborn infant. Lancet 2: 1165–1168

Brenner B, Fishman A, Goldsher D et al 1988 Cerebral thrombosis in a newborn with a congenital deficiency of antithrombin III. American Journal of Hematology 27: 209–211

Brenner B, Tavori S, Zivelin A et al 1990 Hereditary deficiency of all vitamin K-dependent procoagulants and anticoagulants. British Journal of Haematology 75: 537–542

Brettler D B, Brewster F, Levine P H et al 1987 Immunologic abberations, HIV seropositivity and seroconversion rates in patients with hemophilia B. Blood 70(1): 276–281

Brettler D B, Levine P H 1989 Factor concentrates for treatment of hemophilia: which one to choose? Blood 73(8): 2067–2073

Brettler D B, Alter H J, Dienstag J L et al 1990 Prevalence of hepatitis C virus antibody in a cohort of hemophilia patients. Blood 76(1): 254–256

Canale S T, Dugdale M, Howard B C et al 1988 Synovectamy of the knee in young patients with hemophilia. Scottish Medical Journal 81(12): 1480–1486

Capel P, Toppet M, van Remoortel E, Fondu P 1986 Factor VIII inhibitor in mild haemophilia. British Journal of Haematology 62(4): 786–787

Caplan M S, Cohn R A, Langman C B et al 1989 Favourable outcome of neonatal aortic thrombosis and renovascular hypertension. Journal of Pediatrics 115(2): 291–295

Carr J M, McKinney M, McDonagh J 1989 Diagnosis of disseminated intravascular coagulation. American Journal of Clinical of Pathology 91(3): 280–287

Casella J F, Lewis J H, Bontempo F A et al 1988 Successful treatment of homozygous protein C deficiency by hepatic transplantation. Lancet 8583: 435–438

Centres for Disease Control 1982 Pneumocystis carinii

pneumonia among patients with haemophilia A. Morbidity Mortality Weekly Review 31: 365

Chaou W-T, Chou M-L, Eitzman D V 1984 Intracranial hemorrhage and vitamin K deficiency in early infancy. Journal of Pediatrics 105(6): 880–884

Chenaille P J, Horowitz M E 1989 Purpura fulminans. Clinical Paediatrics 28(2): 95–98

Chuansumrit A, Manco-Johnson M J, Hathaway W E 1989 Heparin cofactor II in adults and infants with thrombosis and DIC. American Journal of Hematology 31: 109–113

Comp P C, Doray D, Patton D, Esmon C T 1986 An abnormal plasma distribution of protein S occurs in functional protein S deficiency. Blood 67(2): 504–508

Corrigan J J 1985 Hemorrhagic and thrombotic dieases in childhood and adolescence. Churchill Livingstone, Edingburh, p 150.

Creagh-Kirk T, Doi P, Andrews E et al 1988 Survival experience among patients with AIDS receiving Zidovudine: follow-up of patients in a compassionate plea program. Journal of the American Medical Association 260: 3009–3015

Cumming A M, Fildes S, Cumming R T et al 1990 Clinical and laboratory evaluation of NHS factor VIII concentrate (8Y) for the treatment of von Willebrand's disease. British Journal of Haematology 75: 234–239

Darby S C, Rizza C R, Doll R et al 1989 Incidence of AIDS and excess mortality associated with HIV in haemophiliacs in the United Kingdom: report on behalf of the Directors of Haemophilia Centres in the United Kingdom. British Medical Journal 298: 1064–1068

Darby S C, Doll R, Thakrar B 1990 Time from infection with HIV to onset of AIDS in patients with haemophilia in the UK. Statistics in Medicine 9: 681–689

Deblay M F, Vert P, Andre M, Marchal F 1982 Transplacental vitamin K prevents haemorrhagic disease of infant of epileptic mother. Lancet 1: 1247

Department of Health, Education and Welfare 1972 Pilot study of hemophilia treatment in the United States. National Heart and Lung Institute's Blood Resource Studies, vol 3. Government Printing Office, Washington, US

Donnér M, Holmberg L, Nilsson I M 1987 Type IIb von Willebrand's disease with probable autosomal recessive inheritance and presenting as thrombocytopenia in infancy. British Journal of Haematology 66: 349–354

Ekelund H, Hedner U, Nilsson I M 1970 Fibrinolysis in newborns. Acta Paediatrica Scandinavica 59: 33–43

Elidrissy A T H, Gader A M A 1985 Antithrombin II (ATIII) and fibrinogen levels in nephrotic syndrome in children. Haemostasis 15: 384–388

Emery J L 1962 Pulmonary embolism in children. Archives of Disease in Childhood 37: 591–595

Esteban J I, Esteban R, Viladomiu L et al 1989 Hepatitis C virus antibodies among risk groups in Spain. Lancet 8658: 294–297

Estelles A, Garcia-Plaza I, Dasi A et al 1984 Severe inherited 'homozygous' protein C deficiency in a newborn infant. Thrombosis and Haemostasis 52: 53–56

Feinstein D L 1987 Acquired inhibitors against factor VIII and other clotting proteins. In: Colman R W (ed) Hemostasis and thrombosis. J B Lippincott Inc, Philadelphia, p 825–840

Fennerty A G, Dolben J, Thomas P et al 1987 A comparison of 3 and 6 weeks' anticoagulation in the treatment of venous thromboembolism. Clinical and Laboratory Haematology 9: 17–21

Feusner J H 1980 Normal and abnormal bleeding times in neonates and young children utilizing a fully standardized template technic. American Journal of Clinical Pathology 74: 73–77

Fischer R R, Giddings J C, Roisenberg I 1988 Hereditary combined deficiency of clotting factors V and VIII with involvement of von Willebrand factor. Clinical and Laboratory Haematology 10: 53–62

Fischl M A, Richman D D, Hansen N et al 1990 The safety and efficacy of Zidovudine (AZT) in the treatment of subjects with mildly symptomatic human immunodeficiency virus type 1 (HIV) infection. Annals of Internal Medicine 112(10): 727–737

Foster P A, Zimmerman T S 1989 Factor VIII structure and function. Blood Reviews 3: 180–191

Fricke W A, Wong Yu M-Y 1989 Characterization of von Willebrand factor in factor VIII concentrates. American Journal of Hematology 31: 41–45

Friedland G H 1990 Early treatment for HIV. New England Journal of Medicine 322(14): 1000–1002

Fukui H, Nishino M, Terada S et al 1988 Hemostatic effect of a heat-treated factor VIII concentrate (Haemate P) in von Willebrand's disease. Blut 56: 171–178

Ghirardini A, Mariani G, Iacopino G et al 1987 Concentrated DDAVP: Further improvement in the management of mild factor VIII deficiencies. Thrombosis and Haemostasis 58(3): 896–898

Giannelli F, Choo K H, Rees D J G et al 1983 Gene deletions in patients with haemophilia B and anti-factor IX antibodies. Nature 303: 181–182

Gill J C, Wilson A D, Endres-Brooks J, Montgomery R R 1986 Loss of the largest von Willebrand factor multimers from the plasma of patients with congenital cardiac defects. Blood 67(3): 758–761

Ginsburg D, Konkle B, Gill J et al 1988 Molecular basis of von Willebrand's disease. Blood 72: 297a (abstr. suppl).

Goetzman B W, Stadalnik R C, Bogren H G et al 1975 Thrombotic complications of umbilical artery catheters: a clinical and radiographic study. Pediatrics 56: 374–379

Gordon E M, Ratnoff O D, Saito H et al 1980 Studies on some coagulation factors (Hageman factor, plasma prekallikrein and high molecular weight kininogen) in the normal newborn. American Journal of Pediatric Hematology/Oncology 2: 213–216

Gralnick H R, McKeown L P, Williams S B et al 1988 Plasma and platelet von Willebrand factor defects in uremia. American Journal of Medicine 85: 806–810

Gross R E 1945 Arterial embolism and thrombosis in infancy. American Journal of Diseases of Children 70(2): 61–73

Hambley H, Yates R, McNaughton M C et al 1982 Congenital antithrombin III deficiency: extended use of a pasteurised antithrombin III concentrate in late pregnancy and the puerperium. Proceedings of the British Blood Transfusion Society 11

Han P 1988 Childhood haemostasis III: von Willebrand's disease. Journal of the Singapore Paediatric Society 30(1 & 2): 46–50

Hanada T, Abe T, Takita H 1985 Antithrombin III concentrates for treatment of disseminated intravascular coagulation in children. American Journal of Pediatric Hematology/Oncology 7(1): 3–8

Hanna B D, Bernstein M 1989 Tranexamic acid in the treatment of Kasabach-Merritt syndrome in infants. American Journal of Pediatric Hematology/Oncology

11(2): 191–195

Haroon Y, Shearer M J, Rahim S et al 1982 The content of phylloquinone (vitamin K_1) in human milk, cow's milk and infant formula foods determined by high-performance liquid chromatography. Journal of Nutrition 112: 1105–1117

Harper P L, Luddington R J, Carrel R W et al 1988 Protein C deficiency and portal thrombosis in liver transplantation in children. Lancet 8617: 924–927

Hassan H J, Leonardi A, Guerriero R et al 1985 Hemophilla B with inhibitor: molecular analysis of the subtotal deletion of the factor IX gene. Blood 66(3): 728–730

Hassan H J, Orlando M, Leonardi A et al 1985 Intragenic factor IX restriction site polymorphism in hemophilia B variants. Blood 65(2): 441–443

Hathaway W E 1987 New insights on vitamin K. Hematology/Oncology Clinics of North America 1(3): 367–379

Hathaway W E, Bonnar J 1987 Hemostatic disorders of the pregnant woman and newborn infant. Elsevier Science Publishing Inc, Amsterdam

Hay C R M, Preston F E, Triger D R, Underwood J C E, 1985 Progressive liver disease in haemophilia: An understated problem? Lancet 8444: 1495–1497

Hay C R, Preston F E, Triger D R 1987 Predective markers of chronic liver disease in haemophilia. Blood 69(6): 1595–1599

Hay C R M, Preston F E, Triger D R, Underwood J C E 1985 Liver disease in haemophilia. Lancet 8465: 1187

Hay C W, Robertson K A, Yong S-L et al 1986 Use of a *Bam*HI polymorphism in the factor IX gene for the determination of haemophilia B carrier status. Blood 67(5): 1508–1511

Hedner U, Glazer S, Pingel K et al 1988 Successful use of recombinant factor VIIa in patient with severe haemophilia A during synovectomy. Lancet 8621: 1193

Hennes H, Losek J, Sty J R, Gill J C 1987 Computerized tomography in hemophiliacs with head trauma. Pediatric Emergency Care 3(3): 147–149

Holmberg L, Henriksson P, Ekelund H et al 1974 Coagulation in the human fetus: comparison with term newborn infants. Journal of Pediatrics 85: 860–864

Horgan M J, Bartoletti A, Polansky S 1987 Effect of heparin infusates in umbilical arterial catheters on frequency of thrombotic complications. Journal of Pediatrics 111(5): 774–778

Howard M R, McVerry B A 1987 T-cell lymphoma in a haemophiliac positive for antibody to HIV. British Journal of Haematology 67: 115

Hoyer L W, Rizza C R, Tuddenham E G et al 1983 von Willebrand factor multimer patterns in von Willebrand's disease. British Journal of Haematology 55: 493–507

Hoyle C F, Swirsky D M, Freedman L, Hayhoe F G J, 1988 Beneficial effect of heparin in the management of patients with APL. British Journal of Haematology 68: 283–289

Hudson I R B, Gibson B E S, Brownlie J et al 1990 Increased concentrations of D-dimers in newborn infants. Archives of Disease in Childhood 65: 383–389

Hulac P, Shapiro A, Manco-Johnson M et al 1986 Maternal anticonvulsants and neonatal vitamin K deficiency. Pediatric Research 20: 390a

Imaoka S, Ueda T, Shibata H et al 1986 Fibrinolysis in patients with acute promyelocytic leukaemia and disseminated intravascular coagulation during heparin therapy. Cancer 58: 1736–1738

Ino T, Benson L N, Freedom R M 1988 Thrombolytic therapy for femoral artery thrombosis after pediatric cardiac catheterization. American Heart Journal 115(3): 633–639

Isola L, Forster A, Aledort L M 1984 Desamino-D-arginine vasopression and bleeding time in von Willebrand's disease. Annals of Internal Medicine 101(5): 719–720

Jackson J C, Truog W E, Watchko J F et al 1987 Efficacy of thromboresistant umbilical artery catheters in reducing aortic thrombosis and related complications. Journal of Pediatrics 110(1): 102–105

Jannaccone G, Pasquino A M 1981 Calcifying splenic haematoma in a haemophiliac newborn. Pediatric Radiology 10: 183–185

Johnson C F 1988 Bruising and hemophilia: accident or child abuse? Child Abuse & Neglect. 12: 409–415

Kasper C K 1989 Treatment of factor VIII inhibitors. Progress in Hemostosis and Thrombosis (9): 57–86

Kaufmann H J 1958 Renal vein thrombosis. American Journal of Diseases in Children 95: 377–384

Kessler C M, Schulof R S, Alabaster O et al 1984 Inverse correlation between age related abnormalities of T-cell immunity and circulating thymosin$_1$ levels in haemophilia A. British Joural of Haematology 58: 325–336

Köhler M, Hellstern P, Wenzel E 1985 The use of heat-treated factor VIII-concentrates in von Willebrand's disease. Blut 50: 25–27

Kramer A, Biggar R J, Goedert J J 1990 Markers of risk in HIV-I. New England Journal of Medicine 322(26): 1886–1887

Krasinski S D, Russell R M, Furie B C et al 1985 The prevalence of vitamin K deficiency in chronic gastrointestinal disorders. American Journal of Clinical Nutrition 41: 639–643

von Kries R, Reifenhauser A, Gobel U et al 1985a Late onset haemorrhagic disease of newborn with temporary malabsorption of vitamin K_1. Lancet 8436: 1035

von Kries R, Gobel U, Masse B 1985b Vitamin K deficiency in the newborn. Lancet 8457: 728–729

von Kries R, Maase B, Becker A, Gobel U 1985c Latent vitamin K deficiency in healthy infants? Lancet 8469/70: 1421–1422

von Kries R, Gobel U 1988a Vitamin K prophylaxis: oral or parenteral? American Journal of Diseases of Children 142: 14–15

von Kries R, Shearer M J, Gobel U 1988b Vitamin K in infancy. European Journal of Pediatrics 147: 106–112

Kucuk O, Kwaan H, Gunnar W, Vazquez R M 1985 Thromboembolic complications associated with L-asparaginase therapy. Etiologic role of low antithrombin III and plasminogen levels and therapeutic correction by fresh frozen plasma. Cancer 55(4): 702–706

Lane P A, Hathaway W E 1985 Vitamin K in infancy. Journal of Pediatrics 106(3): 351–359

Lee C A, Phillips A, Elford J et al 1990 Ten-year follow-up of HIV infection in a haemophilic cohort. British Journal of Haematology 75: 623

van Leeuwen E F, Mauser-Bunschoten E P, van Dijken P J et al 1986 Disappearance of factor VIII:C antibodies in patients with haemophilia A upon frequent administration of factor VIII in intermediate or low dose. British Journal of Haematology 64: 291–297

Lenk H, Nilsson I M, Holmberg L, Weissbach G 1988 Frequency of different types of von Willebrand's disease in the GDR. Acta Medica Scandivaca 224: 275–280

Lesko S M, Mitchell A A, Epstein M F et al 1986 Heparin

use as a risk factor for intraventricular hemorrhage in low-birth-weight infants. New England Journal of Medicine 314: 1156–1160

Levine P H 1987 Clinical manifestations and therapy of hemophilia A and B. In: Coleman R W, Hirsh J, Marder V J, Salzman E W (eds) Hemostasis and thrombosis, vol. 6, 2nd edn. J B Lippincott Inc, Philadelphia, p 97–111

Lewis J H, Franklin M D, Bontempo F A et al 1985 Liver transplantation in a hemophiliac. New England Journal of Medicine 312(18): 1189–1190

Leyva W H, Knutsen A P, Joist H 1988 Disappearance of a high response factor VIII inhibitor in a hemophiliac with AIDS. American Journal of Clinical Pathology 89(3): 414–418

Liddell M B, Peake I R, Taylor S A M et al 1989 Factor IX Cardiff: a variant factor IX protein that shows abnormal activation is caused by an arginine to cysteine substitution at position 145. British Journal of Haematology 72: 556–560

Lillicrap D P, Liddell M B, Matthews R J et al 1986 Comparison of phenotypic assessment and the use of two restriction fragment length polymorphisms in the diagnosis of the carrier state in haemophilia B. British Journal of Haematology 62: 557–565

Ludlam C A, Chapman D, Cohen B, Litton P A 1989 Antibodies to hepatitis C virus in haemophilia. Lancet 8662: 560–561

Lusher J M 1987 Management of patients with factor VIII inhibitors. Transfusion Med Rev 1(2): 123–130

Mahasandana C, Suvatte V, Chuansumrit A et al 1990 Homozygous protein S deficiency in an infant with purpura fulminans. Journal of Pediatrics 117(5): 750–753

Mahir W S, Millard R E, Booth J C, Flute P T 1988 Functional studies of cell-mediated immunity in haemophilia and other bleeding disorders. British Journal of Haematology 69: 367–370

Makris M, Preston F E, Triger D R et al 1990 Hepatitis C antibody and chronic liver disease in haemophilia. Lancet 8698: 1117–1119

Malm J, Bennhagen R, Holmberg L, Dahlback B 1988 Plasma concentrations of C4b-binding protein and vitamin K-dependent protein S in term and preterm infants: low levels of protein S-C4-binding protein complexes. British Journal of Haematology 68: 445–449

Manco-Johnson M J, Marlar R A, Jacobson L J et al 1988 Severe protein C deficiency in newborn infants. Journal of Pediatrics 113(2): 359–363

Mannucci P M, Colombo M, Rizzetto M 1982 Nonprogressive course of non-A, non-B chronic hepatitis in multitransfused hemophiliacs. Blood 60(3) 655–658

Mannucci P M, Colombo M 1985 Liver disease in haemophilia. Lancet 8458: 774

Mannucci P M, Lombardi R, Bader R et al 1985 Heterogeneity of type I von Willebrand disease: evidence for a subgroup with an abnormal von Willebrand factor. Blood 66(4): 796–802

Mannucci P M, Tripodi A, Bertina R M 1986 Protein S deficiency associated with 'juvenile' arterial and venous thrombosis. Thrombosis and Haemostasis 55(3): 440

Marciniak E, Wilson H P, Marlar R A 1985 Neonatal purpura fulminans: a genetic disorder related to the absence of protein S-C4b-binding protein complexes. British Journal of Haematology 68: 445–449

Marder V J, Mannucci P M, Firkin B G et al 1985 Standard nomenclature for factor VIII and von Willebrand factor: a

recommendation by the International Committee on Thrombosis and Haemostatis. Thrombosis and Haemostasis. 54(4): 871–872

Marlar R A, Montgomery R R, Broekmans A W 1989 Report of the Working Party on homozygous protein C deficiency of the Subcommittee on Protein C and Protein S, International Committee on Thrombosis and Haemostatis. Diagnosis and treatment of homozygous protein C deficiency. Journal of Pediatrics. 114(4): 528–534

Mauser Bunschoten E P, van Houwelingen J C, Sjamsoedin Visser E J M et al 1988 Bleeding symptoms in carriers of hemophilia A and B. Thrombosis and Haemostatis 59(3): 349–352

McDonald M M, Hathaway W E 1982 Anticoagulant therapy by continuous heparinisation in newborn and older infants. Journal of Pediatrics 101: 451–457

McDonald M M, Koops B L, Johnson M L et al 1984 Timing and antecedents of intracranial haemorrhage in the newborn. Pediatrics 74: 32–36

McNinch A W, Orme R L, Tripp J H 1983 Haemorrhagic disease of the newborn returns. Lancet 1: 1089–1090

McNinch A W, Upton C, Samuels M et al 1985 Plasma concentrations after oral or intramuscular vitamin K$_1$ in neonates. Archives of Disease in Childhood 60: 814–818

McMillan C W, Shapiro S, Whitehurst D et al 1988 The natural history of factor VIII:C inhibitors in patients with hemophilia A: a national cooperative study. II. Observations on the initial development of factor VIII:C inhibitors. Blood 71(2): 344–348

Merion R M, Delius R E, Darrell M D, Campbell Jr D A, Turcotte J G 1988 Orthotopic liver transplantation totally corrects factor IX deficiency in hemophilia B. Surgery 104(5): 929–931

Mibashan R S, Millar D S 1983 Fetal haemostatic value at 17–21 weeks' gestation. British Medical Bulletin 39: 392–398

Miller C H, Graham J B, Goldin L E, Elston R C 1979 Genetics of classic von Willebrand's disease. I. Phenotypic variation within families. Blood 54(1): 117–136

Mills D S, Karpatkin S 1972 Heterogeneity of human adult and fetal fibrinogen: detection of derivatives indicative of thrombin proteolysis. Biochem Biophysia Acta 285: 398–403

Miser A W, Miser J, Newton Jr W A 1986 Intensive factor replacement for management of chronic synovitis on hemophilic children. American Journal of Pediatric Hematology/Oncology 8(1): 66–69

Moake J L, Rudy C K, Troll J H et al 1982 Unusually large plasma factor VIII: von Willebrand factor multimers in chronic relapsing thrombotic thrombocytopenic purpura. New England Journal of Medicine 307(23): 1432–1435

Montgomery R R, Marlar R A, Gill J C 1985 Newborn Haemostasis. Clinics in Haemotology 14: 443–460

Motohara K, Matsukura M, Matsuda I et al 1984 Severe vitamin K deficiency in breast-fed infants. Journal of Pediatrics 105(6) 943–945

Motohara K, Kuroki Y, Kan H et al 1985 Detection of vitamin K deficiency by the use of an enzyme-linked immunosorbent assay for circulating abnormal prothrombin. Pediatric Research 19: 354–357

Motohara K, Endo F, Matsuda I 1986 Vitamin K deficiency in breast-fed infants at one month of age. Journal of Pediatric Gastroenterology and Nutrition 5(6): 931–933

Murphy W G, Moore J C, Barr R D et al 1987 Relationship between platelet aggregating factor and von Willebrand factor in thrombotic thrombocytopenic purpura. British Journal of Haematology 66: 509–513

Neal W A, Reynolds J W, Jarvis C W, Williams H J 1972 Umbilical artery catheterization: demonstration of arterial thrombosis by aortography. Pediatrics 50: 6–13

Ngo K Y, Glotz V T, Koziol J A et al 1988 Homozygous and heterozygous deletions of the von Willebrand factor gene in patients and carriers of severe von Willebrand's disease. Proceedings of the National Academy of Sciences USA 85: 2753

Noel L, Guerois C, Maisonneuve P et al 1989 Antibodies to hepatitis C virus in haemophilia. Lancet 8662: 560

Olson T A, Alving B M, Cheshire J L et al 1985 Intracerebral and subdural hemorrhage in a neonate with hemophilia A. American Journal of Pediatric Hematology/Oncology 7(4): 384–387

O'Neill J A, Neblett W W III, Born M L 1981 Management of major thromboembolic complications of umbilical arterial catheters. Journal of Pediatric Surgery 16(6): 972–978

Parkin J M, Eales L J, Galazka A R, Pinching A J 1987 Atopic manifestations in the acquired immune deficiency syndrome: response to recombinant interferon gamma. British Medical Journal 294: 1185–1186

Pasi K J, Williams M D, Enayat M S, Hill F G 1990 Clinical and laboratory evaluation of the treatment of von Willebrand's disease patients with heat-treated factor VIII concentrate (BPL 8Y). British Medical Journal 75: 228–233

Pauli R M, Lian J B, Mosher D F, Suttie J W 1987 Association of congenital deficiency of multiple vitamin K-dependent coagulation factors and the phenotype of the warfarin embryopathy: clues to the mechanism of teratogenicity of coumarin derivatives. American Journal of Human Genetics 41: 566–583

Payne R M, Martin T C, Bower R J 1989 Management and follow-up of arterial thrombosis in the neonatal period. Journal of Pediatrics 114(5): 853–858

Peake I R, Bowen D, Bignell P et al 1990a Family studies and prenatal diagnosis in severe von Willebrand disease by polymerase chain reaction amplification of a variable number tandem repeat region of the von Willebrand factor gene. Blood 76(3): 555–561

Peake I R, Liddell M B, Moodie P et al 1990b Severe type III von Willebrand's disease caused by deletion of Exon 42 of the von Willebrand factor gene: family studies that identify carriers of the condition and a compound heterozygous individual. Blood 75(3): 654–661

Pettersson H, Gillespy T, Kitchens C et al 1987 Magnetic resonance imaging in hemophilic arthropathy of the knee. Acta Radiologica 28: 621–625

Phelps D L 1984 Vitamin E and CNS haemorrhage (Editorial). Pediatrics 74: 113–114

Piet A A M, Piet B A, Kjell S S et al 1983 Red blood cell size is important for adherence of blood platelets to artery subendothelium. Blood 62: 214–217

Pollack S, Atias D, Yoffe G et al 1985 Impaired immune function in hemophilia patients treated exclusively with cryoprecipitate: Relation to duration of treatment. American Journal of Haemotology 20: 1–6

Pollack S, Etzioni A 1987 Immune function in hemophiliacs, Journal of Pediatrics 110(1): 161–162

Powars D R, Rogers Z R, Patch M J et al 1987 Purpura fulminans in meningococcemia: association with acquired deficiencies of proteins C and S. New England Journal of

Medicine 317(9): 571–572

Priestley B L 1987 Haemorrhagic disease and vitamin K. Archives of Disease in Childhood 62(9): 979

Pui C-H, Chesney C M, Weed J, Jackson C W 1985 Altered von Willebrand factor molecule in children with thrombosis following asparaginase-prednisone-vincristine therapy for leukemia. Journal of Clinical Oncology 3(9): 1266–1272

Ragni M V, Winkelstein A, Kingsley L et al 1986 1986 update of HIV seroprevalence, seroconversion, AIDS incidence, and immunologic correlates of HIV infection in patients with hemophilia A and B. Blood 70(3): 786–790

Ragni M V, Hanley E N 1989 Septic arthritis in hemophilic patients and infection with human immunodeficiency virus (HIV). Annals of Internal Medicine 110(2): 168–169

Ramgren O, Nilsson I M, Blomback M 1962 Haemophilia in Sweden. IV. Hereditary investigations. Acta Medica Scandinavica 171(6): 759–769

Reitsma P H, Bertina R M, Ploos van Amstel J K et al 1988 The putative factor IX gene promoter in hemophilia B Leyden. Blood 72(3): 1074–1076

Rodeghiero F, Castaman G, Dini E 1987 Epidemiological investigation of the prevalence of von Willebrand's disease. Blood 69(2): 454–459

Roggendorf M, Dienhardt F, Rasshofer R et al 1989 Antibodies to hepatitis C virus. Lancet 8658: 324–325

Rothenberg R, Woelfel M, Stoneburner R et al 1987 Survival with the acquired immunodeficiency syndrome: experience with 5833 cases in New York City. New England Journal of Medicine 317(21): 1297–1302

Rugman F P, Mannion P T, Hay C R M et al 1989 Cytomegalovirus serum β_2 microglobulin, and progression to AIDS in HIV-seropositive haemophiliacs. Lancet 8663: 631

Scharrer I, Encke A, Hottenrott C 1988 Clinical cure of haemophilia A by liver transplantation. Lancet 8614: 800–801

Schettini F, De Mattia D, Altomare M et al 1985 Post-natal development of protein C in full-term newborns. Acta Paediatrica Scandinavica 74: 226–229

Schimpf K 1986 Liver disease in haemophilia. Lancet 8476: 323

Schimpf K, Mannucci P M, Krantz W 1987 Absence of hepatitis after treatment with pasteurised factor VIII concentrate in patients with haemophilia and no previous transfusions. New England Journal of Medicine 316: 918–922

Schmidt B, Zipursky A 1984 Thrombotic disease in newborn infants. Clinics in Perinatology 11(2): 461–488

Schmidt B, Zipursky A 1986 Disseminated intravascular coagulation masking neonatal hemophilia. Journal of Pediatrics. 109(5): 886–889

Schmidt B, Andrew M 1988 Neonatal thrombotic disease: prevention, diagnosis, and treatment. Journal of Pediatrics 113(2): 407–410

Schwartz H P, Muntean W, Watzke H et al 1988 Low total protein S antigen but high protein S activity due to decreased C4b-binding protein in neonates. Blood 71: 562–565

Seligshon U, Berger A, Abend M et al 1984 Homozygous protein C deficiency manifested by massive venous thrombosis in the newborn. New England Journal of Medicine 310: 559–562

Sell E J, Corrigan J J Jr 1973 Platelet counts, fibrinogen concentrations, and factor VIII levels in healthy infants according to gestational age. Journal of Pediatrics

82: 1029–1032

Shannon B T, Roach J, Cheek-Lutten M et al 1986 Progressive change in lymphocyte distribution and degree of hypergammaglobulinemia with age in children with hemophilia. Journal of Clinical Immunology 6(2): 121–129

Shapiro A D, Jacobson L J, Armon M E et al 1986 Vitamin K deficiency in the newborn infant: prevalence and perinatal risk factors. Journal of Pediatrics 109(4): 675–680

Shearer M J 1990 Vitamin K and vitamin K-dependent proteins. British Journal of Haematology 75: 156–162

Sheridan-Pereira M, Porreco R, Hays T, Burke M S 1988 Neonatal aortic thrombosis associated with the lupus anticoagulant. Obstetrics & Gynecology 71(6): 1016–1018

Shelton-Inloes B B, Chehab F F, Mannucci P M et al 1987 Gene deletions correlate with the development of alloantibodies in von Willebrand disease. Journal of Clinical Investigation 79: 1459–1465

Shulkin B L, Argenta L C, Cho K J, Castle V P 1990 Kasabach-Merritt syndrome: treatment with epsilon-aminocaproic acid and assessment by indium[111] platelet scintigraphy. Journal of Pediatrics 117(5): 746–749

Siguret V, Amselem S, Vidaud M et al 1988 Identification of a CpG mutation in the coagulation factor-IX gene by analysis of amplified DNA sequences. British Journal of Haematology 70: 411–416

Sills R H, Marlar R A, Montgomery R R et al 1984 Severe homozygous protein C deficiency. Journal of Pediatrics 105: 409–413

Sinha S, Davies J, Toner N, Bogle S, Chiswick M 1987 Vitamin E supplementation reduces frequency of periventricular haemorrhage in very preterm babies. Lancet i: 466–471

Smith G M, Cooper E H, Hall L, McVerry B A 1989 Serum beta 2-microglobulin levels in haemophiliacs. Clinical and Laboratory Haematology 11: 409–410

Sørensen P J, Nielsen A H, Knudsen F, Dyerberg J 1987 Defective protein C in uraemia. Blood Purification 5: 29–32

Sørensen P J, Knudsen F, Nielsen A H, Dyerberg J 1988 Protein C in acute renal failure. Acta Medica Scandinavica 224: 375–380

Sørensen P J, Knudsen F, Nielsen A H, Dyerberg J 1989 Protein C assays in uremia. Thrombosis Research 54: 301–310

Spear M E, Blifeld C, Rudolph A J et al 1984 Intraventricular haemorrhage and vitamin E in the very low birth weight infant: evidence for efficacy or early intramuscular vitamin E administration. Pediatrics 74: 1107–1112

Sthoeger D, Nardi M, Karpatkin M 1989 Protein S in the first year of life. British Journal of Haematology 72: 424–428

Stuart M J 1981 Deficiency of plasma PGI$_2$-like regenerating activity in neonatal plasma. Reversal by vitamin E in vitro. Pediatric Research 15(6): 971–973

Stuart M J, Walenga R W, Sadowitz P D et al 1986 Bleeding time in hemophilia A: potential mechanisms for prolongation. Journal of Pediatrics 108(2): 215–218

Tarby T J, Volpe J J 1982 Intraventricular haemorrhage in the premature infant. Pediatric Clinics of North America 29: 1077–1104

Taylor S A M, Liddell M B, Peake I R et al 1990 A mutation adjacent to the beta cleavage site of factor IX (valine 182 to leucine) results in mild haemophilia B$_m$. British Journal of Haematology 75: 217–221

Townsend C W 1894 The haemorrhagic disease of the newborn. Archives of Pediatrics 11: 559–565

Tripp J H, McNinch A W 1987 Haemorragic disease and vitamin K. Archives of Disease in Childhood 62: 436–437

Tuddenham E G D, Takase T, Thomas A E et al 1989 Homozygous protein C deficiency with delayed onset of symptoms at 7 to 10 months. Thrombosis Research 53: 475–484

Turner T, Prowse C V, Prescott R J, Cash J D 1981 A clinical trial on the early detection and correction of haemostatic defects in selected high-risk neonates. British Journal of Haematology 47: 65–75

Tyson J E, deSa D J, Moore S 1976 Thromboatheromatous complications of umbilical arterial catheterisation in the newborn period: clinicopathological study. Archives of Disease in Childhood 51: 744–754

UK Regional Haemophilia Centre Directors' Committee 1990 Recommendations on choice of therapeutic products for the treatment of non-inhibitor patients with haemophilia A, haemophilia B and von Willebrand's disease. The Haemophilia Society, The Bulletin published by 123 Westminster Bridge Road, London SE1 7HR

Vomberg P P, Breederveld C 1987 Cerebral thromboembolism due to antithrombin III deficiency in two children. Neuropediatrics 18: 42–44

Volberding P A, Lagakos S W, Koch M A et al 1990 Zidoduvine in asymptomatic human immunodeficiency virus infection: a controlled trial in persons with fewer than 500 CD4-positive cells per millimeter. New England Journal of Medicine 322(14): 941–949

Volpe J J 1981 Neonatal intraventricular haemorrhage. New England Journal of Medicine 304: 886–891

Vukovich T, Auberger K, Weil J et al 1988 Replacement therapy for a homozygous protein C deficiency-state using a concentrate of human protein C and S. British Journal of Haematology 70: 534–440

Wang E L, Read S E, Zuliain J, Blanchette V S 1987 Assessment of lymph node size in hemophiliac children: observer agreement and association with serologic status to human immunodeficiency virus I. Pediactric Infectious Disease Journal 6: 383–387

Ware J, Davis L, Frazier D et al 1988 Genetic defect responsible for the dysfunctional protein: factor IX Long Beach. Blood 72(2): 820–822

Warrier I, Brennan C A, Lusher J M 1986 Familial warfarin resistance in a black child. American Journal of Pediatric Hematology/Oncology 8(4): 346–347

Webster A, Lee C A, Cook D G et al 1989 Cytomegalovirus infection and progression towards AIDS in haemophiliacs with human immunodeficiency virus infection. Lancet 8654: 63–65

Weimer R, Schweighoffer T, Schimpf K, Opelz G 1989 Helper and suppressor T-cell function in HIV-infected hemophilia patients. Blood 74(1): 298–302

Weinstein M, Ware J A, Troll J, Salzman E 1988 Changes in von Wilebrand factor during cardiac surgery: effect of desmopressin acetate. Blood 71(6): 1648–1655

Weinstein M J, Blanchard R, Moake J L et al 1989 Fetal and neonatal von Willebrand factor (vWF) is usually large and similar to the vWF in patients with thrombotic thrombocytopenic purpura. British Journal of Hematology 72: 68–72

White G C, Shoemaker C B 1989 Factor VIII gene and hemophilia A. Blood 73(1): 1–12

Wilde J T, Davies J M 1990 Haemostatic problems in acute leukaemia. Blood Reviews 4(4) 245–252

Winship P R, Brownlee G G 1986 Diagnosis of haemophilia B carriers using intragenic oligonucleotide probes. Lancet 8500: 218–219

Winship P R, Rees D J G, Alkan M 1989 Detection of polymorphisms at cytosine phosphoguandine dinucleotides and diagnosis of haemophilia B carriers. Lancet 8639: 631–634

Yonker P G, Graham-Pole J, Mehta P 1985 Presentation of hemophilia A in the newborn period. J Florida M A 72(2): 99–101

Zanetti A R, Mannucci P M, Tanzi E et al 1986 Hepatitis B vaccination on 113 hemophiliacs: lower antibody response in anti-LAV/HTLV-III-positive patients. American Journal of Hematology 23: 339–345

14. Blood and blood product transfusion

G. Dolan

Special considerations must be taken into account when transfusing children with blood or blood products. Their age, size, health and immunological maturity may influence decisions on the choice of appropriate blood product. Blood bank techniques can also be influenced by such problems as the presence of maternal IgG antibodies in neonatal serum, which dictate the selection of compatible blood for transfusion. Despite many extra potential hazards, however, transfusion therapy in paediatric practice remains relatively safe (Luban & Dolan 1984).

The proportion of donated blood being fractionated into various components has greatly increased in recent years. The stimulus for this change has largely been the increased demand for plasma-derived coagulation factors but many other products are also now available (Table 14.1). The resulting dearth of whole blood available for transfusion has led clinicians to become more adept at the use of component therapy. The main indication for use of whole blood remains the restoration of blood volume following acute blood loss.

The quality and safety of blood for transfusion is of prime importance, and various specifications (British Pharmacopoeia in the UK) exist for the collection and processing of donated blood. The risk of infection associated with transfusion has been highlighted in recent years with the advent of the acquired immune deficiency syndrome (AIDS) and the identification of the hepatitis C virus, the aetiological agent responsible for most cases of non-A, non-B hepatitis. At present in the UK, all donations are tested for the presence of syphilis, hepatitis B antigen, and human immunodeficiency virus type-1 (HIV-1) antibody. Plans

Table 14.1 Blood products (From Forman 1987, reproduced by permission of John Wiley & Sons Ltd.)

Cells	Plasma
Whole blood	Fresh frozen plasma
Concentrated red cells	Cryoprecipitate
SAG-M red cells	4.5% Human albumin
Leucocyte-poor red cells	20% Human albumin
Saline-washed red cells	Freeze-dried coagulation
Frozen red cells (some	factor concentrates, e.g.:
centres)	Factor VIII
White cell/granulocyte	Factor IX
concentrates	Antithrombin III concentrate
Platelet concentrates	Immunoglobulin preparations:
	Normal broad spectrum
	Specific, e.g.:
	anti-D
	anti-tetanus
	anti-zoster

are under way to begin screening for hepatitis C (HCV) antibody and human immunodeficiency virus type-2 (HIV-2) antibody in the near future. Some donations are also tested for cytomegalovirus (CMV) antibody.

The greater profile understandably given to transfusion-acquired virus infection in recent years has also heightened the controversy surrounding the use of 'walking' donor panels to provide small volumes of fresh blood on demand for neonatal units. The existence of such panels is strongly discouraged by the transfusion service in the UK. Microbiological screening is a vital part of the quality control of donated blood, and every donation should be tested for HBsAg and HIV antibody. The 'occasional testing' of walking donors is not acceptable (Contreras & Hewitt 1985).

In some centres, some donated blood is collected into specific paediatric multiple-pack systems to minimize the number of donors to which infants are exposed during small-volume top-up

Table 14.2   Red cell products

Product	Volume	Haematocrit (%)
Whole blood*	515 ml ± 10%	35–40
Concentrated red cells	285 ml ± 10%	~60
Optimal additive cells (SAG-M)	335 ml ± 10%	~50

*450 ml donor blood + 63 ml CPD-A solution

transfusions. Up to four aliquots may be made from one single donation in this way. Such multiple packs are expensive, however, and require that the 'mini-units' are used for neonatal transfusion within 5–7 days to be cost effective. Beyond that time, the aged red cells are no longer acceptable for neonatal transfusion and the small volumes are unsuitable for adult transfusion. In centres where demand for 'young blood' is not excessive, the wastage of red cells from complete units may be more acceptable than the expense incurred in providing these special paediatric packs.

USE OF BLOOD AND BLOOD PRODUCTS IN CHILDREN

Red cell transfusion

Red cells may be transfused as whole blood, concentrated red cells or optimal additive cells (Table 14.2). At donation, whole blood is taken into the anticoagulant and preservative solution CPD-A, which contains citrate, phosphate, dextrose and adenine (Table 14.3). Concentrated cells are prepared from whole blood by expressing supernatant plasma into satellite packs. The remaining concentrated red cells will have a haematocrit raised in proportion to the amount of plasma removed, but usually averages around 60% (Table 14.2). The poorer flow rates seen with this product may cause some difficulty and the use of 'optimal additive' solutions may be preferred. The benefits of such solutions include con-

tinued availability of plasma for fractionation, the provision of a red cell concentrate with lower haematocrit and better flow properties, and some improved storage characteristics (Hogman et al 1978, 1983a, 1983b). SAG-M (saline adenine glucose and mannitol) is the most frequently used additive solution and its composition is shown in Table 14.4. The use of optimal additive red cells has some implications for the metabolic sequelae of transfusion. Such red cell concentrates have a lower potassium concentration (1.7 mmol/l) than conventional whole blood (3.5 mmol/l), but this difference is lost by seven days of storage (Herve et al 1980). The reduced citrate content of optimal additive cells also lowers the risk of citrate toxicity, and the addition of mannitol reduces in-vitro haemolysis. Another advantage of this product is that the improved glucose and ATP levels on storage may permit more rapid post-transfusion 2,3-DPG regeneration.

The reduced plasma protein content of SAG-M units also has some advantages, in that the flow properties of red cells are improved and the potential for reaction associated with such proteins is reduced. However, hypoalbuminaemia may occur after large volumes have been transfused, and supplementation with 4.5% human albumin solution is recommended when the transfused volume exceeds 50% of total blood volume. Thus, SAG-M units are probably best avoided for exchange or large volume transfusions in children.

Selection of blood for paediatric transfusion

Potential metabolic effects of transfusion and consequences of the immaturity of the neonatal immune system may govern decisions about the most appropriate choice of red cell preparation. Neonates, especially if premature, are more susceptible to the metabolic effects of high potassium and citrate levels found in transfused blood.

Table 14.3   CPD-A*

Each 100 ml CPD-A solution contains:	
Sodium citrate, Eur. P.	2.63 g
Anhydrous dextrose, B.P.	2.90 g
Citric acid monohydrate, Eur. P	327 mg
Sodium acid phosphate, B.P.	215 mg
Adenine	27.5 mg

*Each 63 ml CPD-A solution contains approximately 18 mmol sodium

Table 14.4   Optimal additive solution SAG-M

Each 100 ml SAG-M solution contains:	
Sodium chloride	877 mg
Adenine	16.9 mg
Glucose	900 mg
Mannitol	525 mg

(Tables 14.2–14.4 from Forman 1987, reproduced by permission of John Wiley & Sons Ltd.)

Hyperkalaemia may provoke serious and potentially fatal cardiac arrhythmias in sick neonates, who may already be acidotic. Hypocalcaemia due to citrate toxicity may develop, particularly in premature neonates whose immature livers cannot handle citrate. This may produce muscle tremors, cerebral irritability, seizures or arrhythmias. The rate of transfusion may also influence the development of citrate toxicity (Cohen et al 1980, Mollison 1987).

The potassium concentration in stored blood rises with time so blood which is less than five days old is usually selected for transfusing neonates. The low potassium and citrate content also make SAG-M blood particularly attractive for neonatal top-up transfusions. Another factor which favours the use of fresh blood in neonates is the preservation of higher 2,3-DPG levels in the transfused red cells, allowing more efficient tissue oxygenation.

The immature immune system of neonates renders them susceptible to unusually severe transfusion-related viral infections. Cytomegalovirus (CMV) infection is a particular hazard, but may be avoided by using only CMV-negative blood and blood products. This is discussed in greater detail later in this chapter.

Immature neonates may also be at risk of graft-versus-host disease following transfusion of fresh blood containing viable lymphocytes, but this may be prevented by irradiation of blood products prior to use (Wolfe et al 1983).

Cross-matching blood for children

The red cells of neonates are deficient in some red cell antigens, the most important of which are the A, B (and H) antigens. The weaker reactions seen with anti-A and anti-B sera may be due to a reduction in the number of antigen sites. Full expression of A and B antigens is reached by the age of 1 year (Mollison 1983). Other antigens not fully expressed in the neonate include Lewis, P and Ii systems. The red cell antigens of the Rhesus, Kell, Kidd and Duffy systems are, however, fully expressed at birth.

IgM anti-A and anti-B antibodies are usually absent in the newborn and do not usually develop until 3–4 months; thereafter, titres may continue to rise beyond the age of 5 years (Mollison 1987). Anti-A and anti-B found in cord sera are

usually IgG and of maternal origin, and can cause ABO haemolytic disease of the newborn if there is ABO incompatibility. Other maternal IgG antibodies can cross the placenta and cause a positive direct antiglobulin test or haemolytic disease of the newborn.

The presence of maternal IgG in the circulation of the neonate explains the need for a maternal clotted sample should a neonate require transfusion. The cells to be transfused must be compatible with any maternal IgG antibody and so the mother's serum is usually used in the cross-match instead of the baby's; not only will her serum be easier to obtain, but also the antibody is often stronger and more readily detectable than in the baby's serum, where it may be missed. Maternal serum can be used for cross-matching infants up to 6 months old. Alternatively, if a maternal antibody screen is negative and the baby's direct antiglobulin test is negative, infants under 4 months can be safely transfused with uncrossmatched ABO and RhD compatible red cells as they are highly unlikely to make alloantibodies.

Exchange transfusion

Hyperbilirubinaemia due to isoimmune haemolytic disease of the newborn is the most common indication for exchange transfusion. Other indications include hyperbilirubinaemia associated with other haemolytic processes, such as G6PD deficiency, severe respiratory distress syndrome and disseminated intravascular coagulation (DIC) (Gross & Melhorn 1971, Guttuso et al 1976). Exchange transfusion for haemolytic disease of the newborn removes antibody-coated red cells, bilirubin and free antibody, and corrects anaemia. Exchange transfusion may be given in utero, immediately after delivery or may be delayed until there are clear signs of increasing unconjugated bilirubinaemia with the associated risk of kernicterus. Most exchange transfusions are still performed for haemolytic disease due to rhesus incompatibility, and this still causes considerable perinatal morbidity and mortality despite the availability of anti-D prophylaxis (Urbaniak 1985).

ABO haemolytic disease of the newborn is rarely sufficiently severe to require exchange transfusion. In that rare event, group O blood should be used either as packed cells or as cells resuspended in albumin or group-specific plasma to the desired haematocrit. The latter manipulation avoids the risk of haemolysis due to lysins in the group O plasma.

Cells selected for exchange transfusion should be rhesus-negative and of the ABO group appropriate to the mother and baby (Table 14.5). The cells should also be cross-match-compatible with maternal serum, but in some instances the suggested group is ABO-incompatible with the maternal serum. In such circumstances, the maternal serum can be treated to neutralize the IgM anti-A or anti-B prior to the match and this can be duplicated with the infant's serum.

Group O cells resuspended in ABO-infant-compatible plasma could be used for all exchange transfusions, but the additional requirements that the blood be rhesus negative, CMV negative and less than 5 days old could place too great a demand on blood supply, and, in practice, appropriate A and B groups are used. Whole blood, unmodified or else partially packed to remove a quantity of plasma to give a higher haematocrit, may be used for exchange transfusion. Packed cells supplemented by fresh frozen plasma may also be used.

It can be calculated that a single volume exchange transfusion will replace 65% of the infant's blood volume, and a double volume exchange, 85% (Allen & Diamond 1958, Cohen et al 1980, Klemperer 1981). Calculations have been based on a neonatal blood volume of 80 ml/kg.

Table 14.5 Choice of ABO group for exchange transfusion

Mother's ABO group	Infant's ABO group			
	O	A	B	AB
O	O	O or A	O or B	–
A	O	A	O or B	AB or A
B	O	O or A	B	AB or B
AB	–	A	B	AB

(From Forman 1987, reproduced by permission of John Wiley & Sons Ltd.)

Calculation of volume for transfusion

When smaller volumes of blood are required, as with top-up transfusions, packed cells are most often used, particularly SAG-M cells which, as indicated already, have better flow properties. Several formulae exist for calculating the appropriate volume to be transfused : most involve the estimated circulating blood volume and the haemoglobin concentration of the product (Klemperer 1981; Table 14.6). These formulae should be treated with caution and as rough guides to the maximum volume per transfusion.

Platelet transfusion

The use of platelet concentrates to control or prevent bleeding has been a major development in the management of children with thrombocytopenia and acquired or congenital platelet dysfunction (see Ch. 6). One unit of platelet concentrate contains the platelets separated from fresh blood suspended in approximately 50 ml of plasma, and

Table 14.6 Calculations for blood and blood product transfusions

Red blood cells

$$\text{Volume transfused} = \frac{\text{circulating blood volume} \times \text{rise in Hb}}{\text{Hb conc. of product}} \quad \text{(Klemperer 1981)}$$

or

Volume of cells = weight (kg) × desired rise in haematocrit (Kevy 1979)

or

Maximum volume (packed cells) of transfusion = 5 ml/pound
If Hb < 5 g/dl then 3 ml/pound (Kevy, 1979)

Granulocytes
Aim for dose of 1×10^{10} neutrophils

Platelets
Adults –   1 unit/10 kg body weight (Menitove & Aster 1983)
             or 1 unit/m^2 to produce rise of 12×10^9/l
Children – 1 unit/5 kg body weight (Sills & Stuart 1980)

Fresh frozen plasma
DIC 15 ml/kg (Gill 1980)

(From Forman 1987, reproduced by permission of John Wiley & Sons Ltd.)

should contain 60×10^9 platelets (Forman 1987). At a storage temperature of $22°C$, they will remain viable for up to 5 days under constant agitation.

The rise in platelet count following transfusion depends on several factors, the most obvious of which, perhaps, is the number of platelets transfused and the size of the child. A satisfactory increment can be achieved by transfusing 1 unit/5 kg body weight in a child, providing there is no clinical problem causing peripheral destruction/ consumption of platelets. A single unit of platelets can raise the platelet count of a neonate by $75–100 \times 10^9/l$ (Sills & Stuart 1980). In practice, many clinicians make judgements on the required dose of platelets on the basis of age and an estimate of size, so that older children and adolescents are given 6 units, infants are given 2 units and those in between are given 4 units (Forman 1987). Platelet requirements may be very much increased in the presence of consumption coagulopathy, splenomegaly and infection, and in these situations, the development of fresh petechiae, bruising or bleeding should be the guide to transfusion requirements.

Children with idiopathic thrombocytopenic purpura rarely require platelet transfusion, but large doses of platelets may very occasionally be effective in controlling bleeding in life-threatening situations, though it must be anticipated that platelet survival will be reduced. Another immune thrombocytopenia, neonatal alloimmune thrombocytopenia, usually caused by maternal anti-P1^{A1} antiplatelet antibodies, may necessitate the transfusion of P1^{A1}-negative platelets in rare circumstances (see Ch. 6).

Platelet survival may be assessed by checking the platelet count one and 24 hours after infusion (Daly et al 1980). Decreased survival may be due to one of the factors described above, or to alloimmunization (see below).

Platelets can be administered through a standard-bore blood giving set of 170-μm pore size, but smaller, specific platelet administration sets are available. Only clear solutions should be administered before and after platelets through the same set.

Granulocyte transfusion

The transfusion of donor granulocytes has been used to help in controlling infection in severely ill children. It may be considered in any situation where a child with marked neutropenia or impairment of neutrophil function has severe infection. In practice, it has been used most commonly in children with bone marrow failure or in septic neonates.

Granulocytes for transfusion may be obtained from single donors by leucapheresis or by single unit or pooled buffy coat layers from fresh blood. Where indicated, a 3–4-day trial of daily transfusion is undertaken. There are no clear data on the minimum number of granulocytes required to produce clinical benefit, but effective doses of 1×10^{10} WBC/transfusion for adults, and $0.2–1 \times 10^9$ WBC/transfusion for infected neonates have been quoted (Hows & Brozovic 1990, Harris 1987). The post-transfusion increment in granulocytes depends on the number of granulocytes transfused, the blood volume of the child, whether the child has been immunized against granulocyte antigens and probably also on the severity of infection.

Several problems are associated with granulocyte transfusions, including alloimmunization, CMV infection, pulmonary infiltration and graft-versus-host disease. The latter problem may be prevented by irradiation of the concentrates prior to transfusion. These are discussed in later sections. Whether granulocyte transfusions are necessary or helpful in the light of newer antibiotics is doubtful.

Plasma products

Fresh frozen plasma, cryoprecipitate and coagulation factor concentrates are obtained by separation of donor blood or by plasmapheresis. The indications for the use of these products is discussed in Chapter 13.

Fresh frozen plasma

Fresh frozen plasma (FFP) is plasma which, after separation from red cells, is frozen within 4 hours of donation. The volume of each unit ranges in volume from 180–200 ml and contains normal levels of clotting factors. The amount of coagulation factor activity in 1 ml of fresh normal plasma is defined as one international unit (i.u.); the actual activity is, however, subject to variation among donors and some activity is lost in the freezing process. FFP should be stored at or below −30°C and thawed at 37°C before use. It should be used as soon as possible and certainly within 4 hours of thawing. It should also be ABO compatible.

FFP may be used in a variety of acquired and congenital coagulation abnormalities, including vitamin K deficiency, liver disease and DIC.

Cryoprecipitate

Cryoprecipitate is formed when FFP is allowed to thaw at 4°C. It contains concentrates of FVIII, fibrinogen, fibronectin and other cold-soluble proteins (Pool & Shannon 1985). Cryoprecipitate contains approximately 80–100 i.u. of FVIII and 25 mg fibrinogen, but the range is relatively wide (Forman 1987). Cryoprecipitate must also be stored at below −30°C and thawed at 37°C before use. ABO compatibility is not required.

Since the advent of factor VIII concentrates which have been subjected to viricidal treatment, cryoprecipitate is now rarely used in the treatment of haemophilia. The use of cryoprecipitate in von Willebrand's disease is also now being superseded by specific concentrates. It retains a role in the management of DIC by providing a source of fibrinogen.

Coagulation factor concentrates

Lyophilized factor concentrates, including concentrates of factor VIII, factor IX, prothrombin complex and antithrombin III, are obtained by fractionation of FFP. These freeze-dried concentrates can be stored at 4°C and reconstituted immediately before use. Their development has revolutionized the care of haemophilia (Ch. 13).

Large-pool plasma products were associated with a high risk of transfusion-acquired viral infection before the advent of specific viricidal treatment of the concentrates (see below).

ALLOIMMUNIZATION DUE TO TRANSFUSION OF BLOOD PRODUCTS

Alloimmunization to red cells, leucocytes and platelets may complicate paediatric transfusion practice. This is especially true for those children requiring multiple transfusion over a prolonged period as, for example, in children with sickle cell disease, thalassaemia or malignant disease. The incidence of alloimmunization appears to depend on the age and functional integrity of the immune system.

Alloimmunization to red cells

Alloimmunization in transfused neonates is rare (Ludvigsen et al 1982, Floss et al 1984) but occasional reports have been made (Smith & Storey 1984). The immaturity of the immune system in young children may prevent antibody formation or allow tolerance to develop to red cell antigens (Diamond et al 1961, Rebulla & Modell 1991, Giacomo et al 1983). Older children have a higher risk of alloimmunization which is greater with multiple transfusions and transfusion from donors of a different racial origin, though those with malignant disease may have a lower incidence of alloimmunization than their peers (Blumberg et al 1984, Kim et al 1984).

Among groups of children with haematological disease, those with sickle cell disease and thalassaemia attract most attention from the point of view of alloimmunization to red cells. In studies of sickle cell disease, the incidence of alloimmunization has ranged from 8–36%, and of these, up to 56% have multiple antibodies (Orlina et al 1978, Coles et al 1981, Fullerton et al 1981). Antibodies to Rhesus antigens are the most common, with anti-Kell and anti-Kidd also being relatively frequent. The range of incidence of alloantibodies in thalassaemic children is wide, but was as high as 70% in one series, with multiple antibodies being found in 15%. Again, Rhesus and Kell antibodies predominate (Coles et al 1981, Rebulla & Modell 1991). There is some evidence that alloantibodies are less common in those children who begin regular transfusion at an early age.

When children requiring long-term transfusion support are first identified, detailed grouping studies should be undertaken to determine probable Rhesus genotype and also to determine Kell, Ss, Kidd and Duffy type (Napier 1987). Although in most circumstances it is impractical to use such extensively cross-matched blood from the outset, information gained prior to regular transfusion will help to identify subsequent antibodies and aid selection of appropriate blood at a later date.

Alloimmunization to platelets

Alloimmunization to platelet antigens is a potentially serious problem and may occur following transfusion of red cells, platelets and granulocytes. The development of platelet antibodies may lead to refractoriness, defined as repeated failure to obtain a satisfactory response to platelet transfusion. The risk factors for alloimmunization and refractoriness are not clearly identified. Up to 70% of multi-transfused individuals may develop antibodies and become refractory, but it is well recognised that many patients never become immunized despite frequent transfusion (Howard & Perkins 1978, Murphy & Waters 1990). Some studies have suggested that the risk of platelet refractoriness is increased with increasing number of transfusions, while others have suggested that immunosuppressed patients with malignant disease are at reduced risk of alloimmunization; both of these generalizations are controversial (Howard & Perkins 1978, Holohan et al 1981, Dutcher et al 1981).

The most frequently occurring platelet alloantibodies are those directed at HLA antigens. These develop in approximately 50% of multi-transfused patients (Howard & Perkins 1978, Murphy & Waters 1990) and appear to be stimulated by contaminating leucocytes in platelet and red cell transfusions. HLA antibodies may cause refractoriness through their affinity for the platelet class I antigens, but many HLA-immunized individuals continue to have a satisfactory response to platelet transfusion. Murphy & Waters (1990) found that only 30% of patients with HLA antibodies were refractory to platelet transfusions, and in these individuals, multi-specific antibodies were found. The remaining, nonrefractory patients had either weak or mono-specific antibodies. Alloimmune HLA antibodies may also disappear when antigenic stimulation is removed either by cessation of transfusion or switching to matched platelets (Murphy et

al 1987). Platelet-specific antibodies may also develop and are associated with a much higher incidence of refractoriness. Such antibodies have been shown to occur in 20–25% of patients with HLA antibodies (Murphy & Waters 1990) and multiple antibodies may develop (Langenscheidt et al 1988).

Several methods for preventing alloimmunization have been investigated, the first and most obvious being the avoidance of unnecessary transfusion. Depleting red cell and platelet concentrates of leucocytes by using either washing techniques or filters can also lead to a significant reduction in alloimmunization (Murphy & Waters 1990). The use of single-donor platelets, thereby limiting the range of antigens to which the recipient is exposed, has also been associated with a lower incidence of alloimmunization, but this effect may only be temporary (Sintnicolaas et al 1981). More recently, the effect of irradiating blood products with ultraviolet light has yielded promising results (Bucholz et al 1988).

When a patient develops refractoriness to platelets, it is essential to first assess whether this may be due to nonimmune causes such as infection. If no such cause is evident, then screening for HLA antibodies should be arranged and matched platelets should be sought using HLA-A and B antigens (C, D and DR antigen compatibility appear to be of little importance). Ideally, children in whom chronic platelet transfusion therapy is anticipated should be HLA-matched at an early stage. In most cases, fully HLA-matched platelets will lead to a satisfactory response. In those with poor response, HLA incompatibility or accompanying platelet-specific antibodies may be present; platelet cross-matching may be helpful in obtaining appropriately matched platelets in this situation. Obtaining matched platelets may not be feasible in an emergency. In such situations, large volumes of fresh platelets from random donors may achieve haemostasis. There is also some evidence that survival of transfused platelets is greater when ABO-compatible donors are used (Duquesnoy et al 1979).

Alloimmunization to granulocytes

Granulocyte concentrates provide a powerful

antigenic stimulus, and HLA- and granulocyte-specific antibodies develop in 70–75% of recipients (Schiffer et al 1979, Ford et al 1982). Alloimmunization may also develop as a result of previous transfusion of platelets and blood. In addition to the hazards of immunological reactions, granulocyte recovery and function may also be impaired in sensitized subjects (Dutcher et al 1983). In alloimmunized subjects, only granulocytes from HLA-matched donors should be transfused while in nonsensitized recipients, conventional cross-matching is sufficient for practical purposes (Napier 1987). Fortunately, perhaps, enthusiasm for granulocyte replacement therapy has waned considerably over recent years, due to lack of evidence of its efficacy and to improvements in antibiotic agents.

Alloimmunization to plasma proteins

Antibodies may develop in response to foreign antigens in donor plasma. Such antibodies include those against pollen or milk proteins, and against IgA in IgA-deficient recipients. These are considered further below.

TRANSFUSION REACTIONS

Transfusion reactions are an important hazard of blood transfusion and may arise in many ways, including both immune and nonimmune phenomena.

Haemolytic transfusion reactions

Haemolytic reactions are associated with increased destruction of red cells following transfusion. The nature of such reactions depends on many factors, including whether they are immune- or nonimmune-mediated the functional integrity of the immune system of the recipient and the nature of antibodies involved.

Immune-mediated haemolytic reactions

Intravascular haemolysis. Acute intravascular haemolysis occurs with complement-binding antibodies, which tend to cause immediate and severe haemolytic reactions. The classic example is the transfusion of ABO-incompatible blood. IgM anti-A and anti-B are powerful complement-fixing antibodies, and give rise to serious reactions which may be fatal in approximately 10% of cases (Contreras & Mollison 1990). The most serious reactions are usually seen in group O individuals, who have the highest titres of anti-A and -B, except in young infants where these antibodies may not develop until 3–4 months of age (Mollison 1987). The vast majority of haemolytic reactions involving the ABO system are due to incorrect recipient identification as a result either of mislabelling the sample or of giving blood to the wrong patient.

Similar, though usually less serious, haemolysis can arise when relatively large volumes of donor plasma containing high-titre anti-A or -B is transfused. This situation is more relevant in paediatric practice, where the recipient's red cell mass is lower in proportion to that of an adult. For this reason, it is wise to avoid giving group O blood unnecessarily and, where possible, to use ABO-compatible fresh frozen plasma, platelet concentrates and cryoprecipitate.

The clinical manifestations of transfusion reactions may depend on the awareness of the recipient. Administrative errors – which, as discussed above, are the most common causes of serious reactions – are more likely to occur in emergency situations where the patient is unconscious or anaesthetized. Conscious patients may develop fever, restlessness, abdominal, loin or substernal pain, headache, sweating and vomiting. In the unconscious patient, the only manifestation may be hypotension or haemorrhage due to associated DIC.

Hypotension is due to the release into the plasma of activated components of the complement system, causing degranulation of mast cells and subsequent release of the vasoactive substances, bradykinin and serotonin. Hypotension is a major contributor to the development of acute renal failure, which is commonly seen after major transfusion reactions. Haemorrhagic problems may occur, as a result of DIC due to the potent thromboplastic effect of disrupted red cell stroma and hypotension. "DIC may occur after transfusion of only small volumes of blood." (Ratnoff 1984).

The management of patients who have suffered

a major transfusion reaction includes immediate cessation of transfusion, maintenance of blood pressure with intravenous fluids, and maintenance of renal function by avoiding hypotension and using diuretics. DIC may be prevented or ameliorated with the use of heparin, and haemorrhagic problems may necessitate transfusion of platelets, cryoprecipitate and fresh frozen plasma.

Extravascular haemolysis. The dramatic symptoms and signs described above are not seen with the slower pace of haemolysis seen in extravascular haemolysis. The antibodies responsible for this type of reaction are usually IgG and do not fix complement. Most such reactions are due to antibodies against the Rhesus, Kell, Duffy and Kidd systems. The transfused, incompatible cells are coated with antibody, and are then removed from the circulation by the reticuloendothelial cells over a period of hours. Initially, the extravascular haemolysis is silent, but within approximately 45 minutes, chills and restlessness develop and, after a period of time, a steady rise in temperature occurs, peaking at around 4 hours after the start of transfusion (Jandl & Tomlinson 1958). The delay in the development of symptoms may lead to difficulty in identifying the unit of blood which actually caused the reaction, since subsequent, innocent blood units may be being transfused when pyrexia develops.

Delayed haemolytic transfusion reaction. This type of transfusion reaction occurs when a recipient has an antibody present at very low levels which is not detected by usual pre-transfusion screening methods. Incompatible blood is then given with no immediate sequelae. However, the concentration of the antibody is boosted by further exposure to the stimulating antigen in transfused blood, and haemolysis occurs between 2 and 10 days after the onset of transfusion, when the titre of the antibody rises. Anti-Kidd antibodies (anti-Jka and -Jkb) are classic examples of those causing delayed transfusion reactions, though other relatively common offenders include Rhesus, Kell and Duffy (Napier 1987).

The clinical effects of this type of reaction depend on the volume of incompatible blood transfused and on the underlying health of the recipient. Haemolysis of a small volume of blood may be clinically silent, but if a large amount of blood is haemolysed, the recipient may develop sudden pallor, jaundice and fever. Renal failure is uncommon but has been described.

Investigation of haemolytic transfusion reaction. When a haemolytic reaction is suspected, investigations should be aimed at determining whether the cause is immune or nonimmune. Plasma and urine samples should be examined for evidence of haemolysis, as should any remaining blood from the transfused unit. All blood units issued for the patient, including empty bags, should be returned to the blood bank for serological and microbiological investigation. Microbiological assessment of the donor unit should also be complemented by blood cultures from the recipient. Full compatibility screening on pre- and post-transfusion samples should then be repeated, and a thorough check for administrative errors should be undertaken. Any other intravenous fluid administered with the transfusion, and the blood administration set, should also be examined to determine whether hypotonic or hypertonic solutions may have caused haemolysis.

Non-immune haemolytic transfusion reactions

Improper handling of blood before and during transfusion may cause haemolysis. Blood stored at too high a temperature or overheated during passage through a blood warmer may result in haemolysis (Sandler et al 1976, Vaughan 1982), as may mixing blood with hypo- or hypertonic solutions (Ryden & Oberman 1975). Infected blood packs, now a rarity though still occasionally encountered, may also cause haemolysis.

Intrinsically abnormal recipient erythrocytes may haemolyse following transfusion; this may be seen in children with paroxysmal nocturnal haemoglobinuria or glucose 6 phosphate dehydrogenase deficiency (see Ch. 9).

Nonhaemolytic transfusion reactions

Febrile reactions

These reactions occur in patients who have antibodies against leucocyte and platelet antigens. Such antibodies may develop after transfusion of granulocyte or platelet concentrates, whole blood, or red cell concentrates contaminated with leucocytes or platelets. A typical febrile reaction begins 30–120 minutes after the start of transfusion and consists of a sensation of coldness followed by chills and an abrupt rise in temperature (de Rie et al 1985). The fever is caused by release of pyrogens from the recipient's granulocytes and monocytes (Contreras & Mollison 1990). HLA antibodies are most commonly involved in such reactions, but granulocyte-specific and platelet-specific antibodies are also implicated (de Rie et al 1985). In patients who have had more than one severe febrile reaction, serological evidence of antibody-mediated reaction should be sought and, if found, further transfusions should be depleted of leucocytes by washing or filtration.

Urticarial reactions

Urticarial reactions are probably the most common adverse reaction associated with the transfusion of any plasma-containing blood product. Such phenomena are thought to be the result of a reaction between a foreign antigen in donor plasma and the corresponding IgE antibody in recipient plasma (Contreras & Mollison 1990). Administration of antihistamines is usually effective and no further investigation is warranted.

Anaphylactic reactions

A severe reaction consisting of flushing, tachypnoea, bronchospasm, hypotension, nausea and vomiting may develop within minutes of starting transfusion. Such allergic reactions are most commonly due to anti-IgA antibodies and may be fatal (Pineda & Taswell 1975). These antibodies usually arise in IgA-deficient individuals who have been exposed to foreign IgA by transfusion. Immediate treatment consists of resuscitation and suppression of the immunological response by corticosteroids. Further transfusion in such individuals should be with IgA-depleted blood or blood products.

Pulmonary infiltrates

These may develop as a result of agglutinating leucocyte antibodies in the donor serum reacting with recipient granulocytes. Fever, cough and dyspnoea may occur and be associated with nodular lung infiltrates (Contreras & Mollison 1990).

IMMUNOLOGICAL ASPECTS OF TRANSFUSION

Immunological abnormality associated with transfusion

A variety of immunological abnormalities have been described in HIV-negative individuals who have received multiple blood transfusions.

Natural killer (NK) activity is inversely related to the number of units transfused (Gascon et al 1985). The CD4:CD8 ratio is usually normal, but evidence of T-cell activation is commonly found and in-vitro T-cell responses to foreign antigens may be impaired (Munn et al 1981). Evidence of B-cell disturbance, such as abnormal immunoglobulin levels, have also been reported (Karpadia et al 1980).

The clinical importance of these abnormalities remain to be determined. In animal models, decreased NK activity is associated with susceptibility to viral infection and tumour engraftment, but there is no clear evidence for this in man (Gascon et al 1985).

Graft-versus-host disease

Post-transfusion graft-versus-host-disease (GVHD) occurs following transfusion of immunocompetent cells in individuals with defective cell-mediated immunity who are incapable of rejecting them (Brubaker 1983).

Several factors conspire to make GVHD difficult to diagnose in the post-transfusion setting; these include the distraction of the underlying disease process, the signs and symptoms of GVHD not being complete, the short and often fatal course of the illness, and a low index of suspicion among clinicians. Table 14.7 illustrates the type of disorder which may make a child susceptible to this potentially devastating illness.

A chronic course has not been reported in transfusion-associated GVHD, all cases having an acute course (Brubaker 1983). Acute GVHD may affect the skin, liver, gastrointestinal tract and bone marrow. Typically, the disease causes high fever, erythematous maculopapular rash, diarrhoea,

Table 14.7 Conditions associated with potential risk of transfusion associated graft versus host disease

---

Congenital
Thymic hypoplasia (Di George syndrome)
Combined immunodeficiency*
  X-linked lymphopenic agammaglobulinaemia (X-linked recessive)
  Swiss-type aggammaglobulinaemia (autosomal recessive) presenting as Letterer-Siwe syndrome
Nezelof's syndrome
Immunodeficiency with enzyme deficiency
Short-limbed dwarfism*
Wiskott-Aldrich syndrome*
Ataxia-telangiectasia
Episodic lymphopenia
Acquired
Thymoma (Good's syndrome)
Chronic mucocutaneous candidiasis
Infections (overwhelming)
Measles
Mumps (and vaccine)
Chickenpox
Influenza
*Premature neonates**
*In-utero haemolytic disease of the fetus**

---

*Indicates the actual diseases and situations in which GVHD resulted from transfusion therapy
From Brubaker 1983. By permission of S Karger A G, Basel.

anorexia, nausea, vomiting, hepatomegaly with abnormal liver function and pancytopenia. The diagnosis is usually made by the clinical findings and skin biopsy appearance. The disease is usually rapidly fatal with bone marrow failure, possibly due to cytotoxic lymphocytes in donor blood attacking haemopoietic stem cells.

GVHD has been reported following transfusion of whole blood, packed red cells, white cell concentrates, fresh plasma and platelets, but not FFP, cryoprecipitate, frozen blood or washed red cells. Irradiating blood products before transfusion has been shown to prevent GVHD, and should be undertaken for any child at risk (Leitman & Holland 1985, Brubaker 1983).

IRON OVERLOAD

For the vast majority of children with congenital anaemia, regular transfusion with red cells is the only means of maintaining a reasonable standard of health. The aims of transfusion regimens should be the prevention or amelioration of the effects of anaemia on growth, development and vital organ function and, in the case of thalassaemia, the inhibition of bone marrow expansion and

hypersplenism. Chronic transfusion creates many difficult problems, one of the more challenging being iron overload.

Accumulation of iron

Each unit of blood contains approximately 200 mg of iron which is not eliminated from the body by normal physiological means. The steady accumulation of iron is therefore an inevitable consequence of chronic transfusion. For children with hypoplastic anaemias, such as aplastic anaemia and Diamond-Blackfan syndrome, transfused iron is the sole cause of overload; in those anaemias associated with erythroid hyperplasia, such as thalassaemia, increased gastrointestinal absorption of iron may also contribute.

Transfused red cells are taken up by the reticuloendothelial system and their iron content is stored in a nontoxic form. However, the capacity of this system is limited and eventually plasma transferrin becomes saturated and iron is thereafter increasingly taken up by hepatic parenchymal cells (Berry & Marshall 1967, Ley et al 1982). Parenchymal iron loading is facilitated by the high plasma iron turnover and increased gastrointestinal absorption seen in the hyperplastic anaemic states, and also by the increased intravascular haemolysis encountered in some congenital anaemias (Marcus & Huehns 1985).

Clinical effects of iron overload

The steady accumulation of iron in tissues leads to structural and functional damage to the myocardium, liver, pancreas and endocrine glands. Clinical complications of iron overload usually become apparent in late childhood and adolescence, but a minority of patients may escape significant problems until their third decade, despite heavy iron burden. It has been suggested that vitamin C deficiency, a recognized feature of iron overload, may confer protection against the toxic effects of iron (Cohen et al 1981).

Disturbance of growth is one of the first and most consistent signs of toxicity due to iron overload (Modell & Berdoukas 1984), and may be related to reduced somatomedin activity as a consequence of hepatic damage (Saenger et al

1980). Delayed sexual development may also be an early clinical manifestation of siderosis, and there is evidence that this may be due to reduced pituitary responsiveness to hypothalamic releasing factors (Woodcock 1987).

Hepatic damage is a serious complication of iron overload and occurs early (Ioncu et al 1977). Hepatomegaly and disturbance of liver function may develop, and advancing liver disease may lead to progressive fibrosis, cirrhosis and portal hypertension. Progression of liver disease may be prevented or controlled with effective chelation therapy.

Cardiomyopathy occurs as a result of the deposition of iron in the cells of the conducting system and myocardium. Progressive cardiac failure and dysrhythmias correlate with the degree of iron overload, and end-stage cardiac failure usually occurs when the iron load rises above 1 g/kg. Echocardiography may detect increased ventricular wall thickness at an early stage, but clinical signs and symptoms, radiological, electrocardiographic and ejection fraction changes occur late (Ley et al 1982). Chelation therapy should be aimed at preventing cardiac damage, but even when such damage already exists, some reversal may occur with intense chelation.

Consequences of iron overload in the pancreas and endocrine glands range from mild biochemical alterations to severe metabolic disturbance, such as hypoparathyroidism and diabetes. Iron-induced endocrinopathies may not improve with chelation therapy. The skin pigmentation seen in iron overload is due to increased melanin deposition and improves with chelation.

Criteria for regular transfusion

The volume and frequency of transfusion should be tailored for each individual child. The aims of transfusion should be clear and will vary according to the underlying disease. In those with anaemia not associated with bone marrow expansion, anaemia may be well tolerated and transfusion may only be necessary if symptoms such as dyspnoea or growth failure develop. The decision about when to start a regular programme of transfusion should therefore be made after a period of careful observation. In others, such as those with

thalassaemia, an additional aim is the suppression of bone marrow expansion, with attendant skeletal abnormalities, and hypersplenism. The decision in this situation is more difficult, since it is clearly undesirable to transfuse children who would otherwise follow the more benign course of thalassaemia intermedia, while the disfiguring skeletal and facial abnormalities which occur in under-transfused children with thalassaemia major are not reversible.

Some authorities have suggested that the age at presentation may be helpful in predicting the severity of the disease (Modell & Berdoukas 1984), with the majority of those children presenting at less than one year having a more severe course. However, age at presentation will be affected by family history, and the awareness of medical attendants and the scoring system proposed by Modell & Berdoukas (1984), using other factors in addition to age, may be more useful. In practice, a haemoglobin level persistently under 7 g/dl is a reasonable indication for regular transfusion, but it is wise to reassess the situation after a few transfusions as intercurrent infection may temporarily worsen anaemia in these children.

The age of red cells in a unit of blood may range from 1–120 days, with a mean of 60 days. It would be advantageous to be able to selectively transfuse younger red cells (neocytes) with a greater life-span as part of a long-term transfusion programme, since this would increase the time interval between transfusions, thereby reducing the iron load. Several methods exist for isolating younger cells from donated blood, including the use of a density gradient using arabinogalactane, centrifugation with cell washers or continuous flow centrifugation (Piomelli et al 1978, Graziano et al 1982, Propper et al 1980, Corash et al 1981). The young cells obtained using these techniques have been shown to have increased survival, with an increased life-span of approximately 40–47 days, compared with 28 days for cells from unfractionated donor units (Bracey et al 1983, Propper et al 1980). Despite considerable interest in the use of young red cells, some workers found only a 16% reduction in transfusion requirements, considerably less than the predicted 50% reduction (Cohen et al 1984). The disappointing clinical trials, and the disadvantages of increased cost, increased preparation time, increased donor exposure and blood wastage have all contributed to the subsequent lack of enthusiasm of widespread use of this therapeutic option to date.

As noted above, for transfusion-dependent children without significant bone marrow expansion, individual management should be aimed at maintaining healthy growth and development while avoiding unnecessary transfusion. However, in children with thalassaemia major, intermittent transfusion will not prevent skeletal and facial deformity and thus they should be regularly transfused to maintain a minimum haemoglobin at which these problems are minimized. Wolman (1964) and Wolman & Ortolani (1969) demonstrated the benefit of maintaining a minimum haemoglobin of between 8–9 g/dl in children with thalassaemia major. This regimen of transfusion every 3–4 weeks was widely adopted even though it produced an associated rise in transfusion requirement (Necheles et al 1974, Piomelli et al 1974).

More recently, increasing the minimum haemoglobin to around 12 g/dl (supertransfusion) has been advocated (Propper et al 1980, Modell & Berdoukas 1984). The theoretical benefits of this are better suppression of erythropoiesis, reduction of hypersplenism, reduction of gastrointestinal absorption of iron, and reduction of bone demineralization. There are conflicting data relating to the clinical value of these cited benefits, and the experience of earlier enthusiasts who found that super-transfusion could be maintained without increasing transfusion requirements is not universal (Propper et al 1980, Gabutti et al 1980, Modell & Berdoukas 1984, Piomelli et al 1985). Clearly, the potential benefits of supertransfusion must be balanced against the possible risk of increasing iron burden through increased transfusion. There is also evidence to suggest that the effectiveness of chelation therapy with desferrioxamine is diminished when maintaining high haemoglobin levels (Pippard et al 1982).

Control of iron overload

The control of iron overload involves several issues. As already discussed, the careful planning of a regime to avoid unnecessary transfusion is essential. The use of young blood (neocytes) for transfusion is an attractive option but, as discussed earlier, there are significant practical limitations. For thalassaemic children with hypersplenism, when transfusion requirements are 1.5 times higher than they otherwise would be, splenectomy will also help to reduce iron loading (Rebulla & Modell 1991). Despite these measures, however, most chronically transfused children need chelation therapy with desferrioxamine (DF).

Desferrioxamine is currently the most effective iron-chelating agent in widespread clinical use. It is a colourless hydroxylamine which binds ferric iron on a 1:1 molecular ratio. The resultant ferrioxamine appears rust-coloured in the urine. It is expensive, and has the additional disadvantage, at present, of having to be given parenterally. Barry et al (1974) were among the first workers who demonstrated that long-term treatment with intravenous desferrioxamine could significantly reduce hepatic iron concentration and arrest hepatic fibrosis in children on a high transfusion regime. They and others found no serious side-effects, despite high doses. Important work which further helped to shape current schedules of chelation therapy showed that continuous subcutaneous administration of desferrioxamine was effective (Hussain et al 1976) and that reducing the infusion time to 12 hours did not appreciably reduce the effectiveness of chelation. Thus, for most transfusion-dependent children with increased iron stores and no significant organ damage, regular subcutaneous infusions with desferrioxamine form the mainstay of chelation therapy.

Dose–response relationships should ideally be determined at the outset to establish an optimal schedule for each child. It is important to remember that although urinary excretion of iron is the main source of removal of chelated iron, faecal iron derived from biliary excretion of hepatic iron may also play an important part (Harker et al 1968, Pippard et al 1982). In children less than 6 years old, the usual dose is less than 1 g/day for 5–6 days per week, while in older children the dose may increase to around 2–4 g/day (Cohen 1987, Hershko et al 1990). Reduction in the iron burden may be further achieved by intermittent high-dose intravenous desferrioxamine at the time of blood transfusion (Hyman et al 1985). For established cardiomyopathy, continuous intravenous infusion of up to 125 mg/kg per day may improve myocardial function (Hersko et al 1990).

Vitamin C may enhance the excretion of iron in subjects receiving chelation with desferrioxamine (Wapnick et al 1969); however, there is evidence that vitamin C deficiency protects against the toxic effects of iron overload (Bothwell et al 1965, Wills 1972), and its use in iron-loaded children should therefore be confined to cases where effective chelation is established and where vitamin C is shown to increase excretion (Nienhuis 1981). In such cases, modest doses of 100–200 mg/day may be appropriate (Pippard & Callendar 1983).

When to start regular chelation therapy is also the subject of some debate. Some prefer to start chelation with the initiation of regular transfusion, based on the findings that parenchymal iron accumulation may occur early (Modell & Berdokas 1984, Pippard & Callendar 1983). However, it may be reasonably argued that introduction of chelation therapy may be delayed until the age of 2–4 years, since permanent organ damage in uncommon at this time and negative iron balance can usually be achieved with desferrioxamine (Cohen et al 1984, Hershko 1990).

Serum ferritin assays are widely used in the assessment of the severity of iron overload and the effectiveness of chelation therapy. In the absence of liver disease, it has been shown that serum ferritin correlates closely with transfused iron burden up to a concentration of 7000 µg/l (Letsky et al 1974). However, there is a high concentration of ferritin in the liver which, when damaged, releases ferritin into the circulation. Thus when there is evidence of liver disease, such as occurs with transfusion-acquired virus infection or advanced siderosis, the serum ferritin becomes less reliable in assessing iron burden (De Virgilis et al 1980). Intercurrent infection may also cause an increase in ferritin levels (Worwood 1990).

As there are limitations in the usefulness of using serum ferritin measurements in the monitoring of iron overload, other investigations may be required. Liver biopsy is a reliable means of assessing iron overload, and the hepatic iron content correlates with the degree of hepatic fibrosis (Risdon et al 1975). Other, less invasive but more expensive, methods of assessing iron burden include computed tomography, magnetic susceptibility measurement (SQUID) and nuclear magnetic resonance measurement (NMR) (Kaltwasser & Werner 1989).

Hazards of desferrioxamine

Although desferrioxamine is of great clinical benefit and has improved the life expectancy in iron-loaded children, there are potentially troublesome complications associated with its long-term use. Many of these unwanted effects are associated with parenteral administration and systemic toxicity and may largely be abolished if the new oral iron-chelators prove to be effective. Local reactions at the site of subcutaneous infusion are fairly common, with swelling, pruritus and wheal formation (Waxman & Brown 1969). When intravenous desferrioxamine is given too rapidly flushing, hyper- or hypotension, tachy- or bradycardia, nausea and vomiting may occur, and patients feel very unwell (Porter & Huehns 1989).

Ocular and ototoxicity are subjects of much concern. There is some debate about whether desferrioxamine causes cataracts. There are some reports of cataracts with no visual loss in thalassaemic patients on long-term treatment, but these are rare in those patients treated with conventional doses (Waxman & Brown 1969, Davies et al 1983). Establishing a causal link in such patients is complicated by the fact that subcapsular lens opacities are known complications of iron overload (Porter & Huehns 1989). There is, however, evidence of such a causal link between cataract formation and desferrioxamine use at higher doses (Davies et al 1983, Modell & Berdoukas 1984). Retinal toxicity is well described, with night blindness, annular field loss and retinal pigmentation, features very similar to those of retinitis pigmentosa (Davies et al 1983, Borgna-Pignatti et al 1984, Oliveri et al 1986). These effects are at least partially reversible on stopping the drug, and iron overload appears to offer some protection against retinal toxicity (Davies et al 1983, Oliveri et al 1986). Children on long-term desferrioxamine therapy should therefore have regular ophthalmic review.

Ototoxicity is a well-recognized-complication of long-term therapy (Marsh et al 1981, Oliveri et al 1986, Wonke et al 1989). Hearing loss, particularly high-frequency sensorineural hearing loss, is the most commonly encountered problem. Again, there is evidence that iron overload confers some protection against ototoxicity, with younger children and those with lower ferritins being most at risk (Oliveri et al 1986, Porter et al 1988). It is therefore wise to check audiometry every 6 months in children on long-term chelation with desferrioxamine, particularly those with ferritins below 2000 µg/l (Porter & Huehns 1989). It has also been suggested that if the ratio of mean dose of desferrioxamine (in mg/kg per day) to mean serum ferritin (in µg/l) is greater than 0.025, the dose of desferrioxamine should be reduced, even if audiometry is normal (Porter & Huehns 1989).

Increased susceptibility to infection has been reported to occur with desferrioxamine therapy. Yersinia infections may be very serious, and should be suspected in the presence of colitis, peritonitis, septicaemia or atypical infection (Lancet editorial 1984, Chiu et al 1986). *Pneumocystis carinii* pneumonia and mucormycosis have also been reported in association with desferrioxamine therapy (Kouides et al 1988). Other rare complications include growth failure (Porter & Huehns 1989), thrombocytopenia in association with renal dialysis (Walker at al 1985, Dickerhoff 1987), pulmonary toxicity (Freedman et al 1989) and renal toxicity (Freedman et al 1989).

INFECTIOUS COMPLICATIONS OF BLOOD TRANSFUSION

Transmission of infectious agents is a well-recognized hazard of blood transfusion. The risk of transmitted disease depends on the prevalence of the infection in the donor population, which is in turn dependent on the geographical variation often seen in these diseases, and also on the number of donors to which the recipient is exposed. The risk may be diminished by attempts to exclude infected individuals from the donor pool, and by anti-infection manipulation of blood products, such as heat-treatment. The features of transfusion-acquired infection may be considered under the broad headings of viral, bacterial and protozoal infections.

Viral infection

Hepatitis

Post-transfusion hepatitis (PTH) is the commonest infectious complication of blood transfusion and there is significant geographical variation in its incidence. Actual figures are difficult to determine, as most estimates were published before the exclusion of high-risk donors and the introduction of surrogate testing. Most such estimates will probably therefore be of little epidemiological value; for example, the much quoted 10% incidence of PTH in the USA in the 1970s has already been reduced to less than 5% (Alter et al 1981, Barabara & Contreras 1990). These estimates are based on the use of single-donor or small-donor-pool products, the risk being considerably higher for large pool plasma products (Kernoff et al 1985).

PTH may be the result of infection with several different viruses:

Hepatitis B. Hepatitis B virus (HBV) is a now a less common cause of PTH than it used to be, but remains an important problem (Conrad 1981). HBV is plasma-borne and can therefore be transmitted by a variety of blood products. The risk of HBV infection is increased with use of large-pool plasma products (Barabara & Contreras 1990). Screening of donors for HBV, exclusion of paid donors and the self exclusion of other high-risk donors have all contributed to the diminishing incidence of transfusion-associated infection (Seef et al 1975, Barabara & Contreras 1990).

The widely employed screening test for hepatitis B surface antigen (HBsAg) is useful but may fail to detect low levels of viraemia in infected donors (Knodell et al 1975), and this at least partially explains why up to 10% of cases of post-transfusion hepatitis are still due to HBV (Bove 1987). The incubation period for HBV infection varies from 2–6 months in the majority of cases, but may be shorter or longer depending on various host factors. The majority of infections are clinically silent and may be realized only if biochemical and serological screening tests are employed. However, 1% of acute HBV infections run a fulminant course with a high mortality rate, and a further 5% may become chronic carriers. Clinical complications include chronic liver disease and hepatocellular carcinoma.

Since vaccination against HBV appears to be effective in preventing infection, all children who require regular transfusion or exposure to large-pool products such as FVIII concentrate should be immunized.

Hepatitis C. Most cases of post-transfusion hepatitis are not associated with infection with either hepatitis A or B viruses. They amount to 90% of all cases of PTH, and are generically classified as non-A, non-B hepatitis (NANBH) (Lancet editorial 1975). Estimates of the incidence of post-transfusion NANBH have varied from 1–2.4%, in the UK (Contreras et al 1991), to 18% in Japan (Watanabe et al 1990). The true incidence may be considerably less than original estimates, since many studies have not taken account of any reduction since the introduction of programmes aimed at excluding high-risk donors.

There is now clear evidence that the majority of cases of post-transfusion NANBH are due to infection with hepatitis C virus (HCV) (Alter et al 1989). HCV is a single-stranded RNA virus with a lipid envelope, and is probably a flavivirus (Choo et al 1989, Kuo et al 1989). HCV infection appears to have an incubation period of approximately 60 days and is usually asymptomatic. The resultant hepatitis may only be discovered by monitoring serum transaminases. Post-transfusion NANBH is usually defined by transaminase levels 2.5 times the upper limit of normal on two or more occasions (Barabara & Tedder 1984). The clinical importance of HCV infection is that chronic infection may develop in approximately 50% of those infected, and this may lead to chronic liver disease and cirrhosis (Underwood 1990). HCV has also been implicated in the pathogenesis of hepatocellular carcinoma (Underwood 1990).

Using enzyme immunoassays for HCV antibody, the frequency of seropositivity among blood donors in various countries varies from 0.3 to 1.4% (Lancet editorial 1990). Some studies have shown that blood from only 14% of such individuals is associated with seroconversion for anti-HCV and NANBH in recipients (Contreras et al

1991). This may explain the low risk of infection with HCV in blood donors in the UK receiving only single-donor unit products (Contreras et al 1991, Dolan et al 1991). This risk is likely to diminish further when large-scale screening of blood donors is introduced.

The risk of infection with HCV is much greater, however, for those individuals who have received large-pool products. The majority (64–85%) of haemophiliacs who have been exposed to non-heat-treated factor VIII and IX concentrates in the past are infected with HCV (Esteban et al 1989, Ludlam et al 1989), and the virus appears to be the cause of most of the chronic liver disease frequently seen in these patients (Makris et al 1990). Fortunately, the risk of HCV infection appears to be greatly reduced by heat treating plasma products (Skidmore et al 1990).

Hepatitis A. Post-transfusion hepatitis due to transmission of hepatitis A virus has been reported but is rare (Hollinger et al 1983). Since the virus is directly cytopathic and incubation period is short, those donors harbouring infection are likely to be symptomatic, thus reducing the chances of donation.

Delta agent. A defective hepatitis virus, the delta agent, may also be transmitted by blood transfusion (Rizetto et al 1977). This agent can only replicate in HBV-infected hosts, and may increase the severity of both acute and chronic HBV infection. Transfusion-associated infection is rare in the UK, and exclusion of HBsAg-positive donors should ensure that it remains so (Barabara & Tedder 1984).

Human immunodeficiency virus

Human immunodeficiency virus (HIV) was first identified in 1983 as the aetiological agent of the acquired immune deficiency syndrome (AIDS) (Gallo et al 1983). Even before this important event, there was already evidence that the disease could be transmitted by blood transfusion (Centres for Disease Control 1982). Since then, it has become clear that transfusion of blood or blood products has been responsible for the infection of many adults and children.

HIV is a retrovirus which selectively invades CD4 helper lymphocytes. Viral replication within the lymphocytes is cytopathic to these cells. The net result is a reduction in the numbers of CD4 helper lymphocytes and marked impairment of cell-mediated immunity. Acute infection with HIV is associated with a mononucleosis-like illness, with fever, arthralgia, pharyngitis, lymphadenopathy and maculopapular rash (Cooper et al 1985). Seroconversion with development of anti-HIV antibodies usually occurs within 8 weeks of infection. The virus is found in most body fluids, and infection is spread via sexual activity involving exchange of such fluids, by transference of infected blood via shared needles and transfusion of blood products, and by vertical transmission to infants of infected mothers. For children, the latter two routes provide the main source of HIV infection. Efforts to control the spread of the virus are based primarily on the exclusion of high-risk groups from donor pools (the definition of such individuals still being under regular review), the screening of donated blood by ELISA assay for anti-HIV antibody, and subjecting large-pool plasma products to viricidal manipulation.

Using such measures, the risk of infection by blood transfusion has decreased significantly and, at present, has been estimated at less than one per million in the UK (Napier 1987). The greatest problem continues to be those donors who deny risk factors and who are in the 'window' period between acquiring the virus and the development of anti-HIV antibodies (Bove 1987). The introduction of screening tests for HIV antigen is likely to further reduce the risk of transfusion-associated HIV infection.

Before the advent of donor exclusion programmes and viricidal treatment of plasma products, many adults and children were infected with HIV. The risk of infection was shown to be much greater for those exposed to multiple donors, as evidenced by the high rate of seropositivity among haemophiliacs treated with non-heat-treated factor VIII and IX concentrates – approximately 35% of the British patients (Evatt et al 1985, Napier 1987). These seropositive haemophiliacs acquired infection via factor concentrates which had not been subjected to viricidal heat treatment, but there is now evidence that heat-treated products, introduced in 1984, are safe in this respect.

HIV infection may result in an asymptomatic but potentially infectious seropositive state, or may progress to symptomatic infection manifesting in many ways (Table 14.8). At present, confirmation of infection is most often achieved by the serological demonstration of HIV antibodies. In the western world, the majority of infection is due to the HIV-1 retrovirus, whereas the other main virus, HIV-2, is a greater problem in West Africa. Although cross-reactivity occurs between

Table 14.8 Revised case definition of AIDS (CDC 1986)

A Without definitive diagnosis of HIV infection but definitive diagnosis of indicator disease
  1. Candidiasis of oesophagus
  2. Extrapulmonary cryptococcosis
  3. Cryptosporidiosis > 1 month diarrhoea
  4. Cytomegalovirus infection (other than liver, spleen or lymph node) in patient older than 1 month
  5. Herpes simplex causing: pneumonitis, oesophagitis, mucocutaneous ulceration for > 1 month
  6. Kaposi's sarcoma in patient < 60 years old
  7. Primary cerebral lymphoma in patient <60 years old
  8. Lymphoid interstitial pneumonia affecting child < 13 years old
  9. *Mycobacterium avium intracellulare* or *M. kansasii* (disseminated)
  10. *Pneumocystis carinii* pneumonia
  11. Progressive multifocal leukoencephalopathy
  12. Toxoplasmosis of brain (patient older than 1 month)

B With definitive diagnosis of HIV infection (indicator disease diagnosis definitively plus diseases above)
  1. Bacterial infection (recurrent) in children
  2. Disseminated coccidiomycosis
  3. HIV encephalopathy
  4. Disseminated histoplasmosis
  5. Isospora diarrhoea >1 month
  6. Kaposi's sarcoma any age
  7. Primary cerebral lymphoma any age
  8. Non-Hodgkin's lymphoma
  9. Any disseminated mycobacterial disease (not *M. tuberculosis*)
  10. Extrapulmonary *M. tuberculosis*
  11. Recurrent *Salmonella* septicaemia (not *S. typhimurium*)
  12. HIV wasting syndrome

C With laboratory evidence of HIV infection but presumptive diagnosis of indicator disease
  1. Oesophageal candidiasis
  2. Cytomegalovirus retinitis with visual loss
  3. Kaposi's sarcoma
  4. Lymphoid interstitial pneumonia in child < 13 year old
  5. Disseminated mycobacterial disease (or species not defined)
  6. *Pneumocystis carinii* pneumonia
  7. Toxoplasmosis of brain

From Gazzard 1990. By permission of Balliére-Tindall, London anti-HIV-1 antibodies and HIV-2 virus, specific assays for the latter agent are likely to become more widely employed (Contreras & Barabara 1990). More accurate methods of confirming infection include isolation of the virus in tissue culture, and demonstration of the viral genome from body fluid or tissue samples.

One situation in which seropositivity does not necessarily indicate infection is in those infants who may have acquired antibody passively via the transplacental route from infected mothers. In such children, antibody may persist for 15 months, and it is recommended that additional proof of infection be sought in these young seropositive infants (Ryan et al 1987; see Table 14.2).

A variety of immunological abnormalities are found in HIV infection, ranging from minimal disturbance to profound suppression of cell-mediated immunity and marked disturbance of B-cell function. The cytopathic effect of virus infection on helper T-cells leads to reduction in absolute numbers of CD4 lymphocytes and reversal of the CD4:CD8 ratio (Amman 1985). This phenomenon is used to monitor progression of HIV infection, but up to 15% of children with progressive disease may have relatively normal CD4 numbers and CD4:CD8 ratios (Ryan et al 1987). Other immunological abnormalities include a variety of functional defects of T-cells and abnormalities of B-cell function, characterized by polyclonal hypergammaglobulinaemia (Scott et al 1984). The development of antinuclear antibodies and antibodies against red cells, neutrophils and platelets is also well described (Scott et al 1984).

The classification system for HIV infection is under continual review, and the one shown in Table 14.8 has made specific provision for the important differences seen in the manifestation of HIV infection between adults and children. Symptomatic HIV infection may manifest in many ways, including opportunistic infection and malignancy. Although there is a paucity of data for children, it has been suggested that the majority of those infected eventually become symptomatic (Ryan et al 1987), and the risk may be greater for neonates (Sandler & Schorr 1987). Furthermore, the incubation period between infection and symptoms appears to be shorter in children (Rogers 1985). A common combination of pre-

senting symptoms in children with symptomatic HIV infection includes interstitial pneumonitis, hepatosplenomegaly and failure to thrive (Shannon & Amman 1985). Notable differences in the manifestations of HIV infection in children, as compared to adults, include: more marked hypergammaglobulinaemia, lymphoid interstitialpneumonitis, chronic parotitis, recurrent bacterial sepsis, candidal infection and progressive neurological disease (Ryan et al 1987, Gazzard 1990). Fewer children present with opportunistic infections (including pneumocystis pneumonia) or malignant disease (Shannon & Ammann 1985, Gazzard 1990).

HTLV-I and HTLV-II

These other retroviruses may also be transmitted by transfusion of blood products containing white blood cells. The risk is greatest in Japan, the Caribbean and parts of Africa. Routine screening for these viruses is likely to be introduced in the UK in the near future. HTLV-I infection is associated with a low attack rate in seropositive individuals. Adult T-cell leukaemia may develop after a long incubation period, and the other recognized illness, HTLV-associated myelopathy (HAM), appears to have a shorter incubation (Contreras & Barabara 1990). The clinical significance of HTLV-II remains to be determined.

Cytomegalovirus

Cytomegalovirus (CMV) is a herpes virus which, in common with other herpes viruses, causes persistent, latent infection. The majority of primary infections are asymptomatic, although a proportion of immunocompetent individuals suffer a glandular-fever-like illness. CMV infection may be acquired by blood transfusion, principally through reactivation of latent virus residing in lymphocytes and monocytes in donated blood. The risk of infection with plasma products appears to be minimal (Barabara & Tegtmeier 1987). Unlike other transfusion-associated viruses, CMV infection is common in donor populations. In developed countries, the prevalence of seropositivity is 40–79% and is higher among older donors (Barabara & Tegtmeier 1987). The risk of infection is therefore relatively high following blood transfusion.

Post-transfusion CMV infection is classified as primary if a seronegative recipient demonstrates serological or virological proof of infection within 12 weeks of transfusion. Recipient-reactivated infection occurs when a recipient with latent infection shows evidence of active infection after transfusion. The third mode of infection, reinfection, is evidenced by shedding of exogenous virus, and may be accompanied by a greater than four-fold rise in antibody titre.

CMV infection may cause significant morbidity and mortality in immunocompromized recipients, including fetuses and neonates. The incidence of transfusion-associated CMV infection in very low birth weight (< 1200 g) seronegative children varies from 10 to 30% (Adler 1988). Symptoms including respiratory distress, apnoea, fever, pneumonia, hepatosplenomegaly, ascites and anaemia. Proving that such symptoms are due to CMV infection in such infants is difficult, because of the need for biopsy evidence of the intranuclear inclusions typically seen in CMV disease, but evidence from autopsy examination suggests that transfusion-acquired infection is associated with a high mortality rate in these children (Yeager et al 1981, Adler 1988).

CMV infection in seronegative infants with birth weight greater than 1300 g, and for seropositive infants with birth weight less than 1200 g, appears to carry a lower risk of fatal outcome, but serious illness may nevertheless develop (Yeager et al 1981, Adler 1988). As it is relatively easy to screen donated blood for CMV antibody, and therefore practical to supply CMV-negative blood, there is a strong case for using only such products for all neonates, regardless of birth weight or serological status. Furthermore, to protect the fetus from serious infection, all seronegative mothers should be transfused with CMV-negative blood.

Although the best way of preventing CMV infection is by screening donors, alternatives, such as frozen deglycerolized red cell concentrates, also appear to be safe. The use of filters to remove leucocytes may also be effective in preventing infection (Adler 1988).

Bacterial infection

Bacterial contamination of blood for transfusion has become rare, through the introduction of rigorous hygienic practice for its collection, storage and transfusion. Introduction of single-use disposable plastic collection bags and disposable administration sets has also contributed to this improvement. Nevertheless, occasional infection does still occur. Clinical consequences of bacterial infection may depend on the general health of the recipient and also on the characteristics of the infective agent. Some organisms may cause only mild pyrexia or rigors, while more serious illness may be caused by organisms such as pseudomonas (Tabor & Gerety 1984). Each suspected case of bacterial infection should be thoroughly investigated by microscopic examination of the contents of the blood pack, cultures from the pack and the recipient's blood, and inspection of the pack for haemolysis and methaemoglobinaemia, the latter two features being suggestive of bacterial contamination.

Treponemal infection

Transfusion-transmitted syphilis was a problem in the early part of this century, when the infection was more common in the community and fresh, unrefrigerated blood was used for transfusion. The decline in prevalence of the disease and the introduction of screening tests have greatly decreased this risk. Furthermore, the exclusion of donors at high risk of venereal disease as a preventative measure against transfusion-acquired HIV infection may further reduce the already small risk. Refrigeration of blood for more than 5 days renders it noninfectious for *Treponema pallidum* (van der Sluis et al 1984), so transmission is likely to be encountered only with the use of fresh blood or platelets (Chambers et al 1969).

Protozoal infection

Malaria

Transfusion-acquired malaria is not limited to endemic areas. Tourists and other travellers may provide a source of infection in nonendemic areas. The infection is transmitted through red cells containing parasites and, thus, the risk with plasma products is minimal. The signs and symptoms of malaria may develop up to 3 months following an infested transfusion. Fever, chills, headache, nausea and vomiting, myalgia, hepatosplenomegaly and abdominal pain may develop. The speed of onset and severity of symptoms appear to depend on the number of parasites, the species of plasmodium, the patient's pre-existing immunity and concurrent administration of antimalarial drugs (Napier 1987). *Plasmodium falciparum* is associated with the most severe cases of transfusion-transmitted malaria, though *P.malaria* and *P.vivax* infections are more common (Sandler & Schorr 1987).

Premature infants and neonates appear to be at greater risk of transfusion-transmitted malaria, as are splenectomized and other immunodeficient recipients (Piccoli et al 1983, Shulman et al 1984, Joishy & Lopez 1980). Fatal infection is more frequent with the transfusion-transmitted route, largely because of delayed treatment through failure to recognize the illness. Treatment with antimalarials depends on the species of plasmodium.

Avoidance of transfusion-transmitted malaria depends on deferring donation from individuals returning from endemic areas and from those previously infected. More specific donor selection may be possible with newer immunoassays.

Other protozoal infections

Trypanosoma cruzi, the agent responsible for Chagas' disease, is a major hazard of blood transfusion in South America, and African trypanosomiasis has also been recognized after blood transfusion (Sandler & Schorr 1987). *Toxoplasma gondii* may be transmitted by cellular blood products, and may cause a glandular-fever-like illness which may be more serious in neonates and immunosuppressed individuals (Napier 1987).

COAGULOPATHY ASSOCIATED WITH BLOOD TRANSFUSION

Transfusion of blood may disturb the equilibrium of the coagulation system in several ways.

Thrombocytopenia

Stored whole blood and red cell concentrates contain very few functioning platelets. Massive transfusion, defined as equivalent to one total volume, or exchange transfusion allow dilutional thrombocytopenia to occur due to excessive loss of platelets and replacement by platelet-poor blood in a time scale where the bone marrow is unable to respond.

Several studies in massively transfused adults and children have shown that dilutional thrombocytopenia is a relatively common occurrence in this setting. In the majority of such cases, the reduction in platelet counts is moderate but may be severe depending on the pre-transfusion platelet count and on the volume of blood transfused (Mannucci et al 1982, Cote et al 1985). Dilutional thrombocytopenia may not be confined to subjects receiving rapid transfusions, and can arise in neonates in the intensive care setting, where thrombocytopenia may occur in up to 60% of such infants. Although no clear cause can be found in the majority of these, it has been suggested that multiple small transfusions may have been responsible (Mehta 1980). The effect of massive transfusion may not be limited to thrombocytopenia, as the functional integrity of platelets may be impaired, increasing the risk of haemorrhagic problems (Lim et al 1973).

Another factor which may increase severity of thrombocytopenia is the coexistence of disseminated intravascular coagulation (DIC). Hypovolaemic shock is a potent stimulus for DIC and subjects whose rate of blood loss warrants massive transfusion may be exposed to this additional hazard through inadequate volume replacement.

Thrombocytopenia is a well recognized complication of exchange transfusion, the physiological basis being similar to that of massive transfusion (Sacher & Lenes 1981). Dilutional thrombocytopenia probably accounts for most of such cases, and the use of fresh blood (less than 72 hours old) or platelet concentrates may prevent bleeding (Christensen et al 1982, Barnard et al 1980). However, the underlying problem for which exchange transfusion is given may also contribute, as evidenced by the study of Chessells & Wigglesworth (1971) in which they suggest that the hypersplenism and DIC seen in some cases of haemolytic disease of the newborn may exacerbate the thrombocytopenia.

The transfusion of relatively small volumes of blood may also cause thrombocytopenia, through the adherence of platelets to infused micro-aggregate debris and their subsequent removal from the circulation by the spleen (Bareford et al 1987, Lim et al 1989). These studies demonstrated a fall of up to 32.5% after transfusion by unfiltered blood. While this transient thrombocytopenia is likely to be clinically insignificant in patients with normal pre-transfusion platelet counts, such a fall in platelet count may precipitate haemorrhage in severely thrombocytopenic children, such as those with bone marrow failure (Lim et al 1989). These studies also showed that filtration of blood using either a 40 μm microaggregate or polyester fibre filter could diminish post-transfusion thrombocytopenia caused by remaining microaggregates, and thus might be considered for use in severely thrombocytopenic individuals.

Post-transfusion purpura – an acute episode of severe immune thrombocytopenia occurring approximately a week after transfusion – is closely associated with alloimmunization by platelet-specific antigens, and is usually seen in a Pl^{A1}-positive pregnancy or transfusion. However, this problem has not been seen thus far in paediatric practice, since the age range of affected individuals to date has been 16–18 years (Waters 1989).

Deficiency of coagulation factors

The extent to which transfused blood causes dilution of coagulation factors also depends on the choice of product used, its volume and the clinical problem prompting its use (Mannucci et al 1982, Collins 1976). Red cell concentrates with reduced plasma volume have reduced concentrations of most coagulation factors and, if used, in large quantities relative to the blood volume of the recipient, may require concomitant administration of fresh frozen plasma. Stored whole blood, often the preparation of choice in massive exchange transfusions, has been shown to contain haemostatic levels of factors II, VII, IX, X, XII, XIII and fibrinogen up to the usual maximum shelf-life of 35 days (Nilssen et al 1983). Depletion of the more labile coagulation factors V and VIII may, however, occur with increasing length of storage.

Factor VIII concentrations fall relatively rapidly to around 50% of the initial value within 24 hours (Urbaniak & Cash 1977, Nilsson et al 1983), but concentration falls more slowly thereafter so that levels of 20% are found at 21 days (Napier 1987). The use of relatively fresh whole blood may therefore avoid significant dilution of these factors.

Abnormalities of coagulation tests have been noted in a relatively high proportion of massively transfused subjects (Mannucci 1982), but most are of doubtful clinical significance. When more serious disturbances are found, there is often evidence of other causes of coagulopathy, such as liver disease or shock-related DIC (Mannucci et al 1982, Lim et al 1973, Miller et al 1971, Collins 1976).

As mentioned previously, inadequate volume replacement during blood loss may cause DIC through hypovolaemic shock. Collins (1976) suggests that the transfusion of large amounts of stored blood containing activated coagulation factors and thromboplastin from disrupted erythrocytes and granulocytes may also contribute. Other, hopefully rare, causes of transfusion-associated DIC include haemolytic transfusion reaction (Ratroff 1984) and septic shock caused by infected blood.

The risk of significant coagulopathy associated with blood transfusion is low in the vast majority of children receiving low volumes of blood in relation to their total body volume. Potential problems exist with massive transfusion, exchange transfusion or in the presence of a pre-existing coagulopathy. Careful evaluation of such children should include early and regular monitoring with appropriate laboratory screening tests of coagulation. Particular care should be exercised in obtaining such samples, especially the avoidance of contamination of heparin from indwelling catheters, and artefactual coagulation abnormalities caused by poor technique. Dilutional coagulopathy may be prevented by correct choice of blood product, such as fresh whole blood in the case of massive transfusion. Where this is not readily available, supplementation by platelet concentrates of fresh frozen plasma should be guided by the results of coagulation tests (Mannucci et al 1982, Napier 1987).

REFERENCES

Adler S P 1988 Cytomegalovirus and transfusions. Transfusion Medicine Reviews 4: 235–244

Allen F H, Diamond L K (eds) 1958 Erythroblastosis fetalis. Little, Brown, Boston

Alter J H, Purcell R H, Holland P V 1981 Donor transaminase and recipient hepatitis : impact on blood transfusion services. Journal of the American Medical Association 246: 630–634

Alter J H, Purcell R H, Shih J W et al 1989 Detection of antibody to hepatitis C virus in prospectively followed transfusion recipients with acute and chronic non-A, non-B hepatitis. New England Journal of Medicine 321: 1494–1500

Ammann A J 1985 The acquired immunodeficiency syndrome in infants and children. Annals of Internal Medicine 103: 734–737

Barabara J A J, Contreras M 1990 Infectious complications of blood transfusion: viruses. In: Contreras M (ed) ABC of Transfusion. British Medical Journal Publications, London p 49–52

Barabara J A J, Tedder R S 1984 Viral infections transmitted by blood and its products. Clinics in Haematology 13: 693–707

Barabara J A J, Tegtmeier G E 1987 Cytomegalovirus and blood transfusion. Blood Reviews 1: 207–211

Bareford D, Changler S T, Hawker R J et al 1987 Splenic platelet sequestration following routine blood transfusions is reduced by filtered/washed blood products. British Journal of Haematology 67: 177–180

Barnard D R, Chapman R G, Simmons M A, Hathaway W E 1980 Blood for use in exchange transfusion in the newborn. Transfusion 20: 401–408

Barry M, Flynn D M, Letsky E A et al 1974 Longterm chelation therapy in thalassaemia major : effect on liver iron concentration, liver histology and clinical progress. British Medical Journal 2: 16–20

Berry C L, Marshall W C 1967 Iron distribution in the liver of patients with thalassaemia major. Lancet 1: 1031–1033

Blumberg N, Peck K, Ross K, Avila E 1983 Immune response to chronic red blood cell transfusion. Vox Sanguinis 44: 212–217

Borgna-Pignatti C, de Stefano P, Broglia A M 1984 Visual loss in patient on high-dose subcutaneous desferrioxamine. Lancet I: 681

Bothwell T H, Abrahams C, Bradlow B A et al 1965 Idiopathic and Bantu hemochromatosis. Archives of Pathology 79:163–168

Bove J R 1987 Transfusion-associated hepatitis and AIDS. New England Journal of Medicine 317: 242–245

Bracey A W, Klein H, Deisseroth A et al 1981 Selective isolation of young erythrocytes for transfusion support of thalassaemia major patients. Blood 57: 599–606

Brubaker D B 1983 Human posttransfusion graft-versus-host-disease. Vox Sanguinis 45: 401–420

Bucholz D H, Miripol J, Aster R H et al 1988 Ultraviolet irradiation of platelets to prevent recipient alloimmunisation. Transfusion 28: 26S

Centres for Disease Control 1982 Possible transfusion-associated acquired immune deficiency syndrome (AIDS) – California. Morbidity and Mortality Weekly Report 31: 652–654

Chambers R W, Foley H T, Schmidt P J 1969 Transmission of syphilis by fresh blood components. Transfusion

9: 32–34

Chessells J M, Wigglesworth J S 1971 Haemostatic failure in babies with rhesus isoimmunization. Archives of Diseases in Childhood 46: 38–45

Chiu H Y, Flynn D M, Hoffbrand A V, Politis D 1986 Infection with Yersinia enterocolitica in patients with iron overload. British Medical Journal 292: 97

Choo Q-L, Kuo G, Weiner A J et al 1989 Isolation of a cDNA clone derived from a blood-borne non-A, non-B viral hepatitis genome. Science 244: 359–362

Christensen R D, Anstall H B, Rothstein G 1982 Use of whole blood exchange transfusion to supply neutrophils to septic neutropaenic neonates. Transfusion 22: 504–509

Cohen A 1987 Management of iron overload in the paediatric patient. Haematology/Oncology Clinics of North America 1(3): 521–544

Cohen A, Martin M, Schwartz E 1981 Response to long term desferrioxamine therapy in thalassaemia. Journal of Pediatrics 99: 689–694

Cohen A, Martin M, Schwartz E 1984 Depletion of excessive liver iron stores with desferrioxamine. British Journal of Haematology 58: 369–373

Cohen A, Sherwood W C, Busen S 1980 Transfusion therapy for hemolytic disease of the newborn. In: Sherwood W C, Cohen A (eds) Transfusion therapy, the fetus, infant and child Masson, New York, p 113–126

Cohen A R, Schmidt J M, Martin M B, Barnsley W 1984 Clinical trial of young red cell transfusions. Journal of Pediatrics 104: 865–868

Coles S M, Klein H G, Holland P V 1981 Alloimmunisation in two multitransfused patient populations. Transfusion 21: 462–466

Collins J A 1976 Massive blood transfusion. Clinics in Haematology 5: 201–222

Conrad M E 1981 Diseases transmissible by blood transfusion : viral hepatitis and other infectious disorders. Seminars in Haematology 18: 122–146

Contreras M, Barabara J A J, Anderson C C et al 1991 Low incidence of non-A, non-B post transfusion hepatitis in London confirmed by hepatitis C serology. Lancet 337: 753–757

Contreras M, Hewitt P E 1985 Prevention of AIDS. Lancet ii: 1362

Contreras M E, Barabara J A J 1990 Retroviruses and blood transfusion. Clinical Haematology 6:1: 65–77

Contreras M, Mollison P L 1990 Immunological complications of transfusion. In: Contreras M (ed) ABC of transfusion. British Medical Journal Publication, London, p 41–44

Cooper D A, Naclean P, Finlayson R et al 1985 Acute AID retrovirus infection. Definition of a clinical illness associated with seroconversion. Lancet i: 538–540

Corash L, Klein H, Diesseroth A et al 1981 Selective isolation of young erythrocytes for transfusion support of thalassaemia major patients. Blood 57: 599–606

Cote C J, Liu M P L, Szyfelbein S K, Goudsousian N G, 1985 Changes in serial platelet counts following massive blood transfusion in paediatric patients. Anaesthesiology 62: 197–201

Crossart Y E, Kirsch S, Ismay S L, 1982 Post-transfusion hepatitis in Australia. Lancet i: 208–213

Daly P A, Schiffer C A, Aisner J, Wiernik P H 1980 Platelet transfusion therapy : one-hour post transfusion increments are valuable in predicting the need for HLA-matched preparations. Journal of the American Medical Association

243: 435–438

Davies S C, Marcus R E, Hungerford J L 1983 Ocular toxicity of high-dose intravenous desferrioxamine. Lancet ii: 181–184

De Alarcon P A, Donovan M E, Forbes G B, Landlow S A 1979 Iron absorption in the thalassaemic syndromes and its inhibition by tea. New England Journal of Medicine 300: 5–8

de Rie M A, van der Plas-van Dalen Engelfriet C P, von dem Borne A E G Kr 1985 The serology of febrile transfusion reactions. Vox Sanguinis 49: 126–134

de Virgilis S, Sanna G, Cornacchia G et al 1980 Serum ferritin, liver iron stores, and liver histology in children with thalassaemia. Archives of Disease in Childhood 55: 43–45

Diamond L K, Allen D, Magill F B 1961 Congenital (erythroid) hypoplastic anaemia. A 25-year study. American Journal of Diseases of Children 102: 403–415

Dickerhoff R 1987 Acute aplasia and loss of vision with desfetrioxamine overdose. American Journal of Pediatric Hematology/Oncology 9: 287–288

Dolan G, Hale J, Bellamy G, Forman K M 1991 Hepatitis C infection in multitransfused children. British Journal of Haematology 77 (suppl 1): 21

Duquesnoy R J, Anderson A J, Tomasulo P A, Aster R H 1979 ABO compatibility and platelet transfusions of alloimmunised thrombocytopenic patients. Blood 54: 595–599

Dutcher J P, Schiffer C A, Aisner J, Weirnik P H 1981 Delayed alloimmunisation following platelet transfusion : the absence of a dose-response relationship. Blood 57: 395–398

Dutcher J P, Schiffer C A, Johnston G S et al 1983 Alloimmunisation prevents the migration of transfused Indium-111-labelled granulocytes to sites of infection. Blood 62: 354–360

Esteban J L, Esteban R, Viladomiu L et al 1989 Hepatitis C virus antibodies among risk groups in Spain. Lancet ii: 294–297

Evatt B L, Gomperts E D, McDougle J S, Ramsey R B 1985 Coincidental appearance of LAV/HTLV III antibodies in hemophiliacs and the onset of the AIDS epidemic. New England Journal of Medicine 312: 483–486

Floss A M, Strauss R G 1984 Multiple transfusions fail to provoke antibodies against blood cell antigens in human infants. Transfusion 24: 429 (abstr)

Ford J M, Brown L M, Cullen M H, Oliver R T D 1982 Combined granulocyte and platelet transfusions. Development of alloimmunization as reflected by decreasing cell recovery values. Transfusion 22: 498–503

Forman K M 1987 Blood and blood product transfusion in children. In: Hinchliffe R F, Lilleyman J S (eds) Practical paediatric haematology. Wiley, Chichester, p 81–102

Freedman M H, Bentur Y, Koreu G 1989 Biological and toxic properties of desferrioxamine. Progress in Clinical and Biological Research 309: 115–124

Fullerton M W, Philippart AI Sarnaik S, Lusher J M 1981 Preoperative exchange transfusion in sickle cell anaemia. Journal of Pediatric Surgery 16: 297–300

Gabutti V, Piga A, Fortina P et al 1980 Correlation between transfusion requirement, blood volume and haemoglobin level in homozygous beta thalassaemia. Acta Haematologica 64: 103–108

Gallo R C, Sarin P S, Gelmann E P et al 1983 Isolation of human T-cell leukaemia virus in acquired immune deficiency syndrome (AIDS). Science 220: 865–67

Gascon P, Zoumbos N C, Young N S 1984 Immunologic abnormalities in patients receiving multiple blood transfusions. Annals of Internal Medicine 100: 173–177

Gazzard B 1990 AIDS: clinical picture and management. Clinical Haematology 3(1): 1–35

Giacomo L, Dell'Osso A, Iannone A et al 1983 Phenotypic immaturity of T & B lymphocytes in cord blood in full term neonates. Biology of the Neonate 44: 303–308

Gill F M 1980 Transfusion therapy for coagulation disorders in the infant. In: Sherwood W C, Cohen A (eds) Transfusion therapy, the fetus, infant and child. Masson, New York, pp 75–94

Graziano J H, Piomelli S, Seaman C et al 1982 A simple technique for preparation of young red cells for transfusion from ordinary blood units. Blood 59: 865–868

Gross S, Melhorn D K 1971 Exchange transfusion with citrated whole blood for disseminated intravascular coagulation. Journal of Paediatrics 78: 415–419

Guttuso M A, Williams M L, Oski F A 1976 The role of exchange transfusions in the management of low birth weight infants with and without severe respiratory distress syndrome. Journal of Pediatrics 78: 279–285

Harker L A, Funk D D, Finch C A 1968 Evaluation of storage iron by chelates. American Journal of Medicine 45: 105–115

Harris M B 1987 Neonatal host-defence mechanisms. In: Kasprisin D O, Luban N L C (eds) Pediatric Transfusion Medicine 1 CRC Press, Boca Raton, p 69–78

Hershko C, Pinson A, Link G 1990 Iron chelation. Blood Reviews 4: 1–8

Herve P, Lamy B, Peters A, Tobin M 1980 Preservation of human erythrocytes in the liquid state : biological results with a new medium. Vox Sanguinis 39: 195–204

Hogman C F, Hedlund K, Zetterstrom H 1978 Clinical usefulness of red cells preserved in protein-poor mediums. New England Journal of Medicine 299: 1377–1382

Hogman C F, Andreen M, Rosen I, Akerblom O 1983a Hemotherapy with red-cell concentrates and a new red-cell storage medium. Lancet i: 269–272

Hogman C F, Akerblom O, Hedlund K, Wiklund L 1983b Red cell suspensions in SAG-M medium. Further experience of in-vivo survival of red cells, clinical usefulness, and plasma-saving effects. Vox Sanguinis 45: 217–223

Hollinger F B, Khan N C, Oefinger P E et al 1983 Post transfusion hepatitis type A. Journal of American Medical Association 250: 2313–2317

Holohan T V, Terasaki P I, Deisseroth A B 1981 Suppression of transfusion-related alloimmunization in intensively treated cancer patients. Blood 58: 122–128

Howard J E, Perkins H A 1978 The natural history of alloimmunisation to platelets. Transfusion 18: 496–503

Hows J M, Brozovic B 1990 Platelet and granulocyte therapy. In: Contreras M (ed) ABC of transfusion. British Medical Journal Publications, London, p 14–17

Hussain M A M, Flynn D M, Green N et al 1976 Subcutaneous infusion and intramuscular injection of desferrioxamine in patients with transfusional iron overload. Lancet ii: 1278–1281

Hyman C B, Agness C I, Rodriguez-Funes R et al 1985 Combined subcutaneous and high dose intravenous desferrioxamine therapy of thalassaemia. Annals of New York Academy of Sciences 445: 293–303

Iancu T C, Landing B H, Neustein H B 1977 Pathogenic mechanisms in hepatic cirrhosis of thalassaemia major :

light and electron microscopic studies. Pathology Annual 12: 171–200

Jandl J H, Tomlinson A S 1958 The destruction of red cells by antibodies in man. II. Pyrogenic, leukocytic and dermal responses to immune hemolysis. Journal of Clinical Investigations 37: 1202–1228

Joishy S K, Lopez C G 1980 Transfusion-induced malaria in a splenectomised beta-thalassaemia major patient and review of blood donor screening methods. American Journal of Haematology 8: 221–229

Kaltwasser J P, Werner E 1989 Diagnosis and clinical evaluation of iron overload. Clinical Haematology 2(2): 363–389

Karpadia A, De Souze M, Markenson A L et al 1980 Lymphoid cell sets and serum immunoglobulins in patients with thalassaemia intermedia : relationship to serum iron and splenectomy. British Journal of Haematology 45: 405–416

Kernoff P B A, Lee C A, Karayannis P, Thomas H C 1985 High risk of non-A non-B hepatitis after a first exposure to volunteer or commercial clotting factor concentrates : effects of prophylactic immune serum globin. British Journal of Haematology 60: 469–479

Kevy S V 1979 Pechatric transfusion therapy. Laboratory Medicine 10: 459–466

Kim H C, Barnsley W, Sweisfurth A W 1984 Incidence of alloimmunisation in multiple transfused pediatric patients. Transfusion 24: 417 (abstr)

Klemperer M 1981 Perinatal and neonatal transfusion. In: Petz L D, Swisher S N (eds) Clinical practice of blood transfusion. Churchill Livingstone, New York, p 659–718

Knodell R G, Conrad M E, Dienstag J L, Bell C J 1975 Etiological spectrum of post transfusion hepatitis. Gastroenterology 69: 1278–1285

Kouides P A, Slapak C A, Rosenwasser L J et al 1988 Pneumocystis carinii pneumonia as a complication of desferrioxamine therapy. British Journal of Haematology 70: 382–384

Kuo G, Choo Q-L, Alter J H et al 1989 An assay for circulating antibodies to a major etiologic virus of human non-A, non-B hepatitis. Science 244: 362–364

Lancet editorial 1984 Yersiniosis today. Lancet i: 84–85

Lancet editorial 1975 Non-A, non-β? Lancet ii: 64–65

Lancet editorial 1990 Hepatitis C upstanding. Lancet 335: 1431–1432

Langenscheidt F, Kiefel V, Santoso S, Mueller-Eckhardt C 1988 Platelet transfusion refractoriness associated with two rare platelet-specific alloantibodies (anti-Bak a and anti-Pl A2) and multiple HLA antibodies. Transfusion 28: 597–600

Leitman S F, Holland P V 1985 Irradiation of blood products. Indications and guidelines. Transfusion 25: 293–300

Letsky E A, Miller F, Worwood M et al 1974 Serum ferritin in children with thalassaemia regularly transfused. Journal of Clinical Pathology 27: 652–655

Ley T J, Griffith P, Nienhuis A W 1982 Transfusion haemosiderosis and chelation therapy. Clinics in Haematology 11: 437–454

Lim R C, Olcott C, Robinson A et al 1973 Platelet response and coagulation changes following massive blood replacement. Journal of Trauma 13: 557–582

Lim S, Boughton B J, Bareford D 1989 Thrombocytopenia following routine blood transfusion : microaggregate blood filters prevent worsening thrombocytopenia in patients with low platelet counts. Vox Sanguinis 56: 40–41

Luban N L C, Dolan M A 1984 Transfusion reactions in pediatric patients. Plasma Therapy and Transfusion Technology 5: 159–172

Ludlam C A, Chapman D, Cohen B, Litton P A 1989 Antibodies to hepatitis C virus in haemophilia. Lancet ii: 560–561

Ludvigsen C, Swanson J, Thompson T, McCullough J 1982 Failure of neonates to form red cell antibodies following transfusion. Transfusion 24: 405 (abstr)

Makris M, Preston F E, Triger D R et al 1990 Hepatitis C antibody and chronic liver disease in haemophilia. Lancet 335: 1117–1119

Mannucci P M, Federici A B, Sirchia G 1982 Hemostasis testing during massive blood replacement. A study of 172 cases. Vox Sanguinis 42: 113–123

Marcus R E, Huehns E R 1985 Transfusional iron overload. Clinical and Laboratory Haematology 7: 195–212

Marsh M N, Holbrook I B, Clark C et al 1981 Tinnitus in a patient with beta-thalassaemia intermedia on long term treatment with desferrioxamine. Postgraduate Medical Journal 57: 582–584

Mehta P, Vasa R, Neumann L 1980 Thrombocytopenia in the high risk infant. Journal of Pediatrics 97: 791–794

Mentinove J E, Aster R H 1983 Transfusion of platelets and plasma products. Clinics in Haematology 12: 239–266

Miller R D, Robbins T O, Tong M J 1971 Coagulation defects associated with massive blood transfusion. Annals of Surgery 174: 794–803

Modell B, Berdoukas V (eds) 1984 The clinical approach to thalassaemia. Grune & Stratton, London

Modell C B, Beck J 1974 Longterm desferrioxamine therapy in thalassaemia. Annals of New York Academy of Sciences 232: 201–210

Mollison P L (ed) 1987 Blood transfusion in clinical medicine, 7th edn. Blackwell Scientific Publications, Oxford

Munn C G, Markenson A L, Karpadia A, DeSousa M 1981 Impaired T-cell mitogen responses in some patients with thalassaemia intermedia. Thymus 3: 119–128

Murphy M F, Waters A H 1990 Platelet transfusions : the problem of refractoriness. Blood Reviews 4: 16–24

Murphy M F, Metcalfe P, Ord J, Lister T A 1987 Disappearance of HLA and platelet-specific antibodies in acute leukaemia patients alloimmunised by multiple transfusions. British Journal Haematology 67: 255–260

Napier J A F (ed) 1987 Transfusion for massive blood loss. In: Napier J A F (ed) Blood transfusion therapy. Wiley, Chichester, 169–179

Necheles R F, Chung S, Sabbah R et al 1974 Intensive transfusion therapy in thalassaemia major : an eight year follow up. Annals of the New York Academy of Science 232: 179–185

Nienhuis A W 1981 Vitamin C and iron. New England Journal of Medicine 304: 170–171

Nilsson L, Hedner U, Nilsson I M, Robertson B 1983 Shelf-life of bank blood and stored plasma with special reference to coagulation factors. Transfusion 23: 377–381

Oliveri N F, Buncic J R, Chew E et al 1986 Visual and auditory neurotoxicity in patients receiving subcutaneous desferrioxamine infusions. New England Journal of Medicine 314: 869–873

Orlina A R, Unger P J, Koshy M 1978 Post transfusion alloimmunisation in patients with sickle cell disease. American Journal of Hematology 5: 101–106

Piccoli D A, Perlman S, Ephros M 1983 Transfusion acquired *Plasmodium malariae* infection in two premature infants. Pediatrics 72: 560–563

Pineda A A, Taswell H F, 1975 Transfusion reactions associated with anti-IgA antibodies : report of four cases and review of the literature. Transfusion 15:10–15

Piomelli S, Seaman C, Reibman J et al 1978 Separation of younger red cells with improved survival in vivo. An approach to chronic transfusion therapy. Proceedings of the National Academy of Sciences USA 75: 3474–3478

Piomelli S, Karpatkin M H, Arzanian M et al 1974 Hypertransfusion regimen in patients with Cooley's anemia. Annals of the New York Academy of Science 232: 186–192

Piomelli S, Hart D, Graziano J et al 1985 Current strategies in the management of Cooley's anaemia. Annals of the New York Academy of Science 445: 256–260

Pippard M, Callendar S T 1983 The management of iron chelation therapy. British Journal of Haematology 54: 503–507

Pippard M J, Callendar S T, Finch C A 1982 Ferrioxamine excretion in iron-loaded man. Blood 60: 99–106

Pool J G, Shannon A E 1985 Production of high-potency concentrates of anti-hemophilic globulin in a closed-bag system : assay in vitro and in vivo. New England Journal of Medicine 273: 1443–1447

Porter J B, Huehns E R 1989 Toxic effects of desferrioxamine. Clinical Haematology 2(2): 459–474

Porter J B, East C A, Jaswon M S, Huehns E R 1988 Audiometric abnormalities in thalassaemia; risk factor associated with the use of desferrioxamine. British Journal of Haematology 69: 107 (abstr)

Propper R D, Button L N, Nathan D G 1980 New approaches to the transfusion management of thalassaemia. Blood 55: 55–60

Ratnoff O D 1984 Disseminated intravascular coagulation. In: Ratnoff O D, Forbes C D (eds) Disorders of hemostasis. Grune & Stratton, Orlando, Florida, p 289–319

Rebulla P, Modell B 1991 Transfusion requirements and effects in patients with thalassaemia major. Lancet 337: 227–280

Risdon R A, Barry M, Flynn D M, 1975 Transfusional iron overload : the relationship between tissue iron concentration and hepatic fibrosis in thalassaemias. Journal of Pathology 116: 83–95

Rizetto M, Canese M G, Arko S et al 1977 Immunofluorescence detection of a new antigen-antibody system [gamma/anti-gamma] associated to the hepatitis B virus in the liver and the serum of HBsAg carriers. Gut 18: 997–1003

Rogers M 1985 AIDS in children: a review of the clinical epidemiologic and public health aspects. Pediatric Infectious Disease Journal 4: 230–236

Ryan B, Connor E, Minnefor A, Desposito F 1987 Human immunodeficiency virus (HIV) infection in children. Hematology/Oncology Clinics of North America 1(3): 381–395

Ryden S E, Oberman H 1975 Compatibility of common intravenous solutions with CPD blood. Transfusion 15: 250–255

Sacher R A, Leues B A 1981 Exchange transfusion. Clinical and Laboratory Medicine 1: 265–283

Saenger P, Schwartz E, Markenson A L et al 1980 Depressed serum somatomedin activity in beta thalassaemia. Journal of Pediatrics 96: 214–218

Sandler G, Berry E, Zlotnick A 1976 Benign hemoglobinuria following transfusion of accidentally frozen blood. Journal of the American Medical Association 235: 2850–2851

Sandler S G, Schorr J B 1987 Acquired immunodeficiency syndrome and other transfusion-transmissible diseases. In: Kasprisin D O, Luban N L C (eds) Pediatric transfusion medicine, vol II. CRC Press, Boca Raton, p 145–165

Schiffer C A, Aisner J, Daly P A, Schimpff S C 1979 Alloimmunisation following prophylactic granulocyte transfusion. Blood 54: 766–774

Scott G B, Buck B E, Leterman J G et al 1984 Acquired immunodeficiency syndrome in infants. New England Journal of Medicine 310: 76–81

Seef L B, Wright E C, Zimmerman H J 1975 VA cooperative study post-transfusion hepatitis, 1969–1974: Incidence and characteristics of hepatitis and possible risk factors. American Journal of Medical Sciences 270: 355–362

Shannon K M, Ammann A J 1985 Acquired immune deficiency syndrome in childhood. Journal of Pediatrics 106: 332–342

Shulman I A, Saxena S, Nelson J M, Furmanski M 1984 Neonatal exchange transfusions complicated by transfusion-induced malaria. Pediatrics 73: 330–332

Sills R H, Stuart M J 1980 Platelet transfusion in the newborn. In: Sherwood W C, Cohen A (eds) Transfusion therapy, the fetus, infant and child. Masson, New York, p 95–111

Sintnicolaas K, Sizoo W, Haije W G et al 1981 Delayed alloimmunisation by random single donor platelet transfusion. A randomised study to compare single donor and multiple donor platelet transfusions in cancer patients with severe thrombocytopenia. Lancet i: 750–753

Skidmore S J, Pasi K J, Mawson S J, Williams M D 1990 Serological evidence that dry heating of clotting factor concentrates prevents transmission of non-A, non-B hepatitis. Journal of Medical Virology 30: 50–52

Smith M, Storey C G 1984 Allo-anti-E in an 18 day old infant. Transfusion 24: 540

Tabor E, Gerety R J 1984 Five cases of pseudomonas sepsis transmitted by blood transfusions. Lancet i: 1403

Underwood J C E 1990 Hepatitis C virus and transfusion transmitted liver disease : review. Journal of Clinical Pathology 43: 445–447

Urbaniak S J, Cash J D 1977 Blood replacement therapy. British Medical Bulletin 33: 273–282

Urbaniak S J 1985 Rh(D) haemolytic disease of the newborn: the changing scene. British Medical Journal 291: 4–6

van der Sluid J J, Onvlee P C, Kothe F C H A et al 1984 Transfusion syphilis, survival of *Treponema pallidum* in donor blood I. Report of an orientating study. Vox Sanguinis 47(3): 197–204

Vaughan R L 1982 Morbidity due to exchange transfusion with heat-hemolized blood. American Journal of Kidney Diseases in Children 136: 646–648

Walker J A, Sherman R A, Eisinger R P 1985 Thrombocytopenia associated with intravenous desferrioxamine. American Journal of Kidney Disease 6: 254–256

Wantanabe J, Minegishi K, Mitsumori T et al 1990 Prevalence of anti-HCV antibody on blood donors in the Tokyo area. Vox Sanguinis 59: 86–88

Wapnick A A, Lynch S R, Charlton R B et al 1969 The effect of ascorbic acid deficiency on desferrioxamine induced urinary iron excretion. British Journal of Haematology

17: 563–568

Waters A H 1989 Post-transfusion purpura. Blood Reviews 3: 83–87

Waxman H S, Brown E B 1969 Clinical usefulness of iron chelating agents. Progress in Haematology vi: 338–373

Wills E D 1972 Effects of iron overload on lipid peroxide formation and oxidative demethylation by the liver endoplasmic reticulum. Biochemical Pharmacology 21: 239–247

Wolfe L, Epstein M, Kevy S V 1983 Blood transfusion for the neonatal patient. Human Pathology 14(3): 256–260

Wolman I J 1964 Transfusion therapy in Cooley's anaemia : growth and health as related to long range haemoglobin levels. A progress report. Annals of the New York Academy of Science 119: 736–747

Wolman I J, Ortolani M 1969 Some clinical features of Cooley's anaemia as related to transfusion schedules. Annals of New York Academy of Science 165: 407–414

Wonke B, Hoffbrand A V, Aldouri M et al 1989 Reversal of desferrioxamine induced auditory neurotoxicity during treatment with G-DPTA. Archives of Disease in Childhood 6: 77–82

Woodcock B E 1987 Iron deficiency and iron overload. In: Hinchliffe R F, Lilleyman J S (eds) Practical paediatric haematology. Wiley, Chichester, p 161–194

Worwood M 1990 Ferritin. Blood Reviews 4: 259–269

Yeager A, Grumet F C, Hafleight E, Arvin A 1981 Prevention of transfusion-acquired cytomegalovirus infections in new born infants. Journal of Pediatrics 98: 281–287

15. Non-haematological disorders with major effects on blood or bone marrow

E. Simpson

INTRODUCTION

The haemopoietic system is affected by many disorders that primarily involve other systems. Abnormalities may exist from presentation of the primary disorder, or evolve during the course of the disease, either directly or as a result of treatment. Haematological features may be sufficiently striking for initial referral to be to a haematologist, or the haematologist may be called upon to perform specialized investigations leading to a diagnosis. Frequently, abnormalities are multifactorial in origin, and the haematological findings reflect circumstances peculiar to an individual patient. Many of the abnormalities found in cardiac, renal, gastrointestinal and respiratory disorders are fully discussed in the appropriate sections of this book. There are, however, some disorders which produce characteristic haematological problems and which are not covered elsewhere. These are considered in more detail below.

ANAEMIA OF CHRONIC DISEASE

Anaemia of chronic disease is a diagnosis of exclusion caused by a wide range of disorders, including malignancy, connective tissue disorders, and infections. Generally, the anaemia is mild, of slow onset with normochromic normocytic red cells, and associated with normal or low reticulocytes. It is characterized by a low serum iron, iron binding capacity and transferrin saturation, but normal or raised serum ferritin and stainable reticuloendothelial iron (Stockman 1987). Hypochromia and microcytosis are seen, but less commonly than is generally supposed. The aetiology is complex. Some conditions produce shortened red cell survival, although the reason for this is unknown. A defective marrow response to anaemia is noted, with one- to two-fold increase in erythropoiesis seen, rather than the normal six- to eight-fold response. It is not known if this is caused by a relative resistance to erythropoietin, or defective release of erythropoietin. A third mechanism is reduced release of iron from reticuloendothelial cells for use in the marrow. Iron absorption in the gut remains normal or low. In chronic inflammation, the rate of fall of haemoglobin has been found to be 1.8 g/dl every 6 days. Other contributing factors in these varied conditions are bleeding, haemolysis, nutritional deficiencies and drug-induced red cell changes.

Connective tissue disorders

Although all connective tissue disorders may have the features of anaemia of chronic disease described above, other more specific haematological features may be observed.

Rheumatoid arthritis

True iron deficiency may be present as a result of gastrointestinal blood loss from analgesics, particularly salicylates, and steroid ingestion. Thrombocytosis may be seen from bleeding, and a neutrophilia is observed in flare-up of the disease requiring differentiation from secondary bacterial infections. Twenty per cent of children with juvenile rheumatoid arthritis have splenomegaly, although not necessarily the triad of rheumatoid arthritis, splenomegaly and neutropenia described by Felty. Neutropenia may result from hypersplenism alone, or be immune-mediated with detectable anti-neutrophil IgG antibodies. It does not always resolve after splenectomy. There is evidence in some patients for a granulocyte maturation arrest, with low levels of granulocyte colony-stimulating activity.

Systemic lupus erythematosus (SLE)

Many haematological changes in addition to anaemia of chronic disease have been described in systemic lupus erythematosus (SLE). Autoantibodies to red cells, neutrophils or platelets result in peripheral destruction, reflected by cytopenias and increased marrow precursors. In contrast, SLE may be the cause of marrow aplasia, or selective granulocyte aplasia. Lymphopenia, with abnormalities of T-cell function proportional to disease activity, is common. Circulating 'lupus anticoagulant', seen in other conditions as well as SLE, is discussed elsewhere (p. 423), but results in a paradoxical tendency to thromboembolic phenomena.

Polyarteritis nodosa

Microangiopathic haemolytic anaemia is seen in association with renal disease or hypertensive crises. Eosinophilia is also prominent.

Wegener's granulomatosis

This is rare in childhood, but presents with fever, cough, haemoptysis, epistaxis, nasal discharge, nodular pulmonary infiltrates and renal failure as the result of widespread necrotizing vasculitis. Haematological features include normochromic, normocytic anaemia, red cell fragmentation typical of microangiopathic haemolytic anaemia, leucocytosis with neutrophilia and eosinophilia, and thrombocytosis.

HAEMATOLOGICAL FEATURES OF INFECTION

Peripheral blood film changes affecting all cell lines are frequent but rarely diagnostic features of infection. Chronic bacterial infections, such as tuberculosis and osteomyelitis, result in anaemia of chronic disease, but other infections can cause an acute and severe anaemia. Haemoglobin may fall precipitously as a result of acute intravascular haemolysis due to haemolysin release in clostridial, staphylococcal, streptococcal and haemophilus infections. Anaemia, following haemolysis and bleeding, is seen in disseminated intravascular coagulation (DIC) due to meningococcal and other septicaemias. *Mycoplasma*, *Listeria* and *Epstein–Barr* viral (EBV) infections can present with immune-mediated haemolytic anaemia with cold agglutinins.

A neutrophilia is usually found in bacterial infections, with morphological findings of toxic granulation, Döhle bodies, and occasional neutrophil vacuolation. The leucocyte alkaline phosphatase score is high, and increased bacterial killing is seen with nitroblue tetrazolium dye testing. Neonates may respond to severe bacterial infection with neutropenia, but other neutrophil features typical of infection are seen. Typhoid fever produces a profound leucopenia and neutropenia early in the course of the disease. Bilobed neutrophils (pseudo Pelger–Huet anomaly) occur in tuberculosis. A monocytosis is usually seen in tuberculosis, syphilis and subacute bacterial endocarditis, and is also seen in the recovery phase following neutropenic episodes for any reason.

Viral infections, such as EBV or hepatitis, are occasionally the suspected cause of aplastic anaemia. Selective red cell aplasia commonly follows parvovirus infection, and patients with underlying increased red cell turnover develop a self-limiting, profound anaemia – the so-called 'aplastic crisis' described in sickle cell anaemia and hereditary spherocytosis. No infectious cause for transient erythroblastopenia of childhood has yet been identified, but it is probably viral in origin.

Viral infections can cause leucopenia (hepatitis B, EBV, rubella, measles, influenza) or lymphocytosis (EBV, cytomegalovirus (CMV), mumps, rubella, hepatitis B). Cat-scratch fever (probably chlamydial in origin) presents with a marked lymphocytosis, as does pertussis. Transplacental infection with 'TORCH' organisms (toxoplasmosis, rubella, CMV, herpes and syphilis) may cause intrauterine death, severe neonatal haemolysis, or failure to thrive associated with pancytopenia and hepatosplenomegaly in addition to the recognized syndromes of fetal damage.

On a global scale, parasitic infections are a

common cause of iron deficiency anaemia, with chronic blood loss from gastrointestinal parasites, such as hookworm, resulting in a chronic debilitating illness throughout the third world. *Schistosoma haematobium* infiltrates the genitourinary tract, causing haematuria and eventual renal failure from fibrotic outflow tract obstruction; other species, particularly *S. mansoni* cause hepatic fibrosis, portal hypertension, hypersplenism, and bleeding from oesophageal varices. Parasitic infestation is also an important cause of eosinophilia; the parasites most commonly responsible are listed in Table 15.1. Eosinophilia may also be seen as an allergic response to fungal infections, particularly *Aspergillus*. Parasitization of red cells with Bartonella species may cause acute, and sometimes fatal, haemolytic anaemia. Malaria and visceral leishmaniasis are discussed below. The aetiology of Kawasaki's disease (mucocutaneous lymph node syndrome) is unknown, but may be infectious; marked thrombocytosis with platelet hyperaggregability is seen.

CONGENITAL INFECTIONS

Transplacental passage of bacterial, viral and protozoal organisms can cause intrauterine infection.

TORCH infections

The organisms commonly involved in intrauterine infections are the so-called TORCH infections – toxoplasma, CMV, herpes, rubella and syphilis (Gray et al 1984, Hinchliffe 1987). Not all infected infants are symptomatic and as few as 10% of CMV-infected babies show signs at birth, although long-term sequelae may become apparent. This contrasts with rubella, where over 95% of babies have generalized features of disease at birth. Infection in the first trimester of pregnancy may cause abortion or fetal damage, whereas later in pregnancy the fetus may become hydropic with preterm delivery or may die in utero. Infants with congenital infections show growth retardation and are often premature and anaemic. This may initially be mild, as in CMV, rubella and herpes infections, but an exaggerated fall in haemoglobin occurs in the first few weeks of postnatal life. In some cases, anaemia may be profound at birth, particularly in toxoplasma and syphilis infections. Jaundice may develop in the first 24 hours of life, and may increase rapidly. Hepatosplenomegaly is usually present, and sometimes a purpuric rash, particularly at areas of pressure during delivery, such as the face and eyelids.

Investigation shows the presence of anaemia with a reticulocytosis, circulating normoblasts, red cell fragments, and some spherocytes. The direct anti-human globulin test is negative. The cause of haemolysis is probably microangiopathic in nature, as infection with the same organisms later in life rarely results in reduced red cell survival. Jaundice may be out of proportion to the degree of haemolysis because of hepatocellular damage by the infecting organism. Exchange transfusion may be necessary to prevent the development of kernicterus from hyperbilirubinaemia. Thrombocytopenia is reported in approximately 50% of infected neonates, and tends to be particularly severe in CMV infections. Extensive haemorrhagic features may be present associated with DIC, particularly in herpes virus infections. Thrombocytopenia is generally due to peripheral consumption, and may take 2–3 months to resolve. An immune defect is described in infants with congenital rubella syndrome, which may mimic severe combined immunodeficiency (SCID). The differential diagnosis of congenital infections in the neonate is from immune causes of neonatal haemolysis, such as Rhesus incompatibility, and from postnatally acquired infections.

Congenital infections may not fully develop until later in infancy, with the late onset of fever,

Table 15.1 Infections causing eosinophilia

Parasitic	Toxocara
	Trichinella
	Echinococcus
	Filaria
	Strongyloides
	Schistosoma
	Ascaris
	Ancylostoma
	Sarcoptes
	Enterobius
Protozoal	Pneumocystis
	Toxoplasma
	Amoeba
	Plasmodium
Fungal	Coccidiomides
	Aspergillus

lethargy, hepatosplenomegaly, jaundice and pan-cytopenia. Clinically, such babies may be difficult to differentiate from infants with storage, histio-cytic or malignant disorders, or those with post-natal infections. Specific features associated with congenital infection syndromes may be present, such as hydrocephaly and choroidoretinitis in toxoplasmosis, or cataracts, deafness and cardiac defects in congenital rubella. Skeletal changes, consisting of periosteal reaction involving the long bones, may be noted on X-ray examination, but these are not specific and have also been reported in cases of infantile acute megakaryoblastic leu-kaemia (Moody et al 1989).

Diagnosis of congenital TORCH infections is by isolation of the causative agent or by serologi-cal testing for specific IgM antibody. Additional evidence of past or present maternal infection confirms the diagnosis. It should be noted that viral shedding of CMV and rubella may continue for as long as a year after birth, which constitutes a potential hazard for pregnant carers of these infants.

HIV infection

Human immunodeficiency virus (HIV) infection in children comprises approximately 1% of the total AIDS population. Twenty per cent of cases acquired the infection through contaminated blood products; the remainder of cases acquired the vi-rus transplacentally (Bakshi et al 1988). Screening of blood products and heat treatment of clotting factor concentrates should reduce the transfusion-related cases, but as female carriers of HIV tend to be of child-bearing age, the problem of transpla-cental infection will continue. Intra-uterine HIV infection has been demonstrated, but teratogeni-city has not. Detailed epidemiology, laboratory diagnosis and clinical presentation is covered elsewhere (see Ch. 11), but HIV should be con-sidered in any infant presenting with failure to thrive, hepatosplenomegaly and lymphadenopathy.

Anaemia, described in 75% of patients, is mul-tifactorial in origin and includes the anaemia of chronic disease, nutritional deficiencies, iatro-genic blood loss for diagnostic tests, and drug-induced marrow depression. Fifty per cent of patients have leucopenia, and 85% have lympho-penia, a striking feature that is a pointer towards HIV infection. The T4:T8 lymphocyte ratio is decreased. Thrombocytopenia is seen in 10–20% of infected children, and may be the presenting feature (Saulsbury et al 1986). The mechanism of this is unclear, with increased platelet-associated immunoglobulin detected in some, but not all patients. Response to steroids or intravenous immunoglobulin is inconsistent. Bone marrow examination of 12 adult AIDS patients (Spivak et al 1984), demonstrated marrow hypoplasia, myelofibrosis and haemophagocytic histiocytes in approximately 50% of their patients, suggesting that the bone marrow is a target organ for HIV.

TROPICAL INFECTIONS

Malaria

Infection with the protozoa *Plasmodium* causes an acute febrile illness; in the western world, this is usually seen in travellers recently returned from malarial areas. The definitive host of *Plasmodium* is the mosquito, with man the intermediate host.

Lifecycle of Plasmodium

The sexual cycle of *Plasmodium* (sporogony) occurs in the mosquito, with the asexual cycle (schizogony) in man. Sporozoites enter the hu-man circulation through the bite of an infected mosquito, and migrate to the liver, where schi-zogony occurs. Metacryptozoites are released into the circulation, red cells are penetrated, and trophozoites form. Division and maturation of trophozoites into schizonts occurs within the red cell, with eventual release of merozoites into the circulation, and reinfection of other red cells. In *P. ovale*, *vivax* and *malariae* infections, some merozoites return to the liver, and a new exo-erythrocytic cycle is set up, providing a reservoir of dormant organisms that cause recurrent epi-sodes of fever over many years, unless appropriate therapy is given. *P. falciparum* does not have this exo-erythrocytic cycle, and treatment with chloro-quin is sufficient to eradicate the infection in those with chloroquin-sensitive disease. Some tropho-zoites do not divide, but form male and female gametocytes, (micro- and macrogametocytes). No further development occurs in man, but if

Table 15.2 Laboratory differentiation of *Plasmodium* species

	P. falciparum	P. vivax	P. ovale	P. malarie
Trophozoites (ring forms)	Small, delicate Double chromatin dots Multiple may be present No Schuffner's dots Maurer's clefts	Intermediate Usually single Schuffner's dots	Thick cytoplasm Half size of RBC Schuffner's dots	Thick cytoplasm Half size of RBC
Trophozoites (maturing)	Not seen in peripheral blood	Amoeboid, vacuolated	Stippled Few granules Few band forms	Compact, band shaped Pigment granules
Schizonts	Rare > 12 merozoites	Fills red cell > 12 merozoites	< 12 merozoites	< 12 merozoites
Gametocytes	Crescent shaped (male – rounded; female – pointed)	Round Fills red cell	Round Fills red cell	Round Fills red cell
RBCs	Normal size and shape	Enlarged	Oval Slightly enlarged	Normal

Adapted from Hall & Malia (1984), with permission

a mosquito is infected, the sexual cycle will restart (Hall & Malia 1984).

Pathology and clinical and laboratory findings

Table 15.2 shows the laboratory findings which help to differentiate between the species, although precise identification may be impossible if only one parasite stage is seen. It should be remembered that infection with more than one species is not uncommon. Examination of a thick film, stained with Giemsa, or Leishman stain, allows a relatively large volume of blood to be examined, and parasites should be identified, even if scanty. Parasites can be seen on MGG staining of thin films, but Giemsa or Leishman staining makes the morphological features much clearer, and aids species identification. Fluorescent microscopy at low power is a further useful test, as malaria parasites fluoresce intensely with acridine orange. A parasite count per 100 red cells is a useful guide to disease severity, 4% being a severe infection likely to be associated with serious complications.

Chronic malaria is a cause of massive splenomegaly, resulting in pancytopenia from hypersplenism. Acute infections may cause anaemia from haemolysis, for which a variety of mechanisms have been described (Woodruff et al 1979). Parasitization of the red cells distorts the cell membrane in certain species, and causes altered membrane permeability with increased osmotic fragility. Intracellular parasite metabolism alters the negative charge normally found on the red cell surface. During passage through the spleen, damaged red cells are either removed, or 'pitted' to remove parasites, leaving microspherocytes. Autoimmune destruction is also described, an IgG antibody forming against the parasite. The resulting immune complex attaches nonspecifically to red cells, complement is activated, and cell destruction occurs. A positive direct antiglobulin test due to IgG is found in 50% of patients with *P. falciparum* malaria. A particularly severe form of acute intravascular haemolysis with acute tubular necrosis is called Blackwater fever. DIC is recognized in malaria, but thrombocytopenia without DIC is a common feature of malaria, now known to be immune mediated (Kelton et al 1983; see also Ch. 6). Malaria antigens are released from lysed red cells, and bind to specific sites on the platelet membrane. IgG antimalarial antibody then bonds to the platelet-bound malaria antigen, and the IgG-platelet-parasite complex is removed in the reticuloendothelial system.

Treatment

Treatment decisions depend on where the malaria was contracted (chloroquin resistance being common on certain areas) and on the infecting species. Recommended treatment and prophylaxis for travellers changes as drug resistance spreads, and advice should be sought from a Tropical Diseases Unit.

The distribution of certain genetic disorders parallels the distribution of malaria that existed before WHO eradication programmes. The heterozygous states for sickle cell anaemia, thalassaemia and G6PD deficiency appear to confer some protection, particularly against cerebral malaria in infancy and early childhood. This protection has resulted in a high incidence of these genes in malaria areas. It has also been noted that the incidence of absence of Duffy blood group antigens is much higher in Negroes (over 70% are Fy{a⁻b⁻}) than in Caucasians (over 95% are Fy{a⁺b⁺}). It is also known that the majority of Negroes are resistant to *P. vivax* infection. The connection was made by Miller et al (1976), who found that the Duffy antigen is a receptor used by the parasite in penetration of the red cell. *P. falciparum* does not use the Duffy antigen as a receptor site, but has been found to bind to glycophorin A or B on the red cell surface. Red cells lacking glycophorin A and B cannot be penetrated by the parasite, suggesting that a specific antibody blocking the receptor could be a therapeutic approach for the future.

Visceral leishmaniasis (kala-azar)

As visceral leishmaniasis usually presents in children with fever, pancytopenia and hepatosplenomegaly, it is not surprising that patients are referred to a paediatric haematologist for investigation and the exclusion of a malignant disorder. The protozoal species *Leishmania* causes a variety of diseases producing cutaneous, mucocutaneous or visceral involvement. Visceral leishmaniasis is known as kala-azar, meaning 'black skin' and referring to the skin hyperpigmentation sometimes seen. The distribution of the disease is worldwide, with cases seen in Central and South America, Asia, Mediterranean regions of Europe and North Africa, subSaharan Africa, and the Middle East. The female sandfly (*Phlebotomous* sp) is the vector, with the dog an important reservoir of infection. In the Mediterranean type, infants and young children are affected, with 80% of patients in Malta presenting under 5 years of age. In contrast, in Asia, man is the only reservoir, and the disease affects mainly older children (Maegraith 1984).

Clinical and laboratory findings

The incubation period may be prolonged to an extent related to the number of protozoa inoculated, with cases reported 2 weeks to 9 years after exposure; however, most cases appear 3–24 months after exposure. Onset may be insidious, but usually there is a 2–3 week history of increasing malaise and lethargy, poor feeding, fever and pallor. Clinical findings are of intermittent fever, massive splenomegaly with a lesser degree of hepatomegaly, and anaemia (Fig. 15.1). Failure to thrive, and oedema from hypoalbuminaemia are seen, but lymphadenopathy is not a feature. Laboratory findings are of anaemia, neutropenia, and thrombocytopenia. Haemorrhagic manifestations appear if thrombocytopenia is profound. Untreated, the disease fluctuates with slow progression, most patients dying within two years.

In an endemic area, the clinical picture is distinctive and diagnosis is rapid. However, cases reported in the European literature have often had delayed diagnosis (Hill & Letsky 1975, Ornvold et al 1989, Kinmond et al 1989) as the problem

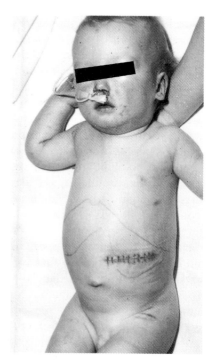

Fig. 15.1 An infant with visceral leishmaniasis, presenting with pancytopenia, fever and pneumonia 4 months after a holiday in Malta.

is rare, and the prolonged incubation period means that the importance of previous travel to endemic areas may be overlooked. A case reported in Austria by Kollaritsch et al (1989) had no known travel to an endemic area, suggesting that infection resulted from an imported infected sandfly. The differential diagnosis includes a range of infections, particularly viral (congenital and acquired), subacute endocarditis, septicaemia or typhoid fever, tuberculosis, syphilis, brucellosis, or tropical diseases such as malaria or schistosomiasis. Malignant disorders, particularly lympho- or myeloproliferative disease, should also be excluded, and storage disorders (Gaucher's and Niemann-Pick disease) and histiocyte disorders should be considered. Leishmaniasis has been described as a trigger infection for the 'infection-associated haemophagocytic syndrome' (IAHS) (Matzner et al 1979).

Diagnosis

The diagnosis is made by finding oval Leishman-Donovan (L-D) bodies, the amastigote stage of *Leishmania*, in cells of the reticuloendothelial system from samples obtained by bone marrow or splenic aspirate (Fig. 15.2). The organism multiplies by fission, is released by cell rupture, and is then taken up by other reticuloendothelial cells. The parasite burden may be high, with numerous macrophages stuffed with L-D bodies seen, but often a prolonged search may be required to identify only a few organisms. Bone marrow is visibly involved in over 50% of cases. Splenic as-

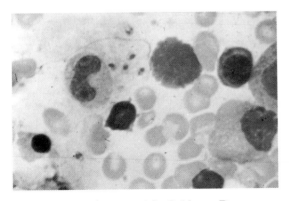

Fig. 15.2 Macrophage containing Leishman–Donovan bodies from the marrow of the child illustrated in Figure 15.1.

pirate is more likely to be diagnostic, but can be a hazardous procedure, and should not be done lightly if platelet counts are less than $50 \times 10^9/l$ or coagulation abnormalities exist. Marrow or splenic aspirates can be cultured for *Leishmania*, using special culture techniques, and antibody may be detected by complement fixation, ELISA, and immunofluorescent antibody tests. Antibody titres may be negative early in the course of the disease, and should not exclude the diagnosis in a clinically typical case with a history of travel to an endemic area.

Treatment

Treatment with pentavalent antimony has been available for the last 40 years. Sodium stibogluconate is given intravenously at a dose of 20–25 mg/kg per day for 3 weeks. Response is prompt, with fever disappearing and correction of haematological abnormalities in the first few days of therapy. Return of hepatosplenomegaly to normal is usually rapid, as relatively little fibrosis develops in response to the infection. Follow-up is essential, as a clinical response can be followed by recurrence of symptoms a few months later. Drug-resistance has been reported in the Mediterranean area and in South America. Multiple courses of antimony are occasionally required, or the addition of amphotericin B. Badaro et al (1990) report the use of combined antimony and human gamma-interferon in resistant and previously untreated disease. It has been demonstrated that an antigen-specific immunosuppression of mononuclear cells exists in leishmaniasis, resulting in defective interferon production in vitro; addition of gamma interferon is believed to enhance the ability of macrophages to clear the intracellular pathogen. Combined interferon and antimony therapy should be reserved for patients with resistant disease, or those who are critically ill at presentation.

HISTIOCYTE DISORDERS

Considerable confusion exists in the literature concerning this rare group of disorders. Greatly varied clinical presentation and natural history, poor understanding of the underlying pathogenesis and inconsistencies in diagnostic criteria have made rational therapy and comparison of outcome impossible. As research into the mononuclear phagocytic system has progressed, it has become possible to classify the histiocytic disorders according to the cell of origin, rather than use eponymous terms based on clinical syndromes, such as Letterer–Siwe disease or Hand–Schuller–Christian syndrome. Precise diagnostic criteria for certain conditions have been defined; however, there are still many areas of controversy, and the currently recommended classification will undergo further modification with time. In 1985, the Histiocyte Society was formed to bring together workers interested in histiocytic disorders, initially to standardize nomenclature and devise a working classification, subsequently to coordinate and critically review research in the field and delineate future research directions, with a view to rationalising treatment (Chu et al 1987). Even with standardized nomenclature, classification and diagnostic criteria, progress in management will be slow, because of the small numbers involved, and because of the diversity of presentation and natural history of the conditions which varies from spontaneous remission through relapsing chronicity to an acute fulminating fatal illness. Patients may be cared for by a range of specialists, both adult and paediatric, and, depending on the organ system primarily involved, may attend physicians, endocrinologists, haematologists, oncologists, dermatologists, general surgeons or orthopaedic surgeons. This further complicates the gathering

Table 15.3 Distinctive features of histiocytes

Features	Ordinary histiocyte	Paracortical interdigitating cell	Langerhans' cell
Nonspecific esterase	+	–	–
α-1 anti-chymotrypsin	+	–	–
α-mannosidase	–	+	+
S-100*	–	+	+
OKT6	–	+	+
Leu M₃†	+	+	+
Birbeck bodies	–	–	+
Peanut lectin binding	Diffuse	Halo and dot	Halo and dot

*S-100 = neuroprotein
† Leu M3 = antigen on monocytes, macrophages and dendritic cells (Becton-Dickinson Inc.)
Reproduced from Favara & Jaffe 1987, with permission

of information, conduction of clinical trials and standardization of therapy.

Histiocytes are cells of the mononuclear phagocytic system (MPS). They are derived from the bone marrow, sharing a common precursor with the granulocyte – the granulocyte-macrophage colony-forming unit (GM-CFU). They leave the marrow as monocytes and remain in the peripheral blood for a relatively short time before populating the tissues as macrophages, predominantly in organs such as skin, lungs, liver and lymph nodes. Histiocytes are a further maturational stage of macrophages. Dendritic cells are also bone-marrow-derived, but are less well understood than macrophages. They are subdivided into Langerhans' cells and paracortical interdigitating cells, based on distribution, and enzymatic and structural differences. Classification of histiocyte disorders depends on the careful identification of the cell line involved, using specialized tests, including electron microscopy. Table 15.3 shows the distinctive features of the main histiocyte cell types. Table 15.4 gives the classification of childhood histiocyte disorders, based on recommendations of the Histiocyte Society.

Langerhans' cell histiocytosis (LCH)

Langerhans' cell histiocytosis (LCH) is a nonmalignant but sometimes pernicious group of syndromes associated with proliferating Langerhans' cells. It includes the range of disorders previously known as histiocytosis X. The previous clinical subdivisions of eosinophilic granuloma, Hand–Schuller–Christian disease and Letterer–Siwe disease have been replaced by consideration of the number of sites and systems involved and the degree of organ failure. Little is known about the underlying aetiology, or why the presentation and clinical course can be so varied. The Langerhans' cell is not normally phagocytic, but functions as an antigen-presenter to T-cells. A reduction in the number of circulating suppressor T-cells has been found in LCH, and it is believed that a primary immuno-regulation defect exists, though research is confused by difficulties in deciding if the subtle immunological defects described are primary or secondary to the disease and its treatment (McLelland et al 1987).

Table 15.4 Classification of childhood histiocyte disorders

1. Langerhans cell histiocytosis (LCH)
   a. Unifocal disease
   b. Multifocal, unisystem disease
   c. Multifocal, multisystem disease

2. Non-Langerhans cell histiocytosis
   a. Reactive˙
      i. Viral-associated haemophagocytic syndrome (VAHS) (EBV, CMV, HSV, HZV, adenovirus, others)
      ii. Infection-associated haemophagocytic syndrome (IAHS) (*Mycobacterium*, treponema, brucella, *Candida*, histoplasma, *Cryptococcus*, *Toxoplasma*, *Leishmania*, *E. coli* etc)
      iii. Sinus histiocytosis with massive lymphadenopathy (Rosai-Dorfman syndrome) (? EBV)
      iv. Familial erythrophagocytic lymphohistiocytosis (FEL) (autosomal recessive)
      v. X-linked lymphoproliferative syndrome (EBV)
      vi. Chediak–Higashi syndrome
      vii. Beryllium, zirconium exposure
   b. Inborn errors of metabolism/lipid storage disorder
      i. Sea blue histiocytosis
      ii. Gaucher's disease
      iii. Niemann–Pick disease
      iv. Fabry's disease
      v. Gangliosidosis type I
      vi. Chronic granulomatous disease
      vii. Cholesterol-ester storage disorder
   c. Malignant disorders
      i. Malignant histiocytosis
      ii. Acute monoblastic leukaemia (FAB M_5)
      iii. True 'histiocytic' lymphoma

LCH is found in all age groups, but 75% of cases are under 15 years at diagnosis. The sex incidence is equal, but a preponderance of cases in population groups of North European origin is noted, and the disorder is relatively rare in Negroes. In a review of patients treated at the Children's Hospital of Philadelphia (Raney & D'Angio 1989), an incidence of 2 cases per million population under 21 years was found. Incidence figures are difficult to assess, as unifocal lesions, particularly bone lesions, may go undiagnosed. The prognosis varies greatly with age, and is also related to organ dysfunction, rather than organ involvement (Lahey 1975, Broadbent et al 1984). Retrospective analysis of 83 patients showed 50 with no organ dysfunction to have a mortality rate of 4%, whereas 66% of the 33 patients with organ dysfunction died. Raney & D'Angio (1989) reported all of 33 patients with unifocal disease to be alive and well at two years, with an actuarial estimate of recurrence-free survival of 93%. Twenty two

patients had multisystem disease but no dysfunction. Of these, 63% had recurrent disease, but only one died of progressive disease, whereas 6 of 9 patients with multisystem disease and organ dysfunction had died.

Other studies report mortality of 50–70% in infants with multisystem disease and dysfunction (Broadbent et al 1984). A scoring system has been devised by Lahey, based on three 'vital' organ systems, failure of which would be life threatening. Liver dysfunction is defined as hypoproteinaemia or hypoalbuminaemia, ascites, oedema, or jaundice not attributable to haemolysis. Pulmonary dysfunction is defined as dyspnoea or tachypnoea, cyanosis, cough or pneumothorax attributable to disease and not infection. X-ray changes alone are not considered evidence for dysfunction. Marrow dysfunction is defined as a haemoglobin of less than 10 g/dl in the absence of iron deficiency, a leucopenia of less than $4 \times 10^9/l$, a neutropenia of less than $1.5 \times 10^9/l$, or thrombocytopenia with lower than $100 \times 10^9/l$ platelets. Marrow infiltration with LCH is evidence of involvement, but not of dysfunction.

Clinical findings

LCH lesions have a predilection for certain sites, in particular, bone, skin, lymph nodes, liver, spleen, lungs, central nervous system and bone marrow. Langerhans' cells are normally found in the skin, and macrophages are present in lymph nodes, bone marrow, liver, spleen and lungs, but the selective involvement of bone and central nervous system remains unexplained. In children, unifocal disease is commonly in the form of a single eosinophilic granuloma of bone. Bones of skull, orbits, and petrous bones are most commonly affected, but any bone can be involved, with the small bones of hands and feet relatively spared. X-rays performed to investigate bone pain or soft-tissue swelling show well-demarcated, 'punched-out' lesions. Multifocal lesions are best detected with conventional radiography rather than radionuclide studies. With healing, the lesion margins become blurred, and lesions at different stages of healing may be observed. Involvement of maxilla and mandible results in gum hypertrophy, and defective dentition with 'floating' teeth, early eruption and loss of teeth. Serum calcium, phosphate and alkaline phosphatase are not greatly altered during the course of the illness.

Cutaneous lesions are common in childhood LCH (Figs 15.3 and 15.4), the lesions ranging from a single nodule to vesicopapular lesions, and eczematous or seborrhoeic eruptions in the post-auricular area, scalp, axillae and groin which may become erythematous, confluent and ulcerated, allowing access to microorganisms and resulting in sepsis. Chronic draining ears are often associated with LCH lesions of skin and external ear canals. In severe cases, the rash may be haemorrhagic and coagulopathy may be present. Infants with generalized cutaneous LCH frequently have multisystem disease, with evidence of marrow, lung and liver failure, fever and systemic upset. However, Lee et al (1988) report a benign cutaneous LCH in infancy which is self-limiting, so careful investigation to exclude multisystem disease is required before deciding on a therapeutic regimen.

In childhood, pulmonary disease is usually part of a multisystem disorder, although it may be the only system involved in young adults. X-rays show a honeycomb pattern, but careful pulmonary function testing may reveal pulmonary involvement in the absence of X-ray changes. Biopsy or the finding of Langerhans cells in bronchoalveolar lavage samples is required for the diagnosis.

The central nervous system may be involved at any site, but there is a predilection for the hypothalamic/pituitary axis, resulting in diabetes insipidus. The incidence is reported as between 5–50% of all childhood cases of LCH (Dunger et al 1989). Clinical signs of diabetes insipidus may be obvious, or water deprivation tests may be required to show minor abnormalities. Diabetes insipidus is usually part of a more generalized disease, but has been described as the only lesion in LCH. Growth hormone deficiency is recognized, as is hypogonadism and delayed puberty. Skull defects need not be present, but CT or MR imaging shows intracerebral or leptomeningeal lesions. Other manifestations include cerebellar dysfunction, seizures, cranial nerve defects, exophthalmos and raised intracranial pressure.

Hepatic involvement may be occult and detected only by liver function tests, or may be the predominant clinical problem, with hepatomegaly and advancing hepatic failure. Cholestatic jaundice may result from fibrosis at a late stage of the disease. Diarrhoea, due to infiltration of gut mucosa, can lead to malabsorption with consequent failure to thrive. Peripheral blood changes are commonest in infants, either pancytopenia secondary to hypersplenism or, more seriously,

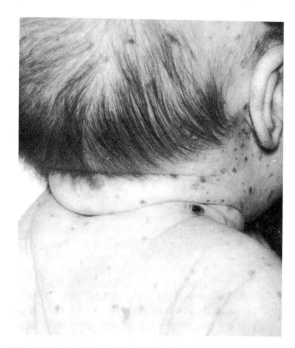

Fig. 15.3 An infant with skin involvement in multisystem Langerhans' cell histiocytosis. In this case, the condition was congenital, progressive and fatal.

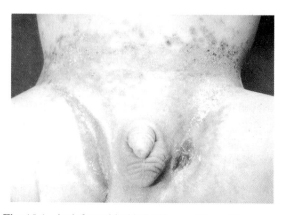

Fig. 15.4 An infant with skin involvement in multisystem Langerhans' cell histiocytosis. The child had been treated for some weeks for nappy rash. Bone and lung involvement was present, but the child made an uneventful recovery.

cytopenias due to marrow infiltration (Berry & Becton, 1987).

Pathology and laboratory findings

All lesions, whether single bone problems or soft tissue involvement found in fulminating multi-system disease, have the same basic pathology. The diagnosis of LCH should always be confirmed by biopsy. A presumptive diagnosis can be made from the typical histological finding of a proliferative, locally destructive lesion, with an infiltrate of Langerhans' cells, lymphocytes and eosinophils. Reactive phagocytic macrophages are present, and variable degrees of necrosis. At a later stage of the disease, lesions are often less cellular, with a reduced number of Langerhans' cells and increasing fibrosis. On conventional staining, Langerhans' cells are large, with homogenous pink cytoplasm, and the nucleus may be grooved or bean-shaped. A higher level of diagnostic confidence is reached with positive staining for two or more of the following features: ATPase, S-100 protein, alpha-D-mannosidase, or characteristic peanut lectin binding. Pathognomonic features are the presence of Birbeck granules (visible only on electron microscopy) in Langerhans' cells within the lesion, or the demonstration of T6 antigenic determinants on the cell surface (Table 15.3). Birbeck granules are membrane-derived, racquet-shaped intracytoplasmic structures, found in normal and LCH Langerhans' cells. The bone marrow is infiltrated with Langerhans' cells in a small percentage of patients with multisystem disease, but diagnosis by marrow aspirate or trephine is difficult, as the cells are not distinctive when stained with normal Romanowsky stains, and the typical nuclear features are lost in air-dried samples. Haemophagocytosis may be present, but this is a reactive process by macrophages, and is not diagnostic of LCH. Occasionally, sheets of infiltrating Langerhans' cells may be seen. Specialized techniques are required to confirm marrow infiltration, including electron microscopy of trephine samples, T6 identification, α-mannosidase staining of air-dried samples, and peanut-lectin binding on alcohol-fixed imprints and aspirates (Favara & Jaffe 1987).

A careful history and clinical examination should cover all systems likely to be involved, probing in particular for evidence of malaise, fever, bone pain or deformity, soft-tissue swellings, lymphadenopathy, skin, ear, gum or dental lesions, respiratory symptoms, polyuria and polydipsia, cerebellar or cranial nerve lesions, hepatosplenomegaly, jaundice, oedema or ascites. Baseline investigations should include biopsy and examination of the presenting lesion by the specialized techniques described above, a full blood count, coagulation screen, liver function tests, chest X-ray, skeletal survey or bone scan, and urine osmolality after overnight water deprivation. Further investigations are required if evidence of organ dysfunction is found, including pulmonary function testing, bronchoalveolar lavage or lung biopsy, liver biopsy, bone marrow aspirate and trephine, and CT or MR imaging (Broadbent et al 1989).

Treatment

The excellent prognosis in unifocal disease is achieved regardless of treatment, and although many types of therapy have been used, controlled clinical trials to evaluate them have not been possible. Healing of bone lesions has been observed after biopsy alone, curettage, low-dose radiotherapy, intralesional steroid injection, systemic steroids, chemotherapy, or no intervention at all. Wide variation in the rate of healing is observed. Some resolution is usually evident within 12–16 weeks, but the process may not be complete for many months (Womer et al 1985). Systemic treatment should not be given for unifocal disease because of the potential side-effects, and local treatment should only be offered for severe pain, if risk of fracture exists, or if the lesion is in an area where deformity or fracture could result in permanent disability, such as spinal involvement. Further bone lesions may appear over the next two years, but overall the prognosis is good, though some patients are left with bone deformity or vertebral collapse.

If mild, skin disease can be left untreated, or steroids or a 20% aqueous solution of mustine may be applied topically (Atherton et al 1986). Superinfection may be present in severe, ulcerated cases.

Multisystem disease without organ dysfunction may be treated conservatively after very careful assessment, but evidence of organ dysfunction requires more aggressive therapy. Chemotherapeutic agents were found to have an effect when Letterer–Siwe disease was thought to be a malignant condition, and they are still used in poor-prognosis patients. Vinblastine and low-dose steroids have been used longterm to establish control, although rapid 'remission' is unusual. More intensive regimes have included high-dose pulsed prednisolone, and CHOP (cyclophosphamide, daunorubicin, vincristine, prednisolone) or methotrexate. Etoposide, which is effective in monocytic/macrophage malignancies, has been widely used as a single agent, either intravenously or orally, with good response rates (Ceci et al 1988, Broadbent et al 1989). Myelotoxic and immunosuppressive treatment should be reserved for children with constitutional symptoms and multisystem disease with organ failure. Such patients are usually under 2 years of age. Full supportive care with blood products and antibiotics will be required. Etoposide has relatively low toxicity and few long-term sequelae, so is preferable to longterm or high-dose steroid regimes.

As LCH is not a malignant disease in the sense of clonal neoplasia, the classical oncological approach of aggressive chemotherapy to achieve rapid complete remission is inappropriate, the aim being to control rather than eradicate the disease, allowing time for spontaneous regression. But many questions remain about the pathogenesis and best management. Multicentre clinical and laboratory studies are required for further progress in this area.

Infection-associated haemophagocytic syndrome (IAHS)

In 1979, Risdall et al described a syndrome of reactive histiocyte proliferation in bone marrow, lymph nodes, liver and spleen, with an acute fulminating course characterized by malaise, fever, lymphadenopathy and hepatosplenomegaly. Rapidly progressive pancytopenia from histiocytic haemophagocytosis, liver dysfunction, and coagulopathy were also described. Many of the original cases had underlying immunoincompetence and evidence of viral infection, resulting in the name viral associated haemophagocytic

syndrome (VAHS). Since then, many case reports (Martin-Moreno et al 1983, Campo et al 1986, Gill & Marrie 1987, Jenkins & Gray 1988) have appeared describing the syndrome and implicating a wide range of infective organisms, including bacterial, fungal, protozoal and parasitic problems, as well as viral infections. All age groups may be affected, with a male preponderance. Mortality rates of 20–42% are reported (Reiner & Spivak 1988).

Clinical and laboratory findings

Symptoms tend to be nonspecific and vague, with fever, chills, sweats, fatigue and anorexia being common. Clinical signs vary with the underlying infection, but fever is present in nearly 100% of patients, and lymphadenopathy and hepatosplenomegaly have been described in 50%. In 1988, Reiner & Spivak reported a series of 23 patients. Seventy five per cent had pancytopenia at presentation, and all had depression of at least two haemopoietic cell lines. Neutropenia and thrombocytopenia may be profound. Atypical vacuolated monocytes or haemophagocytic histiocytes may be seen in the peripheral blood. Fifty per cent of patients have a coagulopathy with a prolonged prothrombin time and partial thromboplastin time, hypofibrinogenaemia, and elevated fibrin degradation products. Liver transaminases are raised in 87%.

Bone marrow aspirate examination shows hypocellular fragments, with prominent haemophagocytic macrophages (Fig. 15.5). Erythroid and myeloid precursors may appear to be reduced, but megakaryocytes are usually easy to find. Plasma cells may be increased. The histiocytes do not have the ultrastructural or immunological features of Langerhans' cells. A marrow trephine biopsy is useful, as hypocellularity may make a diagnostic aspirate difficult to obtain, and histological assessment helps to exclude the presence of an underlying lymphoproliferative disorder. Associated myelofibrosis has been reported by Reiner & Spivak, and other less frequent changes described are dyserythropoiesis, ringed sideroblasts, megaloblastic changes, and granulomas. Occasionally, phagocytosed organisms resembling cell debris or platelets, are seen within the histiocytes, and

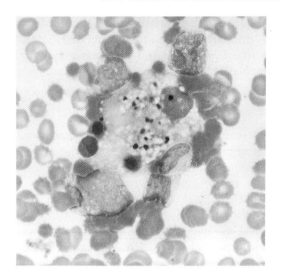

Fig. 15.5 Histiocyte showing haemophagocytosis in the bone marrow of a patient with infection-associated haemophagocytic syndrome.

specialized staining techniques may identify the causative infective organism. Biopsy of other organs shows histiocytic infiltration of sinusoids and medullary cords of lymph nodes, red pulp of the spleen, and sinusoids and portal tracts of the liver. Other organs, such as lungs, heart, adrenals, central nervous system, kidney and gastrointestinal tract, have been reported to contain histiocytic infiltration on postmortem examination of fatal cases. Liver biopsy is hazardous in the face of severe coagulopathy and thrombocytopenia, and should only be undertaken in exceptional circumstances.

Investigations to find the precipitating infection should include direct culture and serology. Multiple organisms are sometimes found, though some may be due to secondary infections arising during the course of the illness. Cytomegalovirus, Epstein Barr virus, herpes simplex, varicella/zoster and adenoviruses are commonly identified, and HIV has also been implicated. From the range of non-viral infectious agents reported, it appears that virtually any infection may trigger the histiocyte proliferative response, although it is not known why this occurs only in certain patients. Fourteen of 19 (74%) of the original VAHS patients described had an underlying acquired immunodeficiency, and 87% of Reiner's patients were also immunosuppressed. Their immunosuppression

varied in origin. Some had received corticosteroids or other immunosuppressives for connective tissue disorders or following renal transplantation; others had been splenectomized, some had acquired immune deficiency syndrome (AIDS), some abused alcohol, and others were receiving cytotoxic agents for a variety of malignant disorders. No evidence of immune disorder was found in the few remaining patients.

Treatment

Management is supportive. In those who do not deteriorate rapidly with multi-organ failure, the condition is self-limiting and nonrecurrent, with resolution of clinical and laboratory abnormalities within a few weeks. The use of cytotoxic agents or immunosuppressives as therapy is not justified.

Familial erythrophagocytic lymphohistiocytosis (FEL)

A rare disorder, with autosomal recessive inheritance, familial erythrophagocytic lymphohistiocytosis (FEL) was first described in 1952 by Farquhar & Claireaux, and until recent years was rapidly and inevitably fatal. Seventy five per cent of patients present in the first 6 months of life, and 90% arise in the first 2 years (Pritchard 1986). The syndrome has many similarities to IAHS, but careful investigation will discriminate between the two conditions. FEL appears to be a recessively inherited disorder. There is a high incidence of parental consanguinity, and complete concordance in reported cases involving identical twins. The diagnosis is often missed in the first affected child, and a family history of previous infant death from an ill-characterized 'infection' is often what suggests the possibility of FEL in the second. From this it can be deduced that the number of missed cases may be quite large, as most afflicted families will have only one child with the disease.

Clinical and laboratory findings

Presentation may be acute or more gradual, but almost all patients have fever, hepatosplenomegaly, anaemia and failure to thrive. Lymphadenopathy is seen in only 10% of patients; skin rashes and bone lesions are rare. Central nervous system involvement is common at presentation, with irritability, vomiting, head retraction or focal seizures. Laboratory tests show pancytopenia, with an infiltration of haemophagocytic histiocytes in the bone marrow. Coagulation abnormalities are common; in particular, prolongation of the prothrombin and partial thromboplastin times, and hypofibrinogenaemia may be present. Sixty per cent of patients have increased cells and protein in the cerebrospinal fluid (CSF) at diagnosis (Fig. 15.6). These cells are mainly mature lymphocytes, with some foamy macrophages, which may exhibit phagocytosis. The incidence of central nervous system involvement increases during the course of the disease. Type IV hypertriglyceridaemia is usual (Brown et al 1987) and is considered to be a cardinal feature of FEL. The reason is obscure. Immunological investigation has produced a variety of results, but the consensus appears to be that a defect in natural killer cell function exists. Ladisch et al (1978) reported that this reverted to normal during periods of quiescence, though more recently Arico et al (1988) have reported persistent abnormalities during remission and also abnormalities in the presumed heterozygote parents and healthy siblings of patients. Culture of blood, urine, swabs and CSF and full serological investigation invariably show

no evidence of bacterial, viral or other infection. The differential diagnosis is from IAHS, multi-system LCH, congenital infections, monocytic/monoblastic leukaemia or neuroblastoma.

Treatment

The treatment of FEL remains unsatisfactory. Early regimens included splenectomy, exchange transfusion, corticosteroids, and various cytotoxic agents, either singly or in combination (Lilleyman 1980, Ladisch et al 1982, Delaney et al 1984). Some brief responses were noted, but long-term survival was extremely rare. The use of etoposide has improved the situation, with good response rates and prolonged survival (Ambruso et al 1980, Fischer et al 1985, Alverado et al 1986), but the course of the disease is recurrent and eventual resistance to etoposide develops, despite dose escalation. Etoposide is also ineffective against central nervous system involvement, but intrathecal methotrexate has been found to be effective. Some workers (Fischer et al 1985, Arico et al 1988) recommend cranial radiotherapy at one year of age. Intensive blood product support is required to correct the coagulopathy, and antibiotics will be needed if secondary infection occurs during neutropenic episodes.

Clinical response sees a settling of fever and reduction in hepatosplenomegaly. Coagulation tests and full blood count parameters return to normal, as does the hyperlipidaemia. CSF abnormalities disappear, as does evidence of marrow haemophagocytosis. It is difficult to decide duration of therapy once clinical remission has been obtained, because rapid reactivation of the disease frequently follows cessation of therapy. As the underlying inherited defect remains unchanged, it seems likely that some sort of maintenance therapy should continue long term. Fischer et al (1986) report a successful allogeneic bone marrow transplant. Arico et al (1988) have reported 10 patients, of whom four are alive and well 10–30 months from diagnosis. Treatment consisted of etoposide, steroids, intrathecal methotrexate and cranial radiotherapy (18 Gy) in the two patients who had attained the age of one year. It is not clear if therapy is continuing in these patients.

Despite these reports, for the majority of patients

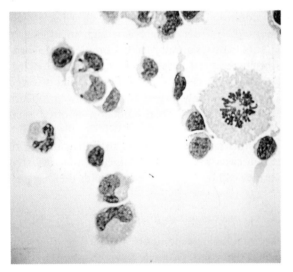

Fig. 15.6 CSF from an infant with familial erythrophagocytic lymphohistiocytosis (cytospin preparation).

the prognosis remains poor. Further elucidation of the underlying immunological defect is essential so that the gene controlling FEL can be identified and, eventually, antenatal screening and diagnosis is made possible. Also, a marker of disease activity would allow intensity and duration of treatment to be rationalized for those achieving initial responses to current therapy. Follow-up of any long-term survivors is important to assess their quality of life, in particular, to assess long-term neurological sequelae of the disease and its therapy.

STORAGE DISORDERS

Many metabolic disorders caused by absence or inactivity of an enzyme result in storage of abnormal or excessive intermediate metabolic products. Lysosomal enzyme defects result in a wide range of disorders, each having a characteristic clinical picture reflecting the pattern of distribution of accumulated metabolites. Sites of storage include:

1. the reticuloendothelial system (RES), resulting in hepatosplenomegaly and bone marrow involvement
2. the central nervous system, with signs of neuronal damage including slow development, regression, fits and blindness
3. skin, bones and cornea causing dysmorphism.

The defective enzyme and exact nature of the stored substance is known for most of the described disorders, so precise diagnosis is possible from enzyme assay of leucocytes, cultured fibroblasts, or biopsy tissue.

Research into enzyme replacement therapy is in progress, with bone marrow transplantation the most promising option; otherwise, there is no effective treatment available for any of these inborn metabolic errors. Attempts to supplement the deficient enzyme with fresh frozen plasma or purified human enzyme have occasionally produced some biochemical improvement, but the half-life of most enzymes is too short to maintain useful concentrations, and usually no clinical improvement seen. In contrast, marrow-derived haemopoietic cells and macrophages (which produce lysosomal enzymes) populate the reticuloendothelial system throughout the body, so enzyme production continues after successful transplantation. This permits correction of biochemical abnormalities, and gradual clinical improvement occurs as stored metabolites are mobilized. Sadly, neither enzyme-producing cells nor free enzyme can cross the blood–brain barrier, so neurological damage persists.

Ideally, bone marrow transplantation should be considered early, before permanent cellular damage and skeletal deformity develop, and before the onset of neurological symptoms. Future improvements in prevention and control of graft-versus-host disease may make matched, unrelated donor (MUD) transplants safer and open this form of treatment to a greater number of patients (Rappeport et al 1984, Barranger 1984).

The majority of disorders are autosomal recessive (exceptions are Fabry's disease and Hunter's syndrome, both X-linked recessive), and recognition of the enzyme defect makes antenatal diagnosis feasible for couples with a previously affected child. Identification of the heterozygous phenotype, important in family studies, is also possible.

Investigations and diagnosis

If a storage disorder is suspected, a full clinical history and examination will suggest the most likely diagnosis, so investigations can be specific rather than pursuing a blanket approach of performing all available enzyme assays in the hope of identifying the defective one. Morphological changes in the peripheral blood film are seen in a number of storage disorders and, while not sufficiently specific to be diagnostic, they can help to determine the direction of further investigation. Pancytopenia, from hypersplenism, is seen in disorders which produce massive splenomegaly. Storage in reticulo-endothelial cells of the bone marrow produces characteristic morphological features in some conditions, although enzyme assay is required for confirmation.

Wherever possible, a diagnosis should be made from easily accessible material (such as peripheral blood or bone marrow) by light and electron-microscopy (EM). Leucocyte enzyme assay can also be carried out on blood or marrow, or fibroblast culture specifically for enzyme assays can be undertaken. Suction rectal biopsy examination will identify diseases with neuronal and smooth

Table 15.5 Storage disorders with haematological abnormalities

1 *Sphingolipidoses*
   a. Gaucher's disease
   b. Niemann–Pick disease
   c. GM1-gangliosidosis (type I or infantile)
   d. GM2-gangliosidosis (Sandhoff variant)

2 *Mucopolysaccharidoses*
   a. Hurler's syndrome, Scheie syndrome
   b. Hunter's syndrome
   c. Sanfilippo syndrome
   d. Morquio's syndrome
   e. Maroteaux-Lamy syndrome

3 *Mucolipidoses*
   a. Mucolipidosis types I–III
   b. Fucosidosis
   c. Mannosidosis

4 *Batten's disease*

5 *Wolman's disease*

muscle involvement, and is a well-tolerated, rapid and simple surgical technique. Liver biopsy may be necessary, particularly in certain glycogen storage diseases, but has more risks and should be avoided if other diagnostic tests are available. Prior to investigation, full coordination between clinicians, histopathologists, biochemists and haematologists is important so that samples obtained are processed appropriately and unnecessary tests are not requested.

Table 15.5 lists the storage disorders which have characteristic haematological features. It is not intended as a complete list of all storage disorders. Abnormalities on Romanowsky-stained peripheral blood films include lymphocyte vacuolation (Table 15.6; Fig. 15.7) and inclusions. These may be in all or a small percentage of lymphocytes, often clustered in the tail of the film where they may be missed. Histochemical staining techniques

Table 15.6 Storage disorders in which vacuolated lymphocytes are found

Small vacuoles	Niemann–Pick, type A
	Wolman's disease
	Pompe's disease
Larger, often numerous vacuoles	GM1-gangliosidosis, type I
	Mucopolysaccharidoses
	Mucolipidoses, types I and III
	I-cell disease (mucolipidosis type II)
	Aspartylglucosaminuria
	Batten's disease (juvenile type)

Adapted from Lake (1989), with permission

may identify the vacuole contents, but lymphocyte electronmicroscopy and leucocyte enzyme assays require special expertise. Dense neutrophil granules (Alder–Reilly bodies) are present in some storage disorders, but neutrophil vacuolation is more likely to be secondary to infection than evidence of storage disorder, although carnitine deficiency has been reported to be associated with neutrophil vacuolation.

Bone marrow aspirate may contain obvious storage cells, and if an adequate cellular sample is obtained, there is little advantage in performing a trephine biopsy, as the histochemical stains to identify the contents of storage cells are best performed on air-dried slides rather than fixed biopsy material. It should be noted that Sudan black staining, as done in haematology laboratories, stains for peroxidase activity characteristic of granulocytes, not for the presence of fat, and so is not useful in the diagnosis of storage disorders unless different histochemical techniques are used (Lake 1989).

The clinical and haematological features of the commoner storage disorders are discussed below; the texts of Kolodny & Boustany (1987), and Brown et al (1984) are also recommended.

Gaucher's disease

Glucocerebroside accumulates in cells of the reticulo-endothelial system and CNS due to a deficiency of the enzyme glucocerebrosidase.

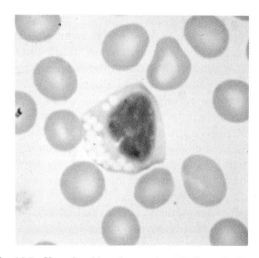

Fig. 15.7 Vacuolated lymphocyte; juvenile Batten's disesae.

Adult onset (type I). The commonest form of the disease, type I Gaucher's may present in late childhood or throughout adult life. The main findings are hepatomegaly and splenomegaly which may be massive, and secondary pancytopenia due to hypersplenism (Fig. 15.8). Haemorrhagic features are occasionally present if thrombocytopenia is severe. Although the liver may be greatly enlarged, liver function remains relatively normal. Lungs and lymph nodes may be infiltrated, and marrow infiltration causes bone pain, deformity and pathological fractures from loss of density and thinning of bone cortex. There are no neurological abnormalities.

Infant onset (type II). The infantile form of Gaucher's is an acute neuropathic disease. It presents early, in the first 6 months of life, with failure to thrive, hepatosplenomegaly, and brain stem disorders. These include dysphagia, laryngospasm, hypertonia and eventual decerebration. Death usually occurs before the age of 2 years.

Juvenile onset (type III). A third type of Gaucher's disease presents in late childhood with hepatosplenomegaly and a slowly progressive neu-ropathic disorder characterized by decreased mental abilities, seizures, incoordination and hypertonia.

Diagnosis

Laboratory diagnosis of all three types of the disease depends on the demonstration of Gaucher's cells in the bone marrow (Fig. 15.9). These are large (50 μm), sometimes multinucleated, with nonvacuolated, bluish-grey, fibrillar cytoplasm, sometimes described as resembling crumpled tissue paper on Romanowsky staining. (Similar cells have also been described in bone marrow from patients with β-thalassaemia and chronic granulocytic leukaemia – so-called pseudo-Gaucher cells). They stain weakly with Sudan black and PAS, but strongly with acid phosphatase. The diagnosis is confirmed by β glucosidase assay in leucocytes or cultured fibroblasts. Heterozygotes can be identified, and antenatal diagnosis can be offered to affected families.

Treatment

Treatment is not effective. The adult, nonneuropathic type is relatively benign, although hypersplenism may cause pancytopenia, thrombocytopenia and bleeding. Splenectomy has been useful in reducing bleeding in some patients, but theoretically may result in increasing bone and hepatic storage,

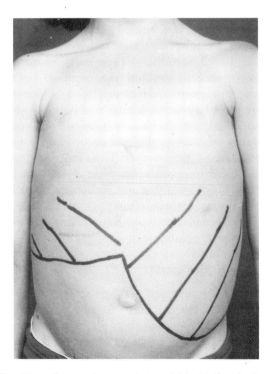

Fig. 15.8 Hepatosplenomegaly in a child with Gaucher's disease, presenting at the age of 6 years.

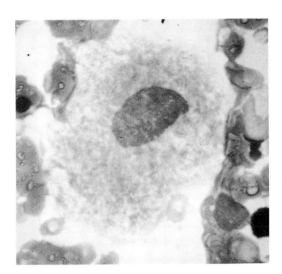

Fig. 15.9 Gaucher cell. Bone marrow (Romanowsky stained).

so accelerating other features of the disease. It remains a controversial issue. Partial splenectomy has been anecdotally successful and may help in some individuals. Supportive treatment only can be offered to infants, but there is a place for bone marrow transplantation in the juvenile type, provided it can be done before the onset of neurological damage as there is no evidence that such damage is reversible even after a successful transplant.

Niemann–Pick disease

Sphingomyelin accumulates due to sphingomyelinase deficiency in Niemann–Pick disease, and foamy storage cells are found in bone marrow, liver, lymph nodes, kidney and central nervous system. Similar clinical features have been described in some patients where sphingomyelinase activity is normal. There are three types:

Acute infantile form, with cerebral involvement (type A). Presentation is at 3–6 months of age with feeding problems, developmental delay and hepatosplenomegaly, the liver being larger than the spleen. The condition progresses with increasing visceromegaly, lymphadenopathy, pulmonary infiltrates, neurological regression, hypotonia, and eventual death in 2–3 years. A cherry-red spot at the macula is present in 50% of cases.

Chronic, visceral type (type B). Onset is at any time during infancy and childhood, with failure to thrive, lymphadenopathy, and hepatosplenomegaly sometimes associated with hypersplenism. Neuronal deposition and damage does not occur. Slow progression results in death in the late teens or early adult life.

Type C. This term covers a variety of conditions clinically similar to Niemann-Pick, but with no demonstrable deficiency of sphingomyelinase. Patients may present in infancy with slowly progressive visceral features, and neurological features appearing later in childhood, or in adults with visceral features only.

Diagnosis and treatment

Haematological abnormalities are seen in both peripheral blood and bone marrow. Type A produces small discrete vacuoles in most peripheral

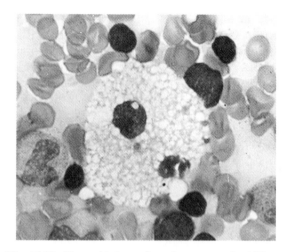

Fig. 15.10 Foamy histiocyte from the marrow of a child with Niemann–Pick disease (type A).

blood lymphocytes, together with large foamy histiocytes in the bone marrow. The histiocyte vacuoles are small and uniform in size; ingested cell debris is rarely seen (Fig. 15.10). The cells stain weakly with Sudan black, are positive with PAS, and strongly positive with acid phosphatase. If the Sudan black preparation is examined in polarized light, a reddish birefringence can be seen. The diagnosis is confirmed by demonstration of absence of sphingomyelinase activity in leucocytes and cultured fibroblasts. Type B shows no lymphocyte vacuolation, but the marrow contains foamy storage cells, as in type A, together with numerous sea-blue histiocytes which may be more prominent than the foamy histiocytes. Type C patients show small discrete vacuoles in a small percentage of lymphoctyes. Their marrow storage cells differ from those in type A, in that the vacuoles vary greatly in size and ingested nuclear debris is frequently present.

There is no effective therapy other than early marrow transplantation.

GM1-gangliosidosis

Type I. This deficiency of β-galactosidase results in failure to thrive from an early age, hepatosplenomegaly, gargoylism, and progression to mental and motor retardation. Death occurs early. Numerous large, coarse vacuoles are seen in the majority of lymphocytes, and foamy macrophages, with no characteristic staining features, appear in the bone marrow. Diagnosis is by demonstration of the absence of β-galactosidase activity in leucocytes or cultured fibroblasts.

Type II. This form of GM1-gangliosidosis has late-infantile onset and does not produce vacuolated peripheral lymphocytes. Marrow storage cells are Gaucher-like, but the cytoplasm is less fibrillar, and stains more intensely blue with MGG stain than does a true Gaucher cell. Enzyme assay is required to make the diagnosis.

GM2-gangliosidosis

In Tay-Sachs disease (type I), absence of hexosaminidase A results in accumulation of ganglioside in neural tissue, with minimal reticuloendothelial storage. Vacuolated lymphocytes have been reported, but not marrow storage cells.

In the Sandhoff variant (type II), both hexosaminidase A and B are absent. The clinical features are as in Tay-Sachs disease, with hypotonia, excessive startle response in the first few months of life, progressive motor weakness, seizures, optic atrophy with a cherry-red spot at the macula together with autonomic dysfunction. Reticuloendothelial storage of ganglioside is more prominent than in type I, with foamy storage cells in the bone marrow, but no hepatosplenomegaly. Diagnosis is by assay of the appropriate enzymes.

Mucopolysaccharidoses

These conditions are disorders of glycosaminoglycan metabolism, an important constituent of connective tissue. Clinical features include coarse features, skeletal dysplasia, limitation of joint movement, growth failure and, in some types, intellectual retardation and corneal clouding (Fig. 15.11). The specific enzyme defect is known in all types, and assays are available. Another diagnostic feature is the excretion of excessive mucopolysaccharides in the urine. Although morphological abnormalities are present in the peripheral blood, they do not distinguish between the subtypes. Occasional lymphocytes contain metachromatic vacuoles, some of which contain small inclusions densely staining with MGG, and these are present in most types but most frequently (over 20% of lymphocytes) in Sanfilippo (type III)

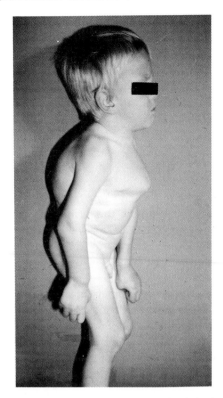

Fig. 15.11   Morquio's disease with extensive skeletal abnormalities.

or Hunter's (type II) syndromes. Five to 20% of lymphocytes with vacuole inclusions suggests Hurler's (type I) or Hunter's syndrome, while less than 5% suggests Hurler's or Scheie's syndromes. Morquio's (type IV) syndrome has no metachromatic vacuolation, but the granulocytes show striking, large, sparsely distributed Alder granules. Maroteaux–Lamy (type VI) syndrome *does* show metachromatic vacuoles, but more striking is the presence of densely packed Alder granulation in the neutrophils. This resembles toxic granulation, but is generally coarser, and stains a reddish-lilac with standard stains. (Toluidine blue staining will differentiate Alder granules from toxic granulation, as Alder granules are basophilic whereas toxic granules remain unstained.) Bone marrow examination shows foamy storage cells in types I–III, but few if any in types IV and VI. Such cells also contain basophilic inclusions within the vacuoles – so-called 'Gasser' cells. Specific diagnosis is by urine analysis and enzyme assay.

Successful bone marrow transplantation has

been reported in a child with Maroteaux–Lamy syndrome, with restoration of absent enzyme and evidence of clearance of storage material (Krivit et al 1984). This form of treatment remains controversial, particularly in those children with impaired intellect. More long-term follow-up is required to assess its effectiveness.

Mucolipidoses

These disorders have the clinical features of Hurler's syndrome and some features of sphingolipidoses, but without the urinary excretion of mucopolysaccharides. Instead, the urine contains oligosaccharides. The peripheral blood contains small numbers of lymphocytes with numerous, large vacuoles in type I. Eighty per cent of lymphocytes contain prominent vacuoles in type II (I cell or inclusion cell disease). Mannosidosis, fucosidosis and aspartylglucosaminuria are all mucolipidoses, with approximately 80% of lymphocytes containing large vacuoles, but marrow foam cells are not a feature (though can be present in some types). Diagnosis is by specific enzyme assay.

Glycogen storage disease

The glycogen storage diseases are characterized by deposition of glycogen in liver and muscle. Patients may present with failure to thrive and hepatomegaly. Most types have no specific haematological features, and liver or muscle biopsy is required for diagnosis. Pompe's disease (type II) is an exception. On peripheral blood examination, every lymphocyte contains one or more small discrete vacuoles, which stain positive for glycogen with PAS. PAS-positivity is seen in normal B-lymphocytes, but this is around the periphery of the cell, not associated with vacuoles, and is present in only a small percentage of lymphocytes. The diagnosis is confirmed by leucocyte or cultured fibroblast assay of acid maltase activity.

Batten's disease

This is a neurodegenerative disorder with accumulation of lipopigments, but its biochemical basis remains unclear. Clinical features vary with different ages of onset; in the types presenting in childhood the main feature is visual impairment progressing to blindness. Neurodegeneration produces seizures, myoclonic jerks, cerebellar signs, intellectual impairment, and eventual death. An adult form presents with insidious-onset dementia without visual disturbance in middle age. In the juvenile-onset type, light microscopy of peripheral blood shows prominent coarse vacuoles in 10–30% of lymphocytes (Fig. 15.7). The vacuole contents are not known, and take up no specific stains. Electronmicroscopy (EM) can be useful in Batten's disease. Infantile-onset disease has no light microscopic changes, but EM shows one or two membrane-bound granular osmiophilic deposits (GROD) in 50% of lymphocytes. Juvenile-onset disease also shows characteristic EM findings, with 'fingerprint bodies' being seen in a very small percentage of lymphocyte vacuoles, but prolonged search is required, making the method unsuitable for routine diagnosis. The late-juvenile-onset type has normal lymphocytes by light microscopy, but EM shows many lymphocytes to contain 'curvilinear' bodies. Confirmation of the diagnosis is by rectal biopsy, with EM and histological examination of neurones and smooth muscle. As neuronal changes are present long before clinical signs develop, rectal biopsy will identify affected siblings of a known case before symptoms develop.

Wolman's disease

A deficiency of acid esterase results in massive accumulation of cholesterol esters and triglycerides. Patients present in the first few months of life with severe vomiting and diarrhoea and rapidly increasing hepatosplenomegaly. Adrenal calcification is seen on abdominal X-ray. Abdominal distension, wasting, low-grade fever and anaemia result in death by one year of age. A less severe juvenile form exists, with onset of hepatomegaly in early childhood. Hepatic fibrosis and oesophageal varices may be seen, but progression is slow, and patients live into adult life. Lymphocytes in the peripheral blood contain small discrete vacuoles, like those in Niemann–Pick type A, or Pompe's disease. The vacuoles contain neutral fat and stain strongly with Oil Red O; their lysosomal origin is shown by staining with acid phosphatase. The bone marrow also contains foamy histiocytes, which stain with Oil Red O, and have a characteristic purple colour on staining with Nile blue. Leucocyte or cultured fibroblast assay for the absence of acid esterase activity confirms the diagnosis.

HEREDITARY HAEMOCHROMATOSIS (HH)

Hereditary haemochromatosis (HH) is an inherited disorder of the regulation of iron absorption which usually presents in middle age with evidence of organ dysfunction due to progressive parenchymal iron overload.

Clinical features and inheritance

The classic triad of haemochromatosis is hepatomegaly, skin hyperpigmentation and diabetes mellitus (bronze diabetes), but many other clinical features may be present, including arthropathy, signs of cirrhosis, splenomegaly, testicular atrophy, cardiac arrhythmias and congestive cardiac failure. Age, sex and alcohol ingestion affect the expression of the disease. By this stage, organ damage is irreversible, although treatment may slow progression. An increased incidence of hepatic and other malignancies has been noted (Bomford & Williams 1976). Reports of children and adolescents with clinical symptoms and signs are rare, but have been reviewed by Kaltwasser et al (1988) and Haddy et al (1988). HH may be the underlying diagnosis in teenagers presenting with cardiac failure or hypogonadism.

Inheritance shows an autosomal recessive pattern, although clinical cases have an increased incidence in males, as premenopausal females lose some excess iron in menstrual blood loss, pregnancy and lactation, thus partially protecting them from iron overload until later in life. The gene for haemochromatosis is closely linked to the histocompatibility gene (HLA) on the short arm of chromosome six. It is particularly associated with HLA types A3, B7 and B14, although these are not the only HLA types found. HLA typing of a proband allows family screening, as a sibling inheriting one haplotype the same as the proband is a heterozygote, and identical HLA type indicates

obligate homozygosity (Simon et al 1977, Escobar et al 1987). The gene incidence in Caucasian populations is surprisingly high, as shown by Cartwright et al (1979), who found a gene frequency of 0.056, corresponding to a homozygote frequency of 0.3% and heterozygote frequency of 10.6%, in a Mormon population. This gene frequency makes hetero/homozygote matings relatively common, and explains the appearance of the disease in successive generations in some family pedigrees.

In childhood, the most frequent cause of iron overload is transfusional iron in patients treated for thalassaemia major, cerebral complications of sickle cell anaemia, or refractory anaemias, but HH is the second most likely cause.

Laboratory findings and diagnosis

Iron balance is achieved by regulation of mucosal absorption, affected through unexplained pathways by iron stores and rates of erythropoiesis. In HH, absorption is inappropriately increased. Haddy et al, (1988) reviewed the literature concerning young patients with HH, diagnosed between 1981 and 1987. 18 patients under the age of 30 years were included, of whom nine were under 15, and the youngest was aged 2. Three children under 15 were clinically affected, with abdominal pain, hepatomegaly, splenomegaly, jaundice, skin pigmentation or amenorrhoea. The other young patients were detected by laboratory testing during family studies. Cardiac abnormalities and diabetes mellitus were seen in the over-15-year-olds, but not in the younger patients. Kaltwasser et al (1988) reviewed 17 patients aged from 4 to 24 years culled from the literature between 1932 and 1983. At the time of that report, 12 had died, eight from cardiac failure. This series contained one child under 15 years who died, aged 4, in a hepatic coma. It seems reasonable to conclude that iron studies should be included in the investigation of children with unexplained hepatosplenomegaly, pancreatic or gonadal dysfunction, or cardiomyopathy.

Definitive laboratory diagnosis is by liver biopsy. Iron deposits are found chiefly in hepatocytes rather than Kupffer cells, although once cirrhosis is present, this distinction is lost. Hepatic iron in normal individuals is generally less than 500 µg/g dry weight of liver, but concentrations many times higher are found in patients with HH. Paediatric normal ranges for hepatic iron are not available, but are likely to be of the same order. Liver biopsy will also allow recognition of developing cirrhosis or fibrosis, or the presence of malignancy. The hazards of liver biopsy mean that it is not ideal as a test for monitoring progress of the disease or effectiveness of therapy. Indirect methods of detecting iron overload are useful in screening programmes and in indicating those family members that require further investigation.

Ferritin and transferrin saturation are raised if iron stores are increased, but both measurements lack both specificity and sensitivity, being affected by the presence of inflammation, infection, malignant disease, liver disease, haemolysis, ineffective erythropoiesis, malnutrition or ascorbic acid deficiency. Nevertheless, a transferrin saturation of over 70% and raised serum ferritin warrants further investigation. Bone marrow examination is not useful, as excess iron in HH is stored in parenchymal rather than reticuloendothelial cells, so it is possible to have normal marrow iron in the presence of massive parenchymal overload. CT scanning and magnetic resonance imaging (MRI) have the potential to measure iron stores in liver by comparison of images obtained at two energy levels, but the modifications and calibrations for the calculations required are not yet available on standard equipment. Magnetic susceptibility measurement (MSM) provides a direct, noninvasive means of determining iron stores based on the ability of all substances, including human tissue, to develop a magnetic field when placed in proximity to a powerful magnet. Iron-loaded liver responds differently from normal liver, and specialized, sensitive equipment can detect and measure that difference, which is directly proportional to the number of iron atoms present. This allows an accurate assay of iron load. The method has been tested in patients with HH and found to be reliable, rapid and safe in both normal and iron-overloaded patients. Eventually, when equipment is more widely available, MSM may provide a method of accurate monitoring of disease progress and effectiveness of therapy (Brittenham 1988).

Treatment

Treatment of patients with established organ dysfunction is symptomatic, together with reduction of iron overload by phlebotomy or chelation. Early organ damage, particularly cardiac, may show some improvement, but hepatic and endocrine damage tends to be irreversible. Effective screening will identify homozygotes before irreversible organ damage occurs, and early diagnosis and treatment could delay or prevent the onset of clinical disease and subsequent malignancy.

Intensive chelation therapy with desferrioxamine is associated with numerous problems, ranging from poor compliance to potential retinal and auditory side-effects and growth failure. It is particularly difficult in childhood and adolescence, and in HH a programme of iron depletion by regular phlebotomy can be equally effective, is often well tolerated and is relatively cheap. Venesection should be performed at approximately 7–10 day intervals, removing 5 ml/kg until excess stores are depleted; the frequency of phlebotomy is then reduced to maintain equilibrium with the abnormal, increased absorption of iron (Escobar et al 1987). Regular assay of iron stores by MSM or CT scanning would be the best method of monitoring response but, in the absence of suitable equipment, response is usually assessed by serial ferritin and transferrin saturation estimations. In patients with cardiac dysfunction, phlebotomy should be undertaken with care. Severe cardiac dysfunction or anaemia are both contraindications to phlebotomy, and desferrioxamine, given in standard subcutaneous doses or short-term high-dose infusion for rapid reduction of iron load, is preferable until venesection can be tolerated. Advice should be given on the avoidance of iron and vitamin C supplements, and in older patients the dangers of alcohol pointed out.

The main role of the paediatric haematologist is in prevention of iron overload in those healthy individuals found by screening to be homozygous for the HH gene.

SOLID TUMOURS

The 'small round cell tumours' of childhood (Table 15.7) are a group of malignancies that cause diagnostic problems; as marrow infiltration

Table 15.7 Incidence of marrow infiltration at presentation in the small round cell tumours of childhood

Tumour	Marrow infiltration (%)
Neuroblastoma	50
Rhabdomyosarcoma	15–20
Ewing's	5–10
Retinoblastoma	< 5
Medulloblastoma	< 5

is not uncommon, they are considered briefly but with no attempt to describe clinical findings or management.

Often, the diagnosis is in no doubt, judged by the site and pathological appearances of the primary tumour. However, as treatment depends on accurate staging, aspirates and trephines, often from multiple sites, are taken to assess the presence and extent of marrow infiltration. The examination may be repeated at intervals to monitor response to therapy and look for recurrence.

Other patients present with nonspecific complaints of malaise, weight loss, fever or bone pain, and are found to have pancytopenia and marrow infiltration with unidentified tumour. Leucoerythroblastic changes may be present in the peripheral blood (though less commonly than in adults with marrow metastases). The differential diagnosis is usually one of acute leukaemia or nonhaemic malignant disease.

It may be difficult to obtain adequate fragments on marrow aspirate, and in such cases a trephine is helpful. Tumour cells usually appear larger than normal haemopoietic precursors, and tend to appear in clumps with poorly defined cell margins (Fig. 15.12). Small cytoplasmic vacuoles are frequently seen, variable amounts of bluish cytoplasm are present, and nuclei are immature. Clumps of tumour cells are best identified by low-power scanning of a number of slides, including the edges of the film. High-power examination usually indicates that the clumps are of nonhaemopoietic origin. Infiltration may be heavy, with normal cells replaced by sheets of tumour cells. Occasionally, tumour cells spread evenly through the marrow, making the differentiation from leukaemia more difficult on morphological grounds (Fig. 15.13), but cytochemical, immunological or cytogenetic studies usually clear any confusion.

Differentiation between the different tumour types is also difficult on marrow cytological examination, but marrow suspended in tissue culture medium, or histological sections of aspirated particles or trephines, can be studied with a panel of monoclonal antibodies directed against the small round cell tumours of childhood. Differentiation between lymphoma and neuroblastoma – the tumours which most commonly infiltrate marrow – is simple, as UJ13A, UJ181.4 and UJ127.11 are positive in the majority of neuroblastomas but negative in lymphoma, whereas pan-leucocyte markers will be positive in lymphoma (Darbyshire et al 1987). Most rhabdomyosarcomas and a small proportion of Ewing's sarcomas take up the

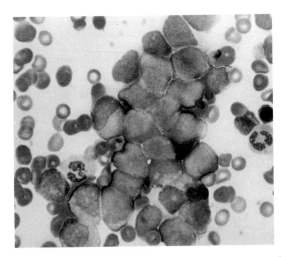

Fig. 15.12 A clump of tumour cells found in the marrow of a child with metastatic Ewing's sarcoma.

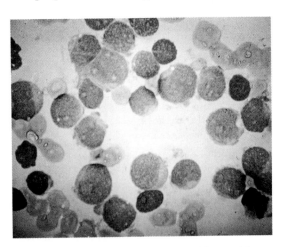

Fig. 15.13 Diffuse marrow involvement with neuroblastoma resembling acute leukaemia.

antibody UJ13A, so it is not specific, but the range of special tests possible with both aspirates and trephines will continue to increase, particularly in the fields of immunocytochemistry, immunohisto-chemistry and in-situ hybridization.

REFERENCES

Alvarado C S, Buchanan G R, Kim T H, Zaatari G, Sartain P, Ragab A H 1986 Use of VP-16-213 in the treatment of Familial erythrophagocytic lymphohistiocytosis. Cancer 57: 1097–1100

Ambruso D R, Hays T, Zwartjes W J, Tubergen D G, Favara B E 1980 Successful treatment of Lymphohistiocytic reticulosis with phagocytosis with epipodophyllotoxin VP16-213. Cancer 45: 2516–2520

Arico M, Nespoli L, Maccario R et al 1988 Natural cytotoxicity impairment in familial haemophagocytic lymphohistiocytosis. Archives of Disease in Childhood 63: 292–296

Atherton D J, Broadbent V, Pritchard J 1986 Topical use of mustine hydrochloride in cutaneous histiocytosis-X. Medical and Paediatric Oncology 14: 112

Badaro R, Falcoff E, Badaro F S et al 1990 Treatment of visceral leishmaniasis with pentavalent antimony and interferon gamma. New England Journal of Medicine 322: 16–21

Bakshi S, Kairam R, Cooper L Z 1988 Acquired immune deficiency syndrome in children. Annals of New York Academy of Sciences 549: 135–146

Barranger J A 1984 Marrow transplantation in genetic disease. New England Journal of Medicine 311: 1629–1631

Berry D H, Becton D L March 1987 Natural history of histiocytosis-X. In: Osband M E, Pochedly C (eds) Histiocytosis-X. Haematology/Oncology Clinics of North America, vol 1,1: 23–34

Bomford A, Williams R 1976 Long-term results of venesection therapy in idiopathic haemochromatosis. Quarterly Journal of Medicine 180: 611–623

Brittenham G M 1988 Non-invasive methods for the early detection of hereditary haemochromatosis. Annals of New York Academy of Sciences 526: 199–208

Broadbent V, Pritchard J, Davies E G et al 1984 Spontaneous remission of multi-system histiocytosis-X. Lancet 1: 253–254

Broadbent V, Pritchard J, Yeomans E 1989a Etoposide (VP16) in the treatment of multisystem Langerhans' cell histiocytosis (histiocytosis X). Medical and Paediatric Oncology 17: 97–100

Broadbent V, Gadner H, Komp D M, Ladisch S 1989b Histiocytosis syndromes in children: II. Approach to the clinical and laboratory evaluation of children with Langerhans cell histiocytosis. Medical and Paediatric Oncology 17: 492–495

Brown J K, Stark G D, Minns R A et al 1984 Disorders of the central nervous system. In: Forfar J O, Arneil G C (eds) Textbook of Paediatrics, 3rd edn. Churchill Livingstone, Edinburgh, p 677–893

Brown R E, Bowman W P, D'Cruz C A, Pick T E, Champion J E 1987 Endoperoxidation, hyperprostaglandinaemia and hyperlipidaemia in a case of erythrophagocytic lymphohistiocytosis. Cancer 60: 2388–2393

Campo E, Condom E, Miro M-J, Cid M-C, Romagosa V 1986 Tuberculosis-associated haemophagocytic syndrome. Cancer 58: 2640–2645

Cartwright G E, Edwards C Q, Kravitz K et al 1979 Hereditary haemochromatosis, phenotypic expression of the disease. New England Journal of Medicine 301: 175–179

Ceci A, Terlissi M, Colella R et al 1988 Etoposide in recurrent childhood Langerhans cell histiocytosis: an Italian cooperative study. Cancer 62: 2528–2531

Chu A, D'Angio G J, Favara B, Ladisch S, Nesbit M, Pritchard J 1987 Histiocytosis syndromes in children. Lancet 1: 208–209

Darbyshire P J, Bourne S P, Allan P M et al 1987 The use of a panel of monoclonal antibodies in paediatric oncology. Cancer 59: 726–730

Delaney M M, Shafford E A, Al-Attar A, Pritchard J 1984 Familial erythrophagocytic reticulosis. Complete response to combination chemotherapy. Archives of Disease in Childhood 1: 173–175

Dunger D B, Broadbent V, Yeoman E et al 1989 The frequency and natural history of diabetes insipidus in children with Langerhans-cell histiocytosis. New England Journal of Medicine 321: 1157–1162

Escobar G J, Heyman M B, Smith W B, Thaler M M 1987 Primary haemochromatosis in childhood. Paediatrics 80: 549–554

Farquhar J W, Claireaux A E 1952 Familial haemophagocytic reticulosis. Archives of Disease in Childhood 27: 519–525

Favara B E, Jaffe R March 1987 Pathology of Langerhans cell histiocytosis. In: Osband M E, Pochedly C (eds) Histiocytosis-X. Haematology/Oncology Clinics of North America, vol 1, No 1.

Fischer A, Virelizier J L, Arenzana-Seisdedos F, Perez N, Nezelof C, Griscelli C 1985 Treatment of four patients with erythrophagocytic lymphohistiocytosis by a combination of epipodophyllotoxin, steroids, intrathecal methotrexate, and cranial irradiation. Paediatrics 76: 263–268

Fischer A, Cerf-Bensussan N, Blanche S et al 1986 Allogeneic bone marrow transplantation for erythrophagocytic lymphohistiocytosis. Journal of Paediatrics 108: 267–270

Gill K, Marrie T J 1987 Haemophagocytosis secondary to Mycoplasma pneumoniae infection. American Journal of Medicine 82: 668–670

Gray O P, Campbell A G M, Kerr M M et al 1984 The newborn. In: Forfar J O, Arneil G C (eds) Textbook of Paediatrics, 3rd edn, Churchill Livingstone, Edinburgh, p 117–258

Haddy T B, Castro O L, Rana S R 1988 Hereditary haemochromatosis in children, adolescents and young adults. American Journal of Paediatric Haematology/ Oncology 10 (1): 23–34

Hall R, Malia R G 1984 Haematology of infections. In: Medical Laboratory Haematology, Butterworths, London, p 461–483

Hill F G H, Letsky E A 1975 Infantile kala-azar in Britain. British Medical Journal 3: 354–355

Hinchliffe R 1987 The haemolytic anaemias. In: Hinchliffe R, Lilleyman J S (eds) Practical paediatric haematology Wiley, Chichester, p 315–357

Jenkins H R, Gray O P 1988 Case report: infection-associated haemophagocytic syndrome in an infant. Journal of Infection 17: 167–170

Kaltwasser J P, Schalk K P, Werner E 1988 Juvenile haemochromatosis. Annals of New York Academy of Sciences 526: 339–341

Kelton J G, Keystone J, Moore J et al 1983 Immune-mediated thrombocytopenia of malaria. Journal of Clinical Investigation 71: 832–836

Kinmond S, Galea P, Simpson E M, Parida S K, Goel K M 1989 Kala-azar in a Scottish child. Lancet 2: 325

Kollaritsch H, Emminger W, Zaunschirm A, Aspock H 1989 Suspected autochthonous kala-azar in Austria. Lancet i: 901–902

Kolodny E H, Boustany R-M 1987 Storage diseases of the reticulo-endothelial system. In: Nathan D G, Oski F A (eds) Haematology of infancy and childhood, 3rd edn. W B Saunders, Philadelphia, p 1212–1247

Krivit W, Pierpont M E, Ayas K et al 1984 Bone marrow transplantation in the Maroteaux-Lamy syndrome (mucopolysaccharidosis type VI). New England Journal of Medicine 311: 1606–1611

Ladisch S, Poplack D G, Holiman B, Blaese R M 1978 Immunodeficiency in familial erythrophagocytic lymphohistiocytosis. Lancet i: 581–583

Ladisch S, Ho W, Matheson D, Pilkington R, Hartman G 1982 Immunologic and clinical effects of repeated blood exchange in familial erythrophagocytic lymphohistiocytosis. Blood 60: 814–821

Lahey M E 1975 Histiocytosis X – an analysis of prognostic factors. Journal of Paediatrics 87: 184–189

Lake B D 1989 Metabolic disorders: general considerations. In: Berry C L (ed) Paediatric pathology. Springer-Verlag, London

Lee C W, Park M H, Lee H 1988 Recurrent cutaneous Langerhans' cell histiocytosis in infancy. British Journal of Dermatology 119: 259–265

Lilleyman J S 1980 The treatment of familial erythrophagocytic lymphohistiocytosis. Cancer 46: 468–470

McLelland J, Pritchard J, Chu A C 1987 Current controversies. In: Osband M E, Pochedly C (eds) Histiocytosis X. Haematology/Oncology Clinics of North America, vol 1, 1: 147–162

Maegraith B 1984 Leishmaniasis In: Maegraith B (ed) Adams and Maegraith: clinical tropical diseases, 8th edn. Blackwell Scientific Publications, Oxford, p 189–210

Martin-Moreno S, Soto-Guzman O, Bernaldo-de-Quiros J, Reverte-Cejudo D, Bascones-Casas C 1983 Pancytopenia due to haemophagocytosis in patients with brucellosis: a report of four cases. Journal of Infectious Disease 147: 445–449

Matzner Y, Behar A, Beeri E, Gunders A E, Hershko C 1979 Systemic leishmaniasis mimicking malignant histiocytosis. Cancer 43: 398–402

Miller L H, Mason S J, Clyde D F, McGinniss M H 1976 The resistance factor to Plasmodium vivax in blacks. New England Journal of Medicine 295: 302–304

Moody A, Simpson E, Shaw D 1989 Florid radiological appearance of megakaryoblastic leukaemia – an aid to earlier diagnosis. Paediatric Radiology 19: 486–488

Ornvold K, Carstensen H, Magnussen P, Nielsen M H, Pedersen F K 1989 Case report: kala-azar in a four-year-old child 18 months after a brief exposure in Malta. Acta Paediatrica Scandinavica 78: 650–652

Pasvol G, Jungery M, Weatherall D J, Parsons S F, Anstee D J, Tanner M J A 1982 Glycophorin as a possible receptor for Plasmodium falciparum. Lancet ii: 947–950

Pritchard J 1986 'Other' histiocytic disorders – clinical aspects (Childhood Histiocytosis Workshop). Medical and Paediatric Oncology 14: 107–108

Raney R B, D'Angio G J 1989 Langerhans cell histiocytosis (histiocytosis X): experience at the Childrens Hospital of Philadelphia, 1970–1984. Medical and Paediatric Oncology 17: 20–28

Rappeport J M, Ginns E I 1984 Bone marrow transplantation in severe Gaucher's disease. New England Journal of Medicine 311: 84–88

Reiner A P, Spivak J L 1988 Haematophagic histiocytosis. Medicine 67: 369–388

Risdall R J, McKenna R W, Nesbit M E et al 1979 Virus-associated haemophagocytic syndrome. Cancer 44: 993–1002

Saulsbury F T, Boyle R J, Wykoff R F, Howard T H 1986 Thrombocytopenia as the presenting manifestation of human T-lymphotropic virus type III infection in infants. Journal of Paediatrics 109: 30–34

Simon M, Bourel M, Genetet B, Fauchet R 1977 Idiopathic haemochromatosis. Demonstration of recessive transmission and early detection by family HLA typing. New England Journal of Medicine 297: 1017–1021

Spivak J L, Bender B S, Quinn T C 1984 Haematologic abnormalities in the acquired immune deficiency syndrome. American Journal of Medicine 77: 224–228

Stockman J A 1987 Haematologic manifestations of systemic diseases. In: Nathan D G, Oski F A (eds) Haematology of infancy and childhood, 3rd edn. W B Saunders, Philadelphia, p 1632–1676

Womer R B, Raney B, D'Angio G 1985 Healing rates of treated and untreated bone lesions in histiocytosis-X. Paediatrics 76: 286–288

Woodruff A W, Ansdell V E, Pettitt L E 1979 Cause of anaemia in malaria. Lancet i: 1055–1057

Index